Molecular Toxicology Protocols

METHODS IN MOLECULAR BIOLOGY™

John M. Walker, SERIES EDITOR

METHODS IN MOLECULAR BIOLOGY™

Molecular Toxicology Protocols

Edited by

Phouthone Keohavong
Stephen G. Grant

Department of Environmental and Occupational Health
University of Pittsburgh, Pittsburgh, PA

HUMANA PRESS ✳ TOTOWA, NEW JERSEY

© 2005 Humana Press Inc.
999 Riverview Drive, Suite 208
Totowa, New Jersey 07512

www.humanapress.com

This publication is printed on acid-free paper. ∞
ANSI Z39.48-1984 (American Standards Institute)

Permanence of Paper for Printed Library Materials.

Cover design by Patricia F. Cleary

Cover illustrations: Detection of mutant K-*RAS* in human colon aberrant crypt foci (Fig. 4, Chap. 24; *see* full caption on p. 269 and discussion on p. 268). Photomicrograph of human lymphocyte in the comet assay (Fig. 1, Chap. 9; *see* full caption and discussion on p. 86).

For additional copies, pricing for bulk purchases, and/or information about other Humana titles, contact Humana at the above address or at any of the following numbers: Tel.: 973-256-1699; Fax: 973-256-8341; E-mail: humana@humanapr.com; or visit our Website: www.humanapress.com

Printed in the United States of America. 10 9 8 7 6 5 4 3 2 1

ISSN: 1064-3745

eISBN:1-59259-840-4

Library of Congress Cataloging-in-Publication Data

Molecular toxicology protocols / edited by Phouthone Keohavong, Stephen G. Grant.
    p. ; cm. -- (Methods in molecular biology ; 291)
  Includes bibliographical references and index.
  ISBN 1-58829-084-0 (alk. paper)
  1. Molecular toxicology--Laboratory manuals. [DNLM: 1. DNA Adducts--analysis. 2. DNA Mutational Analysis. 3. Apoptosis. 4. DNA Repair. QU 58.5 M7185 2005] I. Keohavong, Phouthone. II. Grant, Stephen G. III. Series: Methods in molecular biology (Clifton, N.J.) ; v. 291.
  RA1220.3.M66 2005
  615.9--dc22
                                                                        2004005911

Preface

It seems fashionable today to simply place the word "molecular" in front of a traditional field and consider it reinvented. This, without a clear consensus on what the "molecular" actually means. Certainly chemists working in the field of toxicology have always considered that they worked at the "molecular" level. It has not been so clear on the biological side, however, where there has been a history of ongoing discovery and characterization of toxic mechanisms. In other biological fields, "molecular" really implies using the tools of "molecular" biology, i.e., recombinant DNA. Just as the adoption of molecular biological techniques first invaded, then transformed such biological fields as genetics, physiology, and developmental biology, so too have these new methods begun to transform toxicology.

Molecular Toxicology Protocols is a book about science on the interface, and a science that is about to explode upon the clinical and popular horizon. Toxicology, a subdiscipline of pharmacology, is actually the interface of chemistry and biology. As most practice it, this field also extends into nonchemical "agents" of deleterious biological effects, especially radiation, the purview of the radiobiologist and health physicist. With the huge increase in computational power made available over the last ten years it has become possible to model and predict the potential toxicity of as yet unmade chemicals. Perhaps the greatest change in the practice of toxicology has been application of the the tools of the trade directly to the human population, in what are known clinically as "translational" studies, opening the new frontier of epidemiology through the more conventional portal of biostatistics. These studies expand the traditional public health aspect of toxicology, screening of synthetic agents for toxicological potential prior to their introduction into the environment, attempting to define "normal" or "background," perhaps unavoidable, exposures as mechanisms of human disease, and to design methods of preclinical intervention ("chemo-prevention").

Thus, for our purposes, we will define "molecular" toxicology as either any study of toxicological mechanism, or any translation of toxicological practice into the human population.

Today, such "molecular" toxicology is mostly genetic toxicology, where the genetic material itself, the DNA, is the target molecule. Of course DNA is found throughout the human body, such that all of the traditional modulators of toxicological effect, uptake, distribution, metabolism, and so on, must be taken into account. Although genetic damage can have many outcomes, the one outcome most clearly linking exposure and disease is cancer.

During the past several years, important progress has been made in the understanding of the molecular biology of the cell, the responses of cells to genotoxic agents, and the molecular biology of human cancer. This progress has been achieved thanks to the ongoing development of new state-of-the-art techniques, as well as improvements made upon existing methods to study changes not only in cellular morphology, but also in the cellular genetic material, the DNA, the cellular transcript, the mRNA, and the translated product, proteins. These molecular methods are now opening up many areas to potential clinical applications. Several books are currently available on the applications of molecular methods to various types of technology. However, to our knowledge, there is no book emphasizing the application of molecular methods to genetic toxicology.

Therefore, the aim of *Molecular Toxicology Protocols* is to bring together a series of articles, each describing commonly used methods to elucidate specific molecular aspects of toxicology. With such content, this book addresses not only molecular biologists and molecular toxicologists, but also all individuals interested in applying molecular methods to clinical populations, including geneticists, pathologists, biochemists, and epidemiologists. The volume is divided into seven parts, roughly corresponding to the spectrum of biomarkers intermediate between exposure and disease outcome as proposed in molecular epidemiological models. Thus, Part I includes chapters describing methods of detecting premutagenic lesions in the genetic material, while Part II contains chapters describing the applications of methods to assess gross or macroscopic genetic damage. Parts III and IV focus on detection and characterization of viable mutations, in surrogate markers and cancer-related genes, respectively. The chapters of Part V describe methods for the analysis of the various pathways of DNA repair, an important modulator of genotoxicity. Part VI addresses the application of the new array technologies to genetic toxicology, including methods for the analysis of individual variation in biotransformation and the effects of genotoxic exposure on gene expression. Finally, Part VII describes methods for analysis of cytotoxicity caused by the induction of apoptosis, because cell death can either protect the organism from a transforming cell or cause distinct health effects itself.

We have no doubt that as time goes by "molecular" approaches will play an expanding role in all types of toxicology, not just genetic toxicology. Moreover, genetic toxicology will undoubtedly be found to play a role in many more diseases of aging than cancer alone; it is probably a fundamental mechanism of aging itself. Therefore, while the current focus of *Molecular Toxicology Protocols* is genetic toxicology, and more specifically the genetic toxicology of cancer, we believe this represents just the tip of the iceberg with respect to how the field of molecular toxicology will eventually be understood.

Phouthone Keohavong
Stephen G. Grant

Contents

Contributors

VOLKER M. ARLT • *Section of Molecular Carcinogenesis, Institute of Cancer Research, Sutton, Surrey, UK*

REETAKSHI ARORA • *National Centre of Applied Human Genetics, Jawaharlal Nehru University, Delhi, India*

NARENDRA K. BAIRWA • *National Centre of Applied Human Genetics, Jawaharlal Nehru University, Delhi, India*

RAMESH BAMEZAI • *National Centre of Applied Human Genetics, Jawaharlal Nehru University, Delhi, India*

CHRISTOPHER J. BETTI • *Program in Molecular Biology, Loyola University Chicago Medical Center, Maywood, IL*

WILLIAM F. BLAKELY • *Armed Forces Radiobiology Research Institute, Bethesda, MD*

GRIGORY G. BORISENKO • *Department of Environmental and Occupational Health, University of Pittsburgh, Pittsburgh, PA*

ANNE-LISE BØRRESEN-DALE • *Department of Genetics, The Norwegian Radium Hospital, Oslo, Norway*

SHAMA C. BUCH • *Center for Clinical Pharmacology, University of Pittsburgh, Pittsburgh, PA*

R. C. CHAUBEY • *Genetic Toxicology and Chromosome Studies Section, Radiation Biology and Health Sciences Division, Bhabha Atomic Research Centre, Mumbai, India*

WALTER A. DEUTSCH • *Pennington Biomedical Research Center, Louisiana State University, Baton Rouge, LA*

KAREN H. DINGLEY • *Biology and Biotechnology Research Program, Lawrence Livermore National Laboratory, Livermore, CA*

VASILY N. DOBROVOLSKY • *Division of Genetic and Reproductive Toxicology, National Center for Toxicological Research, US Food and Drug Administration, Jefferson, AR*

JAMES P. FABISIAK • *Department of Environmental and Occupational Health, University of Pittsburgh, Pittsburgh, PA*

ELKE FELDMANN • *Institute of Genetics, University of Essen, Essen, Germany*

JAMES C. FUSCOE • *Center for Functional Genomics, National Center for Toxicological Research, US Food and Drug Administration, Jefferson, AR*

WEIMIN GAO • *Department of Environmental and Occupational Health, University of Pittsburgh, Pittsburgh, PA*

MICHAEL E. GEHRING • *Department of Pediatrics, Wake Forest University School of Medicine, Winston-Salem, NC*

TONY E. GODFREY • *Department of Medicine, Mount Sinai School of Medicine, New York, NY*

WOLFGANG GOEDECKE • *Institute of Genetics, University of Essen, Essen, Germany*

STEPHEN G. GRANT • *Department of Environmental and Occupational Health, University of Pittsburgh, Pittsburgh, PA*

JAN GRAWÉ • *Cell Analysis Core Facility, Uppsala University, Rudbeck Laboratory, Uppsala, Sweden*

KARL OTTO GREULICH • *Department for Single Cell and Single Molecule Techniques, Institute for Molecular Biotechnology Jena, Jena, Germany*

VIBHUTI GUPTA • *National Centre of Applied Human Genetics, Jawaharlal Nehru University, Delhi, India*

KURT W. HAACK • *Center for Accelerator Mass Spectrometry, Lawrence Livermore National Laboratory, Livermore, CA*

ANDREAS HARTMANN • *Novartis Pharma AG, Basel, Switzerland*

MICHAEL HAUSMANN • *Kirchhoff-Institute for Physics, University of Heidelberg, Heidelberg, Germany*

TOMONORI HAYASHI • *Laboratory of Immunology, Department of Radiobiology/ Molecular Epidemiology, Radiation Effects Research Foundation, Hiroshima, Japan*

JOHN B. HAYS • *Department of Environmental and Molecular Toxicology, Oregon State University, Corvallis, OR*

ROBERT H. HEFLICH • *Division of Genetic and Reproductive Toxicology, National Center for Toxicological Research, US Food and Drug Administration, Jefferson, AR*

VIJAY HEGDE • *Pennington Biomedical Research Center, Louisiana State University, Baton Rouge, LA*

ALAN HEWER • *Section of Molecular Carcinogenesis, Institute of Cancer Research, Sutton, Surrey, UK*

STEPHEN R. HEWITT • *Department of Environmental and Molecular Toxicology, Oregon State University, Corvallis, OR*

SAI-MEI HOU • *Department of Biosciences, Karolinska Institute, Huddinge, Sweden*

T. C. HSU • *Department of Cancer Biology, M. D. Anderson Cancer Center, Houston, TX*

MARIA JASIN • *Cell Biology Program, Memorial Sloan-Kettering Cancer Center and Cornell University Graduate School of Medical Sciences, New York, NY*

HILDE JOHNSEN • *Department of Genetics, The Norwegian Radium Hospital, Oslo, Norway*

JENNIFER M. JOHNSON • *Department of Molecular Genetics and Biochemistry, University of Pittsburgh School of Medicine, Pittsburgh, PA*

NINA JOSHI • *Department of Environmental and Occupational Health, University of Pittsburgh, Pittsburgh, PA*

VALERIAN E. KAGAN • *Department of Environmental and Occupational Health, University of Pittsburgh, Pittsburgh, PA*

CRYSTAL M. KELLY • *Department of Obstetrics, Gynecology and Reproductive Sciences, University of Pittsburgh School of Medicine, Pittsburgh, PA*

LORI A. KELLY • *Department of Surgery, University of Pittsburgh School of Medicine, Pittsburgh, PA*

PHOUTHONE KEOHAVONG • *Department of Environmental and Occupational Health, University of Pittsburgh, Pittsburgh, PA*

PATRICK P. KOTY • *Department of Pediatrics, Wake Forest University School of Medicine, Winston-Salem, NC*

STEFFI KUHFITTIG-KULLE • *Institute of Genetics, University of Essen, Essen, Germany*

YOICHIRO KUSUNOKI • *Laboratory of Immunology, Department of Radiobiology/ Molecular Epidemiology, Radiation Effects Research Foundation, Hiroshima, Japan*

SEISHI KYOIZUMI • *Laboratory of Immunology, Department of Radiobiology/ Molecular Epidemiology, Radiation Effects Research Foundation, Hiroshima, Japan*

JEAN J. LATIMER • *Department of Obstetrics, Gynecology and Reproductive Sciences, University of Pittsburgh School of Medicine, Pittsburgh, PA*

GURO ELISABETH LIND • *Department of Genetics, The Norwegian Radium Hospital, Oslo, Norway*

RAGNHILD LOTHE • *Department of Genetics, The Norwegian Radium Hospital, Oslo, Norway*

HITOSHI MAEDA • *Department of Legal Medicine, Osaka City University Medical School, Osaka, Japan*

DHEERAJ K. MALHOTRA • *National Centre of Applied Human Genetics, Jawaharlal Nehru University, Delhi, India*

TOSHINARI MINAMOTO • *Divisions of Diagnostic Molecular Oncology and Surgical Oncology, Cancer Research Institute, Kanazawa University, Kanazawa, Japan*

SHIRLEY MCCREADY • *School of Biological and Molecular Sciences, Oxford Brookes University, Oxford, UK*

PAGE B. MCKINZIE • *Division of Genetic and Reproductive Toxicology, National Center for Toxicological Research, US Food and Drug Administration, Jefferson, AR*

MINAKO NAGAO • *Biochemistry Division, National Cancer Center Research Institute, Tokyo, Japan*

MASAKO OCHIAI • *Biochemistry Division, National Cancer Center Research Institute, Tokyo, Japan*

ANDREA ODERSKY • *Institute of Genetics, University of Essen, Essen, Germany*

IOVANNA PANDELOVA • *Department of Environmental and Molecular Toxicology, Oregon State University, Corvallis, OR*

BARBARA L. PARSONS • *Division of Genetic and Reproductive Toxicology, National Center for Toxicological Research, US Food and Drug Administration, Jefferson, AR*

PETRA PFEIFFER • *Institute of Genetics, University of Essen, Essen, Germany*

DAVID H. PHILLIPS • *Section of Molecular Carcinogenesis, Institute of Cancer Research, Sutton, Surrey, UK*

ANDREW J. PIERCE • *Markey Cancer Center, University of Kentucky, Lexington, KY*

PATAJE G. S. PRASANNA • *Armed Forces Radiobiology Research Institute, Bethesda, MD*

ANAND RANJAN • *National Centre of Applied Human Genetics, Jawaharlal Nehru University, Delhi, India*

ALEXANDER RAPP • *Department for Single Cell and Single Molecule Techniques, Institute for Molecular Biotechnology Jena, Jena, Germany*

MARJORIE ROMKES • *Center for Clinical Pharmacology, University of Pittsburgh, Pittsburgh, PA*

ANJANA SAHA • *National Centre of Applied Human Genetics, Jawaharlal Nehru University, Delhi, India*

JOSEPH G. SHADDOCK • *Division of Genetic and Reproductive Toxicology, National Center for Toxicological Research, US Food and Drug Administration, Jefferson, AR*

KAORI SHINTANI-ISHIDA • *Department of Forensic Medicine, Graduate School of Medicine, University of Tokyo, Tokyo, Japan*

THERESE SØRLIE • *Department of Genetics, The Norwegian Radium Hospital, Oslo, Norway*

GÜNTER SPEIT • *Abteilung Humangenetik, Universitätsklinikum Ulm, Ulm, Germany*

TAKASHI SUGIMURA • *National Cancer Center, Tokyo, Japan*

ROY R. SWIGER • *Midwest Research Institute, Palm Bay, FL*

VLADIMIR A. TYURIN • *Department of Environmental and Occupational Health, University of Pittsburgh, Pittsburgh, PA*

YULIA Y. TYURINA • *Department of Environmental and Occupational Health, University of Pittsburgh, Pittsburgh, PA*

ESTHER A. UBICK • *Biology and Biotechnology Research Program, Lawrence Livermore National Laboratory, Livermore, CA*

P. T. UDHAYASURIYAN • *National Centre of Applied Human Genetics, Jawaharlal Nehru University, Delhi, India*

ANDREW T. M. VAUGHAN • *Department of Radiation Oncology, Loyola University Chicago Medical Center, Maywood, IL*

MICHAEL J. VILLALOBOS • *Program in Molecular Biology, Loyola University Chicago Medical Center, Maywood, IL*

JOHN S. VOGEL • *Center for Accelerator Mass Spectrometry, Lawrence Livermore National Laboratory, Livermore, CA*

PHUONG VU • *Department of Genetics, The Norwegian Radium Hospital, Oslo, Norway*

XIFENG WU • *Department of Epidemiology, M. D. Anderson Cancer Center, Houston, TX*

LIQIANG XI • *Hillman Cancer Center, University of Pittsburgh, Pittsburgh PA*

YUN-LING ZHENG • *Laboratory of Human Carcinogenesis, National Cancer Institute, Bethesda, MD*

BAO-LI ZHU • *Department of Legal Medicine, Osaka City University Medical School, Osaka, Japan*

I

ANALYSIS OF DNA ADDUCTS

1

^{32}P-Postlabeling Analysis of DNA Adducts

David H. Phillips, Alan Hewer, and Volker M. Arlt

Summary

^{32}P-Postlabeling analysis is an ultrasensitive method for the detection of DNA adducts, such as those formed directly by the covalent binding of carcinogens and mutagens to bases in DNA, as well as other DNA lesions resulting from modification of bases by endogenous or exogenous agents (e.g., oxidative damage). The procedure involves four main steps: enzymatic digestion of a DNA sample; enrichment of the adducts; radiolabeling of the adducts by T4 kinase-catalyzed transference of ^{32}P-orthophosphate from [γ-^{32}P]ATP; and chromatographic separation of labeled adducts and detection and quantification by means of their radioactive decay. Using 10 µg or less of DNA, this technique is capable of detecting adduct levels as low as one adduct in 10^9–10^{10} normal nucleotides. It is applicable to a wide range of investigations, including monitoring human exposure to environmental or occupational carcinogens, determining whether a chemical has genotoxic properties, analysis of the genotoxicity of complex mixtures, elucidation of the activation pathways of carcinogens, and monitoring of DNA repair.

Key Words: DNA adducts; ^{32}P-postlabeling; T4 polynucleotide kinase; nuclease P1; complex mixtures; DNA repair; oxidative DNA damage; carcinogens; mutagens; genotoxicity; environmental carcinogens; thin-layer chromatography; HPLC; DNA digestion.

1. Introduction

A common mechanism by which carcinogens initiate the process of malignant transformation is through damaging the DNA in the target organ in such a way that errors in replication can be induced. In many cases, this damage is in the form of a chemical modification of one of the nucleotides in DNA, in which the carcinogen becomes covalently bound to form a stably modified nucleotide (a DNA adduct) (*1*). When a replication error occurs at a critical site in a gene essential for cell cycle control or

From: *Methods in Molecular Biology, vol. 291: Molecular Toxicology Protocols*
Edited by: P. Keohavong and S. G. Grant © Humana Press Inc., Totowa, NJ

genomic integrity, such as a proto-oncogene, tumor suppressor gene, or DNA repair gene, the result can be a progeny cell that lacks the normal growth restraints of that cell's lineage, which can then undergo clonal expansion into a tumor. Thus, the monitoring of DNA adduct formation in human tissues and experimental systems is an important component of studies on the etiology of cancer and on hazard identification for carcinogens and mutagens.

Because of the low levels of DNA adduct formation that can result in tumor initiation, sensitive methods are required for detecting these events. A number of methods are currently available that fulfil some or all of the necessary criteria *(2,3)*. These include earlier approaches in which the carcinogen itself was radiolabeled, so that its binding to DNA could be detected by means of its radioactive decay. However, this method was not applicable to monitoring human exposure to carcinogens, nor to any situation in which exposure occurs over a prolonged period, owing to the economic and safety issues of long-term exposure to radioactive substances. In another approach, antibodies have been prepared to a selected range of carcinogen–DNA adducts, and these have been used to detect adducts of various classes in human and animal tissues *(3)*. Sensitive fluorescence detection methods have also been developed for those classes of carcinogen–DNA adducts that are naturally fluorescent (such as etheno adducts and those formed by polycyclic aromatic hydrocarbons), and mass spectrometry has been applied in a number of instances. The latter method provides the most definitive characterization of adduct structure of all the methods available.

The basis of the ^{32}P-postlabeling method for DNA adduct detection is that the radiolabel is introduced into the adduct *after* it is formed. This overcomes the problem of radioactive containment during the initial experiment and allows retrospective analysis for DNA adducts, which is particularly important for human studies. Furthermore, the use of ^{32}P as the isotope allows for a level of sensitivity not achievable with longer-lived isotopes. For most applications, the principal stages of the ^{32}P-postlabeling assay are digestion of the DNA to nucleoside 3'-monophosphates, enrichment of the adducts to enhance the sensitivity of the assay, 5'-labeling of the nucleotides with ^{32}P-orthophosphate (catalyzed by T4 polynucleotide kinase); chromatographic and/or electrophoretic separation of the labeled species, and their detection and quantitation.

The method was originally developed for simple alkyl-modified DNA adducts *(4)* but was then adapted for the detection of bulky aromatic and/or hydrophobic adducts with high sensitivity *(5)*. One of the two principal enhancement procedures that followed was digestion of the nucleotides with nuclease P_1 prior to labeling, resulting in normal nucleotides, but not many adducts, being converted to nucleosides, not substrates for T4 polynucleotide kinase *(6)*. The other enhancement method involved extraction of the aromatic/hydrophobic adducts into butanol as a means of separating them from the unadducted normal nucleotides *(7)*. For these methods, the labeled adducts are resolved and detected as 3',5'-nucleoside bisphosphates. However, alternative digestion strategies, carried out both before and after ^{32}P-postlabeling, can lead to the production of labeled nucleoside 5'-monophosphates *(8)* (**Fig. 1**). For some appli-

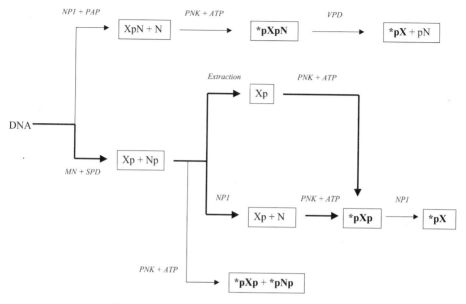

Fig. 1. Methods of ^{32}P-postlabeling. Protocols are given in this article for procedures indicated by bold arrows. X, adducted or modified nucleosides; N, normal nucleosides; p, phosphate; *p,[^{32}P]phosphate; MN, micrococcal nuclease; SPD, spleen phosphodiesterase; NP1, nuclease P$_1$; PAP, prostatic acid phosphatase; PNK, T4 polynucleotide kinase; ATP, [γ-^{32}P]ATP; VPD, venom phosphodiesterase.

cations, the possession of only one charged phosphate group can result in better resolution of carcinogen–DNA adducts and, additionally, improve confidence in the assignment of structures to unknown species on the basis of cochromatography with synthetic standards. Since the earliest days of the assay's use, resolution of DNA adducts has been most commonly performed by multidirectional thin-layer chromatography (TLC), using polyethyleneimine (PEI)-cellulose plates (5). Alternatively, high-performance liquid chromatography (HPLC) offers a technique of higher resolution that is being used more frequently (9,10). For small DNA lesions, such as those resulting from oxidative damage to DNA, polyacrylamide gel electrophoresis (PAGE) of DNA digests has also proved useful for resolving the ^{32}P-postlabeled species (11).

The ^{32}P-postlabeling assay currently has multiple applications that include monitoring human exposure to environmental carcinogens, mechanistic investigations of carcinogen activation and tumor initiation, monitoring DNA repair, testing new compounds for genotoxicity, investigating endogenous DNA damage and oxidative processes, monitoring marine pollution through measurement of DNA adducts in aquatic species, and assessing patient response to cytotoxic cancer drugs (12,13).

There are several advantages of ^{32}P-postlabeling over other methods. It does not require the use of radiolabeled test compounds, making it useful in experiments in which multiple dosing is required, and it is applicable to a wide range of chemicals and types of DNA lesion. Prior structural characterization of adducts is not required, although some assumptions about their likely chromatographic properties may be necessary. It has been used to detect DNA adducts formed by polycyclic aromatic hydrocarbons, aromatic amines, heterocyclic amines (food mutagens), small aromatic compounds (such as benzene, styrene, and alkenylbenzenes), alkylating agents, products of lipid peroxidation, reactive oxygen species, and ultraviolet radiation. It requires only microgram quantities of DNA and is capable of detecting some types of DNA adducts at levels as low as one adduct in 10^{10} normal nucleotides in this amount of material. It can be applied to the assessment of the genotoxic potential of complex mixtures of chemicals, such as environmental airborne combustion products, particulates, and industrial or environmental pollutants.

The method is not without its limitations, however *(14)*. DNA lesions that are not chemically stable as mononucleotides will not be detected reliably. The method does not provide structural information on adducts, and identification of adducts often relies on demonstrating their cochromatography with characterized synthetic standards. Such standards can provide the means for determining the efficiency of labeling and detection, whereas in the absence of standards adduct levels may be underestimated. In the case of complex mixtures, suitable standards often cannot be defined. The method has also been found to detect endogenously derived DNA adducts that may, in some instances, mask the formation of adducts formed by the compound under investigation *(14)*.

In applying ^{32}P-postlabeling to an investigation of the DNA binding activity of a compound or mixture, the investigator is faced with a number of decisions concerning the choice of enhancement procedure to be used and the chromatography conditions to be applied. The protocols given here should be regarded as providing guidance for an initial investigation. In many cases it may be necessary to try several different approaches before the best procedure is found.

Following the adoption of ^{32}P-postlabeling by many laboratories and its use for an increasingly diverse number of applications, it became apparent that protocols varied widely from laboratory to laboratory, even for analysis of the same types of carcinogen–DNA adducts *(15)*. Therefore, an international interlaboratory trial was initiated to establish a set of standardized protocols that would allow comparisons between studies from different laboratories, particularly in the interpretation of human biomonitoring studies *(16)*. Furthermore, validated modified DNA samples, containing adducts derived from benzo[*a*]pyrene, from 4-aminobiphenyl, and from 2-amino-1-methyl-6-phenylimidazo[4,5-*b*]pyridine (PhIP)were prepared, as was DNA containing O^6-methylguanine *(16–18)*, and these standards have been made available to investigators to enable them to determine the efficiency of the ^{32}P-postlabeling assay in their hands.

The protocols described here can be considered an introductory approach to the method and are based on validated studies of known carcinogen–DNA adducts. When a new or unknown type of DNA adduct is being investigated, it cannot be asserted that these conditions will be optimal for its detection and quantitation. Indeed, different carcinogen–DNA adducts have been shown to be postlabeled with different efficiencies *(16,19)*.

2. Materials

2.1. DNA Digestion

1. Use double-distilled water or equivalent throughout.
2. Micrococcal nuclease (MN; cat. no. N3755, Sigma, Poole, Dorset, UK). Dissolve contents in water to give 2 U/μL (*see* **Note 1**).
3. Spleen phosphodiesterase (SPD; from calf spleen, Type II; Calbiochem cat. no. 524711, through CN Biosciences, Nottingham, UK) (*see* **Note 1**).
   Mix to give final concentrations of 36 mU/μL MN and 6 mU/μL SPD (*see* **Note 2**).
4. Digestion buffer: 100 mM sodium succinate, pH 6.0, 50 mM $CaCl_2$.
5. All solutions can be stored at –20°C in small aliquots.

2.2. Nuclease P₁ Digestion

1. 0.25 M Sodium acetate buffer, pH 5.0.
2. 2.0 mM $ZnCl_2$.
3. 1.25 mg/mL Nuclease P_1 (Sigma, cat. no. N8630; *see* **Note 3**).
4. 0.5 M Tris base.
5. All solutions can be stored at –20°C in small aliquots.

2.3. Butanol Extraction

1. Buffer A: 100 mM ammonium formate, pH 3.5.
2. Buffer B: 10 mM tetrabutylammonium chloride.
3. 1-Butanol (redistilled, water-saturated).
4. 1-mL Syringe with blunt-ended needle.
5. 200 mM Tris-HCl, pH 9.5.
6. All solutions should be stored at 4°C.

2.4. DNA Postlabeling

1. T4 polynucleotide kinase (with or without 3'-phosphatase activity; Epicentre, Madison, WI).
2. Kinase buffer: 200 mM bicine, pH 9.0, 100 mM $MgCl_2$, 100 mM dithiothreitol, 10 mM spermidine.
3. [γ-^{32}P]ATP: >3000 Ci/mmol.
4. All solutions must be stored at –20°C in small aliquots.

2.5. Thin-Layer Chromatography

1. 20 × 20 cm PEI-impregnated cellulose TLC sheet (cat. no. 801053 Macherey-Nagel, Middleton Cheney, UK; *see* **Note 4**).
2. Whatman no.1 filter sheets.
3. D1: 1 M sodium phosphate, pH 6.0 (*see* **Note 5**).
4. D2: 3.5 M lithium formate, 8.5 M urea, pH 3.5 (*see* **Notes 6** and **7**).
5. D3: 0.8 M lithium chloride, 0.5 M Tris-HCl, 8.5 M urea, pH 8.0 (*see* **Note 7**).
6. Efficiency solvent: 250 mM ammonium sulfate, 40 mM sodium phosphate.
7. Specific activity solvent: 0.5 M sodium phosphate, pH 6.0.

2.6. Detection and Quantification

1. 2 pmol/μL 2'-Deoxyadenosine 3'-monophosphate, in distilled water.
2. Autoradiography film or an electronic imaging device (e.g., Canberra Packard InstantImager, Downers Grove, IL).

2.7. HPLC Cochromatography

1. 4 M Pyridinium formate, pH 4.5.
2. Ammonium buffer: 2 M ammonium formate, pH 4.5.
3. Acetonitrile.
4. Phenyl-modified reversed-phase column (e.g., 250 × 4.6 mm, particle size 5 mm, Zorbax Phenyl).
5. HPLC system with in-line radioactivity monitor.

3. Methods

3.1. DNA Digestion

1. Take 4 μg DNA solution in a 1.5-mL tube and evaporate to dryness in a Speedvac evaporator.
2. Add 4 μL MN/SPD mix and 0.8 μL digestion buffer/sample. Vortex and centrifuge to ensure complete mixing.
3. Incubate at 37°C overnight.

3.2. Nuclease P₁ Digestion

1. To the above digest add 2.4 μL sodium acetate buffer, 1.44 μL $ZnCl_2$, and 0.96 μL nuclease P₁/sample. Incubate at 37°C for 1 h.
2. Stop the reaction by addition of 1.92 μL Tris base.

3.3. Butanol Extraction

1. Increase volume of DNA digest from 4.8 to 50 μL with water.
2. Premix 15 μL buffer A, 15 μL buffer B, and 70 μL water/sample.
3. Add 100 μL of premix to side of tube.
4. Immediately add 150 μL of butanol and vortex for 60 s at high speed.
5. Microcentrifuge at 8000g for 90 s. Remove upper butanol layer and keep.
6. Repeat **steps 4** and **5**.
7. To pooled butanol extracts add 400 μL butanol-saturated water. Vortex for 60 s. Microcentrifuge as above.
8. Remove water through the butanol layer using a syringe, being careful not to remove any of the butanol.
9. Repeat **step 7** twice, discarding the water each time.
10. Add 3 μL 200 mM Tris-HCl to washed butanol. Vortex briefly.
11. Speedvac to dryness. Redissolve in 50 μL water by vortexing and Speedvac to dryness again.
12. Redissolve in 11.5 μL of water.

3.4. Labeling of Adducts (see Note 8)

1. Premix stock labeling mixture (number of samples + 2) for each sample from: 1.0 μL kinase buffer, 6 U T4 polynucleotide kinase and 50 μCi [γ-^{32}P]ATP/sample. Add appropriate volume to each solution remaining from **Subheadings 3.2.** or **3.3., step 12.**

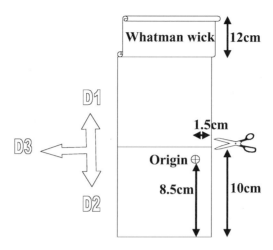

Fig. 2. Diagram showing multidirectional thin-layer chromatography procedures for the resolution of ^{32}P-labeled adducts on polyethyleneimine-cellulose.

2. Incubate at 37°C for 30 min.
3. Staple a 10 × 12-cm Whatman no.1 paper wick to the top edge of a 10 × 20 cm PEI-cellulose TLC sheet as shown in **Fig. 2.** Spot the whole of each sample onto the origin of this sheet. Keep tube for efficiency test (*see* **Subheading 3.5.**).
4. Run in D1 overnight with wick hanging outside tank (*see* **Note 9**).
5. Cut plates down to 10 × 10 cm as shown in **Fig. 2.**
6. Wash plates twice in water and dry plates with cool air.
7. Run in D2 and D3 in directions shown in **Fig. 2.** Before each run, dip lower edge of plate in water to give an even solvent front. Lids should be taken off tanks for 15 min at end of run.
8. Wash plates twice in water and cool air-dry between solvents.

3.5. Test for Efficiency of Enrichment Techniques

1. Wash bottom of tube (*see* **Subheading 3.4.**, **step 3**) with 50 μL water.
2. Vortex and microcentifuge.
3. Spot 5 μL near lower edge of 10 × 20-cm PEI-cellulose TLC sheet.
4. Run in efficiency solvent from **Subheading 2.5.**, **item 6** to top edge (*see* **Note 10**).

3.6. Determining the Specific Activity of [γ-^{32}P]ATP

1. Take 3 μL of 2'-deoxyadenosine 3'-monophosphate (6 pmol) + premix from **Subheading 3.4.**, **step 1.** Incubate at 37°C for 30 min.
2. Dilute to 1.0 mL. Spot 2 × 5 μL 2 cm from the lower edge of a 10 × 20-cm PEI-cellulose TLC sheet. Run in specific activity solvent from **Subheading 2.5.**, **item 7** to top edge.
3. Visualize and count adenosine bisphosphate spot (*see* **Note 11**).
4. This will give you dpm/pmol after allowing for dilution and efficiency of counting. Divide by 2.22×10^3 to give Ci/mmol.

3.7. Imaging and Quantification

1. Adducts can be visualized by placing plates in cassettes with autoradiography film and keeping at –80°C for several h, for up to 4 d. Adduct spots can then be cut from the plate and quantitated in a scintillation counter. Alternatively, an InstantImager can be used, which will give a result in a few minutes.
2. Counts per minute of the adduct should be corrected for efficiency of the counting procedure and divided by the amount of DNA labeled to give dpm/µg. Dividing this by the specific activity figure of dpm/fmol will give fmol of adduct/µg DNA. Results can be expressed in this way or as adducts per 10^8 normal nucleotides. To arrive at this latter figure, divide the number of fmols by 0.03, as 33 adducts per 10^8 nucleotides are equivalent to 1 fmol/µg DNA.

3.8. Extraction of Adducts for HPLC Cochromatography

1. Cut the adduct spot out of the PEI-cellulose TLC sheet and place it in a scintillation vial (*see* **Note 12**).
2. Add 500 µL pyridinium formate and shake gently overnight (*see* **Note 13**).
3. Microcentrifuge extracts at 8000*g* for 90 s to remove small particles.
4. Speedvac to dryness. Redissolve in 100 µL water and methanol (mix 1:1).

3.9. HPLC Cochromatography

1. Analyze aliquots (e.g., 50 µL) of the above extract on a phenyl-modified reversed-phase column with a linear gradient of acetonitrile (from 0 to 35% in 70 min) in aqueous ammonium buffer. Measure the radioactivity eluting from the column by monitoring Cerenkov radiation through a radioactivity detector (*see* **Note 14**).

4. Notes

1. It is necessary to dialyze the MN solution to remove residual oligonucleotides. Use a 10K Slide-A-Lyzer from Pierce (cat. no. 66425, through Perbio Science UK, Tattenhall, Cheshire, UK) suspended in 5 L distilled water at 4°C for 24 h. Change water once. The SPD must also be dialyzed to remove the ammonium salts, which may inhibit the labeling. The enzymes should be stored at –20°C and may be kept for at least 6 mo without loss of enzyme activity.
2. Originally, Roche SPD was used at 2 mU/µL. This product was discontinued in the year 2000, and alternative sources (e.g., bovine phosphodiesterase from Sigma or Worthington) have not proved to be as active. It may be necessary to vary the amount used depending on the type of adducts to be detected.
3. Nuclease P_1 solutions (in water) should be stored at –20°C.
4. Plates should be prerun with distilled water and dried to remove a yellow contaminant, which may lead to an increased background.
5. 1 *M* Sodium phosphate is usually sufficient for many bulky adducts, but smaller or more polar adducts may require higher concentrations (1.7–2.3 *M* sodium phosphate) to avoid streaking.
6. Use lithium hydroxide to adjust pH to 3.5.
7. D2 and D3 are suitable for many lipophilic bulky adducts, but considerable variation is possible in both concentration and content.
8. **Caution:**[γ-^{32}P]ATP is a high-energy β-particle emitter and due regard should be given to handling the material. Exposure to ^{32}P should be avoided by working in a confined laboratory area, with protective clothing, shielding, Geiger counters, and body dosimeter.

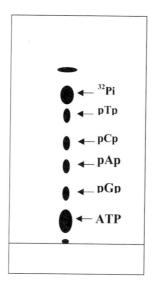

Fig. 3. One-dimensional chromatography of ^{32}P-labeled normal nucleotides on polyethyleneimine-cellulose.

We normally use 1-cm-thick Perspex or glass shielding between the operator and the source material throughout. We routinely wear two pairs of medium-weight rubber gloves and handle the tubes with 30-cm forceps. An appropriate Geiger counter should be on during the whole procedure, and working areas should be monitored before and after work. All apparatus should be checked for contamination and cleaned when appropriate by immersion in a suitable decontamination fluid (RBS 35 or Decon). Waste must be discarded according to appropriate local safety procedures.

9. The top of the tank and the lid should be wrapped around with cling film to avoid contamination with radioactivity.
10. Poor efficiency of either enrichment procedure will be demonstrated by the appearance of the four normal nucleotide spots (*see* **Fig. 3**). If there is no indication of excess ATP, then the sample should be discarded.
11. When quantifying the standard, it is necessary to run a blank using water instead of standard and to subtract the value obtained as background.
12. The origin after D1 can also be cut out of the PEI-cellulose TLC sheet.
13. The extraction can be monitored by measuring Cerenkov radiation in a scintillation counter before and after the extraction procedure.
14. Depending on the adduct type, other HPLC conditions may be more suitable.

References

1. Phillips, D. H. (2002) The formation of DNA adducts, in *The Cancer Handbook* (Allison, M. R., ed.), Macmillan, London, pp. 293–306.
2. Strickland, P. T., Routledge, M. N., and Dipple, A. (1993) Methodologies for measuring carcinogen adducts in humans. *Cancer Epidemiol. Biomarkers Prev.* **2,** 607–619.
3. Poirier, M. C., Santella, R. M., and Weston, A. (2000) Carcinogen macromolecular adducts and their measurement. *Carcinogenesis* **21,** 353–359.

4. Randerath, K., Reddy, M. V., and Gupta, R. C. (1981) ^{32}P-labeling test for DNA damage. *Proc. Natl. Acad. Sci. USA* **78,** 6126–6129.
5. Gupta, R. C., Reddy, M. V., and Randerath, K. (1982) ^{32}P-postlabeling analysis of nonradioactive aromatic carcinogen-DNA adducts. *Carcinogenesis* **3,** 1081–1092.
6. Reddy, M. V. and Randerath, K. (1986) Nuclease P1-mediated enhancement of sensitivity of ^{32}P-postlabeling test for structurally diverse DNA adducts. *Carcinogenesis* **7,** 1543–1551.
7. Gupta, R. C. (1985) Enhanced sensitivity of ^{32}P-postlabeling analysis of aromatic carcinogen:DNA adducts. *Cancer Res.* **45,** 5656–5662.
8. Randerath, K., Randerath, E., Danna, T. F., van Golen, K. L., and Putman, K. L. (1989) A new sensitive ^{32}P-postlabeling assay based on the specific enzymatic conversion of bulky DNA lesions to radiolabeled dinucleotides and nucleoside 5'-monophosphates. *Carcinogenesis* **10,** 1231–1239.
9. Pfau, W., Lecoq, S., Hughes, N. C., et al. (1993) Separation of ^{32}P-labelled 3',5'-bisphosphate adducts by HPLC, in *Postlabelling Methods for Detection of DNA Adducts* (Phillips, D. H., Castegnaro, M., and Bartsch, H., eds.), IARC, Lyon, pp. 233–242.
10. Phillips, D. H., Hewer, A., Horton, M. N., et al. (1999) *N*-demethylation accompanies α-hydroxylation in the metabolic activation of tamoxifen in rat liver cells. *Carcinogenesis* **20,** 2003–2009.
11. Jones, G. D., Dickinson, L., Lunec, J., and Routledge, M. N. (1999) SVPD-post-labeling detection of oxidative damage negates the problem of adventitious oxidative effects during ^{32}P-labeling. *Carcinogenesis* **20,** 503–7.
12. Beach, A. C. and Gupta, R. C. (1992) Human biomonitoring and the ^{32}P-postlabeling assay. *Carcinogenesis* **13,** 1053–1074.
13. Phillips, D. H. (1997) Detection of DNA modifications by the ^{32}P-postlabelling assay. *Mutat. Res.* **378,** 1–12.
14. Phillips, D. H., Farmer, P. B., Beland, F. A., et al. (2000) Methods of DNA adduct determination and their application to testing compounds for genotoxicity. *Environ. Mol. Mutagen.* **35,** 222–233.
15. Phillips, D. H. and Castegnaro, M. (1993) Results of an interlaboratory trial of ^{32}P-postlabeling, in *Postlabelling Methods for Detection of DNA Damage* (Phillips, D. H., Castegnaro, M., and Bartsch, H., eds.), IARC, Lyon, pp. 35–49.
16. Phillips, D. H. and Castegnaro, M. (1999) Standardization and validation of DNA adduct postlabelling methods: report of interlaboratory trials and production of recommended protocols. *Mutagenesis* **14,** 301–315.
17. Beland, F. A., Doerge, D. R., Churchwell, M. I., Poirier, M. C., Schoket, B., and Marques, M. M. (1999) Synthesis, characterization, and quantitation of a 4-aminobiphenyl-DNA adduct standard. *Chem. Res. Toxicol.* **12,** 68–77.
18. Osborne, M. R. and Phillips, D. H. (2000) Preparation of a methylated DNA standard, and its stability on storage. *Chem. Res. Toxicol.* **13,** 257–261.
19. Mourato, L. L. G., Beland, F. A., and Marques, M. M. (1999) ^{32}P-postlabeling of *N*-(deoxyguanosin-8-yl)arylamine adducts: a comparative study of labeling efficiencies. *Chem. Res. Toxicol.* **12,** 661–669.

2

Modification of the ^{32}P-Postlabeling Method to Detect a Single Adduct Species as a Single Spot

Masako Ochiai, Takashi Sugimura, and Minako Nagao

Summary

The original ^{32}P-postlabeling method developed by Randerath and his colleagues has been modified to detect a single type of adduct as a single spot in thin-layer chromatography (TLC), because some types of adducts gave multiple adduct spots by the original method. In the remodified methods, DNA is first digested with micrococcal nuclease and phophodiesterase II and then labeled with [γ-^{32}P]ATP under standard or adduct-intensification conditions. Since the labeled digest includes adducted mono-, di-, and/or oligo-deoxynucleotides, it is further treated with phosphatase and phosphodiesterase prior to TLC. The labeled digest is treated with nuclease P1 (NP1) in method I, and with T4 polynucleotide kinase and NP1 in method II, and then with phosphodiesterase I in both cases, and subjected to TLC. The advantage of these methods is that the number of adduct species formed can be estimated by TLC.

Key Words: Adducted deoxynucleoside 5'-phosphate; nuclease P1; T4 polynucle-otide kinase; phosphatases; phosphodiesterase I; phosphodiesterase II; micrococcal nuclease; intensification method; standard method; method I; method II.

1. Introduction

The ^{32}P-postlabeling method devised by Randerath and his group *(1,2)* is widely used to detect DNA adducts formed in vitro and in vivo with various mutagens and carcinogens. The advantages of this method (and simple modifications like butanol extraction and use of nuclease P1 [NP1] to detect adducts with high efficiency) are introduced in Chapter 1 of this volume. The principle is to detect DNA lesions as adducted deoxynucleoside 3', 5'-diphosphate elements. However, with the established methodology, a single type of adduct is not necessarily detected as a single spot owing to incomplete digestion of adducted DNA.

From: *Methods in Molecular Biology, vol. 291: Molecular Toxicology Protocols*
Edited by: P. Keohavong and S. G. Grant © Humana Press Inc., Totowa, NJ

In this chapter, approaches are introduced that allow for the detection of single adducted forms as single spots, with modifications to the original Randerath method. In these methods, DNA is first digested with microccocal nuclease (MN) and phosphodiesterase II (PDE II), and labeled with $[\gamma\text{-}^{32}P]ATP$ under standard (2) or adduct-intensification conditions (3), the labeled digests obtained are further treated with NP1, T4 polynucleotide kinase (PNK), and phophodiesterase I (PDE I), before analysis of adducted deoxynucleoside 5'-phosphate formation by thin-layer chromatography (TLC).

In some cases, the labeled DNA digests include mono-, di-, and/or oligodeoxynucleotides: $[^{32}P]pX(pN)_np$, where X is an adducted deoxynucleoside, and N is a normal deoxynucleoside. By treatment with NP1, the 3'-phosphate of $[^{32}P]pX(pN)_np$ can be removed to yield $[^{32}P]pX(pN)_n$ (4,5), and further treatment with PDE I may then produce $[^{32}P]pX$ and n(pN). Some types of adducted deoxynucleoside 3', 5'-diphosphate are, however, resistant to the phosphatase activity of NP1, although they are sensitive to that of PNK. Thus, in method I, labeled digests are treated with NP1, and in method II, with PNK and NP1 and then treated with PDE I in both cases, as shown in **Fig. 1**. It is known that the optimum pH for the 3'-phosphatase activity of PNK is 5.9, whereas that for its kinase activity is 6.5–8.5 (6).

To give a concrete example, when DNA from rats treated with the food-borne mutagenic/carcinogenic heterocyclic amine 2-amino-1-methyl-6-phenylimidazo[4,5-b]pyridine (PhIP) was analyzed by the ^{32}P-postlabeling method under standard or intensification conditions, several adduct spots were detected on TLC, and the spot for authentic N-(deoxyguanosin-8-yl)-2-amino-1-methyl-6-phenylimidazo[4,5-b]pyridine 3', 5'-diphosphate (3', 5'-pdGp-C8-PhIP) coincided with a minor adduct spot, although it has been demonstrated to be the sole adduct of PhIP by high performance liquid chromatography (HPLC) analysis using $[^3H]PhIP$ (7,8). The additional spots were demonstrated to be owing to incomplete digestion of DNA (8). A similar result was also obtained with a second heterocyclic amine, 2-amino-3,4-dimethylimidazo[4,5-f]quinoline (MeIQ) (9). Single spots thus were generated with DNA from animals treated with PhIP or MeIQ by method I (8,9).

In the case of the another heterocyclic amine, 2-amino-3-methylimidazo[4,5-f]quinoline (IQ), five spots were detected on TLC by the standard method (10), and for two of them their structures were tentatively identified as N-(deoxyguanosin-8-yl)-2-amino-3-methylimidazo[4,5-f]quinoline 3',5'-diphosphate (pdGp-C8-IQ) (11) and 5-(deoxyguanosin-N^2-yl)-2-amino-3-methylimidazo[4,5-f]quinoline (pdGp-N^2-IQ) (12). However, relatively large amounts of radioactivity were also present in the remaining three spots. When method I was applied for the analysis of IQ-DNA adducts, four spots were detected, and pdGp-N^2-IQ was demonstrated to be resistant to the phosphatase activity of NP1. However, it was converted to pdG-N^2-IQ with PNK, with or without NP1 (10). Thus, for IQ-DNA adducts, method II is appropriate, and by this method, spots of pdG-C8-IQ and pdG-N^2-IQ, as well as a very small radioactive spot representing an unknown form of adduct, could be detected (10).

Recoveries with the modified methods are very close to those with the standard and intensification methods; in other words, very high after treatment with PNK, NP1, and PDE I. These results indicate that ^{32}P-labeled oligonucleotides have modified bases at the 5'-most position.

$$*pXp+*pX(pN)_np+*pYp+*pY(pN)_np \xrightarrow{\text{PNK}} *pX+*pX(pN)_n+*pYp+*pY(N)_np$$

$$\xrightarrow{\text{NP1}} *pX+*pX(pN)_n+*pY+*pY(pN)_n$$

$$\xrightarrow{\text{PDEI}} *pX+*pY+pN$$

Fig.1. Principle of the modified method. *, ^{32}P-label; X and Y, modified deoxynucleosides; N, normal deoxynucleoside. 3' Phosphates of pXp and pX(pN)$_n$p seem to show the same susceptibility to the enzymes. In method I, NP1 and PDE I treatments and in method II, PNK, NP1, and PDE I treatments are performed. NP1, nuclease P1; PDE I, phosphodiesterase I; PNK, T4 polynucleotide kinase.

A major advantage of these methods is that the number of adduct species formed in vivo and/or under in vitro conditions can be estimated by TLC.

2. Materials

2.1. DNA Digestion

1. 0.01X SSC, 0.1 mM EDTA: make as 1X SSC (0.15 M NaCl, 0.015 M Na-citrate), 10 mM EDTA. The solution can be stored at 4°C (*see* **Note 1**).
2. MN (Worthington, Freehold, NJ): dissolve in water to give 4 U/μL (*see* **Note 2**).
3. PDE II from bovine spleen (Worthington): dissolve in water to give 40 mU/μL.
4. Nuclease mixture: mix MN and PDE II solutions at a ratio of 1:1 to give a final concentration of 2 U/μL for MN and 20 mU/μL for PDE II.
5. Digestion buffer: 0.1 M sodium succinate and 0.05 M CaCl$_2$, pH 6.0. This can be stored at 4°C.

2.2. Postlabeling

1. [γ-32P]ATP with a specific activity of approx 260 TBq/mmol (~370 MBq/60 μL, e.g., ICN Biomedical, Irvine, CA).
2. 10 U/μL PNK (e.g., Takara Shuzo, Kyoto, Japan).
3. 10X Kination buffer: 0.3 M Tris-HCl, pH 9.5, 0.1 M dithiothreitol, 0.1 M MgCl$_2$, 0.01 M spermidine.
4. ATP solution: 200 μM ATP.
5. Kination solution A (10 μL used for each tube): 1.5 μL of 10X kination buffer, 1 μL of PNK, 5 μL of [γ-32P] ATP, and 3 μL of ATP solution (*see* **Notes 3** and **4**).
6. Kination solution B (5 μL used for each tube): 1.5 μL of 10X kination buffer, 0.5 μL of PNK, 1.5 μL of [γ-^{32}P] ATP, and 1.5 μL of water.

2.3. Total Nucleotide Analysis

1. 20 mU/μL Potato apyrase (Sigma, St. Louis, MO).
2. Polyethyleneimine (PEI)-cellulose TLC sheets (95-mm height; Polygram CEL 300 PEI, Machery-Nagel, Duren, Germany; *see* **Note 5**).
3. 0.5 M LiCl.
4. Scintillation counter or BioImaging Analyzer (BIA; e.g., BAS2000 Fuji, Tokyo, Japan).

2.4. Digestion of Adducted Oligonucleotides by Method I

1. NP1: dissolve in water to give 1.6 U/µL (Yamasa Shoyu, Choshi, Japan).
2. PDE I: dissolve in water to give 20 mU/µL (Worthington).
3. Digestion buffer I: 0.3 *M* sodium acetate (or 0.13 *M* sodium citrate), pH 5.3. This can be stored at 4°C.
4. 1 m*M* ZnCl$_2$. This can be stored at 4°C.
5. 0.3 *N* HCl. This can be stored at room temperature.
6. 0.5 *M* Tris-base. This can be stored at 4°C.

2.5. Digestion of Adducted Oligonucleotides by Method II

1. NP1: same as in **Subheading 2.4.**, **item 1.**
2. PNK: dissolve in water to give 10 U/µL (New England BioLabs, Beverly, MA).
3. PDE I: same as in **Subheading 2.4.**, **item 2**.
4. Digestion buffer II: 0.2 *M* sodium citrate buffer, pH 5.7. This can be stored at 4°C.
5. 1 m*M* ZnCl$_2$:same as in **Subheading 2.4.**, **item 4**.
6. 0.3 *N* HCl: same as in **Subheading 2.4.**, **item 5**.
7. 0.5 *M* Tris-base: same as in **Subheading 2.4.**, **item 6**.

2.6. Thin-Layer Chromatography of Labeled Adducts

1. PEI-cellulose TLC sheet (Po CEL 300 PEI, Macherey-Nagel), 20 × 20 cm. Keep at 4°C.
2. Whatman no. 1 filter sheets.
3. D1: 2.3 *M* sodium phosphate buffer, pH 6.0.
4. D2: 3.4 *M* lithium formate, 6.4 *M* urea, pH 3.5 (*see* **Note 6**).
5. D3: 0.7 *M* NaH$_2$PO$_4$, 8.5 *M* urea, pH 8.0 (*see* **Note 6**).
6. D4: 1.7 *M* sodium phosphate buffer, pH 6.0

3. Methods

3.1. DNA Digestion

1. Dissolve DNA in 0.01X SSC, 0.1 m*M* EDTA at a concentration of 2 µg/µL.
2. Transfer 5 µL of the DNA solution, 1.5 µL of water, 1.5 µL of the nuclease mixture, and 2 µL of digestion buffer to a 1.5-mL tube.
3. Incubate at 37°C for 3–3.5 h and centrifuge at 12,000*g* for 5 min at 4°C. Dilute a 2-µL aliquot of the supernatant with 58 µL of water (*see* **Note 7**).

3.2. ^{32}P-Postlabeling by the Standard Method or Adduct-Intensification Method

1. Standard condition: transfer an aliquot of 5 µL of the diluted DNA digest and 10 µL of kination solution A to a 1.5-mL tube, and incubate at 37°C for 1 h. Spin down in a microcentrifuge at 4°C (*see* **Note 8**). Proceed to **Subheading 3.3**.
2. Adduct intensification condition: transfer an aliquot of 5 µL of DNA digest, 5 µL of water, and 5 µL of kination solution B to a 1.5-mL tube, and incubate at 37°C for 1 h.

3.3. Total Nucleotide Analysis

1. Transfer an aliquot of 2 µL of the ^{32}P-labeled sample to a 0.5-mL tube, add 5.4 mU (3 µL, 1.8 mU/µL) of apyrase, and incubate at 37°C for 45 min (*see* **Note 9**).
2. Add water to make a total of 250 µL.
3. On a PEI-cellulose sheet, draw 1-cm^2 grids, 3 cm from the base.
4. Spot an aliquot of 5 µL on a PEI-cellulose sheet and dry.

5. Develop with LiCl solution to the top edge.
6. Check separation of nucleotides (origin) from phosphate (Rf: approx 0.2) by exposure to an X-ray film for approx 3 min.
7. Carefully cut out the squares containing nucleotides. Place in scintillation vials, add 3 mL toluene cocktail, and count over the entire energy window (*see* **Note 10**).

3.4. Adduct Analysis by Method I

1. Adjust the pH of the remaining sample (13 μL) of the incubate from **Subheadings 3.2.**, **step 1** or **3.2.**, **step 2** to approx 6.0 by adding 1.8 μL of 0.3 *N* HCl.
2. To the tube, add 1 μL of NP1 solution (1.6 U), 1 μL of $ZnCl_2$ solution, and 1.5 μL of digestion buffer I (pH 5.3) and incubate at 37°C for 10 min (*see* **Note 11**).
3. Adjust the pH to 8.0–9.0 by adding 3 μL of 0.5 *M* Tris-base.
4. Add 1.5 μL of PDE I solution (30 mU) to this tube and incubate at 37°C for 30 min. Proceed to **Subheading 3.6**.

3.5. Adduct Analysis by Method II

The 3'-phosphate of some adducts is resistant to NP1 phosphatase activity. In this case, prior PNK treatment is useful.

1. Adjust the pH of the remaining sample (13 μL) of the incubate from **Subheading 3.2.**, **step 1** or **step 2** to approx 6.0 by adding 1.3 μL of 0.3 *N* HCl.
2. Add 3 μL of PNK solution (30 U) and 1.5 μL of digestion buffer II pH 5.7 (the final concentration of citrate is 16 m*M*) to the tube and incubate at 37°C for 30 min.
3. Add another 1 μL of PNK solution (10 U) and incubate at 37°C for 30 min.
4. Add 0.7 μL of NP1 solution (1.1 U) and 1 μL of $ZnCl_2$ solution, and incubate at 37°C for 10 min.
5. Adjust the pH to approx 8.0 by adding 3 μL of 0.5 *M* Tris-base.
6. Add 1.5 μL of PDE I solution (30 mU), and incubate at 37°C for 30 min.

3.6. TLC Analysis

Almost the same TLC conditions as those described in Chapter 1 are applicable, although migration distances differ from the adducted deoxynucleoside diphosphate case. Run D3 twice (*see* **Note 12**). Run D4 in the same direction as D3 after attaching a 35-mm Whatman filter paper to the top edge of the TLC sheet.

3.7. Imaging and Quantification

1. Visualize and quantify adduct spots as described in Chapter 1, **Subheading 3.7.**, **step 1**.
2. Under standard conditions, calculate relative adduct labeling (RAL) according to the following equation:

$$RAL = \frac{\text{adduct radioactivity (cpm)}}{\text{radioactivity of total deoxynucleotide (cpm)} \times \text{fold dilution}}$$

3. For analysis under intensification conditions, calculate intensification factor (IF) according to the following equation:

$$IF = \frac{RAL_{int}}{RAL_{std}}$$

where RAL_{int} is RAL under intensification conditions, and RAL_{std} is RAL under standard conditions.

4. Notes

1. Ultrapure water prepared by passing through Milli-Q spUF is used.
2. All solutions should be stored at –20°C, except where otherwise stated.
3. To ensure thorough mixing, it is recommended that all tubes containing different components be vortexed and spun down in a microcentrifuge.
4. Protection from radioactivity during handling of radioactive samples is crucially important and should be performed as described in Chapter 1, **Note 8.**
5. Sheets can be stored at 4°C. Plates should be prerun with water overnight after attachment of a 12-cm filter paper wick and dried at room temperature.
6. The solvent used for IQ-DNA adduct analysis is indicated as an example. For D2, 4.5 M lithium formate, 8.5 M urea, pH 3.5 is prepared and diluted appropriately. For MeIQ-adducts 60% and for PhIP-adducts 80% solutions were used. For D3, 1.0 M LiCl, 0.5 M Tris-HCl, 8.5 M urea, pH 8.0, was used for MeIQ and PhIP.
7. When analysis is performed under intensification conditions (*see* **Subheading 3.2., step 2**), it is also necessary to perform the procedure outlined in **Subheading 3.2., step 1**, to determine the IF value of each adduct as written in **Subheading 3.7.**
8. After incubation in a tube, the contents should be spun down at 4°C.
9. Potato apyrase (20 mU/µL) is diluted with water to give a concentration of 1.8 mU/µL.
10. When BIA is used for quantification, a 500X dilution for the standard method (and a 50X dilution for the adduct intensification method), and exposure to X-ray film for approx 30 min are recommended. For BIA analysis, total and adduct analyses should be made on the same imaging plates.
11. This condition is appropriate for PhIP and MeIQ adducts, but the optimum pH may differ depending on specific adducts and it is necessary to check the optimum pH, which should be between 5.3 and 7.0.
12. The background usually becomes clean by running twice. Running once is enough in some cases.

References

1. Randerath, K., Reddy, M. V., and Gupta, R. C., (1981) ^{32}P-Labeling test for DNA damage. *Proc. Natl. Acad. Sci. USA* **78,** 6126–6129.
2. Gupta, R. C., Reddy M. V., and Randerath, K., (1982) ^{32}P-Postlabeling analysis of non-radioactive aromatic carcinogen-DNA adducts. *Carcinogenesis* **3,** 1081–1092.
3. Randerath E., Atrawal H. P., Weaver, J. A., Bordelon C. B., and Randerath K., (1985) ^{32}P-postlabeling analysis of DNA adducts persisting for up to 42 weeks in the skin, epidermis and dermis of mice treated topically with 7,12-dimethylbenz[a]anthracene. *Carcinogenesis* **6,** 1117–1126.
4. Wilson, V. L., Basu, A. K., Essigmann, J. M., Smith, R. A., and Harris, C. C., (1988) O^6-alkyldeoxygunosine detection by ^{32}P-postlabeling and nucleotide chromatographic analysis. *Cancer Res.* **48,** 2156–2161.
5. Randerath, K., Randerath, E., Danna, T. F., van Golden, K. L., and Putaman, L. L., (1989) A new sensitive ^{32}P-postlabeling assay based on the specific enzymatic conversion of bulky DNA lesions to radiolabeled dinucleotides and nucleoside 5'-monophosphates. *Carcinogenesis* **10,** 1231–1239.
6. Cameron, V. and Uhlenbeck, O. C., (1977) 3'-Phosphatase activity in T4 polynucleotide kinase. *Biochemistry* **16,** 5120–5126.

7. Frandsen, H., Grivas, S., Andersson, R., Dragsted, L., and Larsen J. C., (1992) Reaction of the N^2-acetoxy derivative of 2-amino-1-methyl-6-phenylimidazo[4,5-*b*]pyridine with 2'-deoxyguanosine and DNA. Synthesis and identification of N^2-(2'-deoxyguanosin-8-yl)-PhIP. *Carcinogenesis* **13,** 629–635.

8. Fukutome, K., Ochiai, M., Wakabayashi, K., Watanabe S., Sugimura, T., and Nagao, M., (1994) Detection of guanine-C8-2-amino-1-methyl-6-phenylimidazo[4,5-*b*]pyridine adduct as a single spot on thin-layer chromatography by modification of the ^{32}P-postlabeling method. *Jpn. J. Cancer Res.* **85,** 113–117.

9. Tada, A., Ochiai, M., Wakabayashi, K., Nukaya, H., Sugimura T., and Nagao, M., (1994) Identification of *N*-(deoxyguanosin-8-yl)-2-amino-3,4-dimethylimidazo[4,5-*f*]quinoline (dG-C8-MeIQ) as a major adduct formed by MeIQ with nucleotides in vitro and with DNA in vivo. *Carcinogenesis* **15,** 1275–1278.

10. Ochiai, M., Nakagama, H., Turesky, R. J., Sugimura, T., and Nagao, M., (1999) A new modification of the ^{32}P-post-labeling method to recover IQ-DNA adducts as mononucleotides. *Mutagenesis* **14,** 239–242.

11. Snyderwine, E. G., Yamashita, K., Adamson, R. H., et al., (1988) Use of the ^{32}P-postlabeling method to detect DNA adducts of 2-amino-3-methylimidazo[4,5-*f*]quinoline (IQ) in monkeys fed IQ: identification of the *N*-(deoxyguanosin-8-yl)-IQ adduct. *Carcinogenesis* **8,** 1739–1743.

12. Turesky, R. J. and Markovic, J., (1994) DNA adduct formation of the food carcinogen 2-amino-3-methylimidazo[4,5-*f*]quinoline at the C-8 and N^2 atoms of guanine. *Chem. Res. Toxicol.* **7,** 752–761.

3

DNA Isolation and Sample Preparation for Quantification of Adduct Levels by Accelerator Mass Spectrometry

Karen H. Dingley, Esther A. Ubick, John S. Vogel, and Kurt W. Haack

Summary

A protocol is described for the isolation of DNA and subsequent preparation of samples for the measurement of adduct levels by accelerator mass spectrometry (AMS). AMS is a highly sensitive technique used for the quantification of adducts following exposure to carbon-14– or tritium-labeled chemicals, with detection limits in the range of one adduct per 10^{11}–10^{12} nucleotides. However, special precautions must be taken to avoid cross-contamination of isotope between samples and to produce a sample that is compatible with AMS. The DNA isolation method described is based on digestion of tissue with proteinase K, followed by extraction of DNA using Qiagen DNA isolation columns. DNA is then precipitated with isopropanol, washed repeatedly with 70% ethanol to remove salt, and then dissolved in water. This method has been used to generate reliably good yields of uncontaminated, pure DNA from animal and human tissues for analysis of adduct levels. For quantification of adduct levels from ^{14}C-labeled compounds, DNA samples are then converted to graphite, and the ^{14}C content is measured by AMS.

Key Words: Accelerator mass spectroscopy (AMS); DNA damage; adduct; carbon-14; tritium; DNA isolation; risk assessment.

1. Introduction

Most known chemical carcinogens form reactive intermediates that are capable of reacting with DNA, forming covalent adducts. This damage may lead to mutations and ultimately cancer (reviewed in **ref. 1**). Consequently, for risk assessment it is important to establish whether drugs and toxicants are capable of forming DNA adducts, particularly following doses that are encountered in everyday life. Traditional methods used to monitor DNA adducts include ^{32}P-postlabeling (*see* Chap. 1), fluorescence techniques, gas chromatography/mass spectroscopy (GC/MS), and immunoassays (*see* Chaps. 4 and 29), with detection limits typically in the range of one adduct/10^7–10^9 nucleotides (reviewed in **ref. 2**). Accelerator mass spectrometry (AMS) allows one to establish whether chemicals form DNA adducts at even lower

From: *Methods in Molecular Biology, vol. 291, Molecular Toxicology Protocols*
Edited by: P. Keohavong and S. G. Grant © Humana Press Inc., Totowa, NJ

levels (10^{-10}–10^{-12} nucleotides range) through the use of carbon-14 (^{14}C)- or tritium (^{3}H)-labeled compounds (reviewed in **ref. 3**). Thus, DNA adduct levels can be established following low chemical doses or using compounds that have a low covalent binding index (e.g., **refs. 4–7**). Because the amounts of chemicals and radioactivity required are low, such studies can be conducted safely in humans *(4,8,9)*.

AMS is a nuclear physics technique that can measure isotopes with a low natural abundance and a long half-life (e.g., ^{14}C and ^{3}H) with high sensitivity and precision (reviewed in **ref. 10**). It was originally developed for use in the earth sciences but has now found widespread use in biology, with applications in areas such as cancer, nutrition, and pharmaceutical research (for review, *see* **refs. 1, 5, and 11**). However, as AMS is so sensitive, cross-contamination of samples by isotope from equipment and laboratory supplies can be a major problem *(12)*. Therefore, certain methods have been chosen to avoid contamination. For example, we have found that phenol/chloroform extraction, a process that is used frequently in DNA isolations, can be a major source of ^{14}C contamination. All gloves, tubes, forceps, and containers for buffers and other substances used in sample preparation must be disposable. Furthermore, before analysis by AMS, samples must be converted to graphite (for ^{14}C analysis) or titanium hydride (for ^{3}H analysis) *(13,14)*. Therefore, the samples must be compatible with this process. For example, this necessitates the complete removal of sodium salts from the extracted DNA samples by repeated washing with 70% ethanol.

This chapter describes a protocol for extracting DNA from tissues for analysis of ^{14}C or ^{3}H content by AMS. The method is based on the use of Qiagen columns. Procedures for contamination avoidance in samples are included throughout. After the section on DNA isolation, a description of the process for conversion of the biological material to graphite for ^{14}C analysis is presented. AMS is then used to quantitate the amount of ^{14}C in the graphite samples. Owing to the size and cost of an AMS instrument, this technique is not yet a routine tool in many laboratories. However, there are several facilities in the United States where samples can be sent for analysis. One such facility, The Center for Accelerator Mass Spectrometry at Lawrence Livermore National Laboratory, has a compact AMS system for the analysis of biological samples *(15)*.

2. Materials

2.1. Tissue Homogenization and Protein Digestion

1. Plastic wrap (e.g., Saran wrap).
2. Aluminum foil.
3. Parafilm.
4. 50-mL Polypropylene tubes (e.g., Falcon, BD Biosciences, Franklin Lakes, NJ).
5. Hammer and plastic bag to cover.
6. Disposable scalpels.
7. Disposable forceps (Cole-Parmer, Vernon Hills, IL).
8. Lysis buffer: 4 *M* urea, 1% Triton X-100, 10 m*M* EDTA, 100 m*M* NaCl, 10 m*M* Tris-HCl, pH 8.0, 10 m*M* dithiothreitol.
9. 40 mg/mL Proteinase K in double-distilled water.
10. Shaking water bath or other mixer that will incubate at 37°C.

2.2. RNA Digestion

1. RNAse T1: 100 µg/mL in double-distilled water.
2. RNAse A (DNAse-free): 10 mg/mL in double-distilled water.

2.3. Column Purification

1. Qiagen Genomic tip 500 columns (Qiagen, Valencia, CA; *see* **Note 1**).
2. 5 *M* Sodium chloride.
3. 1 *M* 3-Morpholinopropanesulfonic acid (MOPS), pH 7.0.
4. Buffer B: 750 m*M* NaCl, 50 m*M* MOPS, 15% ethanol, 0.15% Triton X-100, pH 7.0.
5. Buffer C: 1 *M* NaCl, 50 m*M* MOPS, 15% ethanol, pH 7.0.
6. Buffer λ: 1.25 *M* NaCl, 50 m*M* MOPS, 15% ethanol, pH 8.0.
7. 50-mL Polypropylene tubes.
8. Holders for 50-mL polypropylene tubes.

2.4. DNA Precipitation, Washing, Redissolution, Concentration, and Purity

1. Isopropanol.
2. Ice-cold 70% ethanol.
3. Double-distilled water.
4. UV spectrophotometer.

2.5. Conversion to Graphite

1. 4 (Inner dimension) × 50-mm quartz sample tube (special order from Scientific Glass of Florida, Sanford, FL).
2. Copper oxide (wire form; Aldrich, Milwaukee, WI).
3. 7 (Inner dimension) × 155-mm quartz combustion tube with breakable tip (Scientific Glass of Florida).
4. 9 (Outer dimension) × 155-mm borosilicate tube with dimple 2 cm from the sealed end (Scientific Glass of Florida).
5. 6 × 50-mm Borosilicate culture tube (Kimble/Kontes, Vineland, NJ).
6. Tributyrin (ICN Pharmaceutical, Costa Mesa, CA).
7. Zinc (powder; Aldrich).
8. Titanium hydride (powder; Aldrich).
9. Cobalt (powder; Aldrich).
10. Vacuum source (Varian, Lexington, MA).
11. Disposable vacuum manifold made from 5/16-inch plastic Y-connector and 1/2-inch outer dimension × 5/16-inch inner dimension plastic tubing (Nalgene, Rochester, NY). For schematic of manifold, *see* **ref. 13**.
12. Torch for tube sealing (oxyacetylene-type preferred).
13. Muffle furnace (e.g., NDI Vulcan 3-550, Neytech, Bloomfield, CT).
14. Vacuum concentrator (e.g., RC 10.10, Jouan, Winchester, VA).
15. Liquid nitrogen bath (consisting of liquid nitrogen in a Dewar flask).
16. Dry ice/isopropanol bath (consisting of a slurry made of dry ice and isopropanol).

3. Methods

3.1. Tissue Homogenization and Protein Digestion

1. Place 400 mg of fresh tissue in the middle of a piece of the plastic wrap and fold the top half of the plastic wrap over the bottom half. Cover the wrapped tissue in a layer of aluminum foil (*see* **Notes 1** and **2**).

2. Cover hammer with a plastic bag or plastic wrap. Pound tissue with the hammer until tissue is well homogenized. Scrape homogenized tissue into a 50-mL polypropylene tube using a clean, disposable scalpel.
3. Add 25 mL fresh lysis buffer.
4. Add 500 µL proteinase K. Mix by vortexing for 5 s.
5. Wrap the top of the tubes with parafilm to prevent leakage and contamination.
6. Place tubes in a 37°C shaking water bath overnight, or until tissue appears to be fully digested (i.e., there are no visible lumps of tissue).
7. Centrifuge at 20°C, 2000*g*, 20 min to remove any undigested tissue.
8. Pour supernatant into a clean 50-mL polypropylene tube. Discard pellet.

3.2. RNA Digestion
1. Add 1.25 mL RNAse A and 1.25 mL RNAse T1 to sample.
2. Mix by vortexing for 5 s.
3. Incubate for 30–60 min at room temperature.

3.3. Column Purification
1. Add 1.25 mL 1 *M* MOPS and 4.5 mL 5 *M* NaCl to the sample.
2. Mix by vortexing for 5 s.
3. Stand the required number of Qiagen columns in a rack, with a disposable 50-mL polypropylene tube under each one.
4. Add 25 mL buffer B to each of the columns.
5. Let the buffer run through the column completely and then discard the buffer.
6. Pour the samples into the columns. Discard the eluate. If column becomes clogged, *see* **Note 3**.
7. Add 25 mL buffer C to each of the columns. Discard the eluate. Repeat and discard the eluate.
8. Add 25 mL buffer λ to each of the columns. Collect the eluate in a clean, new 50-mL polypropylene tube. Keep the eluate, as this will contain the DNA.

3.4. DNA Precipitation
1. Add 25 mL of ice-cold 100% isopropanol to the eluate containing the DNA.
2. Mix by vortexing for 5 s.
3. Wrap the lid in parafilm and place at –20°C overnight to precipitate the DNA.
4. Centrifuge at –4°C, 2000*g* for 3 h.
5. Carefully pour off supernatant. Save the pelleted DNA, and discard the supernatant.

3.5. Sample Washing and Redissolving
1. Add 5 mL 70% ethanol to the pellet.
2. Mix by vortexing for 5 s.
3. Centrifuge at 4°C, 2000*g* for 10 min.
4. Save the pellet, and discard the supernatant.
5. Repeat wash step with 70% ethanol and centrifuge.
6. Carefully pour off the supernatant, taking care not to dislodge the pellet. If the pellet becomes loose, recentrifuge.
7. Carefully invert the tube on laboratory bench paper to drain excess solvent. Leave the tube inverted for 10–15 min.
8. Add double-distilled water to the pellet (*see* **Note 4**).

3.6. DNA Concentration and Purity

1. Dilute an aliquot of the DNA with double-distilled water (*see* **Note 4**).
2. Measure and record the UV absorbance of the diluted DNA at 260 and 280 nm.
3. A 50 μg/mL solution of DNA has a UV absorbance of 1 at 260 nm. Therefore, DNA concentration in μg/mL = absorbance at 260 nm × 50 × dilution factor.
4. DNA purity = absorbance at 260 nm/absorbance at 280 nm. Pure DNA should have a ratio of 1.7–1.9 (*see* **Note 5**).
5. DNA should be prepared for AMS analysis as soon as possible to prevent contamination (*see* **Note 6**).

3.7. AMS Sample Preparation (Conversion to Graphite)

1. Place all quartz components into muffle furnace and heat to 900°C for 2 h. Remove components after they have cooled; handle 6 × 50-mm tubes with disposable forceps only (to prevent contamination).
2. Pipet known amount of DNA into clean, uncontaminated quartz sample tube, and add tributyrin if necessary (*see* **Note 7**). The quartz tube should then be placed within a test tube to protect the sample during vacuum concentration.
3. Remove all volatile components by completely drying with vacuum concentration.
4. Remove quartz sample tube from test tube using disposable forceps. Add 150–200 mg of copper oxide to dried DNA.
5. Place quartz sample tube in larger quartz combustion tube and evacuate. Seal evacuated combustion tube with torch.
6. Place combustion tube in muffle furnace at 900°C for 2 h. Remove after it has cooled.
7. Place all borosilicate components in the muffle furnace and heat to 500°C for 2 h. Remove components after they have cooled; handle 6 × 50-mm tubes with disposable forceps only (to prevent contamination).
8. Place 100–150 mg zinc powder and 10–20 mg titanium hydride powder into larger borosilicate tube.
9. Place 5–8 mg cobalt powder into 6 × 50 mm borosilicate tube.
10. Drop smaller tube into larger tube so that smaller tube rests on dimple in larger tube, thereby suspending it above the zinc and titanium hydride levels.
11. Place disposable vacuum manifold on vacuum source with the arms of the Y hanging down.
12. Push the breakable tip end of the quartz tube into one arm of the Y and push the open end of the borosilicate tube onto the other arm.
13. Evacuate the manifold with the tubes attached.
14. Place the quartz tube into the dry ice/isopropanol bath.
15. Keeping the quartz tube in the dry ice/isopropanol bath, place the borosilicate tube into the liquid nitrogen bath.
16. Isolate the manifold from the vacuum source (do not remove from the vacuum source).
17. Crack the breakable tip of the quartz tube, allowing the carbon dioxide inside to transfer to the borosilicate tube.
18. Evacuate the manifold again without removing the tubes from either bath.
19. Using the torch, seal off the borosilicate tube above level of the top of the 6 × 50-mm tube, trapping the carbon dioxide in the larger borosilicate tube with its other contents.
20. Place the sealed tube in the furnace and heat to 500°C for 4 h. Remove after cooling.
21. Break open the larger borosilicate tube to remove the smaller tube. The black powder in the small tube is the graphite, which can be analyzed by AMS.

22. AMS will establish the $^{14}C/^{12}C$ ratio of the sample. This is then used to calculate the adduct level (*see* **Note 8**).

4. Notes

1. The protocol described is for isolation of up to 400 μg DNA using Qiagen Genomic tip 500 DNA isolation columns. This is approximately equivalent to the amount of DNA obtained from 400 mg wet tissue. Other column sizes are Qiagen Genomic tip 20 for up to 20 μg DNA and tip 100 for up to 90 μg DNA. The protocol can be scaled down for the smaller columns. (Refer to manufacturer's instructions for column loading and wash volumes.)

2. When handling samples, it is essential to avoid cross-contamination of isotope by the use of disposable plastic ware, scalpels, forceps, and gloves. These should be changed in between samples. Liquid samples should be pipeted using filter tips and clean pipets. When homogenizing the tissue, there should be disposable barriers (plastic wrap and foil) in between the sample and hammer.

3. The flow rate of the column will depend on the viscosity of the sample. If the column exhibits a very slow flow rate or becomes completely clogged, the flow can be assisted by attaching a small amount of tubing to the bottom of the column and withdrawing eluate slowly with a syringe. Troubleshooting tips are also described in the Qiagen literature.

4. The volume of water required will depend on the amount of DNA extracted. Typically in this procedure, 300 μL of water will result in well-dissolved DNA with a concentration of 1–2 mg/mL. A 1:20 dilution of this solution should then be within the range suitable for DNA concentration determination by UV spectrophotometry. The AMS sample tubes used in our laboratory have a sample capacity of about 400 μL, so larger samples may need to be concentrated prior to AMS preparation.

5. If A260/A280-nm absorbance ratios are not within the range of 1.7 to 1.9, this is probably because of incomplete removal of protein or RNA. The DNA should be repurified prior to analysis by AMS.

6. We try to submit DNA for analysis by AMS within 24 h of extraction. This reduces the chance of cross-contamination of samples with radioisotope. However, if this is not possible, samples should be stored in a refrigerator or freezer that is not used for storage of high levels of radioisotope.

7. Tributyrin is a nonvolatile hydrocarbon that contains depleted levels of carbon-14. It is used in AMS to increase the size of small samples for efficient graphitization. Typically, using this method, samples that contain less than 0.5 mg carbon require the addition of carrier. For DNA (29% carbon), this would be equal to 1.7 mg. A 40 mg/mL solution of tributyrin in methanol is made, and then 50 μL is added to each DNA sample. Carrier controls should be prepared at the same time (*see* **Note 8**).

8. The isotope ratios determined by AMS are converted to adduct levels first by subtracting the natural radiocarbon content of the sample and the radiocarbon contributed from addition of any carrier. The natural radiocarbon content of the DNA is determined using control DNA samples from subjects or rodents not given the [^{14}C]-labeled compound. Adduct levels (ratio of moles of compound/moles nucleotide) are then calculated based on the percent carbon of DNA (29%) and the compound specific activity *(16)*.

Acknowledgments

The authors thank Kristin Stoker for help with preparation of the manuscript. This work was performed under the auspices of the US DOE (W-7405-ENG-48) with support from the NIH/National Center for Research Resources (RR13461).

References

1. Garner, R. C. (1998) The role of DNA adducts in chemical carcinogenesis. *Mutat. Res.* **402,** 67–75.
2. Poirier, M. C., Santella, R. M., and Weston, A. (2000) Carcinogen macromolecular adducts and their measurement. *Carcinogenesis* **21,** 353–359.
3. Turteltaub, K. W. and Dingley, K. H. (1998) Application of accelerated mass spectrometry (AMS) in DNA adduct quantification and identification. *Toxicol. Lett.* **102–103,** 435–439.
4. Lightfoot, T. J., Coxhead, J. M., Cupid, B. C., Nicholson, S., and Garner, R. C. (2000) Analysis of DNA adducts by accelerator mass spectrometry in human breast tissue after administration of 2-amino-1-methyl-6-phenylimidazo[4,5-*b*]pyridine and benzo[*a*]pyrene. *Mutat. Res.* **472,** 119–127.
5. Turteltaub, K. W. and Vogel, J. S. (2000) Bioanalytical applications of accelerator mass spectrometry for pharmaceutical research. *Curr. Pharm. Design* **6,** 991–1007.
6. Dingley, K. H., Roberts, M. L., Velsko, C. A., and Turteltaub, K. W. (1998) Attomole detection of ^{3}H in biological samples using accelerator mass spectrometry: application in low-dose, dual-isotope tracer studies in conjunction with ^{14}C accelerator mass spectrometry. *Chem. Res. Toxicol.* **11,** 1217–1222.
7. Creek, M. R., Mani, C., Vogel, J. S., and Turteltaub, K. W. (1997) Tissue distribution and macromolecular binding of extremely low doses of [^{14}C]-benzene in B6C3F1 mice. *Carcinogenesis* **18,** 2421–2427.
8. Dingley, K. H., Curtis, K. D., Nowell, S., Felton, J. S., Lang, N. P., and Turteltaub, K. W. (1999) DNA and protein adduct formation in the colon and blood of humans after exposure to a dietary-relevant dose of 2-amino-1-methyl-6-phenylimidazo[4,5-*b*]pyridine. *Cancer Epidemiol. Biomarkers Prev.* **8,** 507–512.
9. Mauthe, R. J., Dingley, K. H., Leveson, S. H., et al. (1999) Comparison of DNA-adduct and tissue-available dose levels of MeIQx in human and rodent colon following administration of a very low dose. *Int. J. Cancer* **80,** 539–545.
10. Vogel, J. S., Turteltaub, K. W., Finkel, R., and Nelson, D. E. (1995) Accelerator mass-spectrometry—isotope quantification at attomole sensitivity. *Anal. Chem.* **67,** A353–A359.
11. Vogel, J. S. and Turteltaub, K. W. (1998) Accelerator mass spectrometry as a bioanalytical tool for nutritional research. *Adv. Exp. Med. Biol.* **445,** 397–410.
12. Buchholz, B. A., Freeman, S. P. H. T., Haack, K. W., and Vogel, J. S. (2000) Tips and traps in the C-14 bio-AMS preparation laboratory. *Nucl. Instr. Methods Phys. Res. B* **172,** 404–408.
13. Vogel, J. S. (1992) Rapid production of graphite without contamination for biomedical AMS. *Radiocarbon.* **34,** 344–350.
14. Roberts, M. L., Velsko, C., and Turteltaub, K. W. (1994) Tritium AMS for biomedical applications. *Nucl. Instr. Methods Phys. Res. B* **92,** 459–462.
15. Ognibene, T. J., Bench, G., Brown, T. A., Peaslee, G. F., and Vogel, J. S. (2002) A new accelerator mass spectrometry system for ^{14}C-quantification of biochemical samples. *Int. J. Mass Spectr.* **218,** 255–264.
16. Vogel J. S., Grant, P. G., Bucholz, B. A., Dingley, K., and Turteltaub, K. W. (2001) Attomole quantitation of protein separations with accelerator mass spectrometry. *Electrophoresis* **22,** 2037–2045.

4

Fluoroimaging-Based Immunoassay of DNA Photoproducts in Ultraviolet-B-Irradiated Tadpoles

Iovanna Pandelova, Stephen R. Hewitt, and John B. Hays

Summary

Sensitive and accurate measurement of photoproducts induced in DNA by natural or artificial ultraviolet-B (UVB; and UVC) light is essential to evaluate the toxic and mutagenic effects of this radiation. Monoclonal antibodies specific for the two major classes of photoproducts—cyclobutane pyrimidine dimers (CPDs) and pyrimidine-[6-4]-pyrimidinone photoproducts ([6-4]PPs)—have made possible highly specific and sensitive assays. Described here is the use of these primary antibodies with fluorescent secondary antibodies to generate 96-spot arrays. Stable fluorescence signals are rapidly and sensitively scored by fluoroimaging and computer analysis of peak-and-valley traces. CPD levels in a series of calibration standards are determined by acid hydrolysis/thin-layer chromatography analyses of radiolabeled bacterial DNA, UV-irradiated to known high fluences, and linear extrapolation to known lower fluences. The nonlinear fluorescence vs CPD curve reflects the effect of photoproduct concentration on single vs double binding by divalent antibody proteins. This technique is applied to photoproducts in whole inbred *Xenopus laevis* tadpoles, chronically irradiated at a series of UVB fluences that reach a lethality threshold when in vivo steady-state photoproduct levels are still quite low. As few as 0.01–0.02 CPDs per DNA kbp can be reliably detected, at signal/noise ratios of roughly 3:1.

Key Words: DNA adducts; UV; cyclobutane pyrimidine dimers (CPD); immunoassay; monoclonal antibody; fluorescent antibody; tadpole; DNA repair; *Xenopus leavis*; [6-4]photoproduct; fluoroimaging.

1. Introduction

Sensitive and accurate detection of photoproducts induced in cellular DNA by ultraviolet (UV) light is essential to interpretation of viability and survival data. Most studies have used cultures of prokaryotic or eukaryotic cells, because of their uniformity and amenability to statistical analyses. Notable exceptions are analyses of photoproduct accumulation and "sunburn" response in outer layers of mammalian skin *(1)*, as well as measurements of photoproducts in thin leaves of alfalfa and *Arabidopsis* seedlings *(2,3)*. To analyze quantitatively ultraviolet-B (UVB) effects on amphibians,

From: *Methods in Molecular Biology, vol. 291, Molecular Toxicology Protocols*
Edited by: P. Keohavong and S. G. Grant © Humana Press Inc., Totowa, NJ

whose drastic global population declines have been linked in some cases with solar UVB radiation *(4,5)*, we have employed cohorts of inbred *Xenopus leavis* tadpoles. Their genetic and chronological homogeneity maximizes biological uniformity, and their small size and semitransparency make even interior organs vulnerable to UV light. When parallel tadpole subpopulations are exposed to UVB light regimes of increasing chronic intensity, survival decreases abruptly at fluences that still induce relatively low levels of photoproducts in DNA *(6)*. Thus, photoproduct assays that are sensitive, accurate, and reasonably reproducible from one animal to another are needed to evaluate lethal UVB thresholds.

Assays that depend on cleavage of DNA strands at photoproduct sites and analysis of the size distributions of the resulting fragments can be highly sensitive. Size distributions are typically measured by alkaline sedimentation of DNA previously radiolabeled in vivo *(2)*, or alkaline gel electrophoresis and electronic imaging *(7)*. Radiolabeling of tadpole DNA in vivo is not practical, since the animals are grown in 1-gallon tanks, and the electrophoresis video-imaging technique requires highly specialized apparatus. Furthermore, extraction of DNA by all but the gentlest techniques breaks DNA, thus distorting size distributions. In any case, determinations of average photoproduct levels from fragment analyses typically involve assumptions about the randomness of photoproduct distribution that may not be warranted for thicker tissues. Lastly, efficient and highly specific incising enzymes are available only for one major class of UV photoproducts, cyclobutane pyrimidine dimers (CPDs); for the other major class, pyrimidine-[6-4']-pyrimidinone photoproducts ([6-4]PPs), precise and efficient incision is difficult to achieve.

In the past few years, polyclonal *(8)* and monoclonal *(9)* antibodies specific for CPDs and [6-4]PPs have been used for photoproduct-specific immunoassays. Radioimmune dilution *(8)* and enzyme-linked immunosorbent assay *(10)* techniques have been employed with considerable success, but the relatively large variability in such measurements has limited sensitivity. More recently, secondary antibodies, able to bind tightly and specifically to photoproduct-specific primary antibodies and themselves linked to signal-generating moieties, have been used for sensitive and reproducible assays *(11,12)*. Antibody-linked horseradish peroxidase can directly generate a color signal on a membrane, which may then be quantitated by densitometry, or can generate a chemiluminescent signal from a proprietary peracid/luminol/enhancer cocktail that registers on film. Disadvantages of the chemiluminescence-film technique are limited linear response and the requirement that membranes must be exposed to film immediately after reactions; the signals slowly decline with time, limiting reproducibility at low signal levels. All these techniques yield signals that can be used for more or less sensitive and reproducible direct comparisons among samples, but absolute determinations of photoproduct frequencies (per DNA bp) require calibration against irradiated DNA standards in which absolute numbers of photoproducts can be determined.

Here we describe a modified photoproduct-immunoassay approach that addresses both sensitivity/reproducibility and calibration issues (*see* **Note 1**). DNA is vigorously extracted from irradiated tadpoles so as to minimize contaminants that might engender spurious fluorescence, and aliquots quantitatively spotted onto membranes, to which anti-CPD or anti-[6-4]PP primary antibodies and fluorescent secondary antibodies are bound. Fluorescence intensities are determined by fluoroimaging of washed membranes, and sample and background signals are analyzed with computer software. CPD signals are calibrated against DNA standards whose CPD contents can be chromatographically determined *(13)*.

2. Materials

2.1. Isolation of Total DNA From Whole Tadpoles

1. Frog tranquilizer (0.1% tricane).
2. Liquid N_2.
3. GenomicPrep Cells and Tissue DNA isolation kit (Amersham, Piscataway, NJ).
4. 20 mg/mL Proteinase K (Worthington, Lakewood, NJ).
5. Phaselock Gel (5 Prime-3 Prime, Inc., Boulder, CO; optional).
6. Phenol/chloroform/isoamyl-alcohol, 25:24:1.
7. Chloroform/isoamyl-alcohol, 24:1.
8. 3 *M* Sodium acetate.
9. Absolute ethanol.
10. TE buffer: 10 m*M* Tris-HCl, pH 7.5, 1 m*M* Na_2EDTA.
11. Filter paper.
12. Mortar and pestle.
13. 1.5-mL Microcentrifuge tubes.
14. Tabletop microcentrifuge.

2.2. Photoproduct Immunoassay

1. Irradiated [^{3}H]DNA standards:

    a. DNA is extracted from thymine-requiring *E. coli* (*thy⁻*, *deo⁻*) cells grown in broth plus [^{3}H]thymidine and then irradiated with UVC light fluences from 15 to 120 J/m^2 (*see* **Note 1**).

    b. Frequencies of T-T cyclobutane dimers (T[CPD]Ts) are determined by acid hydrolysis and thin-layer chromatography, as previously described *(13)*, and total numbers of CPDs are estimated from known or estimated relative frequencies of T[CPD]T, T[CPD]C, C[CPD]T, and C[CPD]C photoproducts *(14)*. The same methods are used to measure sample and standard DNA concentrations, as described in **Subheading 3.1., step 16.**

    c. Standards for [6-4]PPs require a more complicated approach. Treatment of UV-irradiated plasmids with purified CPD-photolyase will leave only [6-4]PPs, whose average density (per plasmid or per DNA bp) can be estimated by transfection of completely repair-incompetent (*uvr⁻*, *phr–*, *recA–*) *E. coli*, or by quantitative polymerase chain reaction (PCR) amplification.

    d. In each case, comparison with unirradiated controls yields the fraction of irradiated targets with no [6-4]PPs, and the Poisson distribution yields the average number per plasmid or per bp.

2. 20X SSPE buffer: 3.6 *M* NaCl, 2 *M* $NaH_2PO_4 \cdot H_2O$, 0.02 *M* $Na_2EDTA \cdot 2H_2O$, pH 7.4 (174 g NaCl, 27.6 g NaH_2PO_4, and 7.4 g Na_2EDTA, dissolved in 800 mL H_2O); pH adjusted to 7.4 with 10 *N* NaOH; volume made up to 1000 mL.

3. 0.4 *M* NaOH.

4. 10X PBS buffer: 1.4 *M* NaCl, 26 m*M* KCl, 10 m*M* Na$_2$HPO$_4$, 17.6 m*M* KH$_2$PO$_4$, pH 7.4 (80 g NaCl, 2 g KCl, 14.48 g Na$_2$HPO$_4$, 2.4 g KH$_2$PO$_4$); pH adjusted to 7.4; volume made up to 1000 mL.
5. Tween-20 detergent.
6. PBS-T buffer: 0.2% Tween-20 in PBS buffer (1000 mL volume).
7. Nonfat dried milk.
8. Primary monoclonal anti-CPD or anti-[6-4]PP antibody (kind gift from T. Mori *[9]*), diluted respectively to 1:2000 or 1:1000 in sterile PBS (1X).
9. Fluorescently labeled secondary antibody, Alexa 568 goat anti-mouse (Molecular Probes, Eugene, OR). The excitation and emission capabilities of the fluoroimager must be taken into account.
10. Microcentrifuge tubes or PCR tubes.
11. Vortex mixer.
12. Slot-blot apparatus (BioRad, Hercules, CA).
13. Hybond N$^+$ membrane (Amersham/Pharmacia).
14. Cellulose filter paper for gel blots, Island Scientific grade 238 or equivalent (Bainbridge Island, WA).
15. Shallow rectangular plastic containers, with lids: two 10-oz containers for soaking of nitrocellulose membrane and for reactions with primary and secondary antibodies; one 48-oz container for incubation with blocking solution.
16. Rocking platform(s) (used at both room temperature and at 4°C, i.e., in the cold room).

2.3. Detection and Quantification of Fluorescent Signal From Bound Secondary Antibody

1. Fluoroimager (Hitachi FMBIOII multiview scanner), with software (FMBIO ReadImage 1.1, FMBIO V.6.0.11, Promega, Madison, WI).
2. Software for data analysis (ImageQuant V.1.2, Molecular Dynamics, Sunnyvale, CA).

3. Methods
3.1. Isolation of Total DNA From Whole Tadpoles

1. Anesthetize tadpole in 0.1% Tricane.
2. Place tadpole on a filter paper to drain excess water.
3. Add liquid N$_2$ to a mortar to chill it, then add more liquid N$_2$ and submerge tadpole.
4. Grind tadpole to a fine powder and transfer into microcentrifuge tube. At this point the sample can be stored at –80°C until further processing.
5. Isolate DNA using GenomicPrep Cells and Tissue DNA isolation kit, supplemented with proteinase K, according to the manufacturer's instructions, beginning with 20–50 mg of frozen sample. Resuspend DNA in 200 μL of TE buffer.
6. Centrifuge samples for 1 min. If a pellet (particulate debris) is formed, transfer the supernatant into a fresh tube and discard the pellet.
7. Add an equal volume of phenol/chloroform/isoamyl-alcohol, and vigorously invert tube 10 times (if using Phase-Lock Gel, add roughly 200 μL to each tube).
8. Centrifuge for 5 min in microcentrifuge at 12,000–14,000 rpm (~12,000*g*).
9. To the supernatant add an equal volume of chloroform/isoamyl-alcohol, and vigorously invert tube 10 times to remove residual phenol from the sample.
10. Centrifuge for 5 min in microcentrifuge at 12,000–14,000 rpm (~12,000*g*).
11. Transfer the supernatant to a fresh tube.

12. Add 0.05 vol of 3 *M* sodium acetate and 2.5 vol of absolute ethanol. Mix well.
13. Centrifuge 1 min in microcentrifuge at 12,000–14,000 rpm (~12,000*g*).
14. Discard the supernatant. Resuspend pellet in 50–100 μL TE buffer.
15. Vortex vigorously and pipet several times up and down with an automatic pipet to shear the DNA. Alternatively, digest DNA with restriction enzyme (*see* **Note 2**). Store samples at 4°C.
16. Determine DNA concentration of each sample (*see* **Note 3**).

3.2. Photoproduct Immunoassay

Sample preparation and blotting

1. Make dilutions so as to place 100 ng of sample or standard DNA (*see* **Subheading 2.2.**, **item 2**) in each tube in a volume of 200 μL or less (if using PCR tubes, 100 μL or less); for [6-4]PP assays, use 1 μg.
2. Boil tubes with samples or standards for 5 min. Use PCR thermocycler, if possible, to avoid condensation and sample contamination.
3. Chill on ice for 5 min.
4. Add equal volumes of 20X SSPE buffer and vortex. Microcentrifuge (1 min at 12,000–14,000 rpm [~12,000*g*]) to remove any particulate matter (*see* **Note 4**).
5. Saturate membrane with deionized water and then with 20X SSPE buffer (*see* **Note 5**).
6. Place membrane on a plastic gasket and cut one corner for orientation. Set up slot-blot apparatus according to the manufacturer's instructions (*see* **Note 6**).
7. Add 200 μL of 20X SSPE buffer to each well, and pull through with a vacuum.
8. Add samples and standards (maximum volume 400 μL to each well; *see* **Note 7**) and let stand for 15 min. Pull through with vacuum, adjusted to slow flow (*see* **Note 8**).
9. Add 200 μL 20X SSPE buffer to rinse wells, and pull through with vacuum.

Fixing and probing of membrane with antibody:

10. Soak filter paper in 0.4 *M* NaOH and pour off excess.
11. Place membrane on NaOH-soaked filter paper for 15 min.
12. Rinse membrane briefly with 5X SSPE buffer.
13. Block membrane by covering with 5% nonfat milk solution in PBS-T buffer (100 mL), in shallow rectangular plastic container with lid.
14. Rock gently at room temperature for at least 2 h, or overnight, at 4°C.
15. Rinse off the milk with PBS-T buffer quickly twice and then for 15 min with rocking.
16. React with primary CPD antibody: place washed membrane in 10 mL of primary antibody solution diluted with PBS buffer, typically 1:2000 for CPDs and 1:1000 for [6-4]PPs (test solutions beforehand with irradiated DNA standards); incubate for 2 h at room temperature in 10-oz plastic container, rocking gently. Remove and store antibody solution at 4°C; solution can be used once more within 2 wk.
17. Wash membrane in PBS-T buffer twice quickly and then once with 20 min of rocking, and twice with 5 min of rocking.
18. React membrane with secondary antibody, diluted 1:2500 in PBS buffer: place washed membrane in 10 mL of secondary antibody solution (*see* **Note 9**). Incubate for 1 h at room temperature, rocking gently. Remove secondary antibody solution and discard.
19. Wash membrane as in **step 17**, but increase the number of 5-min washes (with rocking) to six (*see* **Note 10**).
20. Cover membrane with plastic wrap to keep from drying and with foil to prevent photobleaching.

3.3. Detection and Quantification of Photoproducts (see Note 11)

1. For detection of the fluorescent signal from bound secondary antibody use excitation and emission settings recommended by the antibody supplier and compatible with the fluorimager. Commonly used lasers excite at 405 nm, 488 nm, 543 nm, and 633 nm, with tunability offering some flexibility around each line. Separation between excitation and emission maxima should be maximal, consistent with filtering characteristics of the instrument. Extinction coefficients and quantum yields should be high enough to generate adequate signals. Molecular Probes Inc. describes properties of its wide range of dye-labeled secondary antibodies at http://www.probes.com. Obviously, the immunospecificity of the secondary must match the primary antibody.
2. Membrane must be wet and flattened out on a glass plate. All bubbles must be removed.
3. Place second glass plate on top of the membrane (*see* **Note 12**). Scan according to instructions for fluoroimager (*see* **Notes 13** and **14**).
4. For analysis, scan must first be opened using attached FMBIO Analysis V.6.0.11 software. Invert image under "Mode" dropdown menu and select "Reverse Analysis" option to return to light spots on dark background (*opposite* of membrane shown in **Fig. 1**). Next, "Save Copy As" choosing a unique file name, and change file format to TIFF (Tagged Image File Format). This TIFF file can then be analyzed using ImageQuant software, which gives better control of background and is easier to use. Analyze spots using ImageQuant software. It is usually best to generate a peak and valley trace using a line scan (**Fig. 1**), because backgrounds are determined unambiguously. Comparison of box scans of spots and background (no spot) regions is less reliable.

3.4. Calculations

1. Construct a standard curve of fluorescence (arbitrary units) vs known amounts of CPDs, using irradiated DNA standards (*see* **Subheading 2.2.**, **item 2**; *see* **Note 15**).
2. Use a standard (nonlinear) calibration to determine the CPD amounts from relative fluorescence values of samples (*see* **Note 16**). To determine relative sample fluorescence values, multiple the ratio (observed absolute sample fluorescence)/(observed absolute standard fluorescence) by the appropriate relative standard fluorescence from the standard calibration curve. Using **Fig. 2**, for example, values would be 1.0 for 0.14 CPD/kb and 0.57 for 0.07 CPD/kb. Then read the corresponding CPD values from the calibration curve. Alternatively, use an equation fitted to the curve, e.g. (**Fig. 2**), $y = 2.56 \, x/(0.199 + x)$, where y is relative fluorescence intensity and x is a photoproduct density (CPD/kb), to obtain x for a given y.

4. Notes

1. Linearity between photoproduct induction and UVC or UVB light fluence is well known. Typically only the highest fluences induce enough photoproducts to be measured quantitatively by the acid hydrolysis/TLC technique. Photoproduct levels in lower fluence DNA standards are estimated by linear extrapolation.
2. DNA fragmented to average lengths of 10 kbp or less works best with the slot-blot apparatus.
3. For dsDNA, we use PicoGreen dye (Molecular Probes), with a microplate fluorescence reader. Samples and DNA standards are measured in duplicate or triplicate. Dilute at least 5 μL of sample into a final volume of 200 μL. If DNA concentration is too high, make successive dilutions, always using at least 5 μL.

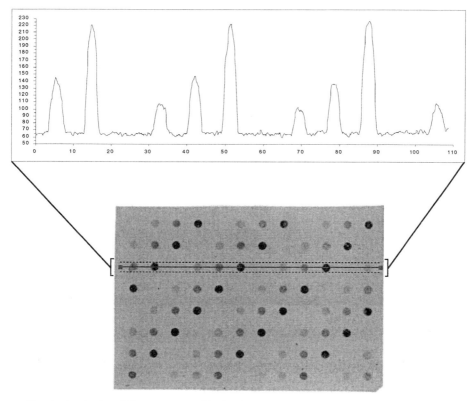

Fig. 1. Analysis of fluorescent-antibody signals. Lower panel: membrane image was obtained by successively binding anti-CPD primary antibody and Alexa 568-labeled secondary antibody to spotted DNA samples, followed by fluoroimaging and analysis with an FMBio scanner and software, as described in the text. Upper panel: light/dark inverted TIFF file from FMBio analysis of indicated row (brackets) of membrane was line-scan-analyzed using ImageQuant software, as described in the text.

4. If particulate matter is observed, pipet off the top 80% (as much as can be cleanly removed from the pellet) of the supernatant and transfer to a clean tube for subsequent processing. Particulate matter to some extent is typical, so this may be done routinely.
5. Never touch membrane with fingers; always use forceps.
6. The slot-blot apparatus should be cleaned with soap and then soaked in 0.4 M NaOH to remove any residual DNA from previous experiments. If this is still a problem, a preliminary membrane can be applied to the apparatus (without sample), washed with 20X SSPE buffer, and then discarded, before applying a new membrane for sample spotting.
7. DNA from each sample (tadpole) is spotted in duplicate or triplicate, along with DNA from unirradiated control tadpoles and a series of irradiated DNA standards (*see* **Subheading 2.2., item 2**). The same amounts of sample and standard DNA are applied, typically 100 ng (CPDs) or 1 µg ([6-4]PPs). When signals are expected to be weak, 150 ng (CPDs) can be used for all spots without loss of linearity.

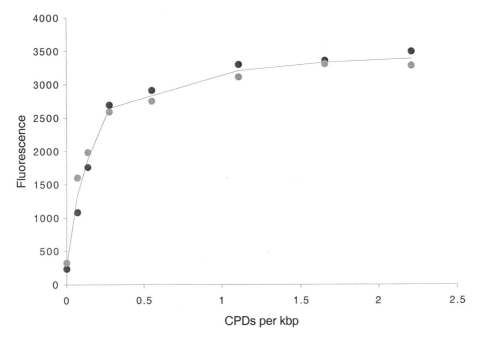

Fig. 2. Fluorescence vs CPD-density calibration. Radiolabeled *E. coli* DNA was UVC-irradi-
ated to various fluences, and CPDs per DNA base from each standard were determined by acid
hydrolysis and TLC analysis of high-fluence standards and linear extrapolation to low-fluence
standards. DNA standards were analyzed using the anti-CPD primary antibody and fluorescent
secondary antibody, as described in the text. Data shown correspond to multiple calibration trials, with each fluorescence signal expressed relative to the signal in that particular strain for the
0.14 CPD/kb standard. The abscissa corresponds to CPDs per *single strand* of DNA. The data
were fitted to a rectangular hyperbola (solid curve) using the GraphPad Prism program: $y =$
$2.56\,x/(0.199 + x)$, where y is relative fluorescence intensity and x is photoproduct density (CPD/kb).
CPD, cyclobutane pyrimidine dimer.

8. Setting the vacuum low, for even, slow distribution of sample to the membrane, results in
    best fluorescent signal distribution.
9. To decrease background, dilute secondary antibody more. (This also decreases signal.)
10. The number of 5-min washes can be increased further, with additional rinses after each
    wash, to reduce nonspecific binding of secondary antibody further.
11. It is important to check the fluorimager filter, laser, and mirror periodically for obstruc-
    tion by dust particle or spilled samples from previous users. Soft lens tissue or air can be
    used to clean these instruments; if necessary, use 70% ethanol.
12. To minimize air bubbles, sparingly wet the membrane on the first glass plate and then
    sandwich the membrane with the second glass plate. To remove trapped air bubbles on
    the other side of the membrane, remove the second glass plate.
13. The appropriate fluoroimager channel should be used (in the case of Alexa 568 dye, Chan-
    nel 1605 nm). Depending on the amount of fluorescence signal, the sensitivity should be
    adjusted. Results are typically best with 15–25% sensitivity.

14. It is very important to turn the auto focus off and to adjust the focus manually. Manual focus is done by scanning a small area (which includes the fluorescence signal), then changing the focus setting up or down in 0.2-mm increments (until the fluorescence signal reaches a maximum and then starts to decline) and then using the setting for maximum signal.

15. Antibody signals show a linear response only at low photoproduct levels (**Fig. 2**), at which presumably one (divalent) primary antibody reacts with one photoproduct. The curvature at higher levels is thought to reflect binding of two neighboring photoproducts by one antibody. For this reason, apparently linear calibration curves obtained by diluting a single heavily irradiated sample (even with unirradiated DNA added to keep total concentrations the same) are spurious.

16. We have routinely determined CPD levels as low as 0.01–0.02 per kbp, at a signal/noise level of roughly 3:1.

Acknowledgments

This work was supported by USEPA grant R-821275 to John B. Hays.

References

1. Freeman, S. E., Hacham, H., Gange, R. W., Maytum, D. J., Sutherland, J. C., and Sutherland, B. M. (1989) Wavelength dependence of pyrimidine dimer formation in DNA of human skin irradiated in situ with ultraviolet light. *Proc. Natl. Acad. Sci. USA* **86,** 5605–5609.

2. Pang, Q. and Hays, J. B. (1991) UV-B-inducible and temperature-sensitive photoreactivation of cyclobutane pyrimidine dimers in *Arabidopsis thaliana. Plant Physiol.* **95,** 536–543.

3. Quaite, F. E., Sutherland, B. M., and Sutherland, J. C. (1992) Action spectrum for DNA damage in alfalfa lowers predicted impact of ozone depletion. *Nature* **358,** 576–578.

4. Blaustein, A. R., Hoffman, P. D., Hokit, D. G., Kiesecker, J. M., Walls, S. C., and Hays, J. B. (1994) UV repair and resistance to solar UV-B in amphibian eggs: a link to population declines? *Proc. Natl. Acad. Sci. USA* **91,** 1791–1795.

5. Blaustein, A. R., Kiesecker, J. M., Hoffman, P. D., and Hays, J. B. (1997) The significance of ultraviolet-B radiation to amphibian population declines. *Rev. Toxicol.* **1,** 147–165.

6. Pandelova, I., Hewitt, S. R., Rollins-Smith, L., and Hays, J. B. UVB-dose toxicity thresholds and steady-state DNA-photoproduct levels during chronic irradiation of inbred *Xenopus laevis* tadpoles. *Photochem. Photobiol.*, submitted.

7. Sutherland, J. C., Monteleone, D. C., Trunk, J. G., Bennett, P. V., and Sutherland, B. M. (2001) Quantifying DNA damage by gel electrophoresis, electronic imaging and number average length analysis. *Electrophoresis* **22,** 843–854.

8. Mitchell, D. L. (1996) Radioimmune assay of DNA damaged by ultraviolet light, in *Technologies for Detection of DNA Damage and Mutation* (Pfeifer, G., ed.), Plenum, New York, pp. 73–85.

9. Mori, T., Nakane, M., Hattori, T., Matsunaga, T., Ihara, M., and Nikaido, O. (1991) Simultaneous establishment of monoclonal antibodies specific for either cyclobutane pyrimidine dimer or (6-4)photoproduct from the same mouse immunized with ultraviolet-irradiated DNA. *Photochem. Photobiol.* **54,** 225–232.

10. Matsunaga, T., Mori, T., and Nikaido, O. (1990) Base sequence specificity of a monoclonal antibody binding to (6-4)photoproducts. *Mutat. Res.* **235,** 187–194.

11. Stapleton, A. E., Mori, T., and Walbot, V. (1993) A simple and sensitive antibody-based method to measure UV-induced DNA damage in *Zea mays. Plant Mol. Biol. Rep.* **11,** 230–236.

12. Crowley, D. J. and Hanawalt, P. C. (1998) Induction of the SOS response increases the efficiency of global nucleotide excision repair of cyclobutane pyrimidine dimers, but not 6-4 photoproducts, in UV-irradiated *Escherichia coli. J. Bacteriol.* **180,** 3345–3352.

13. Hays, J. B. and Hoffman, P. (1999) Measurement of activities of cyclobutane-pyrimidine-dimer and (6-4)-photoproduct photolyases, in *DNA Repair Protocols: Eukaryotic Systems* (Henderson, D. S., ed.), Humana, Totowa, NJ., pp. 133–146.

14. Friedberg, E. C., Walker, A., and Siede, W. (1995) *DNA Repair and Mutagenesis.* American Society of Microbiology, Washington, DC.

5

Analysis of DNA Strand Cleavage at Abasic Sites

Walter A. Deutsch and Vijay Hegde

Summary

Abasic sites in DNA arise under a variety of circumstances, including destabilization of bases through oxidative stress, as an intermediate in base excision repair, and through spontaneous loss. Their persistence can yield a blockade to RNA transcription and DNA synthesis and can be a source of mutations. Organisms have developed an enzymatic means of repairing abasic sites in DNA that generally involves a DNA repair pathway that is initiated by a repair protein creating a phosphodiester break ("nick") adjacent to the site of base loss. Here we describe a method for analyzing the manner in which repair endonucleases differ in the way they create nicks in DNA and how to distinguish between them using cellular crude extracts.

Key Words: DNA abasic sites; oxidative stress; DNA damage; AP endonucleases; AP lyases; base excision repair (BER); tetrahydofuran; DNA oligonucleotides.

1. Introduction

Apurinic/apyrimidinic (AP) abasic sites arise in DNA under a variety of circumstances that, taken together, make them one of the more common lesions found in DNA. For example, free radicals can interact with DNA bases leading to their destabilization and ultimate loss. Free radical attack on DNA can also lead to DNA base modifications, some of which are known to be removed by *N*-glycosylases, resulting in the formation of an AP site as part of the base excision repair (BER) pathway *(1)*. Even in the absence of environmental factors, DNA bases are known to be spontaneously lost *(2)*, leaving behind abasic lesions that, if left unrepaired, can be mutagenic and can also form a blockade to RNA transcription *(3)*.

To illustrate the importance of abasic sites, all organisms that have thus far been tested have the ability to repair these sites by creating an incision adjacent to the AP site to initiate the repair process. The major class of AP endonuclease, at least quantitatively, is one that hydrolytically cleaves 5' and adjacent to an abasic site, producing

From: *Methods in Molecular Biology, vol. 291: Molecular Toxicology Protocols*
Edited by: P. Keohavong and S. G. Grant © Humana Press Inc., Totowa, NJ

nucleotide 3'-hydroxyl and 5'-deoxyribose-5-phophate termini *(4)*. Examples of this activity are the exonuclease lll of *E. coli* and the human multifunctional APE/ref-1 *(5,6)*.

Another kind of activity that acts on abasic sites is part of the BER pathway that is initiated by *N*-glycosylases directed toward a modified or nonconventional base in DNA. Often, these *N*-glycosylases also possess AP lyase activity that cleaves DNA 3' to an abasic site via a β-elimination reaction to leave a 3' 4-hydroxy-2-pentenal-5-phosphate. An example of this type of activity is that possessed by *E. coli* endonuclease lll (endo III), a broad-specificity *N*-glycosylase/AP lyase used for the repair of oxidative damage to DNA *(7,8)*. In some cases, *N*-glycosylases/AP lyases not only cleave DNA via a β-elimination reaction but also are capable of carrying out a second ∂-elimination incision. This results in the removal of the AP site and the formation of a one-nucleotide gap bordered by 3'- and 5'-phosphate termini. The β, ∂-elimination reaction can be concerted, as appears to be the case for the *E. coli* formamidopyrimidine glycosylase (Fpg), which repairs oxidative DNA damage, primarily in the form of 8-oxoguanine (8oxoG) *(9,10)*. On the other hand, repair of 8oxoG by the *Drosophila* S3 *N*-glycosylase/AP lyase activity has been concluded to occur in two distinct steps, catalyzing a ∂-elimination reaction on a second encounter with the lesion after first dissociating from the AP substrate when the β-elimination reaction was completed *(11)*.

There are several ways to monitor enzyme activity on abasic sites present in naturally occurring or synthesized DNA substrates. Originally, we utilized a [^{3}H]-labeled supercoiled phage DNA in a filter-binding assay that accurately measured DNA nuclease activity *(12)*, but this technique was hampered by the tedious and time-consuming preparation of the substrate DNA. Moreover, this assay could only quantify the cleavage of a preprepared abasic DNA substrate, not identify the type of cleavage event unless it was followed up by DNA synthesis to determine whether the incision created a productive 3'-OH terminus *(12,13)*. Recently, we have turned to an assay that utilizes a 5'-end-labeled DNA duplex oligonucleotide containing a single abasic site. After reaction with an AP endonuclease or AP lyase, the products of the reaction are separated on a polyacrylamide gel. Based on the migration of the cleaved product, one can easily visualize the type of strand cleavage possessed by a DNA repair endonuclease by autoradiography *(11,14,15)*. Quantitation of the product(s) formed can be performed either by video densitometric analysis of autoradiograms, or by Phosphorimager analysis and scanning of dried gels. Importantly in this assay, different types of cleavage events generate unique visual images of the products formed by autoradiography; the assay is also adaptable in most cases to the use of both highly purified enzymes as well as cruder preparations.

For the assay described here, a synthetic oligonucleotide is utilized that is 37 bp in length (37-mer). Within the 37-mer is a single uracil (U) residue placed at position 21 during the synthesis of the oligonucleotide. After 5'-end-labeling and gel purification of the single-stranded U-containing oligonucleotide, the complementary strand is annealed to create a duplex 37-mer (*see* **Note 1**). This forms a substrate for uracil-DNA glycosylase *(16)*, which liberates the nonconventional base and forms an abasic site in its place.

Alternatively, tetrahydrofuran can be placed at position 21 within the 37-mer. Tetrahydrofuran is an analog of an abasic site and represents a productive substrate for a

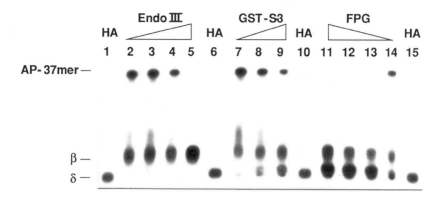

Fig. 1. Mechanisms of nuclease action on abasic site-containing DNA. Reactions contained 1 pmol of AP 37-mer and were incubated for 30 min at 37°C with *E. coli* endonuclease III (Endo III; lanes 2–5) at protein amounts of 100, 150, 200, and 400 pg, respectively, glutathione-S-transferase (GST)-conjugated *Drosophila* S3 (lanes 7–9) at 20, 40, and 80 pg, respectively, or *E. coli* formamidopyrimidine glyosylase (Fpg; lanes 11–14) at 160, 120, 80, and 80 pg, respectively; lanes 1, 6, 10, and 15 contain the products of hot alkali (HA; piperidine) treatment of the AP 37-mer. The reaction products were separated on a 16% polyacrylamide DNA sequencing gel. The electrophoretic mobilities of the uncleaved aburinic/apyrimidine (AP) 37-mer and DNA cleavage products corresponding to β- and ∂-elimination reactions are indicated. (Adapted with permission from **ref. *11*.**)

hydrolytic AP endonuclease *(17)*. It is, however, refractive to cleavage by AP lyases, therefore making it a convenient substrate for measuring hydrolytic AP endonuclease activity in crude preparations that would ordinarily be compromised by AP lyase activity.

To demonstrate the utility of the oligonucleotide assay, the products of three different AP lyases acting on an abasic oligonucleotide DNA substrate are presented in **Fig. 1**. In each case, the migration pattern of the reaction products provides direct information on the type of DNA termini produced by each enzyme. The hot alkali control (HA) provides a landmark for the production of a β, ∂-elimination reaction that reflects the production of a 5'- and 3'-phosphoryl terminus. DNA fragments containing a terminal phosphoryl group migrate faster than those of the same length that lack a terminal phosphate. As can be seen in **Fig. 1**, the reaction products are completely distinct for each of the enzymes tested. Endonuclease III produces a β-elimination product, regardless of the amount of protein added to the assay, as shown in lane 5, where the substrate is totally consumed yet yields only a single product. For *Drosophila* S3, a β-elimination product is also evident at low protein concentrations, yet higher amounts of protein yield what is clearly a ∂-elimination product as well. This suggests that S3 is dissociating from the abasic substrate once the original β-elimination reaction is completed and on a second encounter is then cleaving the remaining AP site via a ∂-elimination reaction. This is in contrast to what is observed for *E. coli* Fpg, which produces equal amounts of β- and ∂-elimination products, regardless of protein concentration (**Fig. 1**) or time of incubation (not shown). This indicates that Fpg is remaining bound to the AP substrate as it carries out both incision activities.

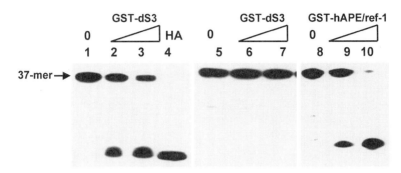

Fig. 2. Activity of GST-dS3 and GST-hAPE/ref-1 on an 8oxoG site and a tetrahydrofuran spacer-containing DNA substrate. Lane 1, 8oxoG 37-mer alone. Lanes 2 and 3, 1 pmol of 8oxoG 37-mer was incubated with 0.2 pmol (lane 2) and 0.4 pmol (lane 3) of purified GST-dS3 at 37°C for 30 min, and the products were separated on a 16% polyacrylamide DNA sequencing gel and analyzed by autoradiography. Lane 4, hot alkali (HA) treatment to generate a β-, ∂-elimination product. Lane 5, 1 pmol tetrahydrofuran-containing 37-mer alone and incubated with 0.2 pmol and 0.4 pmol GST-dS3 (lanes 6 and 7, respectively). Lanes 8–10 are 1 pmol tetrahydrofuran-containing 37-mer alone and incubated with 0.4 pmol and 0.8 pmol purified GST-hAPE/ref-1, respectively.

Another utility of the oligonucleotide assay is that it is amendable to analyzing 5'-acting AP endonucleases in crude extracts without concern over the contribution of contaminating AP lyases that could make interpretation of the actual products formed difficult. This is accomplished by switching from an authentic AP site created in the oligonucleotide substrate by U incorporation to a tetrahydrofuran analog of an AP site that is refractive to cleavage to AP lyases. As seen in **Fig. 2**, the 5'-acting hydrolytic human APE/ref-1 is clearly capable of acting on a 37-mer synthetic DNA substrate with a tetrahydrofuran spacer (lanes 9 and 10), yet the same substrate is totally refractive to cleavage by the AP lyase activity possessed by *Drosophila* S3 (lanes 6 and 7). The same preparation of *Drosophila* S3 is, however, active on a DNA substrate containing a single 8oxoG residue (lanes 2 and 3).

2. Materials

All solutions should be made using molecular biology-grade reagents and sterile distilled water.

2.1. 5'-End-Labeling and Purification of Oligonucleotides Containing a Single Tetrahydofuran or U Residue

The oligonucleotides used in our studies are commercially prepared to our specifications and contain the nonconventional bases U or 8oxoG (Operon Technologies, Alameda, CA) or the abasic spacer tetrahydrofuran (Genosys, Pittsburgh, PA). The single-stranded oligos are deprotected and purified by spin-column chromatography (Gibco-BRL, Grand Island, NY). The individual single-stranded and purified oligonucleotides are then resuspended in distilled water to 10 pmol/μL.

1. 10 U/μL T4 polynucleotide kinase (Stratagene, La Jolla, CA).
2. 10X T4 polynucleotide kinase buffer: 700 m*M* Tris-HCl, pH 7.6, 100 m*M* MgCl$_2$, 50 m*M* dithiothereitol (DTT), 1 m*M* spermidine-HCl.
3. [γ-^{32}P] ATP, 10 mCi/mL, 6000 Ci/mmol (Amersham, Arlington Heights, IL).
4. 10X Annealing buffer: 100 m*M* Tris-HCl, pH 7.6, 100 m*M* MgCl$_2$, 10 m*M* EDTA.
5. Loading buffer: 50% glycerol, 0.5% bromophenol blue, 0.5% xylene cynanol.
6. Phenol, molecular biology grade, neutralized, and equilibrated with 10 m*M* Tris-HCl, pH 8.0, 1 m*M* EDTA.
7. Phenol/chloroform/isoamyl alcohol mixture (25:24:1 by volume).
8. 40% Acrylamide stock: 38:2 acrylamide/*bis*-acrylamide in 100 mL of distilled water.
9. 10X TBE: 890 m*M* Tris-borate, 20 m*M* EDTA, pH 8.0.
10. Nondenaturing 20% polyacrylamide gel (per 100 mL): 50 mL 40% acrylamide stock, 10 mL 10X TBE, 500 μL 10% ammonium persulfate, 60 μL TEMED, distilled H$_2$O to 100 mL final volume.
11. Centrex MF-0.4 microcentrifuge tubes (Schleicher & Schuell, Keene, NH).
12. 35 m*M* HEPES-KOH, pH 7.4.

2.2. Cleavage of Uracil-Containing Oligonucleotides

1. Uracil-DNA glycosylase (Epicentre, Madison, WI).
2. 10X Uracil-DNA glycosylase buffer: 200 m*M* Tris-HCl, pH 8.0, 10 m*M* EDTA, 10 m*M* DTT, 100 μg/mL bovine serum albumin (BSA).
3. 10 m*M* HEPES-KOH, pH 7.4.

2.3. Enzymatic Reactions and Electrophoresis

1. Abasic oligonucleotides (see **Subheadings 3.1.–3.3.**).
2. Purified AP endonuclease or AP lyase (Trevigen, Gaithersburg, MD) *(11)*.
3. 10X *Drosophila* S3 (dS3) buffer: 300 m*M* HEPES, pH 7.4, 500 m*M* KCl, 10 mg/mL BSA, 0.5% Triton X-100, 10 m*M* DTT, 5 m*M* EDTA.
4. 10X *E. coli* Endo lll buffer: 150 m*M* KH$_2$PO$_4$, pH 6.8, 100 m*M* EDTA, 100 m*M* β-mercaptoethanol, 400 m*M* KCl.
5. 10X *E. coli* Fpg buffer: 150 m*M* HEPES, pH 7.5, 500 m*M* KCl, 10 m*M* β-mercapto-ethanol, 5 m*M* EDTA.
6. 10X human APE/ref-1 buffer: 500 m*M* HEPES, pH 7.5, 500 m*M* KCl, 10 μg/mL BSA, 100 m*M* MgCl$_2$, 0.5% Triton X-100.
7. 1 *M* Piperidine.
8. Denaturing polyacrylamide gel: 16% polyacrylamide solution, 7 m*M* urea, 1X TBE.
9. Formamide loading buffer: 96% formamide, 0.05% xylene cyanol, 0.05% bromophenol blue, 10 m*M* EDTA.
10. 15% methanol: 10% acetic acid solution.
11. Whatman 3MM paper.
12. X-ray film (Kodak XAR-5) or Phosphorimager.

3. Methods

Characterization of endonucleases that act at abasic sites existing in DNA can be divided into several parts: first, a 5'-radiolabeled synthetic oligonucleotide containing either a single tetrahydrofuron residue, or one containing a single deoxyU residue, is prepared. Single-stranded oligos are then annealed to their nonradioactive complementary oligonucleotide (*see* **Note 1**). The duplexes are then purified and subsequently further processed by a uracil-DNA glycosylase so as to form an abasic site if necessary. This, or the tetrahydrofuran-containing oligonucleotide, is then employed as a substrate for enzyme reactions using proteins known, or suspected, to act on abasic sites. Upon completion of the enzymatic assays, the reaction products are then separated on a DNA sequencing gel.

3.1. 5' End-Labeling and Purification of Oligonucleotides

Bacteriophage T4 polynucleotide kinase is used to catalyze the transfer of the γ-phosphate of ATP to the 5'-hydroxyl terminus of the oligonucleotide. The following procedure produces sufficient quantities of 5'-end-labeled duplex oligonucleotides for several enzymatic reactions (*see* **Note 2**).

1. Prepare 5'-end labeling reaction mixtures in a 0.5-mL microcentrifuge tube containing the following: 3 μL [^{32}P]ATP, 4 μL 10X kinase buffer, 2 μL oligonucleotide, 2 μL (2 U) of polynucleotide kinase, and 2 μL distilled water.
2. Incubate the reaction mixture for 30 min at 37°C.
3. Extract the reaction mixture once with phenol/chloroform/isoamyl alcohol.
4. Mix for 1 min, and then centrifuge at 12,000*g* for 3 min at room temperature in a microcentrifuge. Transfer the aqueous supernatant to a new tube. Add 2.5 vol of ethanol, mix, and store the tube at –20°C for 1 h.
5. Recover the oligos by centrifugation at 12,000*g* for 15 min at 4°C in a microcentrifuge. Remove the supernatant, and leave the tube open at room temperature until all the ethanol has evaporated.
6. Dissolve the pellet in 20 μL of distilled water.

3.2. Annealing Reaction (see Note 1)

1. Mix together in a microcentrifuge tube the following: 20 μL labeled oligos (1 pmol/mL), 4 μL complementary strand, 4 μL 10X annealing buffer, and 4 μL distilled water to 40 μL final volume.
2. Incubate the annealing mixture at 75°C for 10 min.
3. Slowly cool to room temperature.
4. Add 10 μL loading buffer and mix well.
5. Separate the labeled duplex oligonucleotides on a 20% nondenaturing polyacrylamide gel and then subject to autoradiography.
6. Excise the band corresponding to the labeled duplex oligos from the gel, and transfer to a Centrex MF-0.4 microcentrifuge tube.
7. Crush the acrylamide gel into small pieces against the wall of the tube, add 200 μL 35 m*M* HEPES-KOH, pH 7.4, to the tube, and incubate for 5 h to overnight at 4°C to elute the labeled oligos from the gel. (Typically, < 95% of labeled oligo is eluted.)
8. Collect the duplex oligos by centrifugation at 4000*g* for 3 min in a microcentrifuge.

3.3. Uracil Excision

1. Uracil-DNA glycosylases are used to hydrolyze the *N*-glycosidic bond between the deoxyribose sugar and uracil base. The reaction mixture is as follows: 10 pmol labeled uracil-containing duplex oligo, 4 μL 10X uracil-DNA glycosylase buffer, 1 μL uracil-DNA glycosylase (1 U/μL), and distilled water to 40 μL final volume.

2. Incubate the reaction for 20 min at 37°C. Extract the reaction mixture once with phenol/chloroform/isoamyl alcohol and precipitate the DNA as described in **Subheadings 3.1., steps 3–5**.
3. Dissolve the purified labeled duplex oligonucleotide in 10 m*M* HEPES-KOH, pH 7.4. It can be stored at 4°C for up to 1 wk.

3.4. Enzymatic Reaction

1. Mix together in a microcentrifuge tube: approx 1 pmol of γ-^{32}P abasic oligonucleotide (typically 10,000 cpm), 1 μL 10 X reaction buffer, *X* μL enzyme, and distilled water to 10 μL final volume. Incubate at 37°C for the desired time.
2. Stop the reactions by heating at 75°C for 10 min. Add 2 μL of formamide loading buffer, heat for 4 min at 90°C, cool on ice, and then load immediately on a denaturing polyacrylamide gel.

3.5. Hot Alkali Treatment

1. Add 90 μL of 1 *M* piperidine to 10 μL of 5'-end-labeled abasic oligonucleotide, and incubate for 30 min at 90°C.
2. Lyophilize to dryness using a Speed Vac, and redissolve the pellet in 20 μL of distilled water.
3. Repeat lyophilization step twice more in order to remove all the piperidine.
4. Dissolve the remaining pellet in 50 μL of formamide loading buffer, heat for 4 min at 90°C, cool on ice, and then load immediately on a denaturing polyacrylamide gel.

3.6. Analysis of Endonuclease Activity by Denaturing Gels

1. Load an equal amount of radioactivity (about 5000 cpm) per lane on a pre-electrophoresed 16% denaturing polyacrylamide gel (*see* **Note 3**).
2. Electrophorese in 1X TBE buffer at 45-W constant power until the bromophenol dye front is near the bottom of the gel.
3. Remove the gel plates, pry apart, and transfer the gel to a bath containing 15% methanol and 10% acetic acid for 20 min.
4. With the gel still attached to the glass plate, place a similar sized piece of Whatman 3MM paper on top of the gel, and then carefully peel off the 3MM paper with the gel attached to it.
5. Cover the gel with plastic wrap (Saran Wrap), and dry under vacuum at 80°C for 45 min.
6. Expose the dried gel to X-ray film at 70°C for 12–16 h with an intensifying screen. Alternatively, PhosphorImager cassettes can be used for the same length of time, but at room temperature.

4. Notes

1. One advantage of the oligonucleotide assay is that the sequence can be manipulated so as to determine whether enzyme activity is affected by surrounding DNA bases either adjacent to, or opposite, the target site.
2. Caution should be taken in the preparation of ^{32}P-labeled oligonucleotides when planning assays over a sustained period. We have found that regardless of the method of storage of prepared oligos, degradation products begin to appear in our controls that are presumably owing to radioactive decay that splinters the oligos into smaller fragments. Generally, after 2 wk unused oligos are of little use because of such fragmentation.
3. We have used gels containing 20% polyacrylamide, but to maximize the separation of a β- and ∂-elimination product, 16% gels are preferred.

References

1. Friedberg, E. C., Walker, G. C., and Siede, W. (1995) *DNA Repair and Mutagenesis.* ASM Press, Washington, D.C.
2. Lindahl, T. and Nyberg, B. (1972) Rate of depurination of native deoxyribonucleic acid. *Biochemistry* **11,** 3610–3618.
3. Loeb, L. A. and Preston B. D. (1986) Mutagenesis by apurinic/apyrimidinic sites. *Annu. Rev. Genet.* **20,** 201–230.
4. Doetsch, P. W. and Cunningham, R. P. (1990) The enzymology of apurinic/apyrimidinic endonucleases. *Mutat. Res.* **236,** 173–201.
5. Demple, B. and Harrison, L. (1994) Repair of oxidative damage to DNA: enzymology and biology. *Annu. Rev. Biochem.* **63,** 915–948.
6. Demple, B., Herman, T., and Chen, D. S. (1991) Cloning and expression of APE, the cDNA encoding the major human apurinic endonuclease: definition of a family of DNA repair enzymes. *Proc. Natl. Acad. Sci. USA* **88,** 11,450–11,454.
7. Dizdaroglu, M., Laval, J., and Boiteux, S. (1993) Substrate specificity of the *Escherichia coli* endonuclease III: excision of thymine- and cytosine-derived lesions in DNA produced by radiation-generated free radicals. *Biochemistry* **32,** 12,105–12,111.
8. Kow, Y. W. and Wallace, S. S. (1987) Mechanism of action of *Escherichia coli* endonuclease III. *Biochemistry* **26,** 8200–8206.
9. Dodson, M. L., Michaels, M., and Lloyd, R. S. (1994) Unified catalytic mechanism for DNA glycosylases. *J. Biol. Chem.* **269,** 32,709–32,712.
10. Bailly, V., Verly, W. G., O'Conner, T., and Laval, J. (1989) Mechanism of DNA strand nicking at apurinic/apyrimidinic sites by *Escherichia coli* [formamidopyrimidine] DNA glycosylase. *Biochem. J.* **262,** 581–589.
11. Yacoub, A., Augeri, L., Kelley, M. R., Doetsch, P. W., and Deutsch, W. A. (1996) A *Drosophila* ribosomal protein contains 8-oxoguanine and abasic site DNA repair activities. *EMBO J.* **15,** 2306–2312.
12. Spiering, A. L. and Deutsch, W. A. (1986) *Drosophila* apurinic/apyrimidinic DNA endonucleases. Characterization of mechanism of action and demonstration of a novel type of enzyme activity. *J. Biol. Chem.* **261,** 3222–3228.
13. Warner, H. R., Demple, B. F., Deutsch, W. A., Kane, C. M., and Linn, S. (1980) Apurinic/apyrimidinic endonucleases in repair of pyrimidine dimers and other lesions in DNA. *Proc. Natl. Acad. Sci. USA* **77,** 4602–4206.
14. Yacoub, A., Kelley, M. R., and Deutsch, W. A. (1996) *Drosophila* ribosomal protein PO contains apurinic/apyrimidinic endonuclease activity. *Nucleic Acids Res.* **24,** 4298–4303.
15. Deutsch, W. A. and Yacoub, A. (1999) Characterization of DNA strand cleavage by enzymes that act at abasic sites in DNA. *Methods Mol. Biol.* **113,** 281–288.
16. Lindahl, T. (1980) Uracil-DNA glycosylase from *Escherichia coli. Methods Enzymol.* **65,** 284–295.
17. Wilson, D. M. 3rd, Takeshita, M., Grollman, A. P., and Demple, B. (1995) Incision activity of human apurinic endonuclease (Ape) at abasic site analogs in DNA. *J. Biol. Chem.* **270,** 16,002–16,007.

II

DETECTION OF CHROMOSOMAL AND GENOME-WIDE DAMAGE

6

Premature Chromosome Condensation in Human Resting Peripheral Blood Lymphocytes for Chromosome Aberration Analysis Using Specific Whole-Chromosome DNA Hybridization Probes

Pataje G. S. Prasanna and William F. Blakely

Summary

This paper describes a unique, simple, and rapid method for inducing premature chromosome condensation (PCC) in "resting" human peripheral blood lymphocytes (HPBLs) and also explains an approach to studying numerical changes and/or structural aberrations involving specific chromosomes. HPBLs are isolated from whole blood on a density gradient and, to induce PCC, are incubated at 37°C in cell culture medium supplemented with a phosphatase inhibitor (okadaic acid or calyculin A), adenosine triphosphate (ATP), and p34*cdc2*/cyclin B kinase (an essential component of mitosis-promoting factor [MPF]). PCC spreads are prepared on glass slides after a brief hypotonic treatment of cells and fixing in acetic acid/methanol fixative. Aberrations involving specific chromosomes are analyzed after *in situ* hybridization and chromosome painting by fluorescence microscopy. Normal (undamaged) cells display two fluorescent spots per chromosome, whereas aneuploid cells, or cells with a structural aberration involving the specific chromosome corresponding to the painting probe, may show more than two spots. This method may be used in many biological and toxicological fields that require analysis of numerical and structural aberrations involving specific chromosomes.

Key Words: Premature chromosome condensation; phosphatase inhibitors; p34*cdc2*/cyclin B kinase; chromosome aberration analysis.

1. Introduction

Numerical and structural chromosome aberration analysis is widely used in many fields: in the diagnosis of genetic diseases, in screening of chemical(s) or drug(s) for toxicity, in environmental monitoring for genotoxicity, in biological assessment of radiation dose in accidental or occupational overexposures, in biomonitoring for genotoxic risk assessment, in genomics, and in many other applications. Routine chromosome aberration analysis uses metaphase spreads obtained from either cultured

From: *Methods in Molecular Biology, vol. 291, Molecular Toxicology Protocols*
Edited by: P. Keohavong and S. G. Grant © Humana Press Inc., Totowa, NJ

mammalian cells or from mitogen-stimulated short-term cultures of human peripheral blood lymphocytes (HPBLs). Metaphase spread-based chromosome aberration analysis depends on successful mitogen (e.g., phytohemagglutinin) stimulation of "resting" HPBLs into the cell cycle. Cell cycle progression is then arrested in metaphase using a spindle poison (e.g., colchicine). Chromosome spreads on glass slides are obtained after treatment with a hypotonic solution and fixation in acetic acid/methanol for analysis of quantitative or qualitative changes involving structural and/or numerical aberrations.

Metaphase spread-based chromosome aberration analysis is laborious, requires cytogenetic expertise, and is time-consuming. Confounding factors associated with metaphase spread-based chromosome aberration analysis resulting from cell cycle progression, such as induced cell killing and cell cycle delay, are known to interfere with assay results. In addition, metaphase spread-based quantitative aberration analysis is critically dependent on the availability of a large number of suitable metaphase spreads because often only 3–4% of cells are analyzable. The ability to analyze chromosome aberrations prior to DNA synthesis eliminates most of these inherent problems associated with cell cycle kinetics *(1)*.

A method for inducing premature chromosome condensation (PCC) in "resting" HPBLs so as to obtain chromosome spreads prior to DNA synthesis for chromosome aberration analysis has been described *(2)*. The method involves the fusion of HPBLs with mitotic cells. Mitotic cells are obtained from a mammalian cell culture, and polyethylene glycol (PEG) can be used as a fusogen to allow mitosis-promoting factors (MPFs) to diffuse from mitotic cells into resting lymphocytes and bring about PCC. This method is technically demanding and difficult, and the PCC yield is low and not consistent *(2)*. Therefore, this method of obtaining chromosome spreads prior to DNA synthesis for chromosome aberration analysis has not been widely adopted in cytogenetics.

PCC can also be induced by incubating proliferating cells, such as mitogen-stimulated HPBLs *(3,4)* or human tumor cell lines *(5)*, in cell culture medium containing type 1 and type 2A protein phosphatase inhibitors (e.g., okadaic acid [OA] or calyculin A). This approach, when combined with whole-chromosome-specific hybridization probes, permits both the scoring of chromosomal damage in PCC spreads and the identification of other interphase cells with discrete chromosome domains or spots *(5)*. For autosomes, normal (undamaged) cells display two fluorescent spots, one each corresponding to the paternally and maternally derived homologs, and cells with an aberrant specific chromosome usually show more than two spots. Irradiation, for example, causes a dose-dependent increase in proliferating interphase tumor cells with more than two spots. The method described earlier for inducing PCC in HPBLs using phosphatase inhibitors, such as OA or calyculin A, requires a mitogenic stimulation *(3,4)* and involves a short-term HPBL culture before the PCC spreads are prepared on glass slides for analysis. Stimulation with mitogen results in an asynchronous culture, complicating chromosome-aberration analysis and lengthening the time required to prepare samples for analysis. Differentiated and nonproliferating cells, such as resting HPBLs do not respond to phosphatase inhibitor treatment and do not induce PCC *(6,7)*.

The rationale *(1)*, to be published elsewhere, for developing a method of inducing PCC in resting HPBLs is based on an understanding of the mechanisms of signal transduction events surrounding the regulation of cell cycle phases, DNA replication, chromosome condensation, and mitosis. Briefly, mitosis in proliferating cells is triggered by the specific activation of *cyclin D kinase (cdk)*, and chromosome condensation is regulated by p34*cdc2*/cyclin B kinase activity, the hyperphosphorylation of histone H1, and the phosphorylation of histone H3. For example, treatment of BHK1 cells in G_1 phase with OA alone does not induce PCC *(6)*, apparently owing to a lack of p34*cdc2*/cyclin B kinase activity. Recently, we demonstrated that incubation of resting HPBLs in a special cell culture medium induces PCC without mitogen stimulation *(7)*. The medium contains p34*cdc2*/cyclin B kinase (a component of MPF), a phosphatase inhibitor (OA or calyculin A), and ATP (an enzyme system substrate that increases Ca^{2+}-activated K^+ channels). The method results in a high yield of PCC suitable for fluorescence *in situ* hybridization (FISH) of whole chromosomes and for detection of numerical and structural aberrations involving specific chromosomes. Chromosome aberrations can be rapidly analyzed in a large resting lymphocyte population directly collected from human peripheral whole blood and readily isolated on a density gradient. In this chapter we describe, step by step, this unique, simple, and rapid method for inducing PCC in resting HPBLs as well as an approach to studying numerical changes or structural aberrations involving specific chromosomes.

2. Materials

2.1. Isolation of HPBLs (see Note 1)

1. Biological safety cabinet (clean air station, e.g., NU-425 Labgard, NuAire, Plymouth, MN).
2. Benchtop centrifuge (e.g., Beckman TJ-6 Centrifuge, Beckman, Fullerton, CA).
3. Polystyrene centrifuge tubes (15-mL capacity).
4. Pipets (1-, 2-, 5-, and 10-mL capacities).
5. Vortex mixer.
6. Lymphocyte separation medium (e.g., Histopaque-1077, Sigma, St. Louis, MO; *see* **Note 2**).
7. Dulbecco's phosphate-buffered saline (PBS) without Ca^{2+} and Mg^{2+}.
8. Bone marrow karyotyping medium (e.g., Karyomax, Life Technologies, Rockville, MD; *see* **Note 3**).
9. Disinfectant (e.g., Clorox, Clorox, Oakland, CA).

2.2. PCC Induction

1. Benchtop centrifuge (e.g., Beckman TJ-6 Centrifuge, Beckman).
2. Water bath (e.g., Isotemp 1028P, Fisher Scientific, Pittsburgh, PA).
3. Light microscope (e.g., Leica Phase contrast, Leica Microsystems, Bannockburn, IL).
4. Microscope slides (*see* **Note 4**).
5. Pipets.
6. Polystyrene centrifuge tubes (15-mL capacity).
7. Bone marrow karyotyping medium (e.g., Karyomax, Life Technologies; *see* **Note 3**).
8. ATP (Sigma) (*see* **Note 5**).
9. Colchicine (Sigma) (*see* **Note 6**).

10. OA or calyculin A (Boehringer Ingelheim, Petersburg, VA; *see* **Note 7**).
11. p34^{cdc2}/cyclin B kinase (Cell Signaling Technologies, Beverly, MA; *see* **Note 8**).
12. Potassium chloride (Sigma; *see* **Note 9**).
13. Glacial acetic acid (analytical reagent grade).
14. Methanol (200° proof, analytical reagent grade).

2.3. In Situ *Hybridization, Chromosome Painting, and Fluorescence Microscopy*

1. pH meter.
2. pH papers.
3. Diamond marker.
4. Glass Coplin jars.
5. Microcentrifuge (e.g., Marathon model 16KM, Fisher).
6. Thermalcycler (e.g., DNA Thermalcycler, Perkin-Elmer, Norwalk, CT).
7. *In situ* hybridization machine (e.g., Omnislide Thermo cycler, Thermo Hybaid, Ashford, UK).
8. Water bath (e.g., Isotemp 1028P, Fisher).
9. Micropipets.
10. Cover slips.
11. Rubber cement.
12. Fluorescence microscope and imaging station (e.g., Cytovision, Applied Imaging, Santa Clara, CA).
13. Whole-chromosome–specific probe (e.g., Chromosome 1, Vysis, Downers Grove, IL).
14. 20X SSC solution (*see* **Note 10**).
15. 2X SSC solution (*see* **Note 11**).
16. 2X SSC/0.1% NP-40 wash solution (*see* **Note 12**).
17. 70% Formamide/2X SSC (denaturation) solution (*see* **Note 13**).
18. Ethanol solutions (*see* **Note 14**).
19. 50% Formamide/2X SSC (formamide wash) solution (*see* **Note 15**).
20. 4,6-Diamidino-2-phenyl-indole (DAPI) in a mounting solution (e.g., Vectashield, Vector, Burlingame, CA).

3. Methods

3.1. Isolation of HPBLs From Whole Blood (see Note 16)

1. To a 15-mL conical centrifuge tube, transfer 3 mL of lymphocyte separation media, and carefully layer 3 mL of whole blood such that a density separation of the medium and the blood occurs.
2. Centrifuge at 400g for exactly 30 min at room temperature (~25°C) using a swinging bucket type of rotor.
3. Following centrifugation, carefully aspirate, with a Pasteur pipet, the upper layer to within 0.5 mm of the opaque interface (Buffy coat) containing mononuclear cells. Discard upper layer (*see* **Note 1**).
4. Using a Pasteur pipet, carefully transfer the opaque interface (Buffy coat) to a separate 15-mL centrifuge tube and discard the red blood cells (*see* **Note 17**).
5. Add 10 mL of PBS to the centrifuge tube and gently mix using a pipet.
6. Centrifuge at 200g for 15 min at room temperature.
7. Aspirate the supernatant and discard (*see* **Note 1**).
8. Using a Vortex mixer, gently break up the cell pellet, resuspend with 10 mL of PBS, and mix as above.

9. Centrifuge at 200g for 15 min at room temperature.
10. Repeat **steps 7–9**; discard supernatant (*see* **Notes 1** and **18**).

3.2. PCC Induction (see Note 1)

1. Prepare incubation media: mix 2.96 mL of Karyomax, 30 μL ATP, 12 μL colchicine, 2.25 μL OA (*see* **Note 19**), and p34*cdc2*/cyclin B kinase (*see* **Note 20**).
2. Resuspend lymphocytes at approx 1–1.5 × 10^6 cells per milliliter in the above PCC incubation medium (*see* **Note 21**) in a 15-mL centrifuge tube.
3. Incubate lymphocytes in the above media for 3 h at 37°C in a circulating water bath.
4. Centrifuge at 200g for 8 min.
5. Aspirate the supernatant, gently disrupt the cell pellet by hand vortexing, and add 2 mL of 0.06 M KCl (0.56%).
6. Leave the cell suspension at room temperature for 4–5 min.
7. Centrifuge as in **Subheading 3.2.**, **step 4**, and carefully aspirate supernatant.
8. Gently disrupt the cell pellet by hand vortexing and add 3–4 mL of ice-cold 1:3 acetic acid/methanol fixative carefully down the side of the centrifuge tube (*see* **Note 22**). Leave the cell suspension in a refrigerator at 4°C overnight.
9. Centrifuge, aspirate the supernatant, disrupt the cell pellet, and add 3–4 mL of fresh fixative.
10. Leave the cell suspension at room temperature for 10 min.
11. Centrifuge, aspirate the supernatant, disrupt the cell pellet, and add 3–4 mL of fresh fixative as in **Subheadings 3.3.**, **step 9** and **3.3.**, **step 10** (*see* **Note 23**).
12. Centrifuge, aspirate the supernatant, disturb the cell pellet, and prepare concentrated cell suspension in fresh fixative (*see* **Note 23**).
13. Drop cell suspension onto acid-cleaned microscope slides (*see* **Note 4**).

3.3. In Situ Hybridization, Chromosome Painting, and Fluorescence Microscopy

1. Select an area suitable for hybridization on the slide and mark with a diamond marker.
2. Pipet 40 mL of 70% formamide/2X SSC solution into a Coplin jar (*see* **Note 13**), and place the jar in a water bath at 73°C. Ensure that the temperature inside the Coplin jar is 72 ± 1°C.
3. Immerse the slide in the denaturation solution for 3 min (*see* **Note 24**).
4. Dehydrate the slide in 70, 85, and 100% ice-cold ethanol by immersing the slide for 2 min in each alcohol grade (*see* **Note 25**).
5. Leave the slide immersed in 100% ethanol until the probe is ready.
6. Prepare the probe mixture as follows (*see* **Note 26**):

   a. Bring the probe to room temperature for a complete thaw, and vortex.
   b. In a microcentrifuge tube, mix 7 μL of hybridization buffer, 1 μL of probe, and 2 μL of distilled water.

7. Briefly centrifuge in a microcentrifuge to collect the contents at the bottom of the tube.
8. Denature the probe mixture using a thermalcycler or a water bath at 73°C for 5 min.
9. Hold the tube at 45–50°C until ready to apply to the slide.
10. Remove the slide from 100% ethanol and dry by touching the bottom edge of the slide to blotting paper and wiping the outside of the slide with a clean paper towel, followed by placement of the slide on a slide warmer to evaporate remaining alcohol.

11. Apply 10 μL of the denatured probe mixture (*see* **Subheading 3.3., step 9**) to the target area marked with a diamond maker (*see* **Subheading 3.3., step 1**), immediately apply a cover slip (*see* **Note 27**), and seal with rubber cement.

12. Hybridize at 37°C overnight (8–16 h) either by placing the slide in a prewarmed, humidified box kept in an incubator or by using an *in situ* hybridization machine.

13. To each of three Coplin jars, labeled 1, 2, and 3, transfer 50 mL of 50% formamide/2X SSC and place each in a water bath at 46°C at least 30 min prior to use.

14. Transfer 50 mL of 2X SSC to another Coplin jar, and place it in a water bath at 46°C at least 30 min prior to use.

15. Transfer 50 mL of 2X SSC/0.1% NP-40 to another Coplin jar, and place it in the water bath at 46°C at least 30 min prior to use.

16. Carefully remove the cover slip from the slide, immerse the slide in the 50% formamide/ 2X SSC solution in Coplin jar 1, and agitate the jar frequently to wash the slide.

17. After 10 min, transfer the slide to Coplin jar 2, repeat the procedure as in **step 16**, and subsequently transfer the slide to Coplin jar 3 after 10 min.

18. Immerse the slide in Coplin jar 3, agitate the jar, remove the slide after 10 min, and dry the slide by touching the end of the slide onto blotting paper.

19. Transfer the slide to 2X SSC solution, agitate the jar frequently, and remove the slide after 10 min.

20. Immerse the slide in 2X SSC/0.1% NP-40. Agitate the jar and remove the slide after 5 min.

21. Let the slide dry in total darkness.

22. Apply 10 μL of DAPI (1000 ng/mL) counterstain in mounting medium and apply a cover slip (*see* **Note 26**).

23. These slides are suitable for observation under a fluorescence microscope equipped with filters for DAPI and fluorescin isothiocyanate (FITC). The slides are observed under an oil-immersion objective, at 1000× magnification, for aberrations involving a specific chromosome (*see* **Notes 27 and 28**).

24. The quantitative analysis of chromosome aberrations is based on the following general criteria. The cells included in the analysis should show:

    a. At least a partial separation of chromosomes with condensed chromatin material as determined by DAPI counterstain.

    b. Two or more clearly separated chromosome-specific spots with bright green fluorescent signals (*see* **Note 29**).

    c. Spots that are similar in fluorescent intensity.

    d. An area representing about 15–100% of the area of spots observed in the controls (*see* **Note 30**).

25. Normal (undamaged) cells display two fluorescent spots, which indicate two copies of the chromosome corresponding to the painting probe employed. Cells with aberrant specific chromosomes are characterized by the presence of more than two spots, which possibly reflect fragments, dicentrics, or symmetrical translocations.

4. Notes

1. **Caution:** Adhere to biosafety procedures while carrying out the steps in this protocol. Use of a biological safety cabinet (class II, type A/B3) is required. All liquid wastes should be treated as biologically hazardous. Therefore, liquid wastes should be aspirated into a conical flask containing 50% bleach to sterilize biohazardous liquids. Solid wastes

should be treated as regulated medical wastes and should be disposed of in appropriately labeled burn boxes *(8)*.

2. Store lymphocyte separation medium at 4°C under refrigeration, bringing it up to room temperature (~25°C) before use.

3. Store bone marrow karyotyping medium frozen at –20°C. Thaw it and heat to 37°C before use.

4. Clean microscope slides by immersing them in 4:1 methanol HCl solution for 4 h, rinsing thoroughly in running tap water, washing in soap, and thoroughly rinsing in distilled water five to six times. Store slides in distilled water at 4°C in a refrigerator.

5. Prepare 10 mM stock solution of ATP (molecular weight 551.1) by dissolving 0.0551 g of ATP in 10 mL of Karyomax. Store at 4°C in a refrigerator until used.

6. Prepare 0.25 µg/µL stock solution of colchicine (molecular weight 399.4) by dissolving 2.5 mg in 10 mL of Karyomax. Store it at 4°C in a refrigerator until used. Handle the carcinogen with care.

7. Prepare 1 mM solution of OA (molecular weight 804.9) by dissolving 25 µg in 31.1 µL of 200° proof ethanol. Store at –20°C. Handle the carcinogen with care.

8. Concentration of p34*cdc2*/cyclin B kinase varies with the lot. Therefore, modify the volume of Karyomax accordingly to get a final concentration of 50 U/mL. Store at –70°C. Activity reduces at a rate of about 50% per week.

9. Freshly prepare 0.56% potassium chloride solution by dissolving 0.56 g in 100 mL of distilled water.

10. Adjust pH of 20X SSC solution to 5.3 with HCl. The solution can be stored at room temperature. Discard stock solution after 6 mo, or sooner if found to be cloudy or contaminated.

11. Mix well 100 mL of 20X SSC (pH 5.3) with 850 mL of distilled water. Adjust pH to 7.0 ± 0.2 with NaOH. Add distilled water to bring volume to 1 L. The solution can be kept at room temperature. Discard stock solution after 6 mo, or sooner if the solution appears cloudy or contaminated.

12. Mix well 100 mL of 20X SSC (pH 5.3) with 850 mL of distilled water. Add 1 mL of NP-40. Adjust pH to 7.0 ± 0.2 with NaOH. Add distilled water to bring the volume to 1 L. Solution can be kept at room temperature. Discard after 6 mo, or sooner if it appears cloudy or contaminated.

13. Mix well 49 mL of formamide, 7 mL of 20X SSC, and 14 mL of distilled water in a glass Coplin jar. Measure pH using pH paper to verify a pH of 7.0–8.0. Prepare a fresh mixture for each use.

14. Prepare v/v solutions of 70, 85, and 100% ethanol with distilled water. Prepare a fresh solution for each use.

15. Mix well 105 mL of formamide, 21 mL of 20X SSC, and 84 mL of distilled water. Measure pH using pH paper to verify a pH of 7.0–8.0. Pour equal volumes of the solution into three glass Coplin jars with lids. Prepare the solution fresh every week, and store it covered in a refrigerator at 4°C.

16. Peripheral blood collected from healthy adult donors by phlebotomy into vacutainers containing EDTA is suitable. However, the Human Use Committee may require approved informed consent from the donors, as determined by the policies of the institute where the work will be carried out.

17. Treat solid waste as regulated biomedical waste, and dispose of it in an appropriately labeled burn box.

18. Expected recovery for a healthy adult donor is about 3–4.5 million mononuclear cells from 3 mL of whole blood.
19. The final concentration of OA in the incubation medium is 0.75 μ*M*. Instead of OA, another phosphatase inhibitor, calyculin A, may be used at a final concentration of 50 n*M* and is equally effective in inducing PCC.
20. The concentration of the p34*cdc2*/cyclin B kinase varies with the lot. Therefore, modify the volume accordingly to get a final concentration of 50 U/mL. Although concentrations as low as 5 U/mL induce PCC, the yield is considerably lower *(6)*.
21. Use of a blood cell counter (e.g., Z2 Counter, Beckman Coulter, Miami, FL) for determining lymphocyte count is suggested but not required.
22. Prepare fixative and keep it ice cold until used.
23. After each of these steps involving a wash in fixative, the cells can be monitored for optimum fixation by preparing a test slide and observing under a light microscope. The fixed cells appear highly transparent under low-intensity light.
24. Perform a trial slide denaturation run. Following denaturation, stain with Giemsa and observe under a microscope. If the morphology is altered, then decrease the melting temperature by 2°C, or reduce the denaturation time.
25. The Coplin jars containing alcohol grades should be placed in an ice bucket at least 30–60 min before starting the experiment, to carry out the cold temperature reactions.
26. Aberrations can be studied using any whole-chromosome–specific probe. The manufacturer's original protocol for metaphase chromosomes is modified for applications involving PCC spreads. Protocols may vary for other whole chromosome probes. We suggest following the manufacturer's instructions and suitably modifying the protocol if needed.
27. Care should be taken not to trap air bubbles when applying the cover slip.
28. Alternatively, slides can be stored at –20°C in the dark for up to 1 wk without fading.
29. Cells with single green spots arising because of overlapping signals must not be included.
30. However, the area of spots in the control samples is not always uniform because of differential chromosome condensation and, in a few cases, angular presentation under the microscope. In such cases of ambiguity, cells may be excluded from analysis.

Acknowledgments

The Armed Forces Radiobiology Research Institute (AFRRI) supported this research under work unit AFRRI-02-03. The views expressed are those of the authors; no endorsement by AFRRI has been given and none should be inferred. We thank Dr. D. G. Ledney for critically reviewing the manuscript and D. K. Solyan for expert editorial assistance.

References

1. Prasanna, P. G. S., Hamel, C. J., Escalada, N. D., Duffy, K. L., and Blakely, W. F. (2002) Biological dosimetry using human interphase peripheral blood lymphocytes. *Mil. Med.* **167(suppl. 1)**, 10–12.
2. Pantelias, G. E. and Maillie, H. D. (1983) A simple method for premature chromosome condensation induction in primary human and rodent cells using polyethylene glycol. *Somatic Cell Genet.* **9**, 533–547.
3. Gotoh, E. and Asakawa, Y. (1996) Detection and evaluation of chromosomal aberrations induced by high doses of gamma irradiation using immunogold-silver painting of prematurely condensed chromosomes. *Int. J. Radiat. Biol.* **70**, 517–520.

4. Durante, M., Furusawa, Y., and Gotoh, E. (1998) A simple method for simultaneous interphase-metaphase chromosome analysis in biodosimetry. *Int. J. Radiat. Biol.* **74,** 457–462.

5. Coco-Martin, J. M. and Begg, A. C. (1997) Detection of radiation-induced chromosome aberrations using fluorescence *in situ* hybridization in drug-induced premature chromosome condensation of tumor cell lines with different radiosensitivities. *Int. J. Radiat. Biol.* **71,** 265–273.

6. Yamashita, K., Yasuda, H., Pines, J., et al. (1990) Okadaic acid, a potent inhibitor of type 1 and 2A protein phosphatases, activates cdc2/H1 kinase and transiently induces premature mitosis-like state in BHK21 cells. *EMBO J.* **9,** 4331–4338.

7. Prasanna, P. G. S., Escalada, N. E., and Blakely, W. F. (2000) Induction of premature chromosome condensation by a phosphatase inhibitor and a protein kinase in unstimulated human peripheral blood lymphocytes: a simple and rapid technique to study chromosome aberrations using specific whole-chromosome DNA hybridization probes for biological dosimetry. *Mutat. Res.* **466,** 131–141.

8. Richmond, J. Y. and McKinney, R. W. (eds.) (1993) *Biosafety in Micobiological and Biomedical Laboratories,* CDC NIH, US Department of Health and Human Services, Washington, D.C.

7

Mutagen-Induced Chromatid Breakage as a Marker of Cancer Risk

Xifeng Wu, Yun-Ling Zheng, and T. C. Hsu

Summary

Risk assessment is now recognized as a multidisciplinary process, extending beyond the scope of traditional epidemiologic methodology to include biological evaluation of interindividual differences in carcinogenic susceptibility. Modulation of environmental exposures by host genetic factors may explain much of the observed interindividual variation in susceptibility to carcinogenesis. These genetic factors include, but are not limited to, carcinogen metabolism and DNA repair capacity. This chapter describes a standardized method for the functional assessment of mutagen sensitivity. This in vitro assay measures the frequency of mutagen-induced breaks in peripheral lymphocytes. Mutagen sensitivity assessed by this method has been shown to be a significant risk factor for tobacco-related malignancies, especially those of the upper aerodigestive tract. Mutagen sensitivity may therefore be a useful member of a panel of susceptibility markers for defining high-risk subgroups for chemoprevention trials. This chapter describes methods for and discusses results from studies of mutagen sensitivity as measured by quantifying chromatid breaks induced by chromosome breaking agents, such as the γ-radiation radiomimetic DNA crosslinking agent bleomycin and chemicals that form so-called bulky DNA adducts, such as 4-NQO and the tobacco smoke constituent, benzo[a]pyrene, in short-term cultured peripheral blood lymphocytes.

Key Words: Mutagen sensitivity; chromatid breaks; cancer susceptibility; bleomycin; benzo[a]pyrene; nitroquinoline; γ-irradiation.

1. Introduction

Maintaining the integrity of the genome is essential to normal cell function. Disruption of this normally well-regulated process can lead to cell death or neoplasia. The notion that genetic susceptibility to cancer is related to genomic instability was initially supported by rare autosomal recessive disorders such as ataxia telangiectasia and xeroderma pigmentosum, which are associated with in vivo and in vitro chromosomal instability, defective DNA repair capacity, and increased cancer risk. Hsu *(1)* hypothesized that in the general population, susceptibility to chromosome damage in response to mutagens varies along a continuum, with recognized chromosome fragil-

From: *Methods in Molecular Biology, vol. 291, Molecular Toxicology Protocols*
Edited by: P. Keohavong and S. G. Grant © Humana Press Inc., Totowa, NJ

ity syndromes such as Fanconi's anemia and ataxia telangiectasia being the most extreme. In response to environmental exposures, genetic damage would accumulate more quickly in people with an inherited susceptibility to DNA damage than in other similarly exposed people, and those with the inherited susceptibility might therefore be at higher risk for cancer. Hsu et al. *(2)* developed a phenotypic assay of intrinsic cancer susceptibility, the *mutagen sensitivity assay*.

Mutagen sensitivity is an in vitro assay that gauges host susceptibility by measuring the frequency of induced chromatid breaks in short-term cultured lymphocytes after exposure to an array of mutagens. A series of studies has indicated that mutagen sensitivity is a promising environmental exposure-related cancer risk marker *(3–15)*. This assay has been successfully expanded by replacing the initial test mutagen, bleomycin, with 4-nitroquinoline-1-oxide (4-NQO; a UV mimetic agent), γ-radiation, and benzo[*a*]pyrene diol epoxide (BPDE) to measure risks associated with different types of cancers *(10,14,16–19)*. Different mutagens may act on cells through different molecular mechanisms and may activate different repair pathways. Bleomycin is radiomimetic and generates free oxygen radicals that can induce single-stranded and double-stranded breaks and subsequent mutations. Bleomycin- or γ-radiation-induced DNA damage requires base excision or recombinant DNA repair *(20,21)*. BPDE is a metabolic product of benzo[*a*]pyrene, a major constituent of tobacco smoke. BPDE forms covalent "bulky" adducts upon interaction with DNA *(22,23)*, which require the nucleotide excision repair pathway for their remediation *(24,25)*. DNA damaged by 4-NQO also requires nucleotide excision repair. Because different cancer sites may be associated with different carcinogenic exposures, the relevancy of specific mutagen sensitivity assays might vary from site to site. It has been found that bleomycin sensitivity is associated with increased risk for environmentally related cancers *(2–15)*; BPDE sensitivity is associated with increased risk for smoking-related cancers *(10,14)*; 4-NQO sensitivity is associated with increased risk for skin cancer *(19)*; and γ-radiation sensitivity is associated with increased risk for brain tumors and breast cancer *(17,18)*.

This chapter discusses mutagen sensitivity as measured by quantifying bleomycin-, BPDE-, 4-NQO-, and γ-radiation-induced chromatid breaks in short-term cultured peripheral blood lymphocytes. Chromatid breaks occur in the late S and G_2 phases of the cell cycle and are detected at metaphase. Chromatid breaks are one of five types of chromosomal aberrations, which also include *inter*chromosomal exchange, *intra*chromosomal exchange, interstitial deletions, and chromatid gaps. Briefly, *inter*chromosomal exchanges involve either a symmetrical or an asymmetrical exchange. When a translocation results in two intact, unicentric chromosomes, a symmetrical exchange has occurred, and when it leads to the formation of a dicentric chromosome and an acentric fragment, an asymmetrical exchange has occurred. *Intra*chromosomal exchanges also include symmetrical and asymmetrical exchanges. Symmetrical exchange results in an inversion chromosome but usually causes no mitotic abnormality. An asymmetric exchange produces a ring chromosome and one or two acentric fragments. Interstitial deletion occurs when a chromatid fragment breaks off and the broken ends fuse. These deletions are usually rare. A chromatid *gap* is defined as a small lesion whose size is shorter than the diameter of the chromatid

(26,27). A chromatid gap can occur when two broken ends of a chromatid join together. A chromatid *break* is defined as occurring when the size of the lesion is equal to or larger than the diameter of the chromatid. Using a slightly modified version of the Chatham Barrs Inn Conference (CBIC) nomenclature *(26)*, chromatid breaks are also defined as follows: (1) when the sister chromatid is bent at the point of the lesion (or chromatid gap), or (2) when two "broken" ends do not face each other.

The following protocol provides instructions for conducting mutagen sensitivity assays and for reading and interpreting chromatid breaks.

2. Materials

2.1. Treatment and Culture of Lymphocyte Cells

1. 5 mL Peripheral blood in green-top tube (sodium heparin as anticoagulant; e.g., Vacutainer, Fisher Scientific, Houston, TX).
2. Blood culture media (*see* **Subheading 2.2.**).
3. 25-cm^2 Culture flasks.
4. 37°C Cell culture incubator.
5. Treatment chemical working solutions (*see* **Subheading 2.3.**).

2.2. Blood Culture Medium

1. 1X RPMI-1640 powder (Gibco, Rockville, MD).
2. 20% Fetal bovine serum (FBS; Gibco).
3. 100 U/mL Penicillin, 100 µg/mL streptomycin (Gibco).
4. 2 mM L-glutamine (Gibco).
5. 24 mM (2 g/L) sodium bicarbonate (NaHCO$_3$).
6. 1.25% (v/v) Phytohemagglutinin (PHA; Burroughs Wellcome, Research Triangle Park, NC).
7. 10 U/mL Heparin sodium salt solution (Gibco), reconstituted in distilled, deionized H$_2$O.

2.3. Treatment Chemical Working Solutions

1. 1.5 U/mL bleomycin (Blenoxane, Nippon Kayaku, White Plains, NY) in distilled, deionized H$_2$O. The working solution can be stored at –20°C.
2. BDPE: 12 mM benzo[*a*]pyrene-r-7, t-8-dihydrodiol-t-9,10-epoxide (Midwest Research, Kansas City, MO) in anhydrous tetrahydrofuran (Sigma, St. Louis, MO). Dilute stock solution in dimethyl sulfoxide (DMSO; Sigma) to a final concentration of 0.5 mM immediately before adding it to the blood culture.
3. 1.0 mM 4-NQO (Sigma) in acetone.

2.4. Irradiation Treatment

1. ^{137}Cs source (e.g., Cesium Irradiator Mark 1, model 30, Shepard and Associates, Glendale, CA).

2.5. Harvesting of Lymphocyte Cells and Slide Preparation

1. Colcemid (demecolcine) working solution: 2 µg/mL colcemid (Gibco) in Hanks' balanced salt solution without Ca^{2+} and Mg^{2+} (HBSS; *see* **Note 1**).
2. 15 mL Centrifugation tubes.
3. Centrifuge (e.g., 5804R, Brinkman,Westbury, NY).
4. 0.06 M KCl hypotonic solution.
5. Carnoy's fixative: 3:1 (v/v) methanol and glacial acetic acid, mixed. Prepare fresh every day.

6. Preparative microscope slides (e.g., Erie Scientific, Portsmouth, NH).
7. Giemsa stain working solution: 4% Gurr's Giemsa stain (Bio/Medical Specialties, Santa Monica, CA) in 0.01 M phosphate-buffered saline (PBS) stock solution (pH 7.0).

3. Methods

3.1. Initiation of Lymphocyte Cultures

1. Begin blood culture by adding 1 mL whole blood to 9 mL blood medium (*see* **Note 2**) in 25-cm^2 tissue flask.
2. Culture cells at 37°C for 72–91 h, depending on specific mutagen treatment.

3.2. Treatment of Lymphocyte Cells

1. Bleomycin sensitivity assay: after 91 h, add 200 μL of 1.5 U/mL bleomycin (final concentration of 0.03 U/mL) and incubate cells for an additional 4 h at 37°C. Proceed to **Subheading 3.3.**
2. BPDE sensitivity assay: after 72 h, add 40 μL of BPDE (final concentration of 2 M) and incubate cells for an additional 23 h (*see* **Note 3**) at 37°C. Proceed to section **Subheading 3.3.**
3. 4-NQO sensitivity assay: after 72 h, add 100 μL of 4-NQO (final concentration of 10 μM) and incubate cells for an additional 23 h at 37°C. Proceed to **Subheading 3.3.**
4. γ-Radiation sensitivity assay: after 91 h, irradiate cells with 1.25 Gy from the ^{137}Cs source. To do this, the flasks containing the cell cultures in 10 μL medium are directly exposed to incident γ-radiation at a rate of 15.58 Gy/min (or 0.26 Gy/s) for 4.8 s. Incubate the cells for an additional 4 h at 37°C.

3.3. Harvesting of Lymphocytes

1. After the appropriate length of incubation for the different assays, add 200 μL colcemid (final concentration of 0.04 μg/mL; *see* **Note 4**) to arrest mitotic cells; incubate at 37°C for 1 h.
2. Pour culture into a 15-mL centrifuge tube.
3. Spin for 5 min at 410g.
4. Discard supernatant.
5. Suspend the cell pellet in 8 mL 0.06 M KCl hypotonic solution (*see* **Note 5**); mix thoroughly. Incubate at room temperature for 15 min.
6. Add 1.5 mL Carney's fixative solution to mixture, and mix well.
7. Spin 5 min at 410g.
8. Discard supernatant.
9. Resuspend the cell pellet in fixative twice, bring volume up to 10 mL, spin, and discard supernatant.
10. Wash the cells with fixative twice more.

3.4. Slide Preparation

1. Spin cells down at 410g, discard supernatant, and resuspend the cell pellet in appropriate amount of fixative solution (*see* **Note 6**) to give a slightly cloudy suspension of cells.
2. Rinse the slides with distilled, deionized water.
3. Drop 4–6 drops of the suspension onto each slide; let the suspension air-dry (~1 min).
4. Code the slides (*see* **Note 7**) with laboratory identification numbers and stain with 4% Gurr's Giemsa solution for 2–3 min.

Fig. 1. An example of a chromatid gap. A chromatid strand visibly runs between the broken ends.

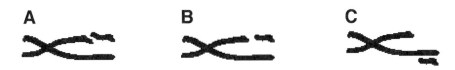

Fig. 2. Examples of chromatid breaks. (**A**) The two "broken" ends do not face each other. (**B**) The fragment is still aligned with the sister chromatid. (**C**) The fragment is displaced at the other side of the intact sister chromatid.

3.5. Reading Chromatid Breaks

1. To view the induced chromatid breaks, two brightfield objectives are needed: low magnification (10–16×) for scanning, and high magnification (100×). Use a 100× dry objective that is specifically designed for preparations lacking cover slips (*see* **Note 8**).
2. When choosing metaphases for scoring chromatid breaks, randomly select full metaphases whose chromosomes are well spread with a minimum amount of overlap (*see* **Note 9**). This can be done at low magnification. At high magnification, avoid chromosomes that have overlapped or chromatids that have been twisted, which can be mistaken for chromatid breaks.
3. Read 50 metaphases per sample and calculate the mean number of breaks. Breaks are recorded as the average number of breaks per cell.

3.6. Recording Chromatid Breaks

1. Before recording chromatid breaks, establish detailed reading criteria and review examples of various types of breakage to ensure high-quality data. When recording chromatid breaks, be conservative (*see* **Note 10**). Record only frank chromatid breaks or exchanges. If multiple breaks are visible on the chromatid, count each break individually. Each chromatid exchange is considered as two breaks. Record the frequency of breakage as breaks per cell. Examples of various types of chromatid aberrations are given in **Figs. 1–8**.
2. Enter the recordings consecutively. Using abbreviations to record the different aberrations is acceptable, but it must be done consistently.
3. Establish a quality control procedure for scoring chromatid breaks (*see* **Note 11**).

4. Notes

1. A premade colcemid working solution can be used, such as KaryoMAX Colcemid Solution (Gibco). However, the final solution should be 10 µg/mL in the blood culture.
2. Take the blood medium from the freezer the day before the experiment and place it in the refrigerator. Do not let it stay in the refrigerator for more than 7 d.
3. The BPDE should be prepared and added to the blood culture in the dark because it is light sensitive.
4. Do not use the colcemid working solution for more than 20 d.
5. The solution lyses the red blood cells, and the suspension will turn brown.

Fig. 3. Example of a chromatid break with the sister chromatid bent at the point of the lesion.

Fig. 4. Example of an isochromatid break. This occurs when the break is visible at identical locations of the sister chromatids.

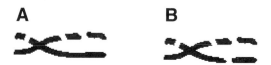

Fig. 5. Examples of chromatids with multiple breaks. (**A**) Three breaks. (**B**) Four breaks.

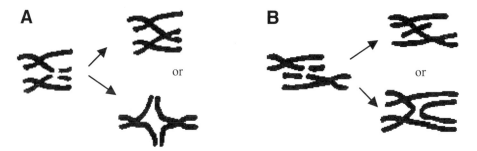

Fig. 6. Examples of *inter*chromosomal exchanges. (**A**) Symmetrical exchange, when a translocated segment leads to two regular chromosomes. (**B**) Asymmetrical exchange, when the exchange leads to the formation of a dicentric chromosome and an acentric fragment.

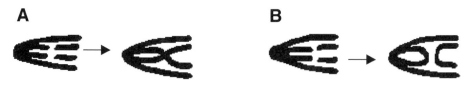

Fig. 7. Examples of *intra*chromosomal exchanges. (**A**) Symmetrical exchange occurs when an inversion in one of the daughter cells causes no mitotic abnormality. (**B**) Asymmetrical exchange will produce a ring chromosome and one or two acentric fragments.

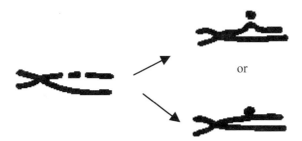

Fig. 8. Example of an interstitial deletion.

6. Depending on the size of the pellet, add 0.5–2 mL of the fixative solution.
7. It is important to code the slides before reading to prevent any introduction of bias. More specifically, the technician reading the slides should not know the case-control status, drug dosage, or duration of treatment related to the slides.
8. The dry 100× objective will have the same resolution as the oil immersion lens. Using the "no cover slip" preparation will prevent the untidiness created by using the oil lens. Make certain that the same field is not observed twice.
9. Do not read cells with incomplete metaphase figures or metaphases with a distorted chromosome arrangement. Avoid reading of prophases and early prometaphases, because chromosomes in these phases show a more beaded morphology and are often more "gappy" than those in full metaphase. Do not read metaphases with crowded chromosomes. It is important to use cells with sister chromatids that are well separated and clearly distinguishable from one another.
10. Be careful when recording chromatid breaks. Breaks usually occur near the ends. If a particular chromosome is difficult to interpret, than consider the chromosome normal. Cells that have been understained tend to show more "gappy" chromosomes, whereas cells that are overstained tend to mask minor chromatid lesions. The heterochromatin regions of chromosomes 1, 9, and 16 usually stain lightly and thus can be misinterpreted as a gap or a break. In approx 1% of bleomycin-treated cultures, metaphases may have extensive (>12) chromatid breaks per cell. These metaphases should be discarded. It might be of interest to record chromatid gaps along with the chromatid breaks; however, they should be recorded separately. The accrued data can be compared with data from other investigators who do not differentiate between chromatid breaks and gaps.
11. It is important to have a well-trained technician to read the slides. The technician should have a basic knowledge of and some experience in cytogenetics. A trained technician will be able to read five to eight slides per day. To become familiar with chromatid breaks, human blood cultures treated with bleomycin (30 µg/mL) for 5 h can be used as test material.

References

1. Hsu, T. C. (1983) Genetic instability in the human population: a working hypothesis. *Hereditas* **98**, 1–9.
2. Hsu, T. C., Johnston, D. A., Cherry, L. M., et al. (1989) Sensitivity to genotoxic effects of bleomycin in humans: possible relationship to environmental carcinogenesis. *Int. J. Cancer* **43**, 403–409.

3. Hsu, T. C., Spitz, M. R., and Schantz, S. P. (1991) Mutagen sensitivity: a biologic marker of cancer susceptibility. *Cancer Epidemiol. Biomarkers Prev.* **1**, 83–89.
4. Spitz, M. R., Fueger, J. J., Beddingfield, N. A., et al. (1989) Chromosome sensitivity to bleomycin-induced mutagenesis, an independent risk factor for upper aerodigestive tract cancers. *Cancer Res.* **49**, 4626–4628.
5. Schantz, S. P., Hsu, T. C., Ainslie, N., and Moser, R. P. (1989) Young adults with head and neck cancer express increased susceptibility to mutagen-induced chromosome damage. *JAMA* **262**, 3313–3315.
6. Spitz, M. R., Fueger, J. J., Halabi, S., Schantz, S. P., Sample, D., and Hsu, T. C. (1993) Mutagen sensitivity in upper aerodigestive tract cancer: a case-control analysis. *Cancer Epidemiol. Biomarkers Prev.* **2**, 329–333.
7. Cloos, J., Steen, I., Joenje, H., et al. (1993) Association between bleomycin genotoxicity and non-constitutional risk factors for head and neck cancer. *Cancer Lett.* **74**, 161–165.
8. Cloos, J., Spitz, M. R., Schantz, S. P., et al. (1996) Genetic susceptibility to head and neck squamous cell carcinoma. *J. Natl. Cancer Inst.* **88**, 530–535.
9. Wu, X., Gu, J., Hong, W. K., et al. (1998) Benzo[*a*]pyrene diol epoxide and bleomycin sensitivity and susceptibility to cancer of upper aerodigestive tract. *J. Natl. Cancer Inst.* **90**, 1393–1399.
10. Spitz, M. R., Hsu, T. C., Wu, X. F., Fueger, J. J., Amos, C. I., and Roth, J. A. (1995) Mutagen sensitivity as a biologic marker of lung cancer risk in African Americans. *Cancer Epidemiol. Biomarkers Prev.* **4**, 99–103.
11. Strom, S. S., Wu, X., Sigurdson, A. J., et al. (1995) Lung cancer, smoking patterns, and mutagen sensitivity in Mexican-Americans. *J. Natl. Cancer Inst.* **18**, 29–33.
12. Wu, X., Delclos, G. L., Annegers, F. J., et al. (1995) A case-control study of wood-dust exposure, mutagen sensitivity, and lung-cancer risk. *Cancer Epidemiol. Biomarkers Prev.* **4**, 583–588.
13. Wu, X., Gu, J., Amos, C. I., Jiang, H., Hong, W. K., and Spitz, M. R. (1998) A parallel study of in vitro sensitivity to benzo[*a*]pyrene diol epoxide and bleomycin in lung cancer cases and controls. *Cancer* **83**, 1118–1127.
14. Wu, X., Gu, J., Patt, Y., et al. (1998) Mutagen sensitivity as a susceptibility marker for human hepatocellular carcinoma. *Cancer Epidemiol. Biomarkers Prev.* **7**, 567–570.
15. Spitz, M. R., Lippman, S. M., Jiang, H., et al. (1998) Mutagen sensitivity as a predictor of tumor recurrence in patients with cancer of the upper aerodigestive tract. *J. Natl. Cancer Inst.* **90**, 243–245.
16. Hsu, T. C., Feun, L., Trizna, Z., et al. (1993) Differential sensitivity among three human subpopulations in response to 4-nitroquinoline-1-oxide and to bleomycin. *Int. J. Oncol.* **3**, 827–830.
17. Bondy, M. L., Kyritis, A. P., Gu, J., et al. (1996) Mutagen sensitivity and risk of glioma: a case-control analysis. *Cancer Res.* **56**, 1484–1486.
18. Buchholz, T. A. and Wu, X. F. (2001) Radiation-induced chromatid breaks as a predictor of breast cancer risk. *Int. J. Radiat. Oncol. Biol. Phys.* **49**, 533–537.
19. Wu, X., Hsu, T. C., and Spitz, M. R. (1996) Mutagen sensitivity exhibits a dose-response relationship in case-control studies. *Cancer Epidemiol. Biomarkers Prev.* **5**, 577–578.
20. Xu, Y. J., Kim, E. Y., and Demple, B. (1998) Excision of C-4'-oxidized deoxyribose lesions from double-stranded DNA by human apurinic/apyrimidinic endonuclease (Ape1 protein) and DNA polymerase beta. *J. Biol. Chem.* **273**, 28837–28844.
21. Dar, M. E., Winters, T. A., and Jorgensen, T. J. (1997) Identification of defective illegitimate recombinational repair of oxidatively-induced DNA double-strand breaks in ataxia-telangiectasia cells. *Mutat. Res.* **384**, 169–179.

22. Arce, G. T., Allen, J. W., Doerr, C. L., et al. (1987) Relationships between benzo(*a*)pyrene-DNA adducts levels and genotoxic effects in mammalian cells. *Cancer Res.* **47,** 3388–3395.

23. Wolterbeek, A. P., Roggeband, R., Steenwinkel, M. J., Rutten, A. A., and Baan, R. A. (1993) Formation and repair of benzo[*a*]pyrene-DNA adducts in cultured hamster tracheal epithelium determined by ^{32}P-postlabeling analysis and unscheduled DNA synthesis. *Carcinogenesis* **14,** 463–467.

24. Shou, M., Harvey, R. G., and Penning, T. M. (1993) Reactivity of benzo[*a*]pyrene-7,8-dione with DNA. Evidence for the formation of deoxyguanosine adducts. *Carcinogenesis* **14,** 475–482.

25. Tang, M. S., Pierce, J. R., Doisy, R. P., Nazimiec, M. E., and Macleod, M. C. (1992) Differences and similarities in the repair of two benzo[*a*]pyrene diol epoxide isomers induced DNA adducts by uvrA, uvrB, and uvrC gene products. *Biochemistry* **31,** 8429–8436.

26. Chatham Workshop Conference (1971) Chatham Workshop Conference on Karyological Monitoring of Normal Cell Populations. International Association of Biological Standardization. Cape Cod, MA.

27. Hsu, T. C., Wu, X., and Trizna, Z. (1996) Mutagen sensitivity in humans—a comparison between two nomenclature systems for recording chromatid breaks. *Cancer Genet. Cytogenet.* **87,** 127–132.

8

Flow Cytometric Analysis of Micronuclei in Erythrocytes

Jan Grawé

Summary

The in vivo micronucleus (MN) test in bone marrow or peripheral blood erythrocytes is widely used as a short-term assay for the detection of agents able to induce chromosome aberrations in somatic cells and has also been shown to have good predictive potential for the identification of carcinogens and germ cell mutagens. The endpoint used is the scoring of micronuclei (MN) in bone marrow or peripheral blood erythrocytes of mice or rats. In this chapter, a detailed description of the flow cytometric micronucleus test will be given, as well as a more general description of the manual micronucleus assay. The DNA of MN is identified using the DNA-specific fluorescent stain Hoechst 33342; discrimination between polychromatic and normochromatic erthrocytes is based on staining with thiazole orange, a fluorescent probe with high RNA affinity. The use of flow-cytometric quantification of micronucleated polychromatic and normochromatic erythrocytes (MNPCE and MNNCE), beyond replacing manual enumeration, provides substantial advantages in terms of speed of analysis, as well as sensitivity. The general description of the MN assay briefly covers choice of animal species and strains, treatment regime, sampling times, and data interpretation. The description of the flow cytometric assay covers in detail erythrocyte preparation and purification, fixation, staining, data acquisition, and data analysis.

Key Words: Micronuclei (MN); erythrocytes; reticulocytes; mouse; rat; flow cytometry; in vivo; micronucleus test; thiazole orange; Hoechst 33342; automation.

1. Introduction

Micronuclei (MN) are small, nucleus-like structures present in the cytoplasm. They are formed by chromosomes, or fragments of chromosomes, that have failed to be incorporated into one of the daughter nuclei during a mitosis or meiosis. This failure occurs because these chromosomes or fragments have lost their connection to a centromere and thus cannot be properly segregated from the metaphase plate to either of the poles during anaphase. The lost material consists either of acentric fragments, formed from chromosome breakage, or whole chromosomes, left behind owing to damage to the mitotic spindle. In telophase, the lost chromosomal material may be enclosed

From: *Methods in Molecular Biology, vol. 291, Molecular Toxicology Protocols*
Edited by: P. Keohavong and S. G. Grant © Humana Press Inc., Totowa, NJ

in a nuclear membrane and, after cytokinesis, then appears as small round nucleus-like structures in either of the daughter cells. MN are present in low frequencies (~1–10 per million) in most cell types. Because they are visible and relatively easily scored in interphase cells, they have become a widely used endpoint for the monitoring of chromosome damage.

The in vivo MN test in bone marrow *(1)* or peripheral blood erythrocytes *(2)* is widely used as a short-term assay for the detection of agents able to induce chromosome aberrations in somatic cells *(3–6)* and has also been shown to have good predictive potential for the identification of carcinogens *(7)* and germ cell mutagens *(8)*. The endpoint involves the scoring of MN in the bone marrow or peripheral blood erythrocytes of mice or rats. MN are formed in bone marrow and, in some cases, spleen erythroblasts, as the result of structural or numerical chromosome damage. During the final maturation of erythroblasts into young or polychromatic erythrocytes (PCE), the main nucleus is expelled (**Fig. 1**). This phenomenon makes the scoring of MN in erythrocytes simpler than in other cell types and also opens the possibility of using automated scoring by flow cytometry. The bone marrow PCE migrate into the peripheral circulation, where they mature into normochromatic erythrocytes (NCE). MN are most often scored in bone marrow PCE or peripheral blood PCE (also termed reticulocytes). The baseline frequency of micronucleated PCE for most strains of mice and rat is between 1 and 3 per million *(9)*.

The kinetics of maturation of a damaged erythroblast is shown in **Fig. 1**. As can be seen, damage induced during the last cell cycle of the erythroblast is, in most cases, best observable about 24 h after damage induction for bone marrow erythrocytes and an additional 20–25 h later in peripheral blood reticulocytes. It is, however, important to note that agent-specific factors such as a requirement for metabolic activation, or delays in cell cycle progression owing to toxic effects, may affect the length of these time spans. It is routine procedure to monitor the ratio of immature bone marrow PCE or peripheral blood reticulocytes as a measure of bone marrow toxicity, because excessive toxicity and concomitant cell cycle delay of damaged erythroblasts may result in false-negative assay results.

In this chapter, a detailed description of the flow cytometric MN test will be given. A full description of the in vivo MN assay is beyond the scope of this paper; however, methodological guidelines for the conduct of this assay are periodically reviewed and published *(3–6)*.

We have developed a flow cytometric approach to enumerating MN in PCE. The DNA of MN is identified using the DNA-specific fluorescent stain Hoechst 33342, and discrimination between PCE and NCE is based on staining with thiazole orange, a fluorescent probe with high RNA affinity. We have shown that the use of flow cytometric quantification of micronucleated polychromatic and normochromatic erythrocytes (MPCE and MNCE), beyond replacing manual enumeration, provides substantial advantages in terms of speed of analysis, as well as sensitivity. Because of the rapidity of the flow cytometric assay, the number of PCE screened per sample may easily be increased by a factor of 100, or from about 1000 to about 100,000, at an assay rate of about 1 sample every 5 min. Assuming a baseline frequency of MN in the population of scored PCE of 2 per million, the expected numbers of MN to be found are 2 and 200, respectively. MN frequencies tend to be Poisson distributed, giving

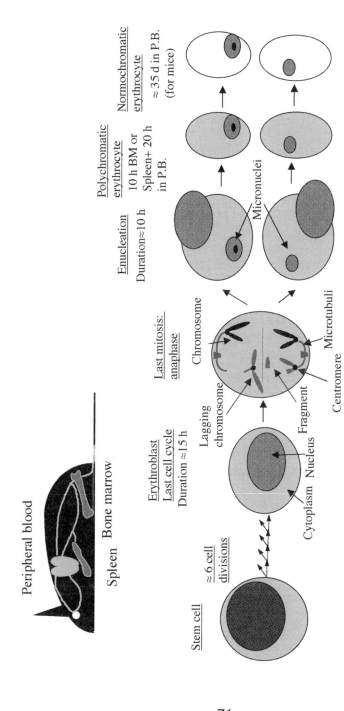

Fig. 1. Kinetics of maturation of erythrocytes and time-course of chromosome damage induced in erythroblasts and expressed as MN. Erythrocytes are formed in the bone marrow and, in some cases (as in young mice), also in the spleen. During a series of cell divisions, the erythroblasts mature from stem cells to their final cell division. Chromosome damage induced during the last cell cycle can be observed in bone marrow (or spleen) polychromatic erythrocytes (PCE) about 24 h after damage induction, or in peripheral blood PCE some 40–48 h after damage induction. MN induced by both chromosome breakage and damage to the mitotic apparatus can be observed. BM, bone marrow; P.B., peripheral blood.

71

standard deviations of about 1.4 and 14 respectively, or 70 and 7% of the number of MN enumerated. Thus, the flow cytometric technique is potentially as much as 10-fold more sensitive than the manual assay. This potentially high sensitivity is also realized in practice. Using both ionizing radiation and diverse chemical agents as inducers of MN, the flow cytometric assay has exhibited a sensitivity increase of about 10-fold in comparison with manual counting *(10–12)*.

The flow cytometric MN assay has recently been adapted for the study of MN in human erythrocytes. Although these studies are still at an early stage, available data indicate that the high sensitivity shown in rodent studies may, to a large degree, be achievable in human studies *(13)*.

2. Materials

2.1. Animal Species and Strains

1. The method has been applied to several strains of mice and rat, as well as wild-living species of rodents, e.g., wood mouse, yellow-necked mouse, and bank and field voles.
2. For the bone marrow erythrocyte test, mouse and rat as well as other species are acceptable; however, only mouse and rat have been extensively validated in the flow cytometric MN assay.
3. For the peripheral blood MN assay, the species used must not remove micronucleated erythrocytes in the spleen, leaving the mouse as the recommended species (*see* **Note 1**).
4. In the mouse, mature erythrocytes are also acceptable for MN analysis when the exposure duration exceeds 4 wk.
5. Among the mouse strains studied using the flow cytometric assay are CBA, C57Bl, Balb-C, and NMRI, and for rats, Fisher 344 and Sprague-Dawley.
6. Animal experiments are subject to local regulations.

2.2. Bone Marrow and Peripheral Blood Sampling

RPMI medium, Percoll, and fixative should be at room temperature at time of use (*see* **Note 2**).

1. Anesthetization equipment (anesthetic ether, CO_2 chamber, or equivalent).
2. Dissection instruments (scalpel, scissors, tweezers).
3. Heparinized blood collection tubes (Vacutainer 367678 or equivalent, BD Biosciences, Franklin Lakes, NJ).
4. 1-mL Syringes with 0.4–0.6-mm needles.
5. RPMI-1640 medium (Invitrogen, Stockholm, Sweden).
6. Conical tubes (11/60 mm, Greiner Labortechnik, Frickenhausen, Germany, or equivalent).
7. Centrifuge with swingout rotor and adaptors for 11/60-mm tubes (e.g., Jouan C3.12, with T4 rotor, Jouan, St. Herblain, France).

2.3. Sample Preparation

1. 1X, 10X Phosphate-buffered saline (PBS; Invitrogen).
2. Percoll (Amersham Biosciences, Uppsala, Sweden).
3. Adjustable micropipets covering 1–1000-µL range (Finnpipette, Thermo Lab Systems, Vantaa, Finland, or equivalent).
4. Percoll density gradient medium: 65% Percoll in PBS (58.5% Percoll, 6.5% 10X PBS, 35% PBS). May be stored for at least 1 wk at 4°C if prepared in a sterile fashion.

5. Centrifuge (as above).
6. Fluorescence-activated cell sorting (FACS) tubes (Falcon 2054, or equivalent; BD Biosciences).
7. Vortex.
8. Sorensen buffer A: 0.5 M KH$_2$PO$_4$ (6.805 g KH$_2$PO$_4$ to 1 L distilled water). Sorensen buffer B: 0.5 M Na$_2$HPO$_4$·2H$_2$O (8.903 g Na$_2$HPO$_4$·2H$_2$O to 1 L distilled water). Both buffers are stable for at least 6 mo at room temperature.
9. 70% Glutaraldehyde (EM grade, Sigma-Aldrich, Stockholm, Sweden).
10. Sodium dodecyl sulphate (SDS; Sigma-Aldrich) stock solution: 1.5 mg/mL in distilled water; filter after preparation; stable for at least 6 mo at room temperature.
11. Fixative: 1% glutaraldehyde, 30 µg/mL sodium dodecyl sulfate (SDS; 50X dilution from stock solution) in 0.05 M PO$_4$ complete Sorensen's buffer, pH 6.8 (for pH 6.8, mix 53.4% Sorensen buffer A and 46.6% Sorensen buffer B). Make fresh every day.
12. 1 mg/mL Thiazole orange (TO; Sigma-Aldrich) stock solution in methanol, stable for at least 1 yr when kept light protected at 4°C.
13. 500 µM Hoechst 33342 (HO342; Molecular Probes, Eugene OR) stock solution in distilled water. Stable for at least 1 yr when kept light protected at 4°C.
14. Staining solution: to 100 mL PBS, add 500 µL HO342 stock solution and 50 µL TO stock solution. Make fresh every day.
15. 37°C water bath.

2.4. Flow Cytometry

1. Flow cytometer capable of simultaneous excitation at UV (minimum power 50 mW) and 488 nm (minimum power 100 mW) lines, preferably with spatially separated beams, e.g., FACSVantage SE (BD Biosciences) equipped with Enterprise dual-wavelength (UV 351–364 and 488 nm) excitation laser (Coherent, Santa Clara, CA). Recent data indicate that benchtop instruments with UV capability, e.g., the LSR from Becton-Dickinson Biosciences equipped with the HeCd UV laser, may also be used.
2. Filter set: 530/30-nm bandpass filter for detection of TO fluorescence emission; 424/44-nm bandpass filter for detection of HO342 fluorescence emission.
3. PBS or equivalent sheath fluid for flow analysis; PBS diluted 1:100–1:300 is recommended for sorting.

3. Methods

3.1. Study Design and Chemical Treatment

For an extensive description of animal care and treatment regimes for the manual in vivo MN assay, as recommended by international expert working groups, *see* **refs. 3–6**. The methods described for animal care and treatment below are based on these recommendations.

Because of the diverse properties of all possible substances that may be subject to testing, no unique treatment schedule can be recommended. Results from extended dose regimens are acceptable if they are positive. For studies showing negative results, there should be either demonstrated toxic effects or the limit dose should be used (*see* **Subheading 3.1.**, **step 3**) and dosing continued until sampling. Some basic recommendations for study design follow.

1. The size of the experiment (i.e., the number of cells scored per animal and the number of animals per group) should be based on statistical considerations: a doubling of the baseline frequency of micronucleated PCE or mature erythrocytes should be detectable compared with a control group with 95% confidence. Minimum recommended requirements for the manual assay are 2000 erythrocytes scored per animal, with at least four animals per dose group (*see* **Note 3**).

2. At least three dose levels should be used. They should be separated by a factor between 2 and the square root of 10. The highest dose tested should be the maximum tolerated dose (MTD). This dose is determined on the basis of mortality, bone marrow cell toxicity as measured by the decrease in PCE frequency, or clinical symptoms such as weight loss or moribund animals. The MTD is usually determined in preliminary range-finding experiments with a smaller number of animals.

3. The highest or limit dose recommended in the absence of any signs of toxicity is 2 g/kg/d for treatment periods of 14 d or less and 1 g/kg/d for treatment periods greater than 14 d.

4. Controls given solvent (vehicle) only should be included at all sampling times (*see* **Note 4**). A concurrent positive control group, i.e., a group given a known MN-inducing agent at an effective dose should be included for each experiment. This is especially important for the interpretation of results in the case of a negative result for the substance being tested. Commonly used positive control substances include cyclophosphamide (monohydrate), mitomycin C, and triethylenemelamine. Positive control substances should be given at doses sufficient to induce a clear increase in MN frequencies but not so high that bone marrow toxicity detected as a reduced PCE frequency is apparent. Although the proper dosage for a positive control must be determined for each laboratory, doses in the range of 50 mg/kg for cyclophosphamide or 1 mg/kg for mitomycin C may give the desired results. These dosages are given for reference only.

5. In a typical experiment, three different dose groups, a vehicle control group, and a positive control group, each consisting of five animals, are treated at the same time. For the bone marrow MN test, animals are sacrificed and bone marrow sampled at 24 and 48 h after treatment. As can be seen in **Fig. 2**, 24 h is the presumed ideal time window for the scoring in bone marrow PCE of MN induced in erythroblasts. The 48-h time is included to allow for delayed effects owing to, for example, the necessity for metabolic activation of the substance. For the peripheral blood MN test, sampling times should be delayed about another 24 h after treatment to allow for the transition of PCE from the bone marrow to the peripheral circulation, with 40–48 and 72 h being possible sampling times.

3.2. Collection of Bone Marrow Cells

1. At time of sampling, anesthetize and sacrifice animals through cervical dislocation.

2. Dissect both femurs. Clean femurs and cut off outermost ends of each.

3. Into one end, insert a syringe filled with 1 mL RPMI-1640 cell culture medium and fitted with a 0.4–0.6-mm gauge needle. Forcefully flush the marrow into a conical tube containing another 1 mL of RPMI. Fill the syringe again with 1 mL of the cell suspension. Flush the femur again into the tube but from the other direction.

4. Repeat with second femur from the same animal.

5. Draw the cell suspension 5–10 times through the syringe to disperse cell aggregates. Let stand for about 1 min.

6. Transfer uppermost approx 1.8 mL to a new tube (*see* **Note 5**).

7. Centrifuge for 5 min at 600*g*.

8. Aspirate all but approx 100 µL of the medium.

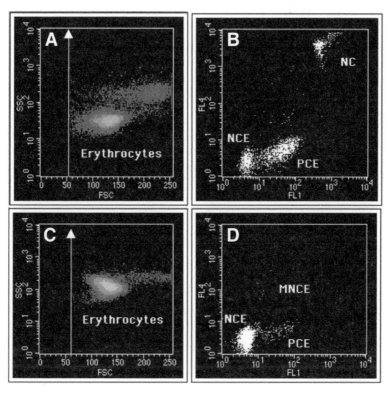

Fig. 2. Plots of flow cytometric data during data acquisition of total erythrocytes for bone marrow (**A, B**) and peripheral blood (**C, D**) samples. Arrows in (A) and (C) indicate threshold levels. The major population in forward scatter–side scatter (FSC-SSC) density plots (A) and (C) represents the erythrocyte population. Dot plots (B) and (D) indicate RNA- (horizontal, Fl1, thiazole orange) and DNA- (vertical, Fl4, HO 342) related fluorescence. (B) and (C) show NC, normochromatic; NCE, NC erythrocytes; MNCE, micronucleated NCE; PCE, polychromatic erythrocytes. 10,000 events.

9. Resuspend cells in remaining medium by gentle vortexing for 1–2 s (repeat if necessary).

3.3. Cell Collection From Peripheral Blood

1. At time of sampling, anesthetize and draw approx 100–300 µL peripheral blood from animals by tail puncture, retro-orbital bleeding, or other suitable means into heparinized blood collection tubes.
2. Mix immediately by gentle vortexing, and again after about 1 min in order to avoid clotting.

3.4. Erythrocyte Purification

1. Prepare 65% Percoll and add 1 mL each to appropriate number of conical test tubes. For each animal, prepare duplicate samples (*see* **Note 6**).
2. For bone marrow samples, layer 50 µL of the bone marrow cell suspension on top of the 65% Percoll in each tube.

3. For peripheral blood samples, add 6 µL of well-mixed peripheral blood on top of the 65% Percoll in each tube.
4. Centrifuge for 20 min at 600*g* with the centrifuge brake turned off.
5. Carefully aspirate the supernatant, including the majority of nucleated cells (*see* **Note 7**), being careful not to aspirate the red cell pellet.
6. Resuspend the pellet of red cells in 30 µL PBS by gentle vortexing.

3.5. Cell Fixation

1. For each sample, add 1.25 mL of freshly made fixative to a FACS tube.
2. Suck the small volume of suspended red cells into an adjustable pipet set to a volume appropriate to accommodate the entire suspension (~50 µL).
3. During vigorous vortexing, quickly expel the cell suspension into the fixative, and continue vortexing for 5 s (*see* **Note 8**).
4. Keep samples at 4°C for at least 24 h and up to 7 d (*see* **Note 9**) before staining.

3.6. Cell Staining

1. Aspirate the fixative.
2. Loosen the cell pellet, which can be tightly packed, by vigorously shaking the test tube rack holding the tubes.
3. Add 1 mL of staining solution (*see* **Note 10**).
4. Stain for 1 h at 37°C in a water bath. Mix samples every 15 min by inverting the tubes.
5. Let stand for at least 2 h or overnight at 4°C before flow cytometric analysis.

3.7. Flow Cytometry (see Note 11)

1. Set UV laser power to at least 50 mW and 488 nm laser power to at least 100 mW for a FACS Vantage instrument.
2. Set the instrument to measure forward light scatter (FSC), side scatter (SSC), 530 nm fluorescence from TO (TOfl) excited by the 488-nm laser (usually the fluorescence isothiocyanate [FITC] channel) and 424 nm fluorescence from HO342 (HOfl) excited by the UV laser.
3. All four signals should be measured in peak height mode. Set the FSC channel to linear amplification, and the other three channels to logarithmic amplification.
4. Run the first sample. Owing to the high cell concentration, a low sample differential pressure is needed (*see* **Note 12**).
5. Set the threshold to FSC. Set the event rate to 3000–5000 events for peripheral blood samples or 1000–2000 events for bone marrow samples.
6. In the data acquisition program, make the following acquisition plots: an FSC-SSC density plot, an FSC-SSC dot plot, and a TOfl-HOfl dot plot. Set the FSC-SSC dot plot to accumulate all events.
7. Set the TOfl-HOfl dot plot to display about 10,000 events. Adjust the FSC and SSC gain to approximately center the cell population in the FSC-SSC plots (**Fig. 2A** and **C**).
8. Set the FSC threshold level to about one-fourth of full scale (~250 on a 1024-channel display).
9. Adjust the TOfl and HOfl gain to place the cell population in the TOfl-HOfl dot plot as shown in **Fig. 2B** and **D**. A bimodal distribution in TOfl should be seen, whereby mature erythrocytes (NCE) have low TO fluorescence, and PCE have a higher fluorescence (**Fig. 2B** and **D**). The division between NCE and PCE should lie at about one-fourth of full scale. The appearance of cells will differ between bone marrow samples, in which PCE constitute some 50% of total erythrocytes (**Fig. 2B**), and peripheral blood samples, in which the PCE frequency is approx 1–3% (**Fig. 2D**). Additionally, a significant amount

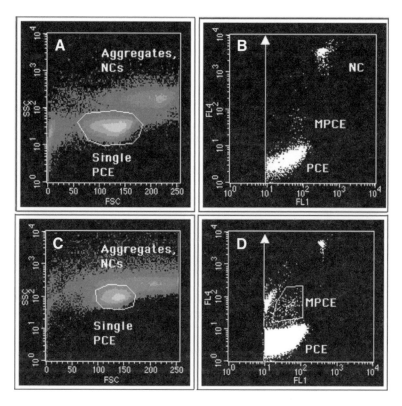

Fig. 3. Plots of flow cytometric data during data acquisition of polychromatic erythrocytes (PCE) for bone marrow (**A, B**) and peripheral blood (**C, D**) samples. Arrows in (B) and (D) indicate threshold levels. The PCE singlet population in the FSC-SSC density plots (A) and (C) has been defined by a region. The corresponding dot plots (B) and (D) for thiazole orange (horizontal) and HO 342 (vertical) fluorescence are gated on the region in the FSC-SSC plots. (B) and (D) show 10,000 events. NC, normochromatic; MPCE, micronucleated polychromatic erythrocytes.

      of residual nucleated cells should be seen in the upper right-hand part of the TOfl-HOfl dot plot in bone marrow samples (**Fig. 2B**).

10. Acquire a list mode file of at least 10,000 events with this setting. These files will be used for the analysis of PCE frequencies in order to detect bone marrow toxicity.

11. Running the same sample, change the threshold to TOfl, and set the threshold level to exclude NCE (**Fig. 3B** and **D**).

12. Adjust the flow rate to about 1000 cells/s for both bone marrow and peripheral blood samples (*see* **Note 13**). In the FSC-SSC dot plot, a bimodal population is now seen (**Fig. 3A** and **C**). One population (lower in FSC and SSC) represents single erythrocytes and one erythrocyte aggregates and nucleated cells.

13. Draw a region of interest around the single erythrocyte population (**Fig. 3A** and **C**, *see* **Note 14**). Gate the TOfl-HOfl dot plot on this region. In the TOfl-HOfl dot plot there should now be three visible populations: PCE, micronucleated PCE (MNPCE) differenti-

ated from the PCE by their higher HO342 fluorescence, and residual nucleated cells in the upper right-hand region (**Fig. 3B** and **D**). Since MNPCE are rare, on the order of 1 per million of the erythrocyte population, only a few will be visible on the dot plot, even if it is set to display 10,000 events.

14. One way of verifying that the dots seen in the presumed MNPCE region are true events is to use so-called backgating. Draw a region around the presumed MNPCE, taking care not to include any PCE without MN (**Fig. 3D**). Gate the hitherto unused FSC-SSC dot plot on this region. As the presumed MNPCE accumulate in this region, a population should form with the same FSC-SSC characteristics as the ungated PCE population in the FSC-SSC density plot. These are the true MNPCE. Events will also be seen with other FCS-SSC properties. These are false events and will be gated out during data analysis. However, if no distinct population appears with the similar population characteristics as the main PCE population, there may be a problem with the sample.

15. Acquire a list mode file of 100,000 events in the single erythrocyte region with this setting. Now run all samples, acquiring both list mode files for each sample. Take care to place the PCE population in the same position for all samples by adjusting amplifier gains, as this greatly simplifies subsequent data analysis.

3.8. Flow Sorting (see Note 15)

It may be desirable to sort micronucleated cells for verification by microscopy or for downstream analysis such as fluorescence *in situ* hybridization (FISH) (*see* **Note 16**).

1. For sorting, the FSC threshold should be used, so that all erythrocytes are "seen" by the instrument; otherwise the sort purity will be very low. This will slow down the sort when sorting MNPCE from peripheral blood, since running PCE at 1000 events/s means that 30,000–40,000 erythrocytes/s pass through the sorter. This rate is too high for sorting for most instruments (*see* **Notes 17** and **18**).

3.9. Data Analysis

Each sample is now represented by two list mode data files, one with all erythrocytes and one with PCE only (and some nucleated cells).

1. For analysis of PCE frequencies, first open a dot plot of HOfl vs TOfl in your flow cytometry data analysis program. Draw a region around all the erythrocytes and another region enclosing the PCE population, and determine the number of events in both regions (**Fig. 4A**).

2. Repeat for all total erythrocyte files.

3. Add the results from duplicate samples from each animal, and use these sums for the calculation of the PCE frequency for each animal. The frequency is generally around 50% in bone marrow and around 1–3% in peripheral blood for control animals, depending on animal strain and age.

4. For analysis of MNPCE frequencies, make an FSC-SSC density plot, and open one of the files containing PCE only. Identify the population of single PCE, and draw a region enclosing it.

5. Make a dot plot of HOfl vs TOfl showing all events. Gate this plot on the PCE region in the FSC-SSC plot in the same way as is done in **Fig. 3A** and **C**.

6. Draw regions identifying PCE and MNPCE, and determine the number of events in these regions (**Fig. 4B** and **C**). When drawing the MNPCE region, take care not to include any PCE without MN.

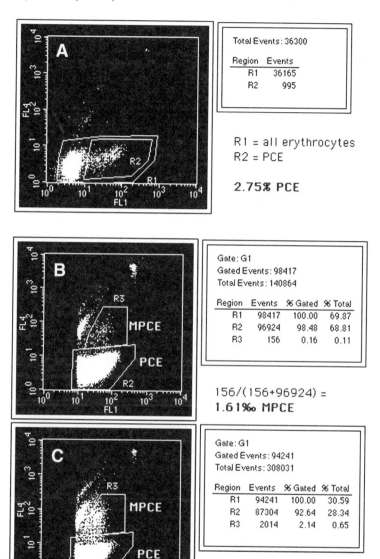

Fig. 4. Data analysis of peripheral blood samples. (**A**) TO-HO342 dot plot of total erythrocytes from a file containing 20,000 events. All events shown. (**B**) TO-HO342 dot plot of PCE from a file containing 300,000 total events. The plot is gated on the PCE singlet population as shown in **Fig. 3C**; about 98,000 events are within the FSC-SSG gate (R1), about 97,000 events are within the PCE region (R2), and 156 events are within the MNPCE region (R3). All events shown. Data from a control animal. (**C**) Same as (**B**) except data from an animal with strongly elevated MNPCE frequency.

7. Add these figures from duplicate samples from each animal, and use these sums for the calculation of the MNPCE frequency for each animal as % MNPCE = number of MNPCE × 1000/(number of PCE + number of MNPCE).

3.10. Data Interpretation

The data evaluation will naturally depend on the design of the experiment. Preliminary data interpretation includes viewing dot plots for samples with abnormal appearance, e.g., strongly deviating positions or shapes of the cell populations. These should be excluded from the evaluation. Determining the existence and nature of a response in the frequency of MNPCE should be based on both biological and statistical considerations. The following proposal is that recommended by Adler et al. *(14)*.

1. In a typical experiment with a control group, three treatment groups, and a positive control group, it should first be determined whether the negative control is within the range (± 3 standard deviations) of the laboratory's historical control data. If the laboratory has not yet generated sufficient control data, published literature values of control data may be of use *(9)*.
2. It should also be determined whether the positive control shows the expected response, with a statistically significant elevation in MN frequency.
3. The dose–response rate of the treatment can then be statistically evaluated using a trend test.
4. Ideally, each treatment group should also be compared pairwise with both the concurrent and the historical controls.
5. For a clear negative result, the trend analysis and the pairwise comparisons should both be without significance. For a clear positive result, the trend test and at least one of the pairwise comparisons should be positive (*see* **Note 19**).

4. Notes

1. However, it is possible to perform the flow cytometric MN assay on rat peripheral blood by using the TO fluorescence intensity to identify the youngest of the peripheral blood PCE *(15)*.
2. Temperature differences among medium, Percoll, and fixative may lead to partial erythrocyte lysis, which in turn gives problems when identifying erythrocytes in the FSC-SSC dot plot during data acquisition and analysis.
3. In general, the use of one gender is adequate for screening. However, if there is evidence indicating differences between males and females in the toxicity of a certain substance, both sexes should be used.
4. Organic solvents such as DMSO are not recommended. Vegetable oils are acceptable as solvents or vehicles. Suspensions (as opposed to solutions) of the test chemicals are acceptable for peroral or intraperitoneal administration, but not for intravenous injection. Freshly prepared solutions or suspensions should be used unless stability data demonstrate the acceptability of storage.
5. Remaining cell aggregates and tissue pieces will thereby be removed, eliminating nozzle clogging problems during flow analysis.
6. Results of parallel samples are pooled for data analysis, reducing the effect of possible variations in sample preparation. In low-dose studies, in which high measurement precision is necessary, triplicate samples are recommended.
7. In bone marrow samples, nucleated cells are visible as a band on top of the Percoll and as a white or pink cloudiness on top of the red pellet. The latter phase can also be removed by careful aspiration, improving the identification of erythrocytes during flow analysis.

8. Immediate and complete mixing is important for a uniform shape after fixation. The SDS in the fixative swells the erythrocytes to uniform spheres for optimal flow analysis.

9. With increasing fixation time, the autofluorescence of the fixed erythrocytes slowly increases, reducing the discrimination between PCE and NCE.

10. Use of 1 mL is standard practice in samples from peripheral blood, as well as for bone marrow when the cell concentration is very similar in all samples. If there are large variations in cell concentration (easily visible in the fixed samples by estimating the size of the sedimented red cell pellet), the amount of staining solution should be adjusted accordingly.

11. A well-aligned instrument is imperative for optimal results.

12. Use of a high cell concentration during sample staining and analysis significantly enhances the quality of the results. High cell concentration when staining reduces nonspecific staining, improving discrimination between MNPCE and PCE. High cell concentration during flow analysis allows a low sample flow rate, which in turn improves especially the precision of the DNA (HO342) measurement.

13. Because of variations between samples, e.g., low PCE frequency in some samples, it may not always be possible to reach speeds of 1000 cells/s.

14. In bone marrow samples, this is usually a discrete population. In peripheral blood samples, the single erythrocyte population often overlaps with the population of doublets and nucleated cells. It is then best to reduce the size of the gate, losing some single erythrocytes, but also most nonspecific events. The shape of this region can be optimized during data analysis, in which the effect of different positions and shapes on the appearance and frequency of the MNPCE population in the HOfl-TOfl dot plot can be evaluated.

15. For a successful sort, one should bear in mind that the MNPCE are very rare. Given a baseline frequency of 2 per million MNPCE among all PCE, and a PCE frequency of 50% among all bone marrow erythrocytes, the frequency of MNPCE among all cells is on the order of 1 per million. In peripheral blood with a PCE frequency of approx 2%, the frequency of MPCE among all cells may be as low as approx 4×10^{-5}.

16. If one is sorting for subsequent probing by FISH an alternative, two-step fixation procedure is required *(16)*. First the pellet is suspended as in **Subheading 3.4.**, **step 7**, and 0.5 mL of PBS containing 5 µg/mL of SDS is added with simultaneous agitation. This step spheres the erythrocytes. After exactly 1 min, 2 mL of Millonig's phosphate-buffered formalin (0.105 M NaOH, 0.137 M KH$_2$PO$_4$ in 10% formalin: 0.42 g NaOH, 1.86 g KH$_2$PO$_4$, 90 mL distilled water, 10 mL 37% formaldehyde) is added. After gentle mixing, the samples are left for 2 h at room temperature (~22°C) before being stored at +4°C for at least 12 h before staining and analysis. The amount of TO stock solution in the staining buffer should then be reduced to 5 µL/100 mL owing to reduced autofluorescence of the fixed cells.

17. To avoid salt buildup when sorting on slides, it is advisable to sort using a low-salt sheath fluid for the sorter. Pure water does not work owing to its low conductivity, but using a standard sorter, it should be possible to use PBS diluted 100–300X with water.

18. Use of silane-coated slides improves the adherence of sorted cells:

    a. Wash slides in detergent solution for 30 min.
    b. Wash slides in running tap water for 30 min.
    c. Wash slides in distilled water for 2 × 5 min.
    d. Wash slides in 95% ethanol for 2 × 5 min.
    e. Air-dry in a dust-free environment for 5 min.
    f. Add 6 mL aminopropyltriethoxysilane solution (Sigma A-3648) to 300 mL acetone.
    g. Dip slides into silane solution for 10 s.

h. Wash twice briefly in distilled water.

i. Dry overnight at 37°C in a dust-free environment.

19. Other alternatives require biological judgment, including control of PCE frequencies, to exclude the possibility of excessive bone marrow toxicity.

References

1. Heddle, J. A. (1973) A rapid in vivo test for chromosomal damage. *Mutat. Res.* **18,** 187–190.

2. MacGregor, J. T. Wehr, C. M., and Gould, D. H. (1980) Clastogen-induced micronuclei in peripheral blood erythrocytes: the basis of an improved micronucleus test. *Environ. Mutagen.* **2,** 509–514.

3. Mavournin, K. H., Blakey, D. H., Cimino, M. C., Salamone, M. F., and Heddle, J. A. (1990) The in vivo micronucleus assay in mammalian bone marrow and peripheral blood. A report of the U.S. Environmental Protection Agency Gene-Tox Program. *Mutat. Res.* **239,** 29–80.

4. Heddle, J. A., Cimino, M. C., Hayashi, M., et al. (1991) Micronuclei as an index of cytogenetic damage: past, present, and future. *Environ. Mol. Mutagen.* **18,** 277–291.

5. Hayashi, M., Tice, R. R., MacGregor, J. T., et al. (1994) In vivo rodent erythrocyte micronucleus assay. *Mutat. Res.* **312,** 293–304.

6. Hayashi, M., MacGregor, J. T., Gatehouse, D. G., et al. (2000) In vivo rodent erythrocyte micronucleus assay. II. Some aspects of protocol design including repeated treatments, integration with toxicity testing, and automated scoring. *Environ. Mol. Mutagen.* **35,** 234–252.

7. Morita, T., Asano, N., Awogi, T., et al. (1997) Evaluation of the rodent micronucleus assay in the screening of IARC carcinogens (groups 1, 2A and 2B): the summary report of the 6th collaborative study by CSGMT/JEMS MMS Collaborative Study of the Micronucleus Group Test. Mammalian Mutagenicity Study Group. *Mutat. Res.* **389,** 3–122. Published erratum appears in *Mutat. Res.* **391,** 259–267, 1997.

8. Waters, M. D., Stack, H. F., Jackson, M. A., Bridges, B. A., and Adler, I. D. (1994) The performance of short-term tests in identifying potential germ cell mutagens: a qualitative and quantitative analysis. *Mutat. Res.* **341,** 109–131.

9. Salamone, M. F. and Mavournin, K. H. (1994) Bone marrow micronucleus assay: a review of the mouse stocks used and their published mean spontaneous micronucleus frequencies. *Environ. Mol. Mutagen.* **23,** 239–273.

10. Zetterberg, G. and Grawé, J. (1993) Flow cytometric analysis of micronucleus induction in mouse erythrocytes by gamma-irradiation at very low dose rates. *Int. J. Radiat. Biol.* **64,** 555–564.

11. Abramsson-Zetterberg, L., Grawé, J., and Zetterberg, G. (1995) Flow cytometric analysis of micronucleus induction in mice by internal exposure to ^{137}Cs at very low dose rates. *Int. J. Radiat. Biol.* **67,** 29–36.

12. Grawé, J., Abramsson-Zetterberg, L., and Zetterberg, G. (1998) Low dose effects of chemicals as assessed by the flow cytometric in vivo micronucleus assay. *Mutat. Res.* **405,** 199–208.

13. Abramsson-Zetterberg, L., Zetterberg, G., Bergström, M., and Grawé, J. (2000) Human cytogenetic biomonitoring using flow-cytometric analysis of micronuclei in transferrin-positive immature peripheral blood reticulocytes. *Environ. Mol. Mutagen.* **36,** 22–31.

14. Adler I. D., Bootman J., Favor J., et al. (1998) Recommendations for statistical designs of in vivo mutagenicity tests with regard to subsequent statistical analysis. *Mutat. Res.* **417,** 19–30.

15. Abramsson-Zetterberg, L., Grawé, J., and Zetterberg, G. (1999) The micronucleus test in rat erythrocytes from bone marrow, spleen and peripheral blood: the response to low doses

of ionizing radiation, cyclophosphamide and vincristine determined by flow cytometry. *Mutat. Res.* **423,** 113–124.

16. Grawé, J., Abramsson-Zetterberg, L., Eriksson, L., and Zetterberg, G. (1994) The relationship between DNA content and centromere content in micronucleated mouse bone marrow polychromatic erythrocytes analyzed and sorted by flow cytometry. *Mutagenesis* **9,** 31–38.

9

The Comet Assay

A Sensitive Genotoxicity Test for the Detection of DNA Damage

Günter Speit and Andreas Hartmann

Summary

The comet assay or single-cell gel (SCG) test is a microgel electrophoresis technique that measures DNA damage at the level of single cells. A small number of cells suspended in a thin agarose gel on a microscope slide is lysed, electrophoresed, and stained with a fluorescent DNA binding dye. Cells with increased DNA damage display increased migration of chromosomal DNA from the nucleus toward the anode, which resembles the shape of a comet. In its alkaline version, which is mainly used, DNA single-strand breaks, DNA double-strand breaks, alkali-labile sites, and single-strand breaks associated with incomplete excision repair sites cause increased DNA migration. On the other hand, crosslinks (DNA–DNA or DNA–protein) can lead to decreased DNA migration. Variations of the comet assay have been established for the detection of specific DNA base modifications. Here we describe the basic methodology of the alkaline comet assay, establishing a sensitive protocol for obtaining reproducible and reliable data. Applications of the comet assay for detecting DNA damage in individual cells are briefly reviewed.

Key Words: Alkaline single-cell electrophoresis; DNA strand breaks; alkali-labile sites; excision repair sites; crosslinks.

1. Introduction

The comet assay (or single-cell gel [SCG]) test permits the sensitive detection of DNA damage at the level of single cells. In this microgel electrophoresis technique, small numbers of cells, such as cultured cells, isolated peripheral lymphocytes or cells isolated from various tissues are suspended in a thin agarose gel on a microscope slide. The cells are lysed with detergent and treated with high salt. Nucleoids are formed, containing non-nucleosomal but still supercoiled DNA. After electrophoresis and staining with a fluorescent DNA-binding dye, cells with increased DNA damage dis-

From: *Methods in Molecular Biology, vol. 291, Molecular Toxicology Protocols*
Edited by: P. Keohavong and S. G. Grant © Humana Press Inc., Totowa, NJ

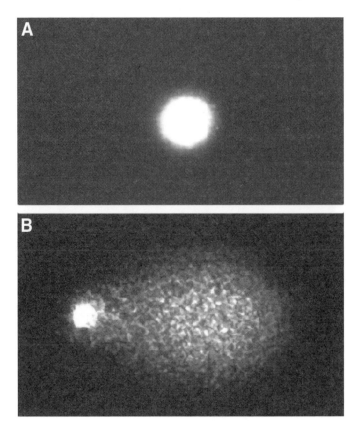

Fig. 1. Photomicrographs of human lymphocytes in the comet assay. (A) Untreated cell (control). (B) Cell exhibiting increased DNA migration after mutagen treatment.

play increased migration of chromosomal DNA from the nucleoid toward the anode, which resembles the shape of a comet (**Fig. 1**). In the alkaline version of the assay which is most often used, DNA strand breaks and alkali-labile sites become apparent, and the amount of DNA migration indicates the amount of DNA damage in the cell. The comet assay combines the simplicity of biochemical techniques for detecting DNA single-strand breaks and/or alkali-labile sites with the single-cell approach typical of cytogenetic assays.

The advantages of the SCG test include its simple and rapid performance, its sensitivity for detecting DNA damage, the analysis of data at the level of the individual cell, the use of extremely small cell samples, and the usability of virtually any eukaryote cell population. Apart from image analysis, which greatly facilitates and enhances the possibilities of comet measurements, the cost of performing the assay is extremely low. The comet assay has already been used in many studies to assess DNA damage and repair induced by various agents in a variety of cells in vitro and in vivo. The test has widespread applications in DNA damage and repair studies, environmental biomonitoring, and human population monitoring (for review, *see* **refs.** *1–4*). The comet assay is widely used in genotoxicity testing in vitro and in vivo, and a proposal for standardized guidelines has recently been published *(5)*.

The alkaline version of the comet assay was introduced by Singh and coworkers *(6)* in 1988. Performing electrophoresis at pH >13.0 enabled the detection of DNA single-strand breaks and alkali-labile lesions. Other versions of the assay were then developed by Olive and coworkers *(7)*, which involved lysis in alkali followed by electrophoresis at either neutral or mild alkaline (pH 12.1) conditions to detect DNA double-strand breaks or single-strand breaks, respectively. Because most genotoxic agents induce many more single-strand breaks and alkali-labile sites than double-strand breaks, the alkaline version (pH >13.0) of the comet assay, although less specific, has the highest sensitivity for detecting induced DNA damage. Important improvements of the test procedure were introduced by Klaude and coworkers in 1996 *(8)*. The use of agarose-precoated slides in combination with drying of gels and fixation of the comets led to a further simplification and a much better handling of the test.

A broad spectrum of DNA-damaging agents cause increased DNA migration in the comet assay. In principal, the alkaline version of the comet assay detects all kinds of directly induced DNA single-strand breaks and any lesion capable of being transformed into a single-strand break at the alkaline pH used (i.e. alkali-labile sites). Breaks introduced into DNA can produce fragments or cause the supercoiled DNA to relax locally. Fragments and/or loops of DNA are then free to migrate toward the anode, thus forming the "comet tail." The alkaline conditions allow DNA strands to unwind and also convert alkali-labile sites, such as apurinic and apyrimidinic sites formed when bases are lost, into DNA breaks. Therefore, the comet assay detects the DNA-damaging effects not only of ionizing radiation and radiomimetic chemicals with high sensitivity but also other types of primary DNA damage such as that induced by hydrogen peroxide and other radical-forming chemicals, alkylating agents, polycyclic aromatic hydrocarbons (PAHs) and other adduct-forming chemicals, various metals and UV irradiation *(1)*. In addition to directly induced strand breakage, processes that introduce single-strand nicks in the DNA, such as incision during excision repair processes, are also detectable. In some cases (e.g., UV, PAHs) the contribution of excision repair to the induced DNA effects in the comet assay seems to be of major importance *(9)*. Some specific classes of DNA base damage can be detected with the comet assay in conjunction with lesion-specific endonucleases. These enzymes, applied to the slides for a short time after lysis, nick DNA at sites of specific base alterations, and the resulting single-strand breaks can be quantified in the comet assay.

Using this modification of the comet assay, the induction and persistence of UV-induced pyrimidine dimers could be monitored in HeLa cells by incubating lysed DNA with a UV-specific endonuclease *(10)*. Oxidized DNA bases have been detected with high sensitivity with the help of endonuclease III or formamidopyrimidine-DNA-glycosylase (FPG) in vitro and in vivo *(11,12)*. Other types of DNA damage, such as pyrimidine dimers and bulky adducts, could be revealed by an indirect immmuno-fluorescence detection using lesion-specific monoclonal antibodies *(13)*. A combination of the comet assay with fluorescence *in situ* hybridization (FISH) makes it possible to investigate the induction and persistence of DNA damage in specific chromosomal regions and genes *(14,15)* (*see* also Chap. 11).

Crosslinks (DNA–DNA or DNA–protein), such as those induced by nitrogen mustard, cisplatin, cyclophosphamide, or formaldehyde, may cause problems in the standard protocol of the test, because crosslinking may stabilize chromosomal DNA and inhibit DNA migration *(16)*. However, the comet assay has also been used to detect crosslinking. One approach is to induce DNA migration with a second agent (e.g., ionizing radiation, methyl methanesulfonate) and to determine the reduced migration in the presence of the crosslinking agent *(17,18)*. Crosslinks can also be detected by increasing the duration of unwinding and/or electrophoresis to such an extent that control cells exhibit significant DNA migration, demonstrating the effect of crosslinking by a retardation in the extent of DNA migration in comparison with the control *(19)*. DNA–DNA and DNA–protein crosslinks can be distinguished by incubating the lysed DNA in proteinase K (PK) prior to electrophoresis. Exposure of crosslinked DNA to PK reduces or eliminates DNA–protein crosslinks and enhances migration, while having no effect on the amount of DNA–DNA crosslinks *(18)*. These modifications of the standard protocol provide additional mechanistic information on the specific types of DNA damage induced by a DNA-damaging agent.

The purpose of this protocol is to provide information on the application of the alkaline comet assay for the investigation of DNA damage in mammalian cells in vitro. For establishing the method, we recommend starting with experiments using blood samples and the induction of DNA damage by a standard mutagen (ionizing radiation or an alkylating agent). The method described here is based on a protocol established by R. Tice according to the original work of Singh et al. *(6)* and includes the modifications introduced by Klaude and coworkers *(8)*. An outline of the protocol is diagrammed in **Fig. 2** (*see* **Notes 1** and **2**).

2. Materials

2.1. Preparation of Slides

1. Microscope slides (with frosted end).
2. Coverslips (24 × 60 mm).
3. Ethanol (absolute).
4. Microcentrifuge tubes.
5. Agarose (low melting point [LMP]).
6. Phosphate-buffered saline (PBS), Ca^{2+}, Mg^{2+} free.
7. Micropipetors and tips.
8. Lysing solution per 1000 mL: 2.5 M NaCl (146.1 g), 100 mM EDTA (disodinar salt; 37.2 g), 10 mM Tris-HCl (1.2 g). Titrate to 10.0 pH with approx 8 g solid NaOH; make up to 890 mL with dH_2O, and store at room temperature. Final lysing solution (100 mL): add fresh 1 mL Triton X-100 and 10 mL dimethyl sulfoxide (DMSO) to 89 mL lysing solution, and then refrigerate (4°C) for 60 min before use.

2.2. Preparation of Cells

1. Heparinized peripheral blood (*see* **Subheading 3.2.** and **Note 3**)
2. RPMI-1640 media (e.g., Gibco, Carlsbad, CA).

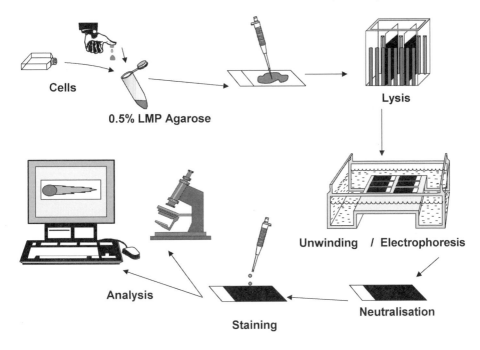

Fig. 2. Scheme for the performance of the comet assay. LMP, low melting point.

3. Ficoll/Hypaque solution (e.g., Pharmacia Biotech, Piscataway, NJ).
4. Centrifuge.

2.3. Electrophoresis and Staining

1. Horizontal gel electrophoresis unit.
2. Electrophoresis buffer: 300 mM NaOH/1 mM EDTA. Prepare from stock solutions: 10 N NaOH (200 g/500 mL dH$_2$O); 200 mM EDTA (14.89 g/200 mL dH$_2$O, pH 10). Store at room temperature. For 1X buffer (made fresh before each run; total volume depends on gel box capacity), mix 45 mL NaOH solution plus 7.5 mL EDTA solution, fill to 1500 mL, and mix well.
3. Neutralization buffer: 0.4 M Tris-HCl (48.5 g). Fill to 1000 mL with dH$_2$O. Set pH to 7.5 with HCl. Store at room temperature.
4. Ethanol (absolute).
5. Staining solution: ethidium bromide (10X stock: 200 μg/mL),10 mg in 50 mL dH$_2$O. Store at room temperature. For 1X stock (20 μg/mL), mix 1 mL with 9 mL dH$_2$O and filter.

2.4. Evaluation of DNA Damage

1. Fluorescence microscope (equipped with an excitation filter of 515–560 nm and a barrier filter of 590 nm).

3. Methods

3.1. Preparation of Slides

1. Clean oily or dusty slides with ethanol before use, and label them with a solvent-resistant marker.
2. Agarose:

    a. For bottom layer, prepare 1.5% normal melting agarose (300 mg in 20 mL PBS) and boil two to three times before use.
    b. Dip the cleaned slides briefly into hot (>60°C) agarose. The agarose should reach halfway up the frosted part of the slide to ensure that the agarose will stick properly to the slide.
    c. Wipe off the agarose from the bottom side of the slide, and place the slide horizontally. (This step has to be performed quickly to ensure a good distribution of the agarose.)
    d. Dry the slides and store them at room temperature until needed. Avoid high-humidity conditions.

3. Prepare 0.5% LMP agarose (100 mg in 20 mL PBS). Microwave or heat until near boiling and the agarose dissolves. Place LMP agarose vial in a 37°C water bath to cool.
4. Add 120 µL of LMP agarose (37°C) mixed with 5000–50000 cells in approx 5–10 µL. (Do not use more than 10 µL). Add cover slip and place the tray in a refrigerator for approx 2 min (until the agarose layer hardens). Using approx 10,000 cells results in approx 1 cell/microscope field (400× magnification). After adding the cells to the slides until the end of electrophoresis, direct light irradiation should be avoided to prevent additional DNA damage.
5. Gently slide off cover slip and slowly lower slide into cold, freshly made lysing solution. Protect from light and place in 4°C refrigeration for a minimum of 1 h. Slides may be stored for extended periods in cold lysing solution (but generally not longer than 4 wk). If precipitation of the lysing solution is observed, slides should be rinsed carefully with distilled water before electrophoresis.

3.2. Preparation and Treatment of Cells (see Note 3)

1. Whole blood: mix approx 5 µL whole blood with 120 µL LMP agarose, and layer onto slide.
2. Isolated lymphocytes:

    a. Mix 40 µL whole blood with 500 µL mL RPMI-1640 in a microcentrifuge tube, and add 150 µL Ficoll below the blood/medium mixture.
    b. Spin for 3 min at 200*g*.
    c. Remove 100 µL of the middle/top of the Ficoll layer, add to 1 mL medium, mix, and spin for 3 min to pellet the lymphocytes.
    d. Pour off the supernatant, resuspend the pellet in 120 µL LMP agarose, and layer onto slide.

3. Cell cultures:

    a. Monolayer cultures: gently trypsinize cells (for about 2 min with 0.15% trypsin; stop by adding serum or complete cell culture medium) to yield approx 1×10^6 cells/mL. Add 10 µL cell suspension to 120 µL LMP agarose, and layer onto slide.
    b. Suspension cultures: add approx 20,000 cells in 10 µL or less volume to 120 µL LMP agarose, and layer onto slide.

3.3. In Vitro Treatment of Cells (see Note 4)

1. For in vitro tests, cells are usually incubated with the test substances for a defined period, then mixed with LMP agarose, and added to the slide *(5)*. A modified protocol, which may be performed in combination with the standard comet assay, suggests treating after cell lysis. Under these conditions, the lysed cells are no longer held under the regulation of any metabolic pathway or membrane barrier *(23)*.

3.4. Standardized Positive Control

For demonstration of a positive effect:

1. Mix 200 μL heparinized whole blood with 50 μL of a 2.5×10^{-4} *M* methyl methanesulfonate (MMS) solution (final concentration: 5×10^{-5} *M*), incubate for 1 h at 37°C and then use 10 μL for the test.
2. Alternatively, cells can be irradiated with 1 Gy γ-irradiation.
3. To evaluate whether the assay is functioning correctly, a treated (e.g., MMS or γ-irradiation), cryopreserved cell sample (e.g., isolated blood lymphocytes or a permanent cell line) can be used.
4. The treated cell population can be stored as 1-mL aliquots (about 10^5 cells/mL) in microcentrifuge tubes. Such a sample can be thawed and processed along with the experimental samples.
5. Data from these samples indicate the interrun variability.

3.5. Electrophoresis and Staining (see Note 5)

1. After at least 1 h at 4°C, gently remove slides from the lysing solution.
2. Place slides on the horizontal gel box near the anode (+) end, sliding them as close together as possible.
3. Fill the buffer reservoirs with freshly made electrophoresis buffer (4°C) until the liquid level completely covers the slides (avoid bubbles over the agarose). Alkaline treatment and electrophoresis are both performed in an ice bath (4°C).
4. Let slides sit in the alkaline buffer for 20–60 min to allow unwinding of the DNA and the expression of alkali-labile damage. For most experiments with cultivated cells, 20 min is sufficient.
5. Turn on power supply to 25 V (~0.8–1.5 V/cm, depending on gel box size), and adjust current to 300 mA by slowly raising or lowering the buffer level. Depending on the purpose of the study and the extent of migration in control samples, allow slides to run for 20–40 min. The goal is to obtain a little migration among the control cells to ensure sensitive test conditions. The optimal electrophoresis duration differs for different cell types and has to be established first.
6. Turn off the power. Gently lift the slides from the buffer, and place on a staining tray. Coat the slides dropwise with neutralization buffer, and let sit for at least 5 min. Repeat two more times.
7. Drain slides, dry the bottom side, incubate for 5–10 min in absolute ethanol, and let them dry (inclined) at room temperature. Slides can be stored for a longer time before staining. To stain, add 50 μL 1X ethidium bromide staining solution, and cover with a cover slip.
8. Slides are stained one by one and evaluated immediately. It is possible to rinse stained (evaluated) slides in distilled water, remove the coverslip, let the slides dry, and stain them at a later time point for re-evaluation.

3.6. Evaluation of DNA Effects (see Note 4)

For visualization of DNA damage, observations are made of ethidium bromide-stained DNA at 400× magnification using a fluorescence microscope equipped with an excitation filter of 515–560 nm and a barrier filter of 590 nm. Generally, 50 randomly selected cells per sample are analyzed. Depending on the size of the cells being analyzed, other magnifications (e.g., 250×) can be used.

In principle, evaluation can be done in four different ways:

1. The percentage of cells with a tail vs those without is determined.
2. Cells are scored visually according to tail size into five classes (from undamaged, 0, to maximally damaged, 4). Thus, the total score for 50 comets can range from 0 (all undamaged) to 200 (all maximally damaged) *(20)*.
3. Cells are analyzed using a calibrated scale in the ocular of the microscope. For each cell, the image length (diameter of the nucleus plus migrated DNA) is measured in microns, and the mean is calculated.
4. An image analysis system linked to a gated CCD camera is used to quantitate DNA image length, head length, tail length, and tail intensity. The statistical variants usually used include DNA migration (image length, tail length), tail intensity, and tail moment. It should be noted that the calculation of tail moment (DNA migration × tail intensity) in different image analysis systems may not be based on the same parameters (*see* Chaps. 10 and 11).

   For the statistical analysis of comet assay data, a variety of parametric and nonparametric statistical methods are used. The most appropriate means of statistical analysis depends on the kind of study and has to take into account the various sources of assay variability. For a powerful statistical analysis of in vitro test data, appropriate replication and repeat experiments have to be performed. When migration length is used as the measure of DNA damage, the median of the 50 cells per experimental point and the mean from repeat experiments should be determined. Mean migration should not be used since a normal size distribution is not observed. Analyses are mainly based on changes in group mean response, but attention should also be paid to the distribution among cells, which often provides additional important information.

4. Notes

1. Many technical variables have been modified, including the concentration and amount of LMP agarose, the composition of the lysing solution and the lysis time, the alkaline unwinding, the electrophoresis buffer and electrophoretic conditions, DNA-specific dyes for staining, and so on (for details, *see* **ref. *1***). Some of these variables may affect the sensitivity of the test. To allow for a comparison obtained in different laboratories and for a critical evaluation of data, it is absolutely necessary to describe the technical details of the method employed clearly.
2. Although the protocol described here detects a broad spectrum of DNA-damaging agents with high sensitivity, modifications have been suggested that further increase the sensitivity and may be advantageous for certain applications *(21,22)*. These modifications include the addition of radical scavengers to the electrophoresis buffer (to reduce damage during prolonged electrophoresis), the addition of PK to the lysing solution (to remove residual proteins that might inhibit DNA migration), and the use of the

DNA dyes SYBR Green-I or YOYO-1 (to increase the sensitivity for the detection of migrated DNA).

3. Many other cell types have been used, and it is a strength of the comet assay that virtually any eukaryote cell population is amenable to analysis. The comet assay is particularly suited for the investigation of organ- or tissue-specific genotoxic effects in vivo (for review, *see* **refs.** *1* and *5*), the only requirement being the preparation of an intact single cell suspension.

4. It is strongly recommended to include some measure of cytotoxicity in every study and to specify the limits of cytotoxicity used in a test. Acute lethal effects can easily be determined by various viability tests such as Trypan blue exclusion, ATP levels, or fluorochrome-mediated assays. However, as cell survival may be significantly reduced in the absence of acute cytotoxicity, tests indicating long-term survivability (e.g., plating efficiency) should also be considered *(24)*. The comet assay has not yet been sufficiently validated and may be sensitive to nongenotoxic cell killing. Upon cell death, elevated DNA migration may be induced by extensive DNA fragmentation. However, data suggest that false-positive results owing to cytotoxicity may be cell type-specific. Although excessive cytotoxicity in V79 Chinese hamster cells *(24,25)* or L5178Y mouse lymphoma cells *(26)* did not result in positive effects in the comet assay, cytotoxicity was reported as a possible confounding effect in TK-6 cells *(27)* or rat lymphocytes *(28)*. However, the comet assay has the advantage that dead or dying cells can be identified on microscope slides by their morphology. Such cells exhibit extensive DNA fragmentation, are without a visible nucleus, and nearly all of their DNA is in the tail *(5)*. For the evaluation of genotoxic effects, it is recommended to record these cells and use them as an additional parameter of cytotoxicity, but to exclude them from evaluation under the principle that they represent dead cells.

5. If specific types of base damage are to determined by using lesion-specific endonucleases, the standard protocol has to be modified in the following way: after at least 1 h at 4°C, gently remove slides from the lysing solution and wash three times in enzyme buffer. Drain slides and cover with 200 μL of either buffer or enzyme in buffer. Seal with a cover slip, and incubate for 30 min at 37°C. Remove the cover slip, rinse slides with PBS, and place them on the electrophoresis box *(11,12)*.

References

1. Tice, R. R. (1995) The single cell gel/comet assay: a microgel electrophoretic technique for the detection of DNA damage and repair in individual cells, in *Environmental Mutagenesis* (Phillips, D. H. and Venitt, S., eds.), βIOS Scientific Publishers, Oxford, pp. 315–339.
2. Rojas, E., Lopez, M. C., and Valverde, M. (1999) Single cell gel electrophoresis assay: methodology and application. *J. Chromatogr. B* **722**, 225–254.
3. Cotelle, S. and Férard, J. F. (1999) Comet assay in genetic ecotoxicology: a review. *Environ. Mol. Mutagen.* **34**, 246–255.
4. Kassie, F., Parzefall, W., and Knasmüller, S. (2000) Single cell gel electrophoresis assay: a new technique for human biomonitoring studies. *Mutat. Res.* **463**, 13–31.
5. Tice, R. R., Agurell, E., Anderson, D., et al. (2000) The single cell gel/comet assay: guidelines for in vitro and in vivo genetic toxicology testing. *Environ. Mol. Mutagen.* **35**, 206–221.
6. Singh, N. P., McCoy, M. T., Tice, R. R., and Schneider, E. L. (1988) A simple technique for quantification of low levels of DNA damage in individual cells. *Exp. Cell Res.* **175**, 184–191.

7. Olive, P. L. (1989) Cell proliferation as a requirement for development of contact effect in Chinese hamster V79 spheroids. *Radiat. Res.* **117**, 79–92.

8. Klaude, M., Erikson S., Nygren J., and Ahnström, G. (1996) The comet assay: mechanisms and technical considerations. *Mutat. Res.* **363**, 89–96.

9. Speit, G. and Hartmann, A. (1995) The contribution of excision repair to the DNA-effects seen in the alkaline single cell gel test (comet assay). *Mutagenesis* **10**, 555–559.

10. Gedik, C. M., Ewen, S. W. B., and Collins, A. R. (1992) Single-cell gel electrophoresis applied to the analysis of UV-C damage and its repair in human cells. *Int. J. Radiat. Biol.* **62**, 313–320.

11. Collins, A. R., Duthie, S. J., and Dobson, V. L. (1993) Direct enzymic detection of endogenous oxidative base damage in human lymphocyte DNA. *Carcinogenesis* **14**, 1733–1735.

12. Dennog, C., Hartmann, A., Frey, G., and Speit, G. (1996) Detection of DNA damage after hyperbaric oxygen (HBO) therapy. *Mutagenesis* **11**, 605–609.

13. Sauvaigo, S., Serres, C., Signorini, N., Emonet, N., Richard, M. J., and Cadet, J. (1998) Use of the single cell gel electrophoresis assay for the immunofluorescent detection of specific DNA damage. *Anal. Biochem.* **259**, 1–7.

14. Santos, S. J., Singh, N. P., and Natarajan, A. T. (1997) Fluorescence in situ hybridization with comets. *Exp. Cell Res.* **232**, 407–411.

15. Rapp, A., Bock, C., Dittmar, H., and Greulich, K. O. (2000) UV-A breakage sensitivity of human chromosomes as measured by COMET-FISH depends on gene density and not on the chromosome size. *J. Photochem. Photobiol.* **56**, 109–117.

16. Hartmann, A., Herkommer, K., Glück, M., and Speit, G. (1995) The DNA-damaging effect of cyclophosphamide on human blood cells in vivo and in vitro studied with the single cell gel test (SCG). *Environ. Mol. Mutagen.* **25**, 180–187.

17. Pfuhler, S. and Wolf, H. U. (1996) Detection of DNA-crosslinking agents with the alkaline comet assay. *Environ. Mol. Mutagen.* **27**, 196–201.

18. Merk, O. and Speit, G. (1998) Significance of formaldehyde-induced DNA-protein crosslinks for mutagenesis. *Environ. Mol. Mutagen.* **32**, 260–268.

19. Fuscoe, J. C., Afshari, A. J., George, M. H., et al. (1996) In vivo genotoxicity of dichloroacetic acid: evaluation with the mouse peripheral blood micronucleus assay and the single cell gel assay. *Environ. Mol. Mutagen.* **27**, 1–9.

20. Collins, A. R., Ai-Guo, A., and Duthie, S. J. (1995) The kinetics of repair of oxidative DNA damage (strand breaks and oxidised pyrimidines) in human cells. *Mutat. Res.* **336**, 69–77.

21. Singh, N. P., Stephens, R. E., and Schneider, E. L. (1994) Modifications of alkaline microgel electrphoresis for sensitive detection of DNA damage. *Int. J. Radiat. Biol.* **66**, 23–28.

22. Singh, N. P. and Stephens R. E. (1997) Microgel electrophoresis: sensitivity, mechanisms, and DNA electrostretching. *Mutat. Res.* **383**, 167–175.

23. Kasamatsu, T., Kohda, K., and Kawazoe, Y. (1996) Comparison of chemically induced DNA breakage in cellular and subcellular systems using the comet assay. *Mutat. Res.* **369**, 1–6.

24. Hartmann, A. and Speit, G. (1997) The contribution of cytotoxicity to effects seen in the alkaline comet assay. *Toxicol. Lett.* **90**, 183–188.

25. Hartmann, A., Kiskinis, E., Fjaellman, A., and Suter, W. (2001) Influence of cytotoxicity and compound precipitation on test results in the alkaline comet assay. *Mutat. Res.* **497**, 199–212.

26. Kiskinis, E., Suter, W., and Hartmann, A. (2002) High-throughput comet assay using 96-well plates. *Mutagenesis* **17,** 37–43.
27. Henderson, L., Wolfreys, A., Fedyk, J., Bourner, C., and Windebank, S. (1998) The ability of the comet assay to discriminate between genotoxins and cytotoxins. *Mutagenesis* **13,** 89–94.
28. Quintana, P. J., de Peyster, A., Klatzke, S., and Park, H. J. (2000) Gossypol-induced DNA breaks in rat lymphocytes are secondary to cytotoxicity. *Toxicol. Lett.* **117,** 85–94.

10

Computerized Image Analysis Software for the Comet Assay

R. C. Chaubey

Summary

Single-cell gel electrophoresis (SCGE) or the *comet assay* is a powerful tool for the detection of DNA single- and double-strand breaks and base damage and for investigating the kinetics of DNA strand break rejoining in human and animal model systems. It is a versatile technique that can be applied in various areas of biomedical research. This chapter highlights the importance of computerized analysis and data processing for the comet assay and describes the criteria used for manual evaluation of comets and their limitations compared with the computer-based analysis. It describes in detail SCGE-Pro, a semiautomatic software developed in our laboratory for comet evaluation and data processing. For comparison, some of the commercially available software for analysis of data from the comet assay is also described.

Key Words: Single-cell gel electrophoresis; comet assay; genotoxicity; DNA strand breaks; DNA base damage; DNA repair; imaging software; SCGE-Pro.

1. Introduction

Single-cell gel electrophoresis (SCGE) or the *comet assay* can be used for detection of DNA damage and repair at the single-cell level and provides a unique opportunity to investigate intercellular differences in any eukaryotic cell population *(1–3)*. During the early development of this assay, the problems inherent in manual evaluation of comets were major stumbling blocks for the widespread acceptance and application of the technique. Measurements of comet characteristics using an ocular micrometer were tedious and time-consuming. Meanwhile, there has been rapid development in the field of imaging devices/sensors, owing to the increasing availability of low-cost, high-speed computational facility and denser memory chips, which has led to the development of a number of imaging techniques and software for biological applications *(4–6)*. Basically, digital image processing (DIP) has four components: image acquisition, processing, storage, and display. During recent years, a number of types of imaging software have been developed for visualization and measurement of various comet characteristics, e.g., total/tail area, DNA content, percentage of DNA in head/tail, head diameter, tail length, and so on. The commercial availability of various imaging soft-

From: *Methods in Molecular Biology, vol. 291, Molecular Toxicology Protocols*
Edited by: P. Keohavong and S. G. Grant © Humana Press Inc., Totowa, NJ

ware packages for evaluation of the comet assay has created considerable interest in laboratories across the world engaged in genotoxicity evaluation of physical and chemical mutagens and carcinogens. This assay has been in applied in many areas of biomedical research, including genetic toxicology, radiation biology, human biomonitoring, clinical and molecular epidemiology, and, as a predictive assay, cancer radiotherapy *(7–9)*.

The comet assay is highly sensitive and can be used to detect DNA double-strand breaks under neutral conditions, as well as DNA single-strand breaks, alkali-labile sites, and incomplete DNA repair sites under alkaline conditions (by converting them to double-strand breaks) *(10)*. In addition, specific types of DNA base damage can be detected and quantified using endonuclease III and formamidopyrimidine-glycosylase (FPG) *(11)*, and UV-induced pyrimidine dimers can be detected and quantified using T4 endonuclease V *(12)*. The assay has been further modified to detect agents that do not produce DNA strand breaks except as transient intermediates during nucleotide excision repair by incubating cells with DNA polymerase inhibitors, such as cytosine arabinoside or aphidicolin *(13)*, and it has also been combined with fluorescence *in situ* hybridization (FISH) to measure gene-specific repair relative to total DNA or loss of heterozygosity (LOH) for a single gene *(14)*.

This chapter describes SCGE-Pro, digital imaging software developed in our laboratory for automated image analysis and data processing of the comet assay *(15)*. It also describes various criteria used for manual scoring of comets and their limitations. Besides SCGE-Pro, a number of other types of software available commercially for evaluation of the comet assay are described and discussed.

2. Materials

2.1. Hardware

A digital imaging system for data capture from the comet assay consists of the following components: a fluorescence microscope, a video camera, a frame grabber (in the case of an analog camera), and a suitable computer with a printer. A high-resolution digital camera can also be used for image acquisition. The various components of the imaging system can be obtained from any reliable vendor. The following examples are derived from our own system.

1. Fluorescence microscope: a Zeiss Axioplan microscope with epifluorescence facility (HBO 50 high-pressure mercury lamp) and suitable filter sets (Zeiss, Göttingen, Germany).
2. Video camera: a high-performance color video camera, JVC KY-F55BE 3CCD (JVC, London, UK). This camera has a 1/3-inch 440,000-pixel CCD with on-chip lens, and it delivers high-quality pictures with a signal-to-noise ratio of 58 dB and sensitivity as high as 2000 lux at F5.6. It has a horizontal resolution of 750 lines. It also incorporates a comprehensive range of automatic functions including automatic level control, continuously variable electronic shutter, and full-time auto white balance. It also has outputs for composite video, RGB, and composite sync signals.
3. Video frame grabber: Integral Flashpoint Intrigue frame grabber (Integral Technologies, Indianapolis, IN). The FlashBus MV uses the PCI bus for real-time transfer of video to system memory. The PCI bus has a theoretical data transfer rate fast enough

for real-time transfer of video data. The actual performance of the FlashBus MV also depends on other factors such as CPU memory, interaction among cards, operating system used, bus implementation, BIOS versions, and so on. The Integral Flashpoint Intrigue frame grabber accepts color composite video output of the camera. It digitizes each of the RGB planes at a tonal resolution of 24 bits per pixel and has a spatial resolution of 768 × 576 per frame.

4. Computer and related accessories: a complete color image requires 640 × 480 × 24 bits (921,600 bytes) of data space. Thus, complex operations on large images require large storage space and a fast computer. For our software, the ideal computer configuration requires a Pentium-III computer with a super VGA 17-inch color monitor, CD-ROM drive, 40 GB hard disk, CD writer for image storage, and printer.

2.2. Software

1. SCGE-Pro: available from the author (contact rchaubey@apsara.barc.ernet.in or kchadda@apsara.barc.ernet.in at the Bhabha Atomic Research Centre, Mumbai 400 085, India).
2. LAI's Automated Comet Analysis System (LACAAS; Loats Associates, Westminster, MD; contact loats@loats.com).
3. Komet 5 (Kinetic Imaging, Bromborough, Wirral, United Kingdom; contact info@kineticimaging.com).
4. Comet Imager and CometScan (MetaSystems, Hard-und Software GmbH, Altlussheim; Germany; contact comet@metasystems.de).
5. Comet assay II (Perspective Instruments, Steeple Bumpstead, Havehill, Suffolk, UK; contact sales@perspective.co.uk).
6. AutoComet (custom software in the context of a complete hardware system; TriTek, Sumerduck, VA; contact sales@TriTekcorp.com).
7. Fenestra Comet (Kinetic Imaging, Durham, NC; contact email@kineticimaging.com).

3. Methods

Exposure of cells to any physical or chemical mutagen produces DNA strand breaks or base damage, which can be easily quantified with the comet assay. The comet assay itself was described in detail in Chapter 9. Briefly, in this assay, the cells of interest (which may have been exposed in vitro or in vivo) are suspended in agarose on microscope slides and lysed with any detergent or high salt solution; then the liberated DNA is electrophoresed under neutral or alkaline conditions. Depending on their size and total negative charge, the DNA fragments migrate different distances toward the anode. After electrophoresis, the cells are stained with a DNA-specific dye and observed under a fluorescence microscope. Under these conditions, individual cells appear as comets with brightly fluorescing nuclei and a "tail" of diminishing fluorescence intensity. The distance migrated by DNA fragments from the nucleus, i.e., tail length (TL), is considered to be a measure of genetic damage. Using digital imaging software, other characteristics of these comets, e.g., tail moment (defined as the product of percentage of DNA in the tail and tail length), percent DNA in the tail (%DNA-T) or head (%DNA-H), can also be measured, which are considered to be more consistent and reliable indicators of DNA damage. **Figure 1** shows a diagrammatic representation of the various steps involved in the comet assay.

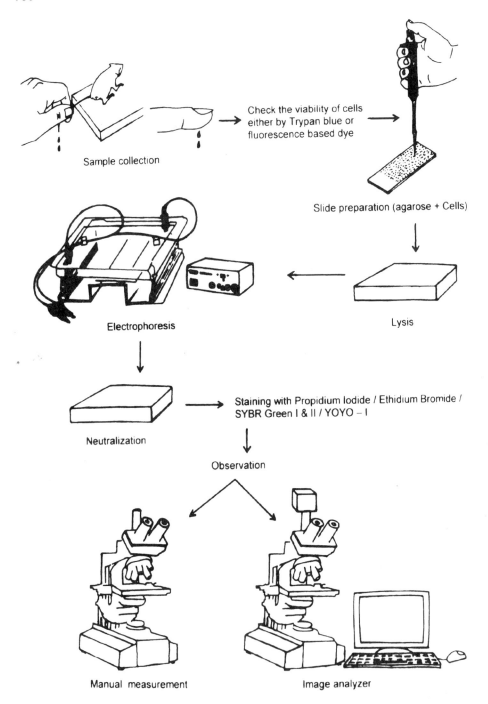

Sample collection

Check the viability of cells either by Trypan blue or fluorescence based dye

Slide preparation (agarose + Cells)

Electrophoresis

Lysis

Neutralization

Staining with Propidium Iodide / Ethidium Bromide / SYBR Green I & II / YOYO – I

Observation

Manual measurement

Image analyzer

Fig. 1. Schematic presentation of comet assay.

3.1. Manual Evaluation of Comets

After staining the cells with a suitable DNA-specific dye, comets are observed at 25× or 40× under a fluorescence microscope with suitable filters. The objectives of the microscope should be calibrated using the stage and ocular micrometer. The length of the comet is measured in microns and recorded. Apoptotic or dead cells should be recorded separately. Some laboratories use visual methods to score comet slides. By this method, the cells are initially classified as undamaged or damaged, and then the degree of damage is estimated by assignment to categories, such as type I (no damage) to type V (highly damaged). This type of visual scoring does not require any software, and it can be performed rapidly by an experienced practitioner. However, observer's bias and subjectivity have been frequently noted.

3.2. Computerized Evaluation and Data Processing for Comet Assay With SCGE-Pro

A typical set of processing operations includes image acquisition, preprocessing, and segmentation analysis of parameters and object classification. The SCGE-Pro software runs on either a Win 95 or a Win NT operating system.

1. Comets are observed at 40× magnification using a fluorescence microscope with Zeiss Filter 15 (BP546/12, FT580, LP590). Images of individual comets are captured using a three-CCD video camera and stored. A PC-based frame grabber board digitizes this signal and stores the images in the computer in separate files. A high-resolution video camera and a frame grabber ensure acquisition of images without loss of useful information from the samples.

2. The system includes several processing functions to process the images sequentially for analysis. These operations can either be performed automatically one after another without any human operator intervention or be carried out interactively by observing the processing results at each stage and modifying the processing parameters. The acquired images have to be preprocessed to remove acquisition artifacts for improving the picture quality. The signal-to-noise ratio is improved by a frame averaging technique. Fluctuations in supplied voltage of a microscope lamp or other illumination sources can cause gray level/color variations in the acquired images. These shading corrections have to be carried out to compensate for nonuniform illumination across the samples.

3. The next step of image processing is to separate the objects of interest from the background using a thresholding technique. The system allows either interactive setting of threshold or a quicker autothresholding method based on a gaussian bimodal histogram model. Measurements performed are in pixel units. The system has to be calibrated to find the scaling factor with respect to the camera and microscope setup.

4. The total Sybr Green II or propidium iodide fluorescence intensity is taken as total DNA content in the comet. The software allows quantitative measurements of total fluorescence of the comet, fluorescence of the tail, and length of migrated DNA fragments, and it calculates tail moment (*16*). **Figure 2** shows nuclei of human leuckocytes exposed to different doses of γ-rays. **Figure 3** shows the image of a comet, a dialogue box for measurements of various comet characteristics, and the result window of SCGE-Pro. **Figure 4** shows various steps involved in the measurement of tail moment. The system has to be calibrated at 25×, 40×, or 100× before making any measurements, depending on the magnification used during image acquisition. **Figure 4A** depicts the selection of the area of

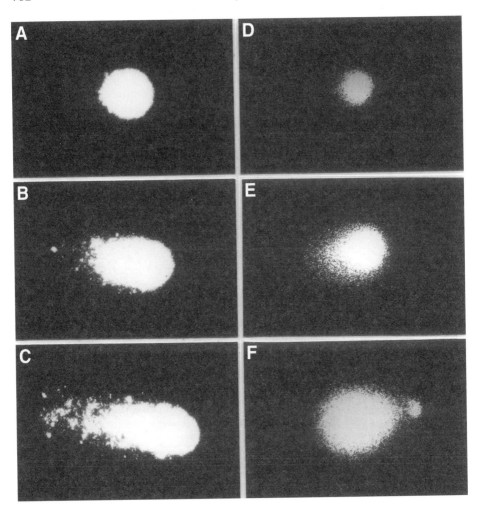

Fig. 2. (**A, D**) Comets from control cells. (**B, C, E**) Comets with different extent of DNA damage. (**F**) An apoptotic cell.

interest (AOI) of the whole comet. **Figure 4B** shows the selection of a fresh AOI, restricted only to the tail region of the comet. For measuring the DNA content in the tail region, both lower threshold and upper threshold have to be set to the same level as in the case of total DNA measurement in the comet. **Figure 4C** shows the measurement of the length of the migrated DNA fragments (µm) by selecting the line mode. **Figure 4D–4F** shows an alternate mode for measuring DNA content in the comet, tail, and TL, respectively. This mode allows more distinct discrimination between the head (nucleus) and tail of the comet. This is a unique feature, allowing for more accurate measurements. The data are automatically stored in an application-specific format in the result file, which can be imported to Microcal Origin version 5 (Origin Lab, Northampton, MA) for various statistical calculations and graphical representations.

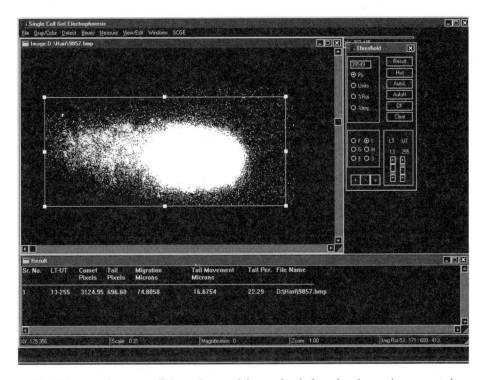

Fig. 3. Image of a comet, dialogue box, and the result window showing various comet characteristics measured by the SCGE-Pro software.

3.3. Overview of Commercially Available Software for Evaluation of the Comet Assay

1. LACAAS is a modular system of hardware and software that provides all the features and components required for efficient and rapid automated analysis of large sets of fluorescent single-cell comets. It has a proprietary image capture system, which provides extended dynamic range capabilities, which are essential for accurate image analysis. Measurements and analysis of cellular fluorescent intensities yield measures of cellular DNA content, distribution, and damage. This software operates under the Windows operating system on Pentium computers. The software eliminates user subjectivity by providing fully automated delineation and analysis of head and tail regions of the comets. It provides multiple quantitative measures of each cell analyzed, e.g., TL, area, moment of inertia, cellular DNA content, percent of cellular DNA in the tail, and so on. It also provides password-protected multilevel access, data audit features, and other features.

2. The Komet system has been designed specifically for image acquisition and sample analysis for the comet assay. This is one of the oldest systems developed for computerized evaluation of the comet assay. Komet 5 is currently the leading DNA damage analysis software for the comet assay. It has the following key features: two-click capture and analysis of comets, fully automatic or interactive computation of head/tail %DNA, Olive tail moment, analysis of the comet at different magnifications, and powerful Microsoft

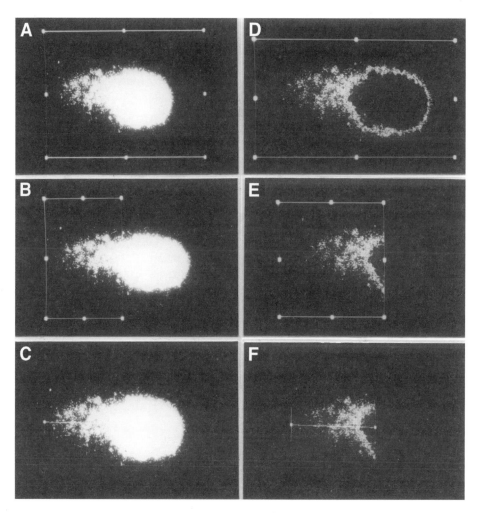

Fig. 4. Various steps involved in measurement of comet parameters using the SCGE-Pro software. (**A**) Measurement of comet total fluorescence. (**B**) Measurement of tail fluorescence. (**C**) Measurement of tail length using the line mode. (**D–F**) Illustrating the clear discrimination of nucleus and tail.

Excel Macros for quick manipulation of data. The system supports a wide variety of video cameras, e.g., Hitachi KMP1 (New York, NY), Cohu 4910 (San Diego, CA), or Pulnix TM745 (Jai Pulnix, Sunnyvale, CA). The user also has the ability to choose from a variety of digital CCD cameras, e.g., PCO SensiCam (Cooke, Auburn Hills MI), Hamamatsu Orca (Hamamatsu Photonics, Hamamatsu City, Japan), or Roper Cool snap/ HQ (Roper Scientific, Tucson, AZ).

3. MetaSystems provides two different products for evaluation of the comet assay, Comet Imager and CometScan. Comet Imager is an interactive system that allows fast and reli-

able analysis of comets under normal lab conditions with moderate throughput and moderately expensive hardware requirements. CometScan is a fully automatic system based on the Metafer automated scanning platform and provides the facility for completely unattended evaluation of comet slides.

4. Comet assay II is an advanced image analysis system developed for quantification of DNA damage by the comet assay. This system consists of an image capture card, a high-sensitivity CCD video camera, and Windows-based software. It has a three-button mouse to position a rectangular frame around the cell to be measured. A single button press then starts analysis, including correction of any variation in background intensity, followed by measurements of head and tail fluorescent intensities of the comet. This system has a special feature that allows the user to perform measurements on live or frozen images, and an interactive editing function that is useful in the case of severely damaged cells. The software provides measurements of various characteristics, such as tail moment, TL, head length, %DNA-H, %DNA-T, cell area, total intensity, and mean gray level. It provides password protection to restrict access to the software and prevent unauthorized changes.

5. AutoComet is a fully automated computer-controlled optical microscopy system for SCGE. The microscope is provided with a motorized stage, motorized focus, and epifluorescence illumination system. The system has been optimized for automatic detection and measurement of comets.

6. Fenestra Comet is an automatic digital imaging software for evaluation of the comet assay. The software allows for a full range of densitometric and geometric parameter measurements. It also allows measurement of two other important parameters; skewness and kurtosis, which provides information on comet morphology.

3.4. Statistical Analysis

Different investigators have used different statistical methods for evaluation of data from the comet assay. If the data have been obtained manually, increase in TL is considered the best criterion of genetic damage. However, mean TL should not be used, because the distribution is not normal; instead, the median TL of 50 cells per experimental point should be used. In our studies, data files from the SCGE-Pro software can be imported to Origin ver.5 for various statistical analyses and graphics. We use one-way ANOVA for statistical analysis. Values are considered significant at $p < 0.05$. There is no general agreement on any specific statistical method to be used for comet assay *(17)*. However, the choice of statistical method depends on the type of distribution obtained with the comet data. In the case of a normal distribution, parametric methods can be used, whereas when the data appear to be Poisson or binomially distributed, nonparametric methods should be used.

References

1. Singh, N. P., McCoy, M. T., Tice, R. R., and Schneider, E. L. (1988) A simple technique for quantitation of low levels of DNA damage in individual cells. *Exp. Cell Res.* **175,** 184–191.
2. Collins, A. R., Ai-Guo. A., and Duthie, S. J. (1995) The kinetics of repair of oxidative DNA damage (strand breaks and oxidized pyrimidines) in human cells. *Mutat. Res.* **336,** 69–77.
3. Rojas, E., Lopez, M. C., and Valverde, M. (1999) Single cell gel electrophoresis assay: methodology and applications. *J. Chromatogr. B.* **722,** 225–254.

4. Gonzalez, R. C. and Wintz, P. A. (1993) *Digital Image Processing*. Addison-Wesley, Boston, MA.

5. Chadda, V. K. (1998) Trends in image processing, in *DAE-BRNS Workshop on Applications of Image Processing in Plant Sciences and Agriculture*, BARC, Mumbai, India, pp 1.1–1.12.

6. Colet, P. (1997) When DSP's and FPGAs meet: optimizing Image Processing architectures. *Adv. Imaging* **Sept,** 14–18.

7. Fairbairn, D. W., Olive, P. L., and O'Neill, K. L. (1995) The comet assay: a comprehensive review. *Mutat. Res.* **339,** 37–59.

8. Kasie, F., Parzefall, W., and Knasmuller, S. (2000) Single cell gel electrophoresis assay: a new technique for human biomonitoring studies. *Mutat. Res.* **463,** 13–31.

9. Collins, A., Dusinska, M., Franklin, M., et al. (1997) Comet assay in human biomonitoring studies: reliability, validation and applications. *Environ. Mol. Mutagen.* **30,** 139–146.

10. Tice, R. R. (1995) The single cell gel/comet assay: a microgel electrophoretic technique for the detection of DNA damage and repair in individual cells, in *Environmental Mutagenesis* (Philips, D. H. and Venitt, S., eds.), BIOS Scientific Publishers, Oxford, UK pp. 315–339.

11. Pouget, J. P., Ravanat, J. L., Douki, T., Richard, M. J., and Cadet, J. (1999) Measurement of DNA damage in cells exposed to low doses of γ-radiation: comparison between HPLC-EC and comet assays. *Int. J. Radiat. Biol.* **75,** 51–58.

12. Gedik, C. M, Ewen, S. W., and Collins, A. (1992) Single-cell gel electrophoresis applied to the analysis of UV-C damage and its repair in human cells. *Int. J. Radiat. Biol.* 62, 313–320.

13. Collins, A. R. (2001) The comet assay: recent advances and applications. *Mutat. Res.* **483(suppl. 1),** S40.

14. Tice, R. R. (2001) The comet assay: novel applications and future directions. *Mutat. Res.* **483(suppl. 1),** S41.

15. Chaubey, R. C., Bhilwade, H. N., Rajagopalan, R., Bannur, S., Kulgod, S. V., and Chadda, V. K. (2000) SCGE-Pro: a fluorescence based Digital Imaging System developed for measuring DNA damage using single cell gel electrophoresis (Comet assay), in *BARC Newsletter* (Kumar, V., ed.), Bhabha Atomic Research Centre, Mumbai, India, **195,** 1–13.

16. Chaubey, R. C., Bhilwade, H. N., Rajagopalan, R., and Bannur, S. V. (2001) Gamma ray induced DNA damage in human and mouse leucocytes measured by *SCGE-Pro*: a software developed for automated image analysis and data processing for Comet assay. *Mutat. Res.* **490,** 187–197.

17. Lovell, D. P., Thomas, G., and Dubow, R. (1999) Issues related to the experimental design and subsequent statistical analysis of in vivo and in vitro comet studies. *Teratogen. Carcinogen. Mutagen.* **19,** 109–119.

11

The Comet–FISH Technique

A Tool for Detection of Specific DNA Damage and Repair

Alexander Rapp, Michael Hausmann, and Karl Otto Greulich

Summary

The comet–FISH technique described in this protocol is a tool to detect genome region-specific DNA damage and repair. It is a combination of two established techniques, the comet assay (or single-cell gel electrophoresis, or the single-cell gel test), to separate highly fragmented from moderately or nonfragmented DNA and to measure it, and fluorescence *in situ* hybridization (FISH), to specifically label DNA sequences of interest. Comet–FISH exists in two versions, based on the neutral and the alkaline comet assays. A detailed description of the comet assay is given in Chapter 9, so readers who are not familiar with this technique can work directly with the protocol described here, without referring to additional protocols reported elsewhere. The neutral version of the comet assay detects double-strand breaks, while the alkaline version detects both double- and single-strand breaks as well as abasic sites or sites of incomplete repair. This chapter also details cell preparation and production of the hybridization probes adapted to the comet–FISH technique. Finally, microscopic analysis of comet–FISH results is described, and possible procedures of quantification of the specific DNA damage are presented.

Key Words: Comet–FISH; comet assay; region-specific DNA damage; DNA probes.

1. Introduction

The comet assay technique is described in detail in Chapter 9. It offers a relatively simple and fast means of measuring the relative amount of DNA damage in individual cells *(1,2)*. The assay can easily be modified to fit the specific requests of the experiment to be performed. For example, comparison of results from the alkaline and neutral versions of the comet assay discriminates between single- and double-strand breaks *(3,4)*. Since semiautomatic, quantitative software has become available and especially since fully automated commercial systems have recently become available *(5)*, the quantitative analysis of DNA damages has become routine *(6,7)* (*see* Chap. 10). The test is highly sensitive, especially with the modifications described by N. P. Singh,

From: *Methods in Molecular Biology, vol. 291, Molecular Toxicology Protocols*
Edited by: P. Keohavong and S. G. Grant © Humana Press Inc., Totowa, NJ

using the alkaline version *(8)*. It is also highly versatile with respect to the cell type amenable to investigation, from mollusk cells to human tissue *(9)* and from bacteria to plant cells *(10,11)*.

The comet assay has several disadvantages. So far, no general protocol can be provided, and the comparison of data from different laboratories is difficult, because no standardization is available *(12)*. Also, numerous parameters affect the results and sensitivity in a comet assay experiment, for example, lysis or electrophoresis conditions and even the geometry of the electrophoresis tank. Therefore, parameters must be kept constant during a series of experiments to reduce possible sources of variation *(13–15)*.

Comet–FISH is a modification of the comet assay that includes a hybridization step after electrophoresis and therefore allows specific labeling of sequences within the comet (**Fig. 1**). The comet assay alone gives information about the level of overall DNA damage, whereas the combination with fluorescence *in situ* hybridization (FISH) allows allocation of the sequence examined to the damaged or undamaged part of the comet and therefore gives additional information on specific sequences or genome regions. The combination of the comet assay with FISH was first published by Santos et al. *(16)* in 1997 and was simultaneously developed in two other laboratories to tackle different experimental questions *(17,18)*. The term *comet–FISH* was coined in **ref. 18**. The FISH protocol has been adapted to the experimental constraints of comets embedded in agarose from standard FISH techniques *(19)*. Therefore, e.g., no thermal denaturation can be used for strand separation (denaturation) of the target DNA *(20)*, but chemical denaturation has to be applied, which does not damage the gel matrix *(21)*. However, even for chemical denaturation, the parameters have to be chosen in such a way that the gel matrix is not damaged. Also, other steps such as posthybridization washes, signal amplification, and microscopic analysis need to be adapted in the comet–FISH technique when specimens are embedded in a 3D gel matrix. Moreover, the hybridization efficiency can be increased using DNA probes optimized for comet–FISH, in such a way that faster probe diffusion into the gel is achieved. These probes need to have a higher DNA concentration and a reduced size compared with the probes used for conventional FISH on metaphase chromosomes.

The comet–FISH technique has been used to tackle a number of different questions. First, it has been used for localization of specific genomic regions on stretched DNA fibers, to gain information on the spatial organization of genomic elements *(16)*. A second application is described in **ref. 17**; this method uses the technique to detect region-specific repair in the comet assay. Also, the site-specific introduction and persistence of radiation-induced damages has been monitored using comet–FISH *(18,22)*. In contrast to DNA sequencing of large genomic loci, comet–FISH is less time- and less cost-intensive, if DNA damage and repair are analyzed. Comet–FISH has been applied not only to animal cell culture but also to plant cells *(20)*. Recently, the comet–FISH technique has been used to discriminate between DNA double-strand breaks and single-strand breaks *(23)* and to study the region-specific effects of oxidative damages induced by different nutrition compounds.

Comet–FISH is still in its infancy. New applications were discussed during the 6th Comet Assay Workshop in Ulm, 2001, for example, the use of comet–FISH to detect

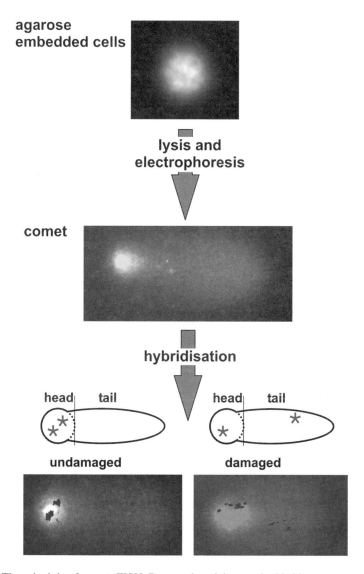

Fig. 1. The principle of comet–FISH. Damaged nuclei are embedded in agarose on a micro-scope slide, cellular protein and membranes are lysed, and the fragmented DNA is separated in an electrophoresis step. Specific sequences are detected after *in situ* hybridization with labeled DNA probes and can be assigned to the head or tail area of the comet (undamaged and dam-aged, respectively). The dark black spots in the comet images are the hybridization signals.

sites where DNA is anchored to the nuclear matrix, screening for chromosomal trans-locations within the comet assay, or enhanced detection of gene-specific DNA dam-age and repair using a two-color approach with one probe flanking the 3' and one flanking the 5' end of a gene of interest. These new applications are supported by modern analysis methods such as (semi-)automated, computer-aided comet evaluation and new quantification parameters to describe the relationship between total DNA damage and the damage of specific sequences *(24)*.

The following protocol describes the two versions of comet–FISH routinely used in our laboratory. The first is based on the alkaline version of the comet assay described by R. Tice et al. *(3)*, and the second is based on the neutral comet assay published by P. Olive *(4)*. These two protocols are additionally given as general guidelines for those who are not very familiar with the comet assay itself. Those readers already experienced with the comet assay should be able to adapt the comet–FISH procedure to their own comet assay protocols. As a complement to this text, the following reviews and guidelines may be helpful: **refs. *9*, *14*, *15*, *25*,** and ***26*** and the Comet Assay Interest Group at www.cometassay.com. A schematic representation of a comet–FISH experiment, including all necessary preparations and accompanying tests is given in **Fig. 2**.

2. Materials

2.1. DNA Probe Preparation

1. Cot-1 DNA (Invitrogen, Karlsruhe, Germany).
2. Polymerase chain reaction (PCR) Core Kit (Roche, Mannheim, Germany).
3. DNase/polymerase mix, or nick translation kit (Invitrogen); store at –20°C.
4. Labeled nucleotides, e.g., digoxigenin-11-dUTP (Roche); store at –20°C.
5. Unlabeled nucleotides (Roche); store at –20°C.
6. Hybridization buffer: 50% formamide, 1X SSC, 10% dextran sulfate; store at room temperature in aliquots of 1 mL.
7. Chromosomes in metaphase state fixed on a slide *(27)*.

2.2. Cell Preparation

1. Phosphate-buffered saline (PBS) buffer (Sigma-Aldrich, Munich, Germany); store at room temperature.
2. Medicon disaggregation system, 50 μm, nonsterile (DakoCytomation, Hamburg, Germany).
3. Ficoll (Biochrom, Germany); store at 4°C.

2.3. Comet Assay and Comet–FISH

1. Fully frosted slides (Labcraft, London, UK).
2. 24 × 60-mm Cover slips.
3. Metal plate size: approx $30 \times 20 \times 2.5$ cm^3, made from aluminum.
4. Ground layer agarose: 0.5% normal melting point agarose (Sigma type II) in PBS (50 mM phosphate).
5. Middle layer agarose: 1.0% normal melting point (Sigma type II) agarose in PBS (100 mM phosphate). Make 50 mL, melt, and store in aliquots of 1 mL at 4°C until use.
6. Top layer agarose: 1.0% low melting point agarose (Sigma Type VII) in water.
7. Neutral lysis buffer: 1% N-lauryl-sarcosinat, 1% Triton X-100, 0.5% dimethyl sulfoxide (DMSO), 10 mM Tris-base, 150 mM NaCl; adjust pH to 8.0.
8. Alkaline lysis buffer (for 1 L): 2.5 M NaCl, 0.1 M EDTA, 0.01 M Tris-base, 0.2 M NaOH, 1% sodium dodecyl sulfate (SDS); adjust pH to 10.0 with NaOH in a volume of 890 mL.

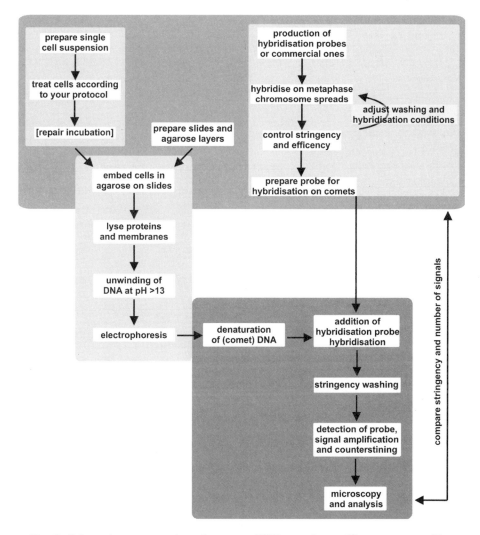

Fig. 2. Schematic representation of a comet–FISH experiment. The upper row of boxes shows the preparations needed. The left light gray box shows the steps of the comet assay technique, and the lower right dark gray box represents the hybridization steps included in the procedure.

This solution can be stored at room temperature for several weeks. Prior to use, mix 1 mL of Triton X-100, 10 mL DMSO with 89 mL of the prepared lysis solution and chill to 4°C. **Caution:** SDS and NaOH may cause skin irritations and eye injuries, wear protective gloves and eye goggles. Alternatively, the lysis solution described in Chapter 9 can be used.
9. Electrophoresis tank e.g., Hofer Supersub with integrated cooling circuit and recirculation (Amersham Biosciences, Freiburg, Germany).

10. Neutral electrophoresis buffer (1X TBE): 90 mM Tris-HCl, 2 mM Na$_2$-EDTA, 90 mM borate: adjust pH to 8.0.
11. Alkaline electrophoresis buffer: 0.3 M NaOH, 1 mM Na$_2$-EDTA; make fresh on the day of use from the stock solutions and chill to 4°C. **Caution:** wear protective gloves and eye goggles.
12. Neutralization buffer: 0.42 M Tris-HCL 0.08 M Tris-base, pH 7.5; store at room temperature for up to 6 mo.
13. SybrGreen fluorescence dye (Molecular Probes, Leiden, The Netherlands). **Caution:** SybrGreen is a potential mutagen; handle with gloves and care.
14. Antifade (Qbiogene, Heidelberg, Germany).
15. Counterstaining solution: 1 μL Sybr Green stock solution, 500 μL water, and 500 μL antifade; store in the dark at –20°C in 500 μL aliquots.
16. Plastic cover slip (Qbiogene).
17. PBD buffer: 94 mM Na$_2$HPO$_4$ · 2 H$_2$O, 6 mM NaH$_2$PO$_4$ · 1 H$_2$O, 0.06% Triton X-100.
18. Posthybridization wash buffer: 0.5–3X SSC buffer depending on the probe (*see* **Note 1**).
19. 1X SSC: 150 mM NaCl, 15 mM Na-citrate, pH 7.0; make as 20X stock and store at room temperature. Stock: 3 M NaCl, 0.3 M Na-citrate.
20. Blocking reagent (Roche).
21. Enzyme-coupled antibodies, e.g., anti-digoxigenin-alkaline peroxidase (DIG-AP), anti-biotin-AP or TUNEL-AP (= anti-fluorescein isothiocyanate [FITC]-AP); all from Roche.
22. HNPP (2-hydroxy-3-naphtoic acid-2'-phenylanilide phosphate) detection kit (Roche):
    a. HNPP buffer 1: 0.1 M Tris-HCl; 150 mM NaCl, pH 7.5.
    b. HNPP buffer 2: 0.5% blocking reagent in HNPP buffer 1.
    c. HNPP buffer 3: 0.05% Tween-20 in buffer 1.
    d. HNPP buffer 4: 0.1 M Tris-HCl, 0.1 M NaCl, 0.01 M MgCl$_2$; adjust to pH 8.0.
    e. Buffers 1 and 4 can be made in larger amounts and stored at room temperature for at least 3 mo.
    f. Buffers 2 and 3 should be made fresh on the day of use.
    g. HNPP solution: 10 mg/mL ready made; 25 mg/mL Fast Red solution in water. (Make small amounts and store in the dark at 4°C for 1 mo.)
    h. HNPP/Fast Red solution: 10 μL Fast Red, 10 μL HNPP solution in 1 mL HNPP buffer 4, sterile-filtered. (Store in the dark at 4°C for 1–2 wk; check for precipitation before use.)
23. Microscope objectives: Plan Neofluar 25×/NA 0.8 oil and Plan Neofluar 40×/NA 1.3 oil (Carl Zeiss, Göttingen, Germany).
24. Filter sets appropriate for the detection of two colors, e.g., filter set no. 10 (FITC) and filter set no. 14 (rhodamine), both from Carl Zeiss.

3. Methods

3.1. Sample Preparations

1. Preparation of a single-cell suspension (*see* **Note 2**).
2. Cell cultures: preparation of samples for the comet assay from blood samples has been described in Chapter 9, Subheading 3.2. (*see* **Note 3**).

3.2. Tissue Preparation

Tissues can be disaggregated in many ways for use in the comet assay, including enzymatic or mechanical techniques. A fast and reliable procedure adapted from flow cytometry is as follows:

1. Wash the Medicon vessel twice with 1 mL of PBS and rotate the blade of the Medicon by hand for 1 min each time.
2. Remove the PBS from the lower part of the vessel, place your pieces of tissue (e.g., four pieces, $3 \times 3 \times 3$ mm^3 each) in the upper Medicon chamber, and rotate by hand for 2 min.
3. Remove the first fraction of the cell suspension from the lower part using a 25-gage needle and a syringe.
4. Rotate again with 1 mL fresh PBS, and remove the suspension cells from the lower part.
5. Filter through a 30-µm nylon mesh (*see* **Note 3**).

3.3. Peripheral Blood

The preparation of samples for the comet assay from blood samples has been described in Chapter 9, Subheading 3.2.

3.4. Slide Preparation

The preparation of slides for comet–FISH is slightly different from the method described in Chapter 9, as the mechanical stress is greater than in the standard comet assay (**Fig. 3**).

1. Boil ground layer agarose and distribute 100 µL of the agarose suspension as a thin layer on the frosted slide using a second slide as a tool.
2. Air-dry completely; slides can be stored in this stage for several months.
3. Add the middle layer the day before the comet assay is performed. Melt the agarose suspension, cool to approx 50°C, drop 400 µL of the suspension carefully on the precoated slides, and quickly cover with a cover slip.
4. Place on a chilled metal plate, in even position (*see* **Note 4**).
5. Store the slides in a moistened chamber at 4°C overnight after solidification of the agarose.

3.5. Preparation of Hybridization Probes

Instead of using self-made DNA probes for *in situ* hybridization, commercially available DNA probes can be used, but a larger amount is required than is usually suggested for metaphase spread hybridizations in the protocols of the suppliers. Otherwise hybridization probes can be self-made if the desired target DNA is available in the form of a clone or can be amplified with PCR *(28,29)*. As short probe lengths are preferred for hybridization on comets, the method of choice for probe labeling is nick translation *(30)*.

1. Prepare cloned DNA or PCR fragments >500 bp by your preferred method (*see* **Note 5**).
2. Dilute DNA to a final concentration of 1 µg/µL in 10 m*M* Tris-base, 1 m*M* EDTA, pH 8.0.
3. Prepare on ice: 5 µg isolated DNA, 20 µL DNase/polymerase I enzyme mixture, 25 µL nucleotide mix (2 m*M* dATP, dCTP, dGTP, 1.8 m*M* dTTP; 0.2 m*M* DIG-dUTP—or equivalent); 25 µL 10X buffer: 500 m*M* Tris-HCl, pH 7.8, 50 m*M* MgCl$_{12}$, 100 m*M* 2-mercaptoethanol, 100 µg/mL nuclease-free bovine serum albumin (BSA) water to 250 µL.
4. Incubate at 37°C for 1–2 h; check the typical probe length of 5-µL aliquots on a 1.5% agarose gel.
5. The optimum is reached when the probe length ranges from 150 to 500 bp and the size of the majority of the probes is around 250 bp.
6. Add 25 µg salmon sperm DNA, 25 µg Cot-1 DNA, 1/10 vol of 4 *M* NaOAc, and precipitate with 2.5 vol ice-cooled ethanol for 2 h minimum in the refrigerator.
7. Spin at maximum speed in a table top centrifuge at 0°C for 30 min.

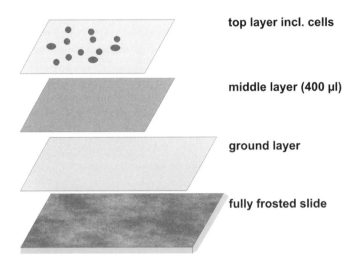

top layer incl. cells

middle layer (400 µl)

ground layer

fully frosted slide

Fig. 3. Schematical representation of the gel sandwich prepared on a slide used in comet–FISH. For details of the preparation, see protocol in **Subheading 3.4.**

8. Remove the supernatant carefully, apply 500 µL 70% ethanol, and spin again at maximum speed for 15 min.
9. Remove the supernatant carefully, dry briefly, and dissolve pellet in 150 µL hybridization buffer. Store in the dark at –20°C
10. Take 15 µL (450 ng) of these probes per hybridization. Before the probes are used, denature them at 72°C for 5 min and prehybridize at 37°C for 20 min.

3.6. Determination of Hybridization Conditions

For a successful experiment it is necessary to control differences in hybridization conditions on metaphase spreads to ensure stringency and selectivity of the comet hybridization. Therefore, hybridize the probe as described above or as suggested by the manufacturer and adjust the posthybridization washes until a reproducible and stringent hybridization pattern is visible on the majority of the metaphase spreads. Optimized washing conditions should be transferred to the comet–FISH procedure.

3.7. Comet Assay

1. Melt the top layer agarose and place in a water bath at 40°C.
2. Adjust the cell density of your cell suspension to 10^6 cells/mL with PBS.
3. Equilibrate the cell suspension to 40°C.
4. Mix 1 vol of cell suspension with 4 vol of agarose, and pipet up and down several times.
5. Carefully remove the cover slip of the slides bearing the middle layer that have been stored in the moistened chamber overnight.
6. Equilibrate the slides briefly to approx 40°C; be sure not to dry the agarose (*see* **Note 6**).
7. Quickly apply 100 µL of the cell suspension to the still moistened middle layer and quickly cover with a cover slip.
8. Place on a chilled metal plate to cool down the slides.
9. Remove the cover slips carefully after 5 min (*see* **Note 7**).

3.8. Alkaline Comet Assay

A detailed protocol for the alkaline version of the comet assay is given in Chapter 9, Subheading 3.6.

3.9. Neutral Comet Assay

1. Place the slides in prechilled lysis solution for 1 h in the fridge.
2. Wash the slides briefly in electrophoresis buffer.
3. Transfer the slides to the electrophoresis tank, and align them perpendicularly to the electrodes.
4. Apply an electric field of 1 V/cm and adjust the current (A) by the buffer level (~2 mm above the slide surface) inside the electrophoresis tank (typical 60 mA, depending on the tank and the buffer level; *see* **Note 8**).

3.10. Hybridization to Comets (Comet–FISH)

1. Store slides in ethanol for 3–15 d at 4°C.
2. Drain the slides briefly and place them in water for 10 min.
3. Denature in 0.5 *M* NaOH at room temperature for 25 min. **Caution:** NaOH causes eye irritation; wear gloves and safety goggles.
4. Dry the slides in an ethanol series (70, 85, 95%) for 5 min each at room temperature.
5. Air-dry the gels completely (*see* **Note 9**).
6. Add the prepared hybridization probe (~450 ng labeled DNA) after the alcohol has completely evaporated.
7. Seal with a plastic cover slip.
8. Place in a moistened chamber at 37°C (*see* **Note 10**).
9. Hybridize overnight. The time needed for hybridization depends on the size of the individual hybridization probe molecules and the amount of probe material added.
10. Prepare a water bath and equilibrate a cuvet with posthybridization washing solution to 72°C.
11. Remove the plastic cover slip carefully.
12. Place the cover slip in the cuvet and incubate for 2 min without agitation.
13. Quench the slides quickly in ice-cooled PBD buffer for 5 min.

3.11. Signal Detection

We recommend using a signal-enhancing system for the detection of the hybridization signals on comets. The strongest enhancement can be achieved using enzyme-coupled antibodies that convert a nonfluorescing substrate to a fluorescing one. Although other detection systems also work, the HNPP fluorescence-enhancing system offers strong enhancement, so even weak signals can be seen under the microscope.

1. Block slides by incubation in PBS containing 1% blocking reagent for 15 min at room temperature.
2. Add 50 μL of the enzyme-coupled antibody; 1:500 diluted in HNPP buffer 2.
3. Seal with a plastic cover slip and incubate in a moistened chamber at 37°C for 1 h.
4. Prepare the HNPP detection mix containing the Fast Red and the HNPP compound: 10 μL Fast Red solution, 10 μL HNPP solution in 1 mL HNPP buffer 4.
5. Remove the cover slip carefully.
6. Wash slides three times in HNPP buffer 3, 10 min each.

7. Wash slides twice in HNPP buffer 2, 10 min each.
8. Drain off excessive buffer, but do not allow the gels to dry.
9. Apply 100 μL of the prepared HNPP mix.
10. Seal with a plastic cover slip and incubate in a moistened chamber at room temperature for 30 min. For small hybridization targets (single-copy gene probes), to enhance the amplification apply in a second step fresh Fast Red/HNPP solution and reincubate the slides.
11. Wash the slides twice for 10 min in HNPP buffer 3 at room temperature.
12. Wash once in water for 10 min at room temperature.
13. Drain off excessive buffer, but do not allow to dry completely.
14. Counterstain the total DNA by adding 30 μL of staining solution.
15. Cover with a glass cover slip.

3.12. Microscopy and Image Analysis

1. Use 25–40× high-aperture oil objectives (*see* **Note 11**).
2. Acquire each color channel as a separate monochrome image using appropriate high-quality bandpass filters. For the procedure described, we use an FITC filter to detect the comet and a Texas Red filter to record the signals (*see* **Note 12**). Overlay image channels in a pseudocolor image.
3. Analyze, if possible, the comet images alone (total DNA stained) with comet assay analysis software; count the number of hybridization signals in the tail (if specific probes are used) of the corresponding image channel (*see* **Note 13**).

4. Notes

1. The concentration of the SSC determines the hybridization stringency. The lower the amount of SSC, the higher the stringency is. A concentration of 1X SSC is a good starting value. Evaluate the hybridization quality on metaphase spreads until the required stringency is achieved, and then transfer the conditions to the comet–FISH experiments. The use of formamide, especially in higher concentrations, in the washing buffer can cause the gels to slip from the slides.
2. For reliable evaluation and interpretation of the comet–FISH results, the use of cells with a stable karyotype during the experiment is required when specific hybridization probes are used (e.g., centromere or gene-specific probes). This is necessary since determination of the hybridization efficiency and stringency requires knowledge of the copy number of a specific sequence.
3. In standard comet assay experiments, it is useful to determine the cell viability and the cell number after cell isolation. Also, microscopic control of the morphology may be useful.
4. Use a water level from the electrophoresis tank to ensure levelled poisoning, as unlevelled placement will lead to uneven gels, which will result in inhomogeneities of the DNA movement and the comets.
5. Target sequences in comet–FISH are similar to those in standard FISH. This means that loci down to 5–10 kbp can be efficiently labeled. Other groups have also reported of the successful use of oligo DNA as a probe to label loci less than 1 kbp.
6. This step is important since a cold middle layer will lead to an unequal distribution of the top layer agarose by untimely gelling. The optimum is achieved when the middle layer is still wet but warm.
7. Check that the top layer still attaches to the gel sandwich by scraping the cover slip over a pipet tip. If top layer does not attach properly to the gel sandwich, increase the gelling time; if necessary, place gels in a refrigerator.

8. Because the current depends on the electrophoresis tank, no specific value can be given, but record the current for one experiment in order to readjust correctly to the same buffer level and ampere values in the following experiments.

9. This is the second critical point during the preparation, as gels may lose contact during drying. We recommend checking this step with some additional slides, so no hybridization probe or specimen is lost if you lose a gel in the beginning.

10. This temperature may differ if you are using commercial probes but should not exceed 42°C.

11. Objectives with higher resolutions and lower working distances lead to weaker signals and complicate the detection of comets if they are distant from the objective inside the agarose layer.

12. The signal may be integrated during recording; therefore a cooled CCD camera with on-chip integration is preferred; alternatively, a video camera connected to a frame grabber can be used, and low-intensity signals can be recorded by computer integration (*see* Chap. 10).

13. Analysis of comet–FISH experiments has not been standardized. Specific hybridization signals are located in the head or tail region and therefore the comets are counted as damaged or undamaged with respect to the specific sequence *(24)*. Diffuse hybridization results have been analyzed by performing a second comet analysis on the signal channel. Semiautomated systems are currently under development, e.g., Komet++ from Kinetic Imaging (Bromborough, Wirral, UK), for the quantification of specific DNA damage using comet–FISH.

References

1. Ostling, O. and Johanson, K. J. (1984) Microelectrophoretic study of radiation-induced DNA damages in individual mammalian cells. *Biochem. Biophys. Res. Commun.* **123**, 291–298.

2. Singh, N. P., McCoy, M. T., Tice, R. R., and Schneider, E. L. (1988) A simple technique for quantitation of low levels of DNA damage in individual cells. *Exp. Cell Res.* **175**, 184–191.

3. Tice, R. R., Andrews, P. W., Hirai, O., and Singh, N. P. (1991) The single cell gel (SCG) assay: an electrophoretic technique for the detection of DNA damage in individual cells. *Adv. Exp. Med. Biol.* **283**, 157–164.

4. Olive, P. L. and Banath, J. P. (1995) Radiation-induced DNA double-strand breaks produced in histone-depleted tumor cell nuclei measured using the neutral comet assay. *Radiat. Res.* **142**, 144–152.

5. Ashby, J., Tinwell, H., Lefevre, P. A., and Browne, M. A. (1995) The single cell gel electrophoresis assay for induced DNA damage (comet assay): measurement of tail length and moment. *Mutagenesis* **10**, 85–90.

6. Bocker, W., Bauch, T., Muller, W. U., and Streffer, C. (1997) Image analysis of comet assay measurements. *Int. J. Radiat. Biol.* **72**, 449–460.

7. Frieauff, W., Hartmann, A., and Suter, W. (2001) Automatic analysis of slides processed in the comet assay. *Mutagenesis* **16**, 133–137.

8. Singh, N. P., Danner, D. B., Tice, R. R., McCoy, M. T., Collins, G. D., and Schneider, E. L. (1989) Abundant alkali-sensitive sites in DNA of human and mouse sperm. *Exp. Cell Res.* **184**, 461–470.

9. McKelvey-Martin, V. J., Green, M. H., Schmezer, P., Pool-Zobel, B. L., De Meo, M. P., and Collins, A. (1993) The single cell gel electrophoresis assay (comet assay): a European review. *Mutat. Res.* **288**, 47–63.

10. Singh, N. P., Stephens, R. E., Singh, H., and Lai, H. (1999) Visual quantification of DNA double-strand breaks in bacteria. *Mutat. Res.* **429**, 159–168.

11. Angelis, K. J., McGuffie, M., Menke, M., and Schubert, I. (2000) Adaptation to alkylation damage in DNA measured by the comet assay. *Environ. Mol. Mutagen.* **36**, 146–150.

12. Sasaki, Y. F., Sekihashi, K., Izumiyama, F., et al. (2000) The comet assay with multiple mouse organs: comparison of comet assay results and carcinogenicity with 208 chemicals selected from the IARC monographs and U.S. NTP Carcinogenicity Database. *Crit. Rev. Toxicol.* **30**, 629–799.

13. Tice, R. R., Agurell, E., Anderson, D., et al. (2000) Single cell gel/comet assay: guidelines for in vitro and in vivo genetic toxicology testing. *Environ. Mol. Mutagen.* **35**, 206–221.

14. Cotelle, S. and Ferard, J. F. (1999) Comet assay in genetic ecotoxicology: a review. *Environ. Mol. Mutagen.* **34**, 246–255.

15. Fairbairn, D. W., Olive, P. L., and O'Neill, K. L. (1995) The comet assay: a comprehensive review. *Mutat. Res.* **339**, 37–59.

16. Santos, S. J., Singh, N. P., and Natarajan, A. T. (1997) Fluorescence in situ hybridization with comets. *Exp. Cell Res.* **232**, 407–411.

17. McKelvey-Martin, V. J., Ho, E. T., McKeown, S. R., et al. (1998) Emerging applications of the single cell gel electrophoresis (comet) assay. I. Management of invasive transitional cell human bladder carcinoma. II. Fluorescent in situ hybridization comets for the identification of damaged and repaired DNA sequences in individual cells. *Mutagenesis* **13**, 1–8.

18. Bock, C., Monajembashi, S., Rapp, A., Dittmar, H., and Greulich, K. O. (1999) Localisation of specific sequences and DNA single strand breaks in individual UV-A irradiated human lymphocytes observed by COMET FISH. *SPIE Proc.* **3568**, 207–217.

19. Clark, M., ed. (1996) *In Situ Hybridization 3.* Chapman & Hall, Weinheim.

20. Menke, M., Angelis, K. J., and Schubert, I. (2000) Detection of specific DNA lesions by a combination of comet assay and FISH in plants. *Environ. Mol. Mutagen.* **35**, 132–138.

21. Rauch, J., Wolf, D., Hausmann, M., and Cremer, C. (2000) The influence of formamide on thermal denaturation profiles of DNA and metaphase chromosomes in suspension. *Z. Naturforsch. C.* **55**, 737–746.

22. Rapp, A., Bock, C., Dittmar, H., and Greulich, K. O. (1999) COMET-FISH used to detect UV-A sensitive regions in the whole human genome and on chromosome 8. *Neoplasma* **46(suppl. 1)**, 90–101.

23. Fernandez, J. L., Vazquez-Gundin, F., Rivero, M. T., Genesca, A., Gosalvez, J., and Goyanes, V. (2001) DBD-fish on neutral comets: simultaneous analysis of DNA single- and double-strand breaks in individual cells. *Exp. Cell Res.* **270**, 102–109.

24. Rapp, A., Bock, C., Dittmar, H., and Greulich, K. O. (2000) UV-A breakage sensitivity of human chromosomes as measured by COMET-FISH depends on gene density and not on the chromosome size. *J. Photochem. Photobiol. B* **56**, 109–117.

25. Speit, G. and Hartmann, A. (1999) The comet assay (single-cell gel test). A sensitive genotoxicity test for the detection of DNA damage and repair. *Methods Mol. Biol.* **113**, 203–212.

26. Collins, A., Dusinska, M., Franklin, M., et al. (1997) Comet assay in human biomonitoring studies: reliability, validation, and applications. *Environ. Mol. Mutagen.* **30**, 139–146.

27. Celeda, D., Aldinger, K., Haar, F. M., et al. (1994) Rapid fluorescence in situ hybridization with repetitive DNA probes: quantification by digital image analysis. *Cytometry* **17**, 13–25.

28. Lichter, P., Cremer, T., Borden, J., Manuelidis, L., and Ward, D. C. (1988) Delineation of

individual human chromosomes in metaphase and interphase cells by in situ suppression hybridization using recombinant DNA libraries. *Hum. Genet.* **80**, 224–234.

29. Lichter, P. (1997) Multicolor FISHing: what's the catch? *Trends Genet.* **13**, 475–479.
30. Rigby, P. W., Dieckmann, M., Rhodes, C., and Berg, P. (1977) Labeling deoxyribonucleic acid to high specific activity in vitro by nick translation with DNA polymerase I. *J. Mol. Biol.* **113**, 237–251.

12

DNA Double-Strand Break Damage and Repair Assessed by Pulsed-Field Gel Electrophoresis

Nina Joshi and Stephen G. Grant

Summary

This assay quantifies the amount of DNA double-strand break (DSB) damage in attached cell populations embedded in agarose and assayed for migratory DNA using pulsed-field gel electrophoresis (PFGE) with ethidium bromide staining. The assay can measure pre-existing damage, as well as induction of DSB by chemical (e.g., bleomycin), physical (e.g., X-irradiation), or biological (e.g., restriction enzymes) agents. By incubating the cells under physiological conditions prior to processing, the cells are allowed to repair DSB, primarily via the process of nonhomologous end joining. The amount of repair, corresponding to the repair capacity of the treated cells, is then quantified by determining the ratio of the fractions of activity released in these repaired lanes in comparison with the total amount of DNA fragmentation following determination of a optimal exposure for maximum initial fragmentation. Repair kinetics can also be analyzed through a time-course regimen.

Key Words: DNA double-strand breaks (DSB); double-strand break repair; nonhomologous end joining; pulsed-field gel electrophoresis; DNA fragmentation; genotoxicity; clastogenicity.

1. Introduction

Of all the forms of DNA damage, double-strand breaks (DSBs) induced from exogenous sources, such as ionizing radiation and chemical agents, or endogenous sources, such as oxidative stress, may be the most deleterious, for if they are unrepaired or misrepaired, they can lead to carcinogenic transformation or cell death.

DSBs (and some proportion of single-strand breaks, when they are clustered closely enough) result in high-molecular-weight DNA fragments that can be liberated from the cell and resolved by electrophoresis. This technique can be thought of as a bulk method for performing the comet assay *(see* **ref. *1***, and Chaps. 9–11), although with several advantages over that assay: (1) thousands to millions of cells are analyzed, rather than hundreds; (2) a single measurement for the population is derived, rather

From: *Methods in Molecular Biology, vol. 291, Molecular Toxicology Protocols*
Edited by: P. Keohavong and S. G. Grant © Humana Press Inc., Totowa, NJ

than hundreds; and, (3) multiple samples, including controls, can be analyzed on the same gel. Application of pulsed-field gel electrophoresis (PFGE) also allows for a greater separation of DNA sizes, giving a better characterization of the nature of the underlying DNA damage.

Both the comet assay and the PFGE assay have been used extensively to study DNA repair, by observing the reduction in migrating DNA when cells are allowed a period of repair following genotoxic insult. These assays are therefore functional measures of DNA DSB repair *(2,3)*.

From experiments using cell extracts from *Xenopus* eggs *(4,5)*, Chinese hamster ovary cells *(6)*, and human cells *(7–9)* to repair plasmids containing breaks (e.g., the prokaryotic *lacZ* gene *[8]*), as well as the transfection of damaged plasmids into DNA repair-deficient/proficient cell lines, two distinct DSB pathways—homologous recombination (HR) and nonhomologous end joining (NHEJ)—have been identified. In HR, the major DSB repair pathway in yeast, a homologous chromosome, or more frequently, a sister chromatid, is used as a template to repair the damaged copy of the sequence in an error-free manner *(10)*. In contrast, NHEJ, the most prevalent pathway for DSB repair in vertebrates *(11)*, is independent of sequence homology *(12)*. In this process, the two ends of the breakpoint are religated together after limited modulation at the termini. Thus, small inserted sequences, as well as deletions, are often introduced by this repair process, making NHEJ an inherently error-prone pathway.

Although these cell extract and transfection techniques have provided valuable information, results from the cell extract experiments are often inconsistent *(13)*, and there is always the possibility that repair processes in plasmids do not reflect normal DSB repair in genomic DNA in intact cells *(14)* (*see* also Chap. 18). Thus, an in vitro assay has been developed that quantifies the amount of repaired genomic DNA DSBs in attached mammalian cells *(15,16)*. Repair capacity is only measured under conditions of maximum damage, which are likely to differ between cell lines and cell types. Thus, an optimal dose for DSB damage is initially determined, and then, after applying this optimal dose, DSB repair can be examined over time by determining the ratio of remaining DNA fragmentation in comparison with the unrepaired control.

Cells with deficiencies in DNA protein kinase (DNA-PK; believed to regulate the accessibility of DNA ends and possibly recruit repair factors in the NHEJ pathway *[16]*), as well as mouse fibroblasts deficient in Ku80 (another NHEJ-related protein involved in the protection and alignment DNA ends *[17]*), have decreased repair capacity in this assay. Deficiencies in the *BRCA2* gene, associated with HR pathways through Fanconi's anemia genes *(18,19)*, have not been detected using this assay *(20)*. Whether patients with Fanconi's anemia, ataxia telangiectasia, Bloom's syndrome, Nijmegen breakage syndrome, Berlin breakage syndrome, and Werner's syndrome, cancer-prone syndromes attributed to deficiencies in DNA DSB repair, are associated with the NHEJ pathway is unknown. Characterization of these processes is critical to our understanding of human disease as well as cellular responses to genotoxic stress. A technique for analysis of the other type of mammalian DSB repair, HR, is given in Chapter 31 (a variant of the host cell reactivation assay described in Chap. 28).

Finally, there are two modifications that might allow the PFGE assay to analyze other types of DNA damage. Taking a cue from the comet assay, this assay could be extended to analysis of the majority of single-strand breaks by converting them to DSBs by alkaline treatment *(21)*. By running cell samples processed under both neutral and basic pH side by side, the contribution of single-strand breaks can be observed as the quantitative difference in DNA migration. Next, by allowing a longer period between in vitro exposure and analysis, this assay could be used to quantitate the amount of "complex" or irreparable DNA damage associated with high-energy radiation *(22)*.

2. Materials

2.1. Generation of Double-Strand Breaks

1. T-25 (25-cm) cell culture flasks (Fisher Scientific, Pittsburgh, PA).
2. Appropriate growth media for each cell type, with appropriate amount and type of serum.
3. Cell culture incubator (e.g., ThermoForma Series II Water Jacketed CO_2 Incubator, Forma Scientific, Marietta, OH).
4. Irradiation source (e.g., cesium source, model 143-45A, JL Shepard, San Francisco, CA; *see* **Note 1**).

2.2. Cell Sample (Agarose Plug) Preparation

1. Trypsin (or other means of harvesting cells; Invitrogen, Carlsbad, CA).
2. 15-mL Conical tubes (BD Falcon, BD Biosciences, Bedford, MA).
3. Appropriate cell culture medium (serum-free).
4. Hemocytometer (Fisher) or Coulter counter (Beckman Coulter, Fullerton, CA).
5. 1-, 5-, and 10-mL Pipets and pipet aid.
6. 20-, 200-, and 1000-µL Micropipetors (Rainin, Woburn, MA) and appropriate pipet tips (Fisher).
7. Benchtop centrifuge (e.g., Sorval RT 6000D, Kendro Lab Products, Asheville, NC).
8. 50–56°C shaking water bath.
9. 1% InCert agarose solution (BioWhittaker, Rockland, ME). Incubate at 50–56°C to prevent solidification.
10. 100-µL Plastic plug molds taped on the bottom (Bio-Rad, Hercules, CA).
11. Lysis solution: 10 m*M* Tris-HCl, pH 8.0, 50 m*M* NaCl, 0.5 *M* EDTA, 2% *N*-lauryl sarcosyl (all Sigma, St. Louis, MO), 0.1 mg/mL proteinase K (Invitrogen).
12. Wash buffer: 10 m*M* Tris-HCl, pH 8.0, 0.1 *M* EDTA.
13. RNase solution (Invitrogen): 10 m*M* Tris-HCl, pH 7.5, 0.1 *M* EDTA, 0.1 mg/mL RNase. Make 2.5 mL per sample fresh each time.

2.3. Pulsed-Field Gel Electrophoresis (PFGE)

Although a number of PFGE apparatus have been developed, clamped homogenous electric field (CHEF) and asymmetric field inversion gel electrophoresis (AFIGE) are most often used for DSB analysis (*see* **Note 2**).

1. CHEF: CHEF DRII apparatus (Bio-Rad) with refrigerated water bath and circulating pump.
   AFIGE: Horizontal gel electrophoresis system, model H4 (Invitrogen) with refrigerated water bath and circulating pump.

2. Seakem agarose (BioWhittaker).
3. 0.5X TBE: 45 m*M* Tris-HCl, pH 8.0, 45 m*M* boric acid, 1 m*M* EDTA. Prepare a 5X stock solution in large volumes (~500 mL); can be stored indefinitely at room temperature.
4. 10 mg/mL Ethidium bromide (made up in 10-mL lots, kept wrapped in aluminum foil in the refrigerator).
5. FluorImager (Bio-Rad)

3. Methods

3.1. Generation of Double-Strand Breaks (see Notes 1, 3, and 4)

1. Cells should be firmly attached, semiconfluent, and in log phase growth when exposed to ionizing radiation (IR). Thus, they should be plated at least 48 h prior to exposure and the T-25 flasks seeded with the appropriate number of cells to attain these conditions (*see* **Note 5**).
2. Cool cells on ice to 4°C prior to irradiation.
3. Expose cells in T-25 flasks to a source of ionizing radiation at doses ranging from 10 to 100 Gy (or at optimized dose, if this has been predetermined). Include one flask as an unexposed control to determine background DNA fragmentation levels.

3.2. Cell Sample (Agarose Plug) Preparation

1. Harvest cells, by trypsinization or other appropriate technique on ice in 15-mL conical tubes (*see* **Note 6**). This process may take 5–10 min. Centrifuge the cells for 5 min at 800*g*. Wash the cells once in serum-free medium.
2. Resuspend the cells in serum-free medium and count the cells, using a hemocytometer or Coulter counter. Aliquot the cells at a concentration of 1×10^6 or multiples of 1×10^6 (e.g., 2×10^6, 3×10^6) into 15-mL conical tubes and spin for 5 min at 800*g*.
3. Remove excess media with a pipet without disrupting the cell pellet. Add 30 µL of serum-free media to the 15-mL conical tubes for each 1×10^6 cells. Triturate the cell suspension to ensure that no clumps are present.
4. Mix the cell suspension with an equal volume of 1% agarose incubated at 50°C. The final concentration of agarose should be 0.5% with 1×10^6 cells per 60 µL of serum-free medium and agarose solution.
5. Pipet the 60 µL (or 60-µL aliquots) into the precooled 100 µL plastic plug molds, and incubate on ice for 5 min until the plugs solidify.
6. Extrude the solidified plugs from the molds into a 15-mL conical tube by removing the tape from the bottom of the molds and pipeting lysis buffer directly over the plug.
7. Add 2 mL lysis solution and incubate at 4°C for 45 min.
8. Transfer the plugs to 50°C for 16–18 h in a moderately shaking water bath.
9. Wash the plugs once with 2 mL washing buffer. Incubate in 2 mL of fresh washing buffer for 1 h at 37°C in a moderately shaking water bath.
10. Transfer the plugs to 2 mL RNase solution and incubate for 1 h at 37°C.
11. Plugs can then be stored in 5 m*M* EDTA buffer at 4°C indefinitely.

3.3. Preparation for Plug Gel Electrophoresis

1. Cast a 0.8% agarose gel in 0.5X TBE with the appropriate comb when using the Bio-Rad CHEF-DRIII or a 0.5% agarose gel when using AFIGE. Allow the gel to solidify for approx 1 h.

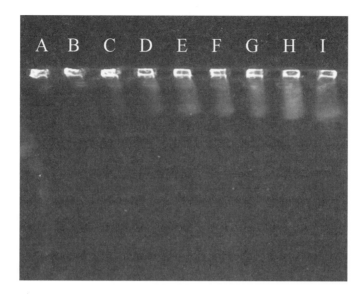

Fig. 1. DNA fragmentation following irradiation. lane A, unirradiated control; lane B, 5 Gy; lane C, 10 Gy; lane D, 20 Gy; lane E, 30 Gy; lane F, 40 Gy; lane G, 50 Gy; lane H, 60 Gy; lane I, 70 Gy. The dose yielding the maximum amount of DSB DNA damage is 60 Gy.

2. Remove the comb after solidification, and load the plugs into the wells. Seal the wells with agarose to ensure that the plugs are not released from the wells during electrophoresis.
3. Place the gel into a precooled (10°C) electrophoresis box with 0.5X TBE.
4. Electrophorese for 23 h at 200 V with 60-s pulses for the first 8 h, followed by 120-s pulses for 15 h with the Bio-Rad CHEF-DRIII *(23)*. Using AFIGE, cycles of 1.25 V/cm for 900 s in the forward direction and 5 V/cm for 75 s in the reverse direction *(23)* should be used (*see* **Note 7**).
5. Stain the gel for 1 h with 0.5 μg/mL ethidium bromide (*see* **Note 8**).
6. Expose the gel to a FluorImager for analysis.
7. Quantitate the DSBs present by determining the ratio between the fraction of activity released from the plug (FAR) vs the total DNA in both the plug and in the lane: FAR = lane counts/(plug + lane) counts *(23)*.
8. For quantification of damage, FAR should be compared with a standard control or curve. For quantification of repair, the amount of migratory DNA in the experimental lane may be subtracted directly from that in the control (no repair incubation), provided that the total amounts of DNA in both plugs/lanes are similar.
9. To examine repair capacity, first determine the optimal dose of radiation (the dose that provides the maximum fragmentation), and then plot dose vs FAR (**Figs. 1** and **2**).

3.4. Analysis of the Time-Course of DSB Repair

1. Prewarm medium supplemented with serum to 42°C (sufficient to replace media in all experimental flasks).
2. Cool cells on ice prior to irradiation and expose each flask to the optimal IR dose determined in **Subheading 3.3.**, **step 9**.

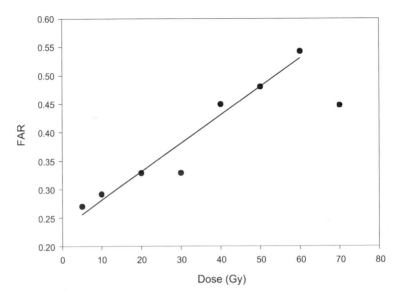

Fig. 2. Regression analysis of DNA fragmentation, quantified as the fraction of activity in the lane, vs dose to determine the optimal dose to be used to examine repair kinetics. A dose of 60 Gy provided optimal damage. FAR, fraction of activity released.

3. Replace medium in each flask with prewarmed medium (which rapidly restores the cultures to 37°C, at which temperature repair is activated):

 a. Return flasks to the incubator for various times to allow for repair (time points: 0, 10, 20, 30, 60, 120, 128, 240, and 360 min).
 b. After the predetermined repair incubation periods, remove the flasks, harvest the cells, and place on ice for 5–10 min.
 c. Process samples as in **Subheadings 3.2.** and **3.3.**

An example of the resulting gel is given in **Fig. 3.**

4. Notes

1. Direct DSB agents such as bleomycin, toposimerase II inhibitors, and carcinostatin, as well as enzymes that cleave DNA, such as *Bam*H1, *Pvu*11, *Hinf*1, and *Hae*III transfected into cells can be utilized as alternate sources of DBS damage *(23,24)*.
2. PFGE separates larger DNA pieces than standard constant field electrophoresis by alternating the direction of the electric field at regular intervals, forcing the DNA to reorient itself constantly in new directions, resulting in far superior size separation. A number of PFGE apparatus have been developed, including orthogonal field agarose electrophoresis (OFAGE), transverse alternating field electrophoresis (TAFE), CHEF, and AFIGE *(24)*. The choice depends on the type of equipment available, keeping in mind that CHEF and AFIGE have been most often used for DSB analysis. The AFIGE apparatus produces more uniform DNA fragments and should be used when the analysis does not require the precise size of DNA fragmentation *(23,25)*. The CHEF gel apparatus should be used when size detection is important.

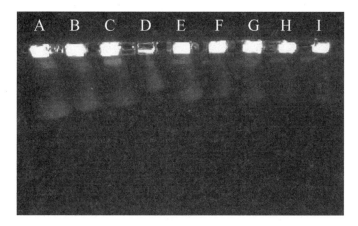

Fig. 3. DNA fragmentation resulting from repair of DSB damage induced by exposure of Ishikawa endometrial cancer cells to 60 Gy ionizing radiation (*see* **Figs. 1** and **2**) and repair for: lane A, 0 min; lane B, 10 min; lane C, 20 min; lane D, 30 min; lane E, 60 min; lane F, 120 min; lane G, 180 min; lane H, 240 min; lane I, 360 min.

3. If the intent of the assay is simply to quantify existing DNA damage, it may not be necessary to induce DSB. To allow for variability between gels, however, we recommend that, rather than using the absolute amount of migratory DNA as a measure of such damage, that experimental samples always be compared with known controls (such a comparison is inherent if the assay is used as a measure of repair, since migratory DNA from the cells allowed to undergo repair is considered relative to the same cells with no opportunity for repair). We have not yet established a control cell type with a stable level of "uninduced" DSB, so we recommend using radiated cells as controls. This also allows for exposures to different doses of radiation and/or for different incubation times for repair, as well as the establishment of a standard curve for the control cells.

4. If the intent of the assay is to measure repair capacity, an induction dose for maximum DNA DSB damage must first be determined by processing samples subjected to a range of IR dosages, as given in **Subheading 3.1., step 3.**, then optimizing the incubation time for repair according to the protocol given in **Subheading 3.4.**
Using this maximum dose provides damage and a damage signal (migratory DNA) on PFGE that makes sure the entire repair capacity of the cells is engaged. This dose is always a lethal dose, however, and it would be useful to confirm results from such experiments at sublethal levels of exposure and DNA damage.

5. DNA from cells in S phase migrate three to four times more slowly than from cells in G_1 or G_2 phase (*26*). Thus, cells should be analyzed once they reach the plateau phase, increasing the number of cells in G_1/G_0 and decreasing the variability in fragmentation. This phenomenon occurs not only in this assay but also in other techniques that measure DNA fragmentation (*24*).

6. Cells and plugs used during this assay should remain on ice at all times to decrease repair except during the predetermined repair incubation period in **Subheading 3.4., step 4**.

7. These electrophoresis conditions have been optimized for resolution of migratory DNA after a maximal induction of DSB (**Figs. 1** and **2**). Different conditions may need to be

developed for the lesser damage observed in unexposed cells or cells exposed to less efficient inducing agents than IR.

8. Cells and migratory DNA can also be detected using incorporation of radiolabeled thymidine (Sigma Aldrich, Maryland Heights, MO) and a Phosphoimager (STORM, Amersham Biosciences, Piscataway, NJ) or a scintillation counter (MicroBeta, Boston, MA) *(16)*.

References

1. Singh, N. P., McCoy, M. T., Tice, R. R., and Schneider, E. L. (1988) A simple technique for quantification of low levels of DNA damage in individual cells. *Exp. Cell Res.* **175,** 184–191.
2. Speit, G. and Hartmann, A. (1995) The contribution of excision repair to the DNA-effects seen in the alkaline single cell gel test (comet assay). *Mutagenesis* **10,** 555–559.
3. DiBiase, S. J., Guan, J., Curran, W. J. Jr., and Iliakis, G. (1999) Repair of DNA double-strand breaks and radiosensitivity to killing in an isogenic group of p53 mutant cell lines. *Int. J. Radiat. Oncol. Biol. Phys.* **45,** 743–751.
4. Pfeiffer, P. and Vielmetter, W. (1988) Joining of nonhomologous DNA double strand breaks *in vitro. Nucleic Acids Res.* **16,** 907–924.
5. Lehman, C. W., Clemens, M., Worthylake, D. K., Trautman, J. K., and Carroll, D. (1993) Homologous and illegitimate recombination in developing Xenopus oocytes and eggs. *Mol. Cell Biol.* **13,** 6897–6906.
6. Feldmann, E., Schmiemann, V., Goeddecke, W., Reichenberger, S., and Pfeiffer, P. (2000) DNA double-strand break repair in cell-free extracts from Ku80-deficient cells: implications for Ku serving as an alignment factor in non-homologous DNA end joining. *Nucleic Acids Res.* **28,** 2585–2596.
7. North, P., Ganesh, A., and Tacker, J. (1990) The rejoining of double-strand breaks in DNA by human cell extracts. *Nucleic Acids Res.* **18,** 6205–6210.
8. Ganesh, A., North, P., and Tacker, J. (1993) Repair and misrepair of site-specific DNA double-strand breaks by human cell extracts. *Mutat. Res.* **299,** 251–259.
9. Boe, S. O., Sodroski, J., Helland, D. E., and Farnet, C. M. (1995) DNA end-joining in extracts from human cells. *Biochem. Biophys. Res. Commun.* **215,** 987–993.
10. Khanna, K. K. and Jackson, S. P. (2002) DNA double-strand breaks: signaling, repair and the cancer connection. *Nat. Genet.* **27,** 247–254.
11. Weaver, D. T. (1995) What to do at an end: DNA double-strand-break repair. *Trends Genet.* **10,** 388–392.
12. Valerie, K. and Povirk, L. F. (2003) Regulation and mechanisms of mammalian double-strand break repair. *Oncogene* **22,** 5792–5812.
13. Rathmell, W. K. and Chu, G. (1998) Mechanisms for DNA double-strand break repair in eukaryotes, in *DNA Damage and Repair*, vol. II: *DNA Repair in Higher Eukaryotes* (Nickoloff, J. A. and Hoekstra, M. F., eds.), Humana, Totowa, NJ, pp. 299–316.
14. Cheong, N., Perrault, A. R., and Iliakis, G. (1998) In vitro rejoining of DNA double-strand-breaks: a comparison of genomic DNA with plasmid DNA-based assays. *Int. J. Radiat. Biol.* **73,** 481–493.
15. Iliakis, G., Metzger, L., Denko, N., and Stamato, T. D. (1991) Detection of DNA double-strand breaks in synchronous cultures of CHO cells by means of asymmetric field inversion gel electrophoresis. *Int. J. Radiat. Biol.* **59,** 321–341.
16. DiBiase, S. J., Zeng, Z. C., Chen, R., Hyslop, T., Curran, W. J., and Iliakis, G. (2000) DNA-dependent protein kinase stimulates an independent active, nonhomologous, end-joining apparatus. *Cancer Res.* **60,** 1245–1253.

17. Nachsberger, P. R., Li, W. H., Guo, M., et al. (1999) Rejoining of DNA double strand breaks in Ku80-deficient mouse fibroblasts. *Radiat. Res.* **151**, 398–407.

18. Howlett, N. G., Taniguchi, T., Olson, S., et al. (2002) Biallelic inactivation of BRCA2 in Fanconi anemia. *Science* **297**, 606–609.

19. D'Andrea, A. D. and Grompe, M. (2003) The Fanconi anaemia/BRCA pathway. *Nat. Rev. Cancer* **3**, 23–34.

20. Xia, F., Taghian, D. G., Defrank, J. S., et al. (2001) Deficiency of human BRCA2 leads to impared homologous recombination but maintains normal non-homologous end joining. *Proc. Natl. Acad. Sci. USA* **98**, 8644–8649.

21. Olive, P. L. (1989) Cell proliferation as a requirement for development of contact effect in Chinese hamster V79 spheroids. *Radiat. Res.* **117**, 79–92.

22. Pastwa, E., Neumann, R. D., Mezhevaya, K., and Winters, T. A. (2003) Repair of radiation-induced DNA double-strand breaks is dependent upon radiation quality and the structural complexity of double-strand breaks. *Radiat. Res.* **159**, 251–261.

23. Kinashi, Y., Okayasu, R., Iliakis, G., Nagasawa, H., and Little, J. B. (1995) Induction of DNA double-strand breaks by restriction enzymes in X-ray-senstive mutant Chinese hamster ovary cells measured by pulse-gel electrophoresis. *Radiat. Res.* **141**, 153–159.

24. Olive, P. L. (1998) Molecular approaches for detection of DNA damage, in *DNA Damage and Repair,* vol. II: *DNA Repair in Higher Eukaryotes* (Nickoloff, J. A. and Hoekstra, M. F., eds.), Humana, Totowa, NJ, pp. 539–557.

25. Blocher, D. and Pohlit, W. (1982) DNA double strand breaks in Ehrlich ascites tumors cells at low doses of X-rays. II. Can cell death be attributed to double strand breaks? *Int. J. Radiat. Biol.* **42**, 329–338.

26. Loucas, B. D. and Geard, C. R. (1994) Kinetics of chromosome rejoining in normal human fibroblasts after exposure to low- and high-LET radiation. *Radiat. Res.* **138**, 352–360.

III

DETECTION AND CHARACTERIZATION
OF SURROGATE GENE MUTATION

13

Analysis of In Vivo Mutation in the *Hprt* and *Tk* Genes of Mouse Lymphocytes

Vasily N. Dobrovolsky, Joseph G. Shaddock, and Robert H. Heflich

Summary

Determining mutant frequencies in endogenous reporter genes is a tool for identifying potentially genotoxic environmental agents and discovering phenotypes prone to genomic instability and diseases, such as cancer. Here we describe a high-throughput method for identifying mouse spleen lymphocytes having mutations in the endogenous X-linked hypoxanthine-guanine phosphoribosyltransferase (*Hprt*) gene and the endogenous autosomal thymidine kinase (*Tk*) gene. The selective expansion of mutant lymphocytes is based on the phenotypic properties of *Hprt*- and *Tk*-deficient cells. The same procedure can be utilized for quantitating *Hprt* mutations in most strains of mice (and, with minor changes, in other mammalian species), whereas mutations in the *Tk* gene can be determined only in transgenic mice that are heterozygous for inactivation of this gene. Expanded mutants can be further used to classify the types of mutations in the *Tk* gene (small intragenic mutations vs large chromosomal mutations) and to determine the nature of intragenic mutation in both the *Hprt* and *Tk* genes.

Key Words: Hypoxanthine-guanine phosphoribosyltransferase; *Hprt*; thymidine kinase; *Tk*; alamarBlue™; mutation; loss of heterozygosity.

1. Introduction

Mutations in key genes may significantly alter signal processing cascades and control of cellular proliferation and may contribute to the initiation and progression of cancer (*1*). Intragenic mutations, such as base substitutions, small deletions, and insertions, can result in permanent activation of proto-oncogenes and inactivation of cell-cycle regulators. Large size mutations, such as multilocus deletions and homologous and nonhomologous recombination, can result in loss of heterozygosity (LOH) of tumor suppressor genes. As it is often difficult to quantify mutant frequencies in genes relevant to carcinogenesis, surrogate targets (reporter genes) can be used that have easily selected mutant phenotypes. A significant body of knowledge has accumulated from studies of mutation in vitro, although the kinetics and specificity of metabolic

From: *Methods in Molecular Biology, vol. 291, Molecular Toxicology Protocols*
Edited by: P. Keohavong and S. G. Grant © Humana Press Inc., Totowa, NJ

processing and DNA repair in cultures of established cell lines may not be the same as those occurring in vivo. The endogenous hypoxanthine-guanine phosphoribosyl-transferase (*Hprt*) and thymidine kinase (*Tk*) genes were among the first reporter genes used for detection of mutations in vitro *(2–6)*. Later, a number of models were proposed for studying in vivo mutation in *Hprt (7–9)* and other endogenous genes *(10–16)*, as well as in transgenic targets in genetically manipulated laboratory rodents *(17–23)* (*see* Chap. 14).

The endogenous X-linked *Hprt* gene participates in the purine nucleotide salvage pathway. Mammalian somatic cells have a single functional copy of the *Hprt* gene, since the gene is not present on the Y chromosome in male cells, and participates in X-chromosome inactivation in female cells. Cells having a mutation in the gene that inactivates Hprt function can be grown in the presence of the toxic purine analog 6-thioguanine (6-TG). In nonmutant cells, the wild-type Hprt enzyme converts 6-TG into a product that interferes with DNA synthesis and kills the cells.

The product of the endogenous autosomal *Tk* gene is another participant in nucleotide salvage and can also be used as a target for the detection of mutation. *Tk* mutations, however, can be effectively detected only in cells that are heterozygous for this gene. *Tk* mutants grow in the presence of the thymidine analog 5-bromodeoxyuridine (BrdUrd), whereas nonmutant cells die because the functional Tk enzyme metabolizes BrdUrd into a toxic nucleotide analog that incorporates into nascent DNA. Recently, an in vivo model for mutation detection in the *Tk* gene was developed by disrupting one copy of the endogenous wild-type gene in embryonic stem cells and producing *Tk*$^{+/-}$ transgenic mice *(21)* (*see* **Note 1**).

Although in vivo *Tk* mutation can be effectively detected only in heterozygous transgenic mice, *Hprt* mutation has been detected and studied in a variety of transgenic and nontransgenic mammalian species, including laboratory rodents and humans *(7–9)* (*see* Chaps. 15 and 16). The autosomal *Tk* gene is sensitive to mutations resulting in LOH *(24,25)*, whereas the *Hprt* gene and most transgenic reporter gene models are not. Unfortunately, the detection of in vivo mutation in the *Tk* and *Hprt* genes is limited to tissues that produce primary cell cultures with a reasonable potential for clonal expansion, and for this reason spleen lymphocytes have been used in the overwhelming majority of studies in the mouse.

In general, the procedure for determining the frequency and types of mutations in the *Hprt* and *Tk* genes of spleen lymphocytes from *Tk*$^{+/-}$ mice consists of the following steps:

1. T lymphocytes are isolated from the spleen, purified by density gradient centrifugation, and stimulated to proliferate by the mitogen concanavalin-A (Con A).
2. Cultures of lymphocytes are established in 96-well plates using selective medium (for selection of mutant clones) and nonselective medium (for determining cloning efficiencies).
3. Surviving clones are scored (using either an inverted microscope for visual counting or a fluorescent plate reader for computer-assisted automated counting *[25]*), and the frequencies of mutant cells are calculated.
4. Mutations in the *Hprt* and *Tk* genes of drug-resistant clones are characterized using molecular techniques, such as allele-specific polymerase chain reaction (PCR) for determin-

ing LOH at the *Tk* gene or reverse transcriptase (RT)-PCR/sequencing for analysis of intragenic mutation in both the *Hprt* and *Tk* genes.

Primary T cells have limited proliferation potential in vitro; nevertheless, a significant fraction (30–70%) of *Hprt* mutant clones can be expanded beyond 96-well plates, to produce up to 1×10^6 cells. The expanded cell populations make a better template for the RT-PCR amplification of *Hprt* mRNA and sequencing of the resulting cDNA fragments.

2. Materials

2.1. Medium for Culture and Propagation of T Lymphocytes (see Note 2 and ref. 26)

1. 249 mL RPMI-1640 (Gibco, Carlsbad, CA; for 500 mL total).
2. 12.5 mL HEPES, (1 *M* stock, Gibco; final concentration: 25 m*M*).
3. 12.5 mL L-Glutamine, (200 m*M* stock; Gibco; final concentration: 5 m*M*).
4. 5 mL Minimum essential medium (MEM) nonessential amino acids (10 m*M* stock; Gibco; final concentration 0.1 m*M*).
5. 5 mL Sodium pyruvate (100 m*M* stock; Gibco; final concentration: 1 m*M*).
6. 1 mL Penicillin-streptomycin (100X stock; Gibco; final concentration: 0.2X).
7. 0.175 mL 2-Mercaptoethanol (143 m*M* stock; Sigma, St. Louis, MO; final concentration: 50 μ*M*).
8. 100 mL HL-1™ medium (BioWhittaker, Walkersville, MD; final concentration in propagation medium: 20%).
9. 65 mL Fetal bovine serum (Atlanta Biologicals, Norcross, GA; final concentration: 13%).
10. 0.5 mL Mouse interleukin-2 (IL-2; 10,000 U/mL stock; Roche, Basel, Switzerland; final concentration: 10 U/mL).
11. 50 mL Rat T-STIM™ culture supplement (Collaborative Biomedical Products, Bedford, MA; final concentration: 10%).

2.2. Isolation and Priming of T Lymphocytes

1. Surgical instruments: two 4-inch curved microdissecting sharp scissors, two 4-inch Adson forceps (with teeth), and one 4-inch microdissecting curved forceps.
2. Laminar flow hood.
3. 75-cm^2 Tissue culture flasks.
4. Phosphate buffered saline (PBS; Gibco).
5. Con A (Worthington Biochemical, Lakewood, NJ); prepare a 1 mg/mL stock solution in PBS, filter-sterilize, and kept as 2-mL aliquots at –20°C for up to 1 yr.
6. 12-Well tissue culture plates.
7. 15-mL Disposable polystyrene tubes.
8. Lympholyte®-M (Accurate Chemical & Scientific, Westbury, NY).
9. Spray bottle with 70% ethanol.
10. 10-mL Individually packaged disposable syringes with serrated plungers (BD Biosciences, Franklin Lakes, MA, cat. no. 309604).
11. 25-Gage syringe needles.
12. Lab centrifuge with swinging bucket rotor (e.g., IEC PR-7000M, Thermo, Milford, MA).
13. 5- and 10-mL Pipets.
14. Humidified CO_2 cell culture incubator (37°C, 95% humidity, 5% CO_2; e.g., Forma 3120, Forma Scientific, Marietta, OH).

2.3. Lymphocyte Primary Culture

1. 6-TG (Sigma, cat. no. A-4882).
2. BrdUrd (Calbiochem, San Diego, CA).
3. Disposable 15-mL polystyrene tubes.
4. 1-, 0.2-, and 0.02-mL micropipetors and appropriate tips.
5. Counting vials, e.g., Dilu-Vial® (Elkay Products, Shrewsbury, MA).
6. Isotonic diluent, e.g., Hematall® (Fisher Scientific, Pittsburgh, PA).
7. Zap-oglobin®II lytic reagent (Coulter, Miami, FL).
8. Coulter®Z1 cell counter (Coulter).
9. Disposable 50-mL polypropylene tubes.
10. γ-Ray source, e.g., ^{60}Co irradiator (model 109, J.L. Shepherd, Glendale, CA).
11. Impact2™ 12-channel pipetor and matching tips and 100-mL reagent reservoirs (Matrix Technologies, Lowell, MA).
12. 96-Well round-bottomed tissue culture plates (Corning, Acton, MA).

2.4. Scoring Clones and Determining Mutant Frequencies

1. Inverted microscope, 40–100× magnification, e.g., TMS (Nikon, Melville, NY).
2. 12-Channel pipetor, tips, and reagent reservoirs.
3. AlamarBlue™ viability indicator (Trek Diagnostics, Chicago, IL).
4. SPECTRAFluor fluorometer (Tecan, Research Triangle Park, NC).
5. 1.5-mL Microcentrifuge tubes.
6. Dry ice.
7. –70°C Freezer.
8. 24-Well tissue culture plates (Corning).
9. Benchtop centrifuge, e.g., Eppendorf 5415C (Brinkmann Instruments, Westbury, NY).

2.5. Molecular Analysis of Mutations

1. Cell lysis buffer: 10 m*M* Tris-HCl, pH 7.5, 2.5 m*M* MgCl$_2$, 0.5% Triton X-100 (Sigma), 0.5% Tween-20 (Sigma), and 0.4 mg/mL Proteinase K (Gibco).
2. Disposable PCR tubes.
3. HotStarTaq™ DNA polymerase kit (Qiagen, Valencia, CA).
4. dNTP mix (10 m*M*; Applied Biosystems, Foster City, CA).
5. Primers for *Tk* LOH analysis:

   a. TK14: 5'-CTTGTAACTGTGTAGCTGCCTCGAG-3'.
   b. TK16: 5'-GGTGCAAGGCTGGGGGTCCTT-3'.
   c. NEO4: 5'-GGAGAACCTGCGTGCAATCCATCTT-3'.

6. Primers for *Hprt* cDNA amplification:

   a. HPRT1: 5'-CTCACTGCTTTCCGGAGC-3'.
   b. HPRT2: 5'-GGCCACAGGACTAGAACACC-3'.

7. Primers for *Hprt* nested PCR:

   a. Zee1: 5'-GGCTTCCTCCTCAGACCGCT-3'.
   b. M902R: 5'-GGCAACATCAACAGGACTCC-3'.

8. Primers for *Tk* cDNA amplification:

   a. FwdTK-RTPCR: 5'-TAACTAAGGTTTGCACAGCAG-3'.
   b. TK10: 5'-GGTACATTGTCCATTAGGAATG-3'.

9. Primers for *Tk* nested PCR:

    a. FwdTK-RTPCR: 5'-TAACTAAGGTTTGCACAGCAG-3'.
    b. RevTK-RTPCR: 5'-AGTCCAACCTGGGTAGGAG-3'.

10. Primers for actin cDNA amplification:

    a. m-Actin-F: 5'-TGGGTCAGAAGGACTCCTATG-3'.
    b. m-Actin-R: 5'-CAGGCAGCTCATAGCTCTTCT-3'.

11. PCR Thermocycler, e.g., GeneAmp® PCR System 9700 (Applied Biosystems).
12. Nonidet P40 (Gibco).
13. RNasin® ribonuclease inhibitor (Promega, Madison, WI).
14. Access RT-PCR System (Promega).
15. Purescript® RNA Isolation Kit (Gentra, Minneapolis, MN).
16. Disposable 1.5-mL microcentrifuge tubes.
17. Microcentrifuge.
18. Oligo(dT) primer (Ambion, Austin, TX).
19. Isopropanol.
20. 70% and 100% ethanol.
21. RETROScript™ RT buffer (Ambion).
22. RNaseOUT™ ribonuclease inhibitor (Gibco).
23. SuperScript™ reverse transcriptase (Gibco).
24. Proteinase K (Gibco).
25. Electrophoresis grade agarose gels (Gibco, cat. no. 15510-027)
26. Horizontal gel electrophoresis apparatus (e.g., Horizon 58; Gibco) and power supply (e.g., PowerPac 300, Bio-Rad, Hercules, CA).

3. Methods

3.1. Isolation of Lymphocytes

1. Prior to necropsy, sterilize surgical instruments and prepare sterile growth medium containing IL-2 and T-STIM (at least 20 mL of medium for each animal assayed).
2. In a laminar flow hood:

    a. Dispense 15 mL of growth medium into 75-cm^2 tissue culture flasks (one flask for each animal), and add 80 μL of sterile 1 mg/mL Con A to each flask.
    b. Dispense 3 mL RPMI-1640 into each well of the required number of 12-well plates (1 well for each animal).
    c. Dispense 3 mL of Lympholyte-M into sterile 15-mL tubes (one tube for each animal); dispense 5 mL of RPMI-1640 into sterile 15-mL tubes (one tube for each animal).

3. Sacrifice animals using methods approved by your Institutional Animal Care and Use Committee (e.g., CO_2 asphyxiation).

    a. In an aseptic environment on the lab bench, place sacrificed animal on its right side, and soak the left side with 70% ethanol.
    b. Pinch the skin below the rib cage on the left side with forceps, and make a small lateral incision.
    c. Using a pair of Adson forceps, grab the skin above and below the incision and pull apart toward the head and tail to expose the abdominal cavity.
    d. Identify the spleen under the body wall by its characteristic dark red color.

    e. Use separate sets of scissors and forceps for external and internal surgical procedures.

    f. Lift the peritoneum with small curved forceps and make a 5–7-mm incision over the area where the spleen is located.

    g. Gently pull the spleen from the abdomen through the incision with small forceps; cut out the intact spleen, trimming off as much connecting tissue and fat as possible.

    h. Place the spleen into an individual well of a 12-well plate containing RPMI-1640.

    i. Move the plate with the spleens to the laminar flow hood.

4. Crush the spleen, using several squeeze-and-twist motions with the serrated butt end of the syringe plunger:

    a. Slowly aspirate the cloudy medium containing released lymphocytes into a sterile 10-mL syringe fitted with a 25-gage needle.

    b. Holding the needle against the tube wall, slowly layer the contents of the syringe on top of the Lympholyte-M in a 15-mL tube.

5. Centrifuge the tubes in the swinging bucket rotor for 20 min at $1500g$ at room temperature. T lymphocytes will concentrate at the interface of the clear Lympholyte-M and the pink RPMI-1640 medium. Transfer the lymphocyte fraction into the tube with 5 mL of RPMI-1640, mix the contents by a few gentle inversions, and centrifuge for 10 min at $800g$ at room temperature.

6. Discard the supernatant, resuspend the cell pellet in 5 mL of complete growth medium, and transfer the entire contents into a 75-cm^2 tissue culture flask containing 15 mL of growth medium and Con A. The final Con A concentration is 4 µg/mL.

7. Place the flasks into the CO_2 incubator, standing them at a 45° angle to allow the cells to concentrate in the corner of the flask between the wall and bottom. Leave screw caps loose, and incubate at 37°C overnight.

3.2. Limiting Dilution Culture of Lymphocytes

1. Continuing from **Subheading 3.1.**, **step 7** the next morning, prepare up to 100 mL of growth medium for each mouse assayed. Depending on the assays to be performed, make 2 mL of fresh 1000X 6-TG stock solution at 2 mg/mL in water and 10 mL of fresh 200X BrdUrd stock solution in RPMI-1640 at 10 mg/mL (*see* **Note 3**). Sterilize both working solutions by filtration.

2. Dispense 3 mL of growth medium into 15-mL tubes (one tube for each animal).

3. Remove the flasks with the splenocyte cultures from the CO_2 incubator:

    a. Resuspend the settled cells by gentle agitation, and transfer 0.5 mL of the cell suspension into a counting vial filled with 24.5 mL of isotonic diluent.

    b. Add a few drops of Zap-oglobin II to the vial, cap the vial, and mix the contents by vigorous inversion.

    c. Count the cell suspension in a cell counter.

    d. Determine the cell concentration in the overnight cultures using the counts returned by the counter and the dilution factors (*see* **Note 4**).

4. Transfer 30 µL of the cell suspension from the flask (**Subheading 3.1.**, **step 7**) into the 15-mL tube containing 3 mL of growth medium to make a 1:100 dilution of cells for determining cloning efficiency (CE) in the absence of selective agents.

5. In 50-mL tubes (one tube for each animal), mix 13.2×10^6 cells from each overnight culture (*see* **Subheading 3.1.**, **step 7**) with fresh growth medium to make up a cell suspension with a final concentration of 4×10^5 cells/mL in a final volume of 33 mL. (These

cells will be used for *Hprt* mutation detection.) Add 33 μL of the 1000X stock of 6-TG to each tube with 33 mL of cells to give a final 6-TG concentration in the selection cultures of 2 μg/mL. Cap the tubes and mix by inversion.

6. In another 50-mL tube, make 53 mL of a 1×10^5 cells/mL cell suspension for each overnight culture in **Subheading 3.1., step 7**. (These cells will be used for *Tk* mutation detection; this step is omitted if mutation is to be determined only for the *Hprt* gene.) Add 265 μL of the 200X stock of BrdUrd to each tube with 53 mL of cells, giving a final BrdUrd concentration in these selection cultures of 50 μg/mL. Cap the tubes and mix by inversion.

7. Combine the unused cells from the overnight cultures (*see* **Subheading 3.1., step 7**) into one 75-cm² flask and determine the resulting cell concentration as described above. (These cells will be used as feeders for the CE plates; alternatively, a few dedicated mice can be used as a source of feeder cells.)

   a. Irradiate these cells with 90 Gy of γ-radiation by exposure to ^{60}Co or another source of ionizing radiation.

   b. In a 50-mL tube, mix growth medium, cells from the tube with the 1:100 dilution (*see* **Subheading 3.2., step 4**), and irradiated feeder cells to make up a final volume of 23 mL with a nonirradiated, target cell concentration of 80 cells/mL and an irradiated, feeder cell concentration of either 4×10^5 cells/mL (if only *Hprt* mutant frequency is determined) or 1×10^5 cells/mL (if *Tk* mutant frequency is to be determined separately or concurrently with *Hprt* mutant frequency).

8. Pour the cell suspension for determining CE (*see* **Subheading 3.2., step 7**) from its 50-mL tube into a 100-mL reagent reservoir:

   a. Using the 12-channel pipetor, dispense 100 μL of cell suspension into each well of two 96-well plates.

   b. Discard any leftovers.

   c. Continue processing the remaining CE cultures. Using the same approach, dispense each 6-TG–containing culture (*see* **Subheading 3.2., step 5**) into three 96-well plates, and each BrdUrd-containing culture (*see* **Subheading 3.2., step 6**) into five 96-well plates.

   d. Replace the reservoirs and pipet tips between the dispensing of the CE, 6-TG, and BrdUrd cultures.

   e. With the suggested concentrations of cells and dispensing volumes, each well in the CE plates will contain eight target cells (N_{CE}) and 4×10^4 or 1×10^4 irradiated feeder cells; each well in the 6-TG selection plates will contain 4×10^4 cells (N_{TG}); each well in the BrdUrd selection plates will contain 1×10^4 cells (N_{BU}; *see* **Note 5**).

9. Load the 96-well plates into the CO_2 incubator and incubate for 10–11 d at 37°C.

3.3. Scoring Lymphocyte Clones in 96-Well Plates

3.3.1. Manual Method

1. After 11 d of culture (*see* **Note 6**), inspect all wells of each plate using an inverted microscope at 40× magnification.

2. Mark wells that contain growing clones (positive wells). Growing clones have common characteristic features: the overall size of the cell mass in positive wells is relatively large; elongated or rounded cells are present on the periphery of the cell mass; and most individual cells on the periphery have sharp refractive membranes. Dead cells are small, without a distinct refractive membrane; and the overall amount of the cell mass in a negative well is smaller.

3. Switch the microscope to 100× magnification if needed for detailed examination of the cells on the periphery of the cell mass.

3.3.2. Automated Method

1. After 10 d of culture, make a 5% solution of alamarBlue (v/v) in growth medium (2.5 mL for each plate).
2. Using the 12-channel pipetor, add 25 µL of alamarBlue-containing medium to each well of all plates (*see* **Note 7**).
3. Return plates to the CO_2 incubator for an additional overnight culture.
4. The next day, read all plates with the fluorometer using a 530-nm excitation filter and a 590-nm emission filter, a gain of 47, and four flashes per well.
5. Using the fluorescence data array generated by the reader, identify the well with the minimum fluorescence (MIN) for each plate.
6. Determine the wells that produce fluorescence at least twofold higher than the MIN; these are scored as positive wells for this plate (*see* **Note 8**).

3.4. Calculating Mutant Frequencies

1. For each animal, count the total number of positive wells in two CE plates (P_{CE}), the total number of positive wells in three 6-TG selection plates (P_{TG}), and the total number of positive wells in five BrdUrd selection plates (P_{BU}).
2. Calculate the CE of cells without selection (CE_0) using the formula $CE_0 = 1/N_{CE} \times \ln([T_{CE} - P_{CE}]/T_{CE})$, where T_{CE} is the total number of wells seeded with target cells in the medium without selection (the number of CE plates multiplied by 96 wells per plate, or 2 × 96 in our case).
3. Calculate the CE of cells grown in 6-TG selection medium (CE_{TG}) using the formula $CE_{TG} = 1/N_{TG} \times \ln([T_{TG} - P_{TG}]/T_{TG})$, where T_{TG} is the number of 6-TG selection plates multiplied by 96 (3 × 96 in our case).
4. Calculate the CE of cells grown in BrdUrd selection medium (CE_{BU}) using the formula $CE_{BU} = 1/N_{BU} \times \ln([T_{BU} - P_{BU}]/T_{BU})$, where T_{BU} is the number of BrdUrd selection plates multiplied by 96 (5 × 96 in our case). Determine the *Hprt* mutant frequency (MF_{Hprt}) using the formula $MF_{Hprt} = CE_{TG}/CE_0$. Determine the *Tk* mutant frequency (MF_{Tk}) using the formula $MF_{Tk} = CE_{BU}/CE_0$ (*see* **Note 9**).

3.5. Preservation of Cells for Future Analysis

1. Resuspend the cells in individual wells of the 96-well plate by gentle pipeting, and divide the cell suspension from each well between two 1.5-mL microcentrifuge tubes filled with 0.5 mL PBS.
2. One tube will contain cells for RT-PCR analysis, and the other will contain cells for LOH analysis.
3. Centrifuge the tubes for 10 min at 800*g*, remove the supernatant without disturbing the cell pellets (often almost invisible), quick-freeze the pellets on dry ice, and store the tubes at −70°C.

3.6. Expansion of 6-TG-Resistant Lymphocytes Beyond 96-Well Plates

1. Transfer the entire contents of a positive well into an individual well of a 24-well tissue culture plate containing 0.5 mL of growth medium supplemented with 4 µg/mL Con A.
2. After incubating the plate in the CO_2 incubator overnight (angled at 30°), add another 0.5 mL of growth medium (without Con A), and continue the incubation for additional 2–5 d.

3. Examine the wells for cell growth. For freezing expanded cells, resuspend the cells in the well medium by pipeting, and transfer the cell suspension into two 1.5-mL microcentrifuge tubes containing 0.5 mL PBS. Spin the tubes for 10 min at 800*g*, remove the supernatant, freeze the cell pellets on dry ice, and store the tubes at –70°C.

3.7. Molecular Analysis of Isolated Mutants

3.7.1. Tk *LOH Analysis of Frozen Cells Collected From 96-Well Plates*

1. Thaw one of the two tubes containing the cell aliquots derived from each mutant clone (produced as in **Subheading 3.5.**) at room temperature and resuspend in 50 μL of cell lysis buffer.
2. Incubate cell pellets for 1 h at 60°C and 15 min at 95°C.
3. For three primer allele-specific PCR using the HotStarTaq DNA polymerase kit, combine: 2 μL of 10X buffer, 4 μL of Q-solution, 1 U of HotStarTaq DNA polymerase, 2 μL of dNTP mix, 2 μL of 10X primer mixture (TK14, TK16, and NEO4, 10 μ*M* each), 4 μL of released genomic DNA, and water to a final volume of 20 μL in a PCR tube.
4. Process the samples using a temperature profile of 95°C × 15 min + (95°C × 1 min + 65°C × 1 min + 72°C × 3 min) × 35.
5. Analyze 6 μL of PCR products by electrophoresis on 1% agarose gel (*see* **Note 10**) *(27)*.

3.7.2. RT-PCR Analysis of Frozen Cells Collected From 96-Well Plates

1. Thaw one of the cell pellets aliquoted from each mutant clone to be analyzed on ice, resuspend each in 50 μL of cold buffer containing 2.5% Nonidet P40 and 0.4 U/μL RNasin, and release total RNA on ice for 20 min.
2. In fresh tubes, combine the cell lysate and primers with the components of the Access RT-PCR System: 4 μL of reaction buffer, 0.4 μL of dNTP mix, 0.8 μL of MgSO$_4$ stock, 0.4 μL AMV reverse transcriptase, 0.4 μL *Tfl* DNA polymerase, 4 μL of released total RNA, each of the two primers to a concentration of 1 μ*M* and water to final volume of 20 μL. For amplification of the *Hprt* cDNA, use primers HPRT1 and HPRT2; for amplification of the *Tk* cDNA, use primers FwdTK-RTPCR and TK10.
3. Process the mixtures using a PCR temperature profile of: 48°C × 45 min + 94°C × 2 min + (94°C × 30 s + 60°C × 1 min + 68°C × 2 min) × 40 + 68°C × 7 min.
4. Analyze 5 μL of the RT-PCR products on a 1% agarose gel *(27)*. The full size of the amplified *Hprt* cDNA fragment is 823 bp, and the full-sized *Tk* cDNA fragment is 815 bp.

3.7.3. Nested PCR

If the amount of amplified cDNA appears to be low, a nested PCR can be performed. Dilute the RT-PCR product 1:100 with water and use 1 μL in the second round of PCR with primers Zee1 and M902R for the *Hprt* gene and FwdTK-RTPCR and RevTk-RTPCR for the *Tk* gene. The expected sizes of the amplified products are 754 bp and 764 bp, respectively.

3.7.4. RNA Extraction From Expanded Hprt *Mutant Clones*

1. Prepare RNA using the Purescript RNA isolation kit following the manufacturer's instructions.
2. Resuspend the cell pellet (*see* **Subheading 3.3.**) in 100 μL of cell lysis solution, add 33 μL of protein–DNA precipitation solution, and leave on ice for 5 min.
3. Microcentrifuge for 3 min at full speed, transfer the supernatant into a new tube, and precipitate the RNA with 100 μL of isopropanol.

4. Pellet the RNA by spinning the tube for 3 min at full speed, remove the supernatant fluid, and wash the pellet with 100 µL of 70% ethanol.
5. Air-dry the pellet and rehydrate the RNA in 15 µL of hydration solution from the kit; store the RNA at –70°C (*see* **Note 11**).

3.7.5. RT-PCR Analysis of Expanded Hprt Mutant Clones

1. Combine: 2 µL oligo(dT), 4 µL of dNTP mix, 8 µL of water, and 2 µL of RNA (from **Subheading 3.7., step 4**).
2. Denature the RNA at 75°C for 3 min, followed by cooling on ice.
3. Add 2 µL of RETROScript buffer, 1 µL of RNaseOUT inhibitor, and 1 µL of SuperScript polymerase.
4. Incubate for 1 h at 42°C and 3 min at 97°C; store the cDNA at –20°C.
5. Amplify the *Hprt* cDNA using the HotStarTaq kit. In a PCR tube, combine 3 µL of the 10X buffer, 6 µL of Q-solution, and 0.3 µL HotStarTaq polymerase; add 3 µL of dNTP mix, 3 µL of HPRT1 primer (10 µ*M*), 3 µL of HPRT2 primer (10 µ*M*), 8.7 µL water, and 3 µL of cDNA.
6. Process the samples using a PCR temperature profile of 95°C × 15 min + (95°C × 1 min + 52°C × 1 min + 72°C × 3 min) × 35 + 72°C × 7 min.
7. As a template quality control, mouse β-actin cDNA may be amplified in parallel using the primers m-Actin-F and m-Actin-R. The expected size of the amplified actin cDNA product is 591 bp.

3.7.6. Sequencing Amplified cDNA

Perform sequencing of amplified cDNA products using your favorite protocol *(28)*.

4. Notes

1. *Tk*[+/–] mice are available from the Jackson Laboratory through the MMRRC (Mutant Mouse Regional Resource Centers) program (http://www.mmrrc.org/strains/14/0014.html), or in limited quantities from the authors.
2. Prepare growth medium from sterile components or sterilize by filtration through a 0.2-µm filter; may keep at 4°C for up to 2 wk before use.
3. Use yellow light while handling solutions containing BrdUrd.
4. Most automated cell counters are configured to count cells in a 0.5 mL volume. The cell count for 0.5 mL should be multiplied by 2 and by the dilution factor 50 (0.5 mL of cell suspension in 24.5 mL of isotonic diluent). The resulting cell concentration is expressed in cells/mL. A range of $1–3 × 10^6$ cells/mL is typical for untreated mice. Cell counts may be lower in animals affected by a specific genotype or the experimental regimen.
5. Example: the counter detected 10,500 events for an experimental sample and 15,600 for the feeder cells. The concentrations are calculated to be $1.05 × 10^6$ cells/mL for the experimental cells and $1.56 × 10^6$ cells/mL for the feeder cells. A 1:100 dilution of the experimental cells is $1.05 × 10^4$ cells/mL. For three plates with 6-TG selection, use 12.57 mL of cells and 20.43 mL of medium. For five plates with BrdUrd selection, use 5.05 mL of cells and 47.95 mL of medium. For two CE plates, use 175 µL of the 1:100 dilution, 1.47 mL of irradiated feeder cells, and 21.53 mL of medium (or 175 µL of dilution, 5.9 mL of irradiated feeders and 17.1 mL of medium, if only *Hprt* mutants are analyzed).
6. If the animals are sacrificed on a Thursday, then cell plating occurs on Friday, alamarBlue is added on Monday (of the second week), and clone scoring is done on Tuesday.
7. Final concentration of alamarBlue in the wells is 1%.

8. With computerized support, a 8 × 12 fluorescence data array for each plate can be processed either by software supplied with the plate reader or exported to a spreadsheet processor. The plate reading, finding MIN, calculating the cutoff value, and determining the total number of positive wells on each plate are achieved in one step.

9. Example: two CE plates, three 6-TG-containing plates, and five BrdUrd-containing plates were established for an experimental animal, with the following concentrations of target cells: 8 cells/well in CE plates, 4×10^4 cells/well in TG plates, and 1×10^4 cells/well in BrdUrd plates. The total number of identified positive wells in the CE plates was 89, in the 6-TG selection plates, 23, and in the BrdUrd selection plates, 32. The T-cell cloning efficiency in the absence of selection was calculated to be 7.78%, the frequency of *Hprt* mutants was 26.7×10^{-6}, and the frequency of *Tk* mutants was 88.6×10^{-6}.

10. Dead $Tk^{+/-}$ cells are always present in the wells containing growing *Tk* mutants. In allele-specific PCR, these dead cells produce a background amplification of both Tk^+ and Tk^- alleles, even when cells from negative wells are analyzed. A BrdUrd-resistant clone that produces PCR products having two distinct bands with sizes of approx 350 and 700 bp is classified as having an intragenic *Tk* mutation. A clone that produces a faint 700-bp band and a distinct 350-bp band is classified as having undergone LOH at the *Tk* locus. Cells from negative wells produce two faint bands. The number of cycles in allele-specific PCR can be decreased in order to diminish the background level of allele amplification from the dead cells.

11. This is a scaled-down protocol suggested by the manufacturer.

References

1. Bertram, J. S. (2000) The molecular biology of cancer. *Mol. Aspects Med.* **21,** 167–223.
2. Szybalski, W. (1959) Genetics of human cell lines. II. Methods or determination of mutation rates to drug resistance. *Exp. Cell Res.* **18,** 588–591.
3. Chu, E. H. Y. and Malling, H. V. (1968) Mammalian cell genetics. II. Chemical induction of specific locus mutations in Chinese hamster cells in vitro. *Proc. Natl. Acad. Sci. USA* **61,** 1306–1312.
4. Chasin, L. A. (1972) Non-linkage of induced mutations in Chinese hamster cells. *Nature* **240,** 50–52.
5. Clive, D., Flamm, W. G., Machesko, M. R., and Bernheim, N. J. (1972) A mutational assay system using the thymidine kinase locus in mouse lymphoma cells. *Mutat. Res.* **16,** 77–87.
6. Adair, G. M., Carver, J. H., and Wandres, D. L. (1980) Mutagenicity testing in mammalian cells. I. Derivation of a Chinese hamster ovary cell line heterozygous for the adenine phosphoribosyltransferase and thymidine kinase loci. *Mutat. Res.* **72,** 187–205.
7. Jones, I. M., Burkhart-Schultz, K., and Carrano, A. V. (1985) A method to quantify spontaneous and in vivo induced thioguanine-resistant mouse lymphocytes. *Mutat. Res.* **147,** 97–105.
8. Aidoo, A., Morris, S. M., and Casciano, D. A. (1997) Development and utilization of the rat lymphocyte *hprt* mutation assay. *Mutat. Res.* **387,** 69–88.
9. Albertini, R. J., Castle, K. L., and Borcherding, W. R. (1982) T-cell cloning to detect the mutant 6-thioguanine-resistant lymphocytes present in human peripheral blood. *Proc. Natl. Acad. Sci. USA* **79,** 6617–6621.
10. Mendelsohn, M. L., Bigbee, W. L., Branscomb, E. W., and Stamatoyannopoulos, G. (1980) The detection and sorting of rare sickle-hemoglobin containing cells in normal human blood, in *Flow Cytometry IV* (Laerum, O. D., Lindmo, T., and Thorud, E., eds.), Universitetsforlaget, Oslo, pp. 311–313.

11. Griffiths, D. F. R., Davies, S. J., Williams, D., Williams, G. T., and Williams, E. D. (1988) Demonstration of somatic mutation and colonic crypt clonality by X-linked enzyme histochemistry. *Nature* **333,** 461–463.
12. Janatipour, M., Trainor, K. J., Kutlaca, R., et al. (1988) Mutations in human lymphocytes studied by an HLA selection system. *Mutat. Res.* **198,** 221–226.
13. Kyoizumi, S., Akiyama, M., Hirai, Y., Kusunoki, Y., Tanabe, K., and Umeki, S. (1990) Spontaneous loss and alteration of antigen receptor expression in mature CD4+ T cells. *J. Exp. Med.* **171,** 1981–1999.
14. Hakoda, M., Yamanaka, H., Kamatani, N., and Kamatani, N. (1991) Diagnosis of heterozygous states for adenine phosphoribosyltransferase deficiency based on detection of in vivo somatic mutants in blood T cells: application to screening of heterozygotes. *Am. J. Hum. Genet.* **48,** 552–562.
15. Grant, S. G. and Bigbee, W. L. (1993) *In vivo* somatic mutation and segregation at the human glycophorin A *(GPA)* locus: phenotypic variation encompassing both gene-specific and chromosomal mechanisms. *Mutat. Res.* **288,** 163–172.
16. Meydan, D., Nilsson, T., Tornblom, M., et al. (1999) The frequency of illegitimate TCRbeta/gamma gene recombination in human lymphocytes: influence of age, environmental exposure and cytostatic treatment, and correlation with frequencies of t(14;18) and hprt mutation. *Mutat. Res.* **444,** 393–403.
17. Okada, N., Masumura, K., Nohmi, T., and Yajima, N. (1999) Efficient detection of deletions induced by a single treatment of mitomycin C in transgenic mouse *gpt* delta using the Spi⁻ selection. *Environ. Mol. Mutagen.* **34,** 106–111.
18. Burkhart, J. G., Burkhart, B. A., Sampson, K. S., and Malling, H. V. (1993) ENU-induced mutagenesis at a single A:T base pair in transgenic mice containing phi X174. *Mutat. Res.* **292,** 69–81.
19. Dycaico, M. J., Provost, G. S., Kretz, P. L., Ransom, S. L., Moores, J. C., and Short, J. M. (1994) The use of shuttle vectors for mutation analysis in transgenic mice and rats. *Mutat. Res.* **307,** 461–478.
20. Gossen, J. and Vijg, J. (1993) Transgenic mice as model systems for studying gene mutations in vivo. *Trends. Genet.* **9,** 27–31.
21. Dobrovolsky, V. N., Casciano, D. A., and Heflich, R. H. (1999) *Tk*⁺/⁻ mouse model for detecting in vivo mutation in an endogenous, autosomal gene. *Mutat. Res.* **423,** 125–136.
22. Wijnhoven, S. W., Van Sloun, P. P., Kool, H. J., et al. (1998) Carcinogen-induced loss of heterozygosity at the *Aprt* locus in somatic cells of the mouse. *Proc. Natl. Acad. Sci. USA* **95,** 13759–13764.
23. Liang, L., Deng, L., Shao, C., Stambrook, P. J., and Tischfield, J. A. (2000) In vivo loss of heterozygosity in T-cells of B6C3F1 *Aprt*⁺/⁻ mice. *Environ. Mol. Mutagen.* **35,** 150–157.
24. Dobrovolsky, V. N., Chen, T., and Heflich, R. H. (1999) Molecular analysis of in vivo mutations induced by *N*-ethyl-*N*-nitrosourea in the autosomal *Tk* and the X-linked *Hprt* genes of mouse lymphocytes. *Environ. Mol. Mutagen.* **34,** 30–38.
25. Dobrovolsky, V. N., Shaddock, J. G., and Heflich, R. H. (2000) 7,12-Dimethylbenz[*a*]anthracene-induced mutation in the *Tk* gene of *Tk*⁺/⁻ mice: automated scoring of lymphocyte clones using a fluorescent viability indicator. *Environ. Mol. Mutagen.* **36,** 283–291.
26. Meng, Q., Skopek, T. R., Walker, D. M., et al. (1998) Culture and propagation of *Hprt* mutant T-lymphocytes isolated from mouse spleen. *Environ. Mol. Mutagen.* **32,** 236–243.
27. Voytas, D. (1988) Resolution and recovery of large DNA fragments, in *Current Protocols in Molecular Biology*, vol. 1 (Jannssen, K., ed), Wiley, New York, pp. 2.5.1–2.5.9.
28. Ausubel, F. M., Albright, L. M., Slatko, B. E., et al. (1988) DNA sequencing, in *Current Protocols in Molecular Biology*, vol. 1 (Jannssen, K., ed), Wiley, New York, pp. 7.0.1–7.7.31.

14

Quantifying In Vivo Somatic Mutations Using Transgenic Mouse Model Systems

Roy R. Swiger

Summary

This chapter describes the use of the bacteriophage *cII* positive selection assay with the Muta™Mouse transgenic model system. The assay is similar to others involving a transgenic target, including the *cII* and *lacI* assays in the Big Blue® Mouse, *lacZ* in the MutaMouse, and the *gpt* delta assay. Briefly, high-molecular-weight DNA is purified from the tissue of interest and used as substrate during in vitro packaging reactions, in which the λ transgenes are excised from the genome and assembled into viable phage. Phage containing the mutational targets are then adsorbed into an appropriate bacterial host, and mutations sustained in vivo are evidenced by either standard recombinant screening or selection assays. Mutant frequencies are reported as the ratio of mutant phage to total phage units analyzed. The λ-based transgenic mouse assays are used to study and characterize in vivo mutagenesis, as well as for mutagenicity assessment. The models permit the enumeration of mutations sustained in virtually any tissue of the mouse and are sensitive and robust. Application of the assays is simple, not requiring resources beyond those commonly found in most academic laboratories.

Key Words: *cII*; *gpt*; *lacZ*; *lacI*; assay; Big Blue; induced; MutaMouse; mutagen; mutation; somatic; spontaneous; tissue.

1. Introduction

Few endogenous loci are suitable for in vivo mutational analysis. Furthermore, those that are used for such a purpose are limited with respect to quantification, tissue in which analysis can be conducted (tissue type), or developmental stage requirements (*see* Chaps. 13, 15, 18, and 19). The mouse is recognized as a useful experimental surrogate for human beings. Transgenic technology has revolutionized many areas of biological research, including molecular toxicology. To date, several λ-based transgenic mouse mutational model systems have been described, involving the *SupF* and *lacZ* genes (MutaMouse), the *lacI* gene (Big Blue Mouse), and the *gpt* gene *(1–4)*.

These in vivo models are founded on different genetic background strains, have transgenic loci mapping to different chromosomes, and differ in transgene copy number. Additionally, the sizes of the target loci differ by nearly an order of magnitude, typically

From: *Methods in Molecular Biology, vol. 291, Molecular Toxicology Protocols*
Edited by: P. Keohavong and S. G. Grant © Humana Press Inc., Totowa, NJ

consisting of bacterial sequences (such as *cII* and *lacZ*) cloned into λ phage arms. The λ sequences are heavily methylated and exist as high-copy-number, reiterated sequences, integrated at a single site, and are organized in so-called "head-to-tail" arrays.

These transgenic mutation assays are quantitative. Despite their differences, the systems have been characterized as having similar spontaneous mutant frequencies in most tissues, with the notable exception of the gametes *(5–7)*. The assays are robust and sensitive, having the ability to quantify rare spontaneous events occurring at a frequency no greater than 3–9 in every 100,000 loci screened. Additionally, the dynamic range of detection exceeds three orders of magnitude.

Transgene expression in the small intestine and in blood lymphocytes permits the comparison of mutant frequency between transgenes and the endogenous loci *Dlb-1* and *Hprt*, respectively. When such comparisons have been conducted, the loci are reported as having generally similar spontaneous and induced mutant frequencies *(8–10)*, with some important exceptions *(11–13)*.

Application of the transgenic mutation assays is elegant. The transgenic animals contain the bacteriophage transgene loci in all tissues, so tissue-specific analysis or whole-animal analysis can be conducted. The process includes the use of standard mammalian genomic DNA purification methods, followed by in vitro packaging reactions. The packaging extract can be purchased or made in the laboratory and contains phage catalytic and structural proteins that selectively excise the λ sequences, pack the sequences into phage heads, and assemble viable phage. Subsequently, the phage are incubated and adsorbed into their bacterial hosts, usually in the presence of $MgSO_4$. The bacterial mixture is then plated under nonselective (titers) and selective (or screening) conditions to identify mutants and enumerate total phage plated. The ratio of mutant to total phage plated is expressed as the mutant frequency.

The models are continually being characterized, validated for use, and improved. Notable improvements include better packaging extracts, selection substrates, and reduction of the size (bp) of the mutational target, to make molecular characterization more efficient. The bacteriophage *cI* and *cII* loci are present on most λ cloning vectors. In wild-type bacteriophage λ, these loci are essential components in the lysogenic life cycle pathway. Although the structural lysogeny-specific sequences have been removed or replaced (with stuffer fragments) in many cloning vectors, the lytic vs lysogenic decision-making pathways are still present. In the case of the λ *gt*10 vector used to construct the transgene in the MutaMouse system, the CI protein is inactivated by the insertion of the *lacZ* gene into the *cI* coding sequence.

The phage lytic vs lysogenic life cycle is codependent on bacterial host loci. Specific to this discussion are the high-frequency lysogeny *Hfl* A and B loci coding for proteins that, when functioning properly, digest and hydrolyze the CI and CII phage proteins. Bacteria containing mutations at these loci are referred to as lysogenic or *Hfl* strains and result in forfeiting the bacterial contribution to the lytic vs lysogenic pathway chosen by phage upon adsorption into the host.

The 294 bp *cII* locus was first used as a mutational target in the Big Blue Mouse assay *(14)* and subsequently incorporated to the MutaMouse system *(15)*. More recently, a *cII* transgenic fish (*Medaka*) has been described for use in environmental toxicology *(16)*. The *cII* assay has been characterized as similar to the *lacI* assay in the Big Blue Mouse and rat 2 cell line *(17–20)* and equivalent to the *lacZ* assay in the MutaMouse *(7,15,21–23)*. The use of *cII* as the target gene addresses different deficiencies associated with each system, notably the labor and cost of *lacI* analysis (Big Blue Mouse) and the large target size (3.1 kb) of the *lacZ* gene in MutaMouse, which is difficult to sequence routinely. Moreover, when the *cII* and either the *lacI* or *lacZ* assays are applied to the same sample(s), "jackpot" mutations, or outliers in datasets owing to developmental mutations or artifacts can be identified without the use of sequencing *(15)*.

This chapter outlines the *cII* selection assay for use with the commercially available MutaMouse transgenic system (Covance, Princeton, NJ). The assay is similar to that described originally for the Big Blue Mouse system (Stratagene, La Jolla, CA).

2. Materials

2.1. Preparation of High-Molecular-Weight DNA From Whole Tissue

1. Distilled water.
2. Proteinease K (Sigma Aldrich, St. Louis, MO).
3. ProK lysis buffer containing 1% sodium dodecyl sulfate (SDS) (*see* **Note 1**).
4. Water bath (55°C).
5. 15-mL Serological screw-cap centrifuge tubes.
6. Vortex.
7. 25:24:1 Phenol/chloroform/isoamyl alcohol (PCI), molecular grade, or DNA RecoverEase™ DNA isolation kit (Stratagene; *see* **Note 2**). PCI should be stored at 4°C. **Caution**: Phenol is caustic, and staff should use double gloving, wear protective eyewear, and work in a chemical fume hood.
8. Tabletop serological or equivalent centrifuge.
9. Phenol waste disposal container.
10. Ethanol, molecular grade.
11. 1.5-mL Microcentrifuge tubes (sterile).
12. Glass capillary tubes.
13. Disposable 5-mL squeeze top pipets.
14. 25-mL Disposable serological pipet and pipetor.
15. UV grade spectrophotometer cuvets.
16. P20, P100 or P200, P1000 micropipetor set and micropipet tips.
17. Spectrophotometer.

2.2. In Vitro Packaging Reaction

1. Packaging extract (e.g., Stratagene or Epicentre, Madison, WI; *see* **Note 3**).
2. 1.5-mL Microcentrifuge tubes (sterile).
3. 1.5-mL Microcentrifuge tube rack.
4. Vortex.
5. Phage SM buffer *(24)*.
6. 30°C Water bath or incubator.
7. Timer.
8. P20, P100 or P200, P1000 micopipetor set and micropipet tips.

2.3. Bacterial Culture, Adsorption, and Plating

1. High-frequency lysogenization bacteria strain (*Hfl* A/B; *see* **Note 4**).
2. TB media (*see* **Notes 5–8**):

   a. TB top agar plates containing 7.5 g/L agar. TB top agar may be made up to 2 wk prior to use and stored at room temperature until needed.
   b. TB bottom agar plates containing 15.0 g/L agar. TB bottom plates should be made within days of plating.

3. Microbiological grade agar.
4. Standard bacterial 100-mm plates.
5. Casein peptone (essential reagent; *see* **Note 6**).
6. Vitamin B$_1$ (thiamine; essential reagent).
7. Kanamycin, molecular grade.
8. 100X (200 m*M*) MgSO$_4$ for preparation of TB media and agar (*see* **Notes 7** and **8**).
9. 100X (20%) Maltose for preparation of TB media and agar (*see* **Notes 8** and **9**). If desired, can also prepare a joint 100X solution of 20% maltose, 200 m*M* MgSO$_4$.
10. 10 m*M* MgSO$_4$, specifically for resuspension of bacterial pellets. Should be made fresh weekly and sterilized prior to use.
11. 50-mL Serological screw-cap centrifuge tubes.
12. 15-mL Serological screw-cap centrifuge tubes.
13. Disposable 1.0-mL or visible grade (VIS) spectrophotometric cuvets.
14. Vortex.
15. 37°C Shaking water bath.
16. 15-mL Serological tube rack.
17. Timer.
18. Digital thermometer to record selection incubation temperature.
19. P20, P100 or P200, P1000 micropipetor set and micropipet tips.

3. Methods

3.1. Preparation of High-Molecular-Weight DNA From Whole Tissue (see *Note 10*)

1. Place chopped, ground tissue into 15-mL serological screw-cap centrifuge tubes.
2. Fill centrifuge tubes to 4–5 mL with Pro K lysis and digestion buffer containing Proteinase K and SDS (*see* **Note 11**).
3. Vortex gently or invert to mix.
4. Place at 55°C for 1–2 h (*see* **Note 12**).
5. Vortex gently or invert to mix every hour until complete solubilization of tissue (may require 8 h to overnight).
6. Perform PCI extraction in chemical fume hood:

   a. Add equal volume (4–5 mL) PCI and vortex gently.
   b. Spin in serological centrifuge at full speed for 5–10 min.
   c. Remove aqueous phase (top) and place into new 15-mL serological screw-cap centrifuge tubes.
   d. Repeat extraction with PCI up to four times, until aqueous phase is clear and the interface is no longer turbid.

7. Perform one chloroform extraction phase to remove residual phenol (optional).

8. Ethanol-precipitate using twice the volume of sample (100% ethanol).
9. Invert tubes gently.
10. Spool out DNA with glass hook.
11. Place DNA in dry 1.5-mL centrifuge tube and dry for 5 min to remove volatile ethanol.
12. Add 200–500 mL distilled water, or Tris-EDTA, pH 8.0 (TE), and resolubilize for 1 h at 50°C or overnight on benchtop.
13. Quantify OD_{260} DNA concentration using spectrophotometric analysis (*see* **Note 13**).

3.2. In Vitro Packaging Reaction (see Note 14)

1. Place 5–10 µL resolubilized DNA into the first reaction tube and mix with micropipetor.
2. Place labeled reaction(s) at 30 or 37°C as specified by commercial supplier of packaging extract for 1.5 h.
3. Thaw second reaction just prior to adding and add specified amount of second reaction in each packaging reaction.
4. Place labeled reaction(s) at 30 or 37°C as specified by commercial supplier of packaging extract for 1.5 h.
5. Arrest the packaging reaction by adding 830 µL SM phage buffer, and vortex immediately.
6. Place reactions on ice, or store at 4°C (*see* **Note 15**).
7. Make titer tubes for each sample and label accordingly. Remove 20 µL packaged phage in SM buffer and conduct serial dilutions (1:10 and 1:100) using SM phage buffer. Vortex vigorously and place on ice.

3.3. Bacterial Culture, Adsorption, and Plating (see Note 16)

1. Grow an overnight culture the night *before* plating (*see* **Note 17**).

   a. Place 5 mL TB media containing 25 µg/mL kanamycin, 10 mM $MgSO_4$, and 0.2% maltose into a 15-mL serological screw-cap centrifuge tube.
   b. From a TB kanamycin (50 µg/mL) master plate, graze an *Hfl* colony using a sterile loop or pipet tip.
   c. Place the colony into the 5 mL of liquid TB kanamycin (25 µg/mL) and place 15-mL serological centrifuge tube into shaking incubator at 30–37°C.

2. Pour TB top and bottom plates (*see* **Note 18**).
3. Grow multiple same-day cultures:

   a. Place 20 mL TB media containing maltose and the lower concentration of kanamycin (25 µg/mL) into multiple 50-mL serological screw-cap centrifuge tubes. Alternatively, kanamycin can be omitted from same-day cultures.
   b. Add 200–400 µL of each overnight culture to 20 mL of TB media (containing 10 mL 10 mM $MgSO_4$ and 0.2% maltose) in 4 × 50-mL serological screw-cap centrifuge tubes.
   c. Place same-day cultures in 30°C shaking water bath, at 225 rpm for up to 5–6 h. The temperature may be raised to increase cell division.
   d. Begin checking the optical density for the cultures (OD_{600}) after 4–5 h. Blank with media, and use disposable visible (VIS) grade 1.0 mL cuvets.

4. Adjust the OD_{600} of the same-day cultures to 0.5 using 10 mM $MgSO_4$:

   a. Remove the same-day cultures from the incubator when the OD_{600} = 0.5–0.8.
   b. Centrifuge cultures for 5–10 min using a table top serological (1/2 speed) or equivalent centrifuge, and spin at 3000g to form a visible pellet, ensuring that the supernatant is clear.

c. Decant media and dab dry with a Kimwipe.

d. Resuspend the bacterial pellets with 10 mM MgSO$_4$ to OD$_{600}$ = 0.5.

e. Place resuspended bacteria on ice.

5. Perform phage adsorptions (*see* **Note 18**):

   a. Place 10 labeled 15-mL screw-cap serological centrifuge tubes per animal into a rack.

   b. Label titer tubes accordingly (two to four per animal).

   c. Aliquot 200 µL of resuspended same-day culture into 15-mL screw-cap serological centrifuge tubes.

   d. Place 80–100 µL of packaged phage into each 15-mL screw-cap serological centrifuge tube containing 200 µL of resuspended same-day culture.

   e. For titers, place 20–80 µL of diluted packaged phage into each labeled titer 15-mL screw-cap serological tube.

   f. Incubate at 30°C or on benchtop for 15–30 min.

6. Plate bacteria (*see* **Note 19**):

   a. Add 2–4 mL of top agar to each 15-mL screw-cap serological centrifuge tube containing 200 µL of resuspended same-day culture and phage aliquots.

   b. Quickly vortex, or invert twice and immediately pour onto TB bottom plates.

   c. Let plates stand for 5–15 min with lid ajar to permit evaporation without condensation.

   d. Invert plates and place titers at 37°C overnight.

   e. Place selection plates at 23.5°C for 48 h (*see* **Note 20**).

3.4. Calculating Mutant Frequency (see Note 21)

1. Count the number of plaques in titer plates and take the average. Multiply the average by the dilution factor and divide by the volume plated. The resulting value is the pfu/µL package reaction.

2. The total pfu screened or plated on selection plates is determined by multiplying the pfu/µL package reaction by the total volume of the package reaction plated on selection plates.

3. Mutant frequency is determined as the total pfu counted on all *selection* plates for a given sample divided by the total pfu screened for that sample.

4. The relative packaging efficiency is determined by multiplying the pfu/µL package reaction by the volume (in µL) of DNA sample packaged. If the A$_{260}$ of the sample has been determined, then the packaging efficiency pfu/µg may be determined.

4. Notes

1. Standard formulation: 100 mM NaCl, 25 mM EDTA, 10 mM Tris-HCl, pH 8.0 *(25)*. The NaCl concentration can be reduced to as low as 20 mM.

2. RecoverEase™ DNA isolation kit is recommended for liver samples.

3. Commercial extract is recommended and typically yields greater packaging efficiencies and reproducibility. Although protocols for producing in vitro packaging extract are simple in principle, preparing high-quality packaging extract *repeatedly* is difficult and should not be taken lightly. It is highly recommended that different or new lots of packaging extract be compared. Test each new lot of packaging extract by selecting five reactions randomly and package a DNA sample that has previously yielded high titers. If commercial extracts cannot be used, the method of Poustka *(26)* is recommended for optimal isolation of packaging extract in the laboratory.

4. *Hfl* strains suitable for use are commercially available from Stratagene or Epicentre. To ensure that the strain is working properly, save cored *cII* mutant and *cII* wild-type plaques

as controls. Routinely assay the bacteria with the stocks under selective and nonselective conditions.

5. TB recipes are provided with commercial bacterial strains and can be found in any microbiological methods manual, or in most molecular biology protocol manuals *(24)*.

6. Casein peptone obtained from various sources should be assessed in the laboratory for effectiveness before selecting a supplier. If plates appear mottled, titers drop substantially, or if things "go wrong," begin troubleshooting by purchasing fresh casein peptone, or switch suppliers.

7. The use of 2 mM MgSO$_4$ in the preparation of TB media and TB bottom agar is optional and should be evaluated in the laboratory. It is essential in the preparation of TB top agar, however. MgSO$_4$·7H$_2$O must be used. Stock solutions should be autoclaved. Stocks of 10 or 20X MgSO$_4$·7H$_2$O are stable for months at room temperature.

8. Do not add MgSO$_4$ or maltose to top agar until immediately prior to plating, after TB top agar has cooled to 55°C and while it is still molten.

9. A final concentration of 0.2% maltose in TB media and top agar is used to induce expression of the bacterial LamB receptor, the port of entry for bacteriophage λ. Sterile stocks (100X) of maltose or maltose/MgSO$_4$ may be stored for several weeks at 4°C. Maltose solutions are labile and therefore should be filter-sterilized and handled aseptically. Maltose is not generally required in the bottom agar.

10. Tissue samples should be stored in 15-mL serological centrifuge tubes and placed in liquid nitrogen or ethanol/dry ice baths immediately upon dissection. All tissues should be stored at –80°C until performing DNA extractions. Samples should be treated somewhat delicately when one is attempting to isolate high-molecular-weight DNA. It is essential to minimize "DNA shearing" during the preparation. The use of wide-bore pipets, and rocking, or inverting, samples to mix is recommended.

11. Proteinase K recommended concentrations vary and may be adjusted according to the surface to volume ratios of the tissue. A reasonable starting concentration is 0.1 mg/mL.

12. Water bath temperatures may be increased to 60°C, to reduce incubation time.

13. The quality of extractions may often vary. Also, packaging efficiency may not necessarily correspond to DNA quantity. Many researchers no longer bother to quantify DNA and instead have established standard operating procedures in their laboratories based on historical observation. Remember that each sample has its own titer plate(s) set to verify pfu plated. Overdigesting with proteinase K may result in loss of packaging efficiency. Dialysis of the DNA against TE buffer can often increase packaging efficiency from poor packaging samples.

14. Packaging reactions are simple and require two successive 1.5-h incubations. Therefore, fresh plates may be poured while simultaneously packaging samples.

15. The packaging reactions may be stored at 4°C for days without loss of viability. To extend the half-life, add a droplet of chloroform.

16. No more than 300,000 pfu should be plated on a selection plate. Therefore, it is advisable to plate titers 1 d before plating selection plates (storing remaining packaging reactions at 4°C). This will minimize waste, or overplating reactions with poor packaging efficiency, and will optimize plate usage for high-titer samples. New titer dilutions should be made the following day at the time of plating the remaining reaction (selection plates).

17. This culture may be stored at 4°C and used for up to 1 wk if necessary.

18. The protocol assumes blind titers. Make appropriate adjustment to the number of selection plates if titers have been determined prior to selection plating, as discussed in **Note 15**, above.

19. Top agar may be stored at room temperature for up to 1–2 wk. Two hours prior to plating bacteria, microwave the top agar to boil (place in secondary container in water) and vent

often. Place melted liquid top agar in water bath at 55°C until needed. Prior to plating top agar and after cooling to 55°C, add fresh $MgSO_4$ and maltose. The final concentrations should be 2 mM $MgSO_4$ and 0.2% maltose.

20. The selection temperature is critical, and therefore it is advisable to record it using a sensitive thermometer. Additionally, many groups find that placing a water-jacketed incubator into a 4°C walk-in cold room is optimal for maintaining the selection temperature at 23.5°C.

21. Four titer plates at each dilution are desirable. Because spontaneous mutations occur far less frequently than induced mutations, more plaques must be screened for spontaneous samples than induced.

Acknowledgments

I wish to thank Professor John A. Heddle, York University, for introducing and educating me on the transgenic models. Thanks to Ms. Lorien Newell for useful comments.

References

1. Leach, E. G., Narayanan, L., Havre, P. A., Gunther, E. J., Yeasky, T. M., and Glazer, P. M. (1996) Tissue specificity of spontaneous point mutations in lambda supF transgenic mice. *Environ. Mol. Mutagen.* **28,** 459–464.

2. Gossen, J. A., de Leeuw, W. J. F., Tan, C. H. T., et al. (1989) Efficient rescue of integrated shuttle vectors from transgenic mice: a model for studying mutations in vivo. *Proc. Natl. Acad. Sci. USA* **86,** 7971–7975.

3. Kohler, S. W., Provost, G. S., Fieck, A., et al. (1991) Spectra of spontaneous and mutagen-induced mutations in the lacI gene in transgenic mice. *Proc. Natl. Acad. Sci. USA* **88,** 7958–7962.

4. Nohmi, T., Katoh, M., Suzuki, H., et al. (1996) A new transgenic mouse mutagenesis test system using Spi- and 6-thioguanine selections. *Environ. Mol. Mutagen.* **28,** 465–470.

5. Douglas, G. R., Jiao, J., Gingerich, J. D., Gossen, J. A., and Soper, L. M. (1995) Temporal and molecular characteristics of mutations induced by ethylnitrosourea in germ cells isolated from seminiferous tubules and in spermatozoa of *lacZ* transgenic mice. *Proc. Natl. Acad. Sci. USA* **92,** 7485–7489.

6. Zhang, X. B., Urlando, C., Tao, K. S., and Heddle, J. A. (1995) Factors affecting somatic mutation frequencies in vivo. *Mutat. Res.* **338,** 189–201.

7. Swiger, R. R., Cosentino, L., Masumura, K. I., Nohmi, T., and Heddle, J. A. (2001) Further characterization and validation of gpt delta transgenic mice for quantifying somatic mutations in vivo. *Environ. Mol. Mutagen.* **37,** 297–303.

8. Tao, K. S., Urlando, C., and Heddle, J. A. (1993) Comparison of somatic mutation in a transgenic versus host locus. *Proc. Natl. Acad. Sci. USA* **90,** 10681–10685.

9. Walker, V. E., Gorelick, N. J., Andrews, J. L., et al. (1996) Frequency and spectrum of ethylnitrosourea-induced mutation at the *hprt* and *lacI* loci in splenic lymphocytes of exposed *lacI* transgenic mice. *Cancer Res.* **56,** 4654–4661.

10. Cosentino, L. and Heddle, J.A. (1999) A comparison of the effects of diverse mutagens at the *lacZ* transgene and *Dlb-1* locus in vivo. *Mutagenesis* **14,** 113–119.

11. Shaver-Walker, P. M., Urlando, C., Tao, K. S., Zhang, X. B., and Heddle, J. A. (1995) Enhanced somatic mutation rates induced in stem cells of mice by low chronic exposure to ethylnitrosourea. *Proc. Natl. Acad. Sci. USA* **92,** 11470–11474.

12. Skopek, T. R., Kort, K. L., Marino, D. R., et al. (1996) Mutagenic response of the endogenous *hprt* gene and *lacI* transgene in benzo[*a*]pyrene-treated Big Blue B6C3F1 mice. *Environ. Mol. Mutagen.* **28,** 376–384.

13. Cosentino, L. and Heddle, J. A. (2000) Differential mutation of transgenic and endogenous loci in vivo. *Mutat. Res.* **454,** 1–10.
14. Jakubczak, J. L., Merlino, G., French, J. E., et al. (1996) Analysis of genetic instability during mammary tumor progression using a novel selection-based assay for in vivo mutations in a bacteriophage lambda transgene target. *Proc. Natl. Acad. Sci. USA* **93,** 9073–9078.
15. Swiger, R. R., Cosentino, L., Shima, N., Bielas, J. H., Cruz-Munoz, W., and Heddle, J. A. (1999) The *cII* locus in the MutaMouse system. *Environ. Mol. Mutagen.* **34,** 201–207.
16. Winn, N. R., Norris, M. B., Brayer, K. J., Torres, C., and Muller, S. L. (2000) Detection of mutations in transgenic fish carrying a bacteriophage λ*cII* transgene target. *Proc. Natl. Acad. Sci. USA* **97,** 12655–12660.
17. Zimmer, D. M., Harbach, P. R., Mattes, W. B., and Aaron, C. S. (1999) Comparison of mutant frequencies at the transgenic lambda *LacI* and *cII/cI* loci in control and ENU-treated Big Blue mice. *Environ. Mol. Mutagen.* **33,** 249–256.
18. Watson, D. E., Cunningham, M. L., and Tindall, K. R. (1998) Spontaneous and ENU-induced mutation spectra at the *cII* locus in Big Blue Rat2 embryonic fibroblasts. *Mutagenesis* **13,** 487–497.
19. Harbach, P. R., Zimmer, D. M., Filipunas, A. L., Mattes, W. B., and Aaron, C. S. (1999) Spontaneous mutation spectrum at the lambda *cII* locus in liver, lung, and spleen tissue of Big Blue transgenic mice. *Environ. Mol. Mutagen.* **33,** 132–143.
20. You, Y. H. and Pfeifer, G. P. (2001) Similarities in sunlight-induced mutational spectra of CpG-methylated transgenes and the *p53* gene in skin cancer point to an important role of 5-methylcytosine residues in solar UV mutagenesis. *J. Mol. Biol.* **305,** 389–399.
21. Shima, N., Swiger, R. R., and Heddle, J. A. (2000) Dietary restriction during murine development provides protection against MNU-induced mutations. *Mutat. Res.* **470,** 189–200.
22. Suzuki, T., Wang, X., Miyata, Y., et al. (2000) Hepatocarcinogen quinoline induces G:C to C:G transversions in the cII gene in the liver of lambda/lacZ transgenic mice (MutaMouse). *Mutat. Res.* **456,** 73–81.
23. Kohara, A., Suzuki, T., Honma, M., et al. (2001) Mutation spectrum of o-aminoazotoluene in the *cII* gene of lambda/lacZ transgenic mice (MutaMouse). *Mutat. Res.* **491,** 211–220.
24. Sambrook, J., Fritsch, E. F., and Manniatis, T. (eds.) (1989) *Molecular Cloning: A Laboratory Manual,* vol. 1, 2nd ed. Cold Spring Harbor Laboratory Press, Cold Spring Harbor, NY.
25. Straus, W. M. (1994) Preparation of genomic DNA from mammalian tissue, in *Current Protocols in Molecular Biology,* vol. 1, suppl. 13 and 25 (Ausubel, F. M., Brent, R., Kingston, R. E., et al., eds.), Wiley Interscience, New York, pp. 2.2.1–2.2.3.
26. Poustka, A. (1993) Construction and use of chromosome jumping libraries. *Methods Enzymol.* **217,** 358–378.

15

Methods for Detecting Somatic Mutations In Vitro

The Human T-Cell Cloning Assay Selecting for HPRT *Mutants*

Sai-Mei Hou

Summary

The T-cell cloning assay, which detects mutations in the gene for hypoxanthine-guanine phosphoribosyltransferase (*HPRT*), is the most well-developed reporter system for studying specific locus mutation in human somatic cells. The assay is based on a mitogen- and growth factor-dependent clonal expansion of peripheral T lymphocytes in which the 6-thioguanine-resistant *HPRT* mutants can be selected, enumerated, and collected for molecular analysis of their mutational nature. The assay provides a unique tool for studying in vivo and in vitro mutagenesis and for investigating the functional impact of common polymorphisms in metabolism and repair genes. The present chapter presents a simple and reliable method for the enumeration of *HPRT* mutant frequency induced in vitro without using any source of recombinant interleukin-2. The other main feature is that only truly induced and unique mutants are collected for further analysis.

Key Words: Cloning assay; T lymphocytes; *HPRT* gene; mutations.

1. Introduction

The T-cell cloning assay, which enables the enumeration and molecular analysis of peripheral T lymphocytes with mutations in the X-linked hypoxanthine-guanine phosphoribosyl transferase (*HPRT*) gene, has been extensively used for studying human somatic gene mutation in vivo. The assay combines mitogen- and growth factor-dependent expansion of lymphocyte clones with 6-thioguanine (TG) selection of mutant cells. Resistance to TG identifies cells lacking the *HPRT* enzyme owing to inactivation or loss of the *HPRT* gene *(1)*. Knowledge of the entire human *HPRT* gene sequence has further enabled analysis of the molecular nature of *HPRT* mutations and the establishment of background and induced mutational spectra in various cell types *(2)*. Inherited mutations in the *HPRT* gene can also be studied in patients with the Lesch-Nyhan syndrome, which makes it possible to compare the mechanisms for mutagenesis in somatic and germline cells. Methods for molecular analysis of *HPRT* mutations have been described in detail *(3)* (*see* also Chap. 16).

From: *Methods in Molecular Biology, vol. 291, Molecular Toxicology Protocols*
Edited by: P. Keohavong and S. G. Grant © Humana Press Inc., Totowa, NJ

A wide range of mean background *HPRT* mutant frequencies (MFs) have been reported for normal nonexposed adult donors ($1.1–16.5 \times 10^{-6}$) *(4)*. Much of the considerable variation can be explained by interlaboratory variation in experimental methodologies and donor attributes such as age and smoking. The age effect may be associated with a decrease in DNA repair capacity, an increase in the mutation rate, or an accumulation of mutations over time. Differences in individual susceptibility to environmental mutagens owing to common inherited polymorphisms in metabolism and repair enzymes may also contribute to such variation *(5)*. The assay may thus provide a unique tool for studying the functional impact of common polymorphisms in metabolism and repair genes, especially under controlled treatment conditions in vitro.

For example, human *N*-acetyltransferase (NAT2) and glutathione S-transferase μ (GST-μ) are known to exhibit marked genetic polymorphisms. At least 50% of most Caucasian populations are slow acetylators or completely lack GST-μ activity (GSTM1 null genotype). NAT2 is involved in the metabolic activation of 2-nitrofluorene to the known carcinogen *N*-acetyl-2-aminofluorene. Further metabolism results in deactivation through glutathione conjugation. We obtained a clear dose-related increase in the *HPRT* mutant frequency after treating mitogen-stimulated lymphocytes isolated from a normal blood donor with 2-nitrofluorene (up to fivefold at 400 μg/mL, 24-h exposure; **Fig. 1**). No such mutant induction was seen when using cells from another donor. The susceptible cells turned out to have the NAT2 rapid and GSTM1 null genotype combination (capable of activation, with insufficient deactivation), whereas the resistant cells had NAT2 slow and GSTM1-positive genotypes (incapable of activation). This finding suggests that functional polymorphisms in metabolism and repair genes may indeed affect mutant induction in T cells, both in vitro and in vivo.

The possibility of using primary T lymphocytes for in vitro mutational analysis has only been utilized in a few studies *(6–9)*. Many attempts have been made to improve the T-cell cloning assay *(*reviewed in **refs. 5** and *10)*. Most laboratories use different concentrations of recombinant interleukin-2 (IL-2) with or without addition of conditioned medium or lymphokine-activated killer cell (LAK) supernatant (10–20% in growth medium). The LAK supernatant is basically used in culture medium with a large amount of recombinant IL-2 added to stimulate the proliferation of "killer" cells from cancer patients. However, this medium is not available in most laboratories. The present chapter describes a T-cell cloning protocol *(5)* using only a conditioned medium that is easily prepared from X-irradiated lymphocytes with lethally irradiated TK6 cells as allogenic stimulators (modified from **ref. 11**). The procedure for the enumeration and collection of *HPRT* mutants induced in vitro has been described recently *(9)*. In brief, pre-existing in vivo *HPRT* mutants are removed before in vitro treatment, and independent mutants are collected from different subcultures for molecular analysis. The mutational spectra obtained should thus be considered as the true in vitro spontaneous or induced spectra in the T cells of the blood donor without any in vivo background mutants or in vitro sibling mutants.

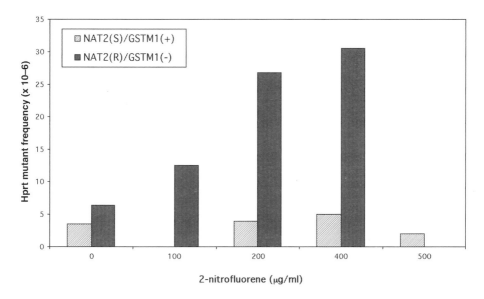

Fig. 1. *Hprt* mutant frequency in human peripheral lymphocytes exposed in vitro to 2-nitrofluorene. Different dose responses were obtained using cells from blood donors with different genotypes. Donor 1, *N*-acetyltransferase 2 (NAT2) slow and glutathione *S*-transferase M1 (GSTM1)-positive; Donor 2, NAT2 rapid and GSTM1-null.

2. Materials

2.1. Cells

1. Buffy coats (leukocyte preparations, each from 0.5 L whole blood centrifuged at 2700*g* for 10 min; obtained from hospital blood center).
2. TK6 cells (kindly provided by Dr. William Thilly at the Massachusetts Institute of Technology, Center for Environmental Health Sciences, Cambridge, MA).
3. Feeder cells: lymphoblastoid RJK853 cells (kindly provided by Dr. Richard Gibbs at Baylor College of Medicine, Houston, TX), lethally X-irradiated (40 Gy) prior to use.

2.2. Culture Media

1. Basic medium (BM): RPMI-1640 (Dutch modification) supplemented with 0.3 mg/mL *L*-glutamine, 150 IU/mL benzylpenicillin, and 150 µg/mL streptomycin (all from Gibco-BRL, Life Technologies, Gaithersburg, MD).
2. Nutrient medium (NM): BM with 5% heat inactivated (56°C, 30 min) fetal calf serum (FCS; Gibco BRL, Life Technologies) and 5% heat-inactivated human AB serum (HS; supplied by hospital blood center, pooled).
3. Growth medium (GM): NM with 0.3% (3 µg/mL) phytohemagglutinin (PHA; BD Biosciences, Franklin Lakes, NJ) and 20% T cell growth factor-enriched conditioned medium (CM; prepared according to **Subheading 3.2.**).

2.3. Hprt *Assay*

1. Phosphate-buffed saline (PBS).
2. 50X Concentrated hypoxanthine, aminopterin, and thymidine (HAT) supplement (Gibco BRL, Life Technologies).
3. Stock solution of 6-TG (Sigma): 1 mg/mL in 0.01 M NaOH made immediately before use.
4. Microplates (96 wells, 7-mm round bottom; Nunc, Weisbaden, Germany).
5. 24-Well plates (Nunc).
6. UNI-SEP tubes with Ficoll-Paque (Wak-Chemie Medical, Steinbach, Germany).

3. Methods

3.1. Preparation of Mononuclear Cells

1. Obtain a buffy coat from a hospital blood center.
2. Dilute the content threefold with PBS.
3. Isolate the mononuclear cell fraction by Ficoll-Paque density separation in UNI-SEP tubes, according to the manufacturer's instructions.
4. Wash the cells twice in PBS.
5. Resuspend the cells in nutrient medium.

3.2. Preparation of Conditioned Medium

1. Isolate mononuclear cells from three buffy coats according to **Subheading 3.1.**
2. Resuspend the cells in BM to 3×10^6 cells/mL.
3. Irradiate with 10 Gy of X-rays.
4. Mix these cells with an equal volume of lymphoblastoid TK6 cells that have been X-irradiated at the same density in BM, but with 40 Gy.
5. Dilute the cell mixture three times with BM to make the final density of each type of cells 5×10^5/mL.
6. Supplement with 2% FCS.
7. Stimulate with 1% PHA.
8. Incubate the cells for 72 h at 37°C with 5% CO_2 in the air.
9. Collect the supernatant by centrifugation at 1500 rpm for 30 min.
10. Store at –80°C.

3.3. Testing for Quality of Conditioned Medium and Human Serum

1. Use a T-cell culture that has been grown in GM for 10 d or more to test for the ability of CM or HS to promote the long-term proliferation of activated T cells on a microplate.
2. Seed each well with 1×10^4 cells in 200 µL GM containing 0.3% PHA and various concentrations of CM or HS. Use an internal laboratory standard batch that has been prepared previously as control.
3. Incubate the plate for at least 1 wk.
4. Compare the cell growth between different wells, both visually by using an inverted microscope and quantitatively by Trypan blue staining and cell counting.

3.4. Mutant Induction

1. Purify lymphocytes from the buffy coat of a healthy blood donor according to **Subheading 3.1.**
2. Wash and resuspend the cells in NM supplemented with 0.3% PHA to a density of 1.5×10^6 cells/mL.

3. Incubate for 20 h.
4. Remove pre-existing in vivo *HPRT* mutants by treating the cells with 2% HAT for 24 h.
5. Wash the cells with PBS and resuspend them in GM to a cell density of 1.5×10^6/mL.
6. Expose the cells to the chemical agent over a day or night.
7. Wash the cells with PBS and resuspend them in GM to a cell density of 1.5×10^6/mL.
8. Seed two 96-well plates with two test cells and 2×10^4 feeder cells per well in GM for determination of relative cloning efficiency (CE: relative survival, treated vs control).
9. Subculture the remaining cells on 24-well plates, in 2 mL GM/well.
10. Incubate for 8 d for mutant expression. Keep approx 2×10^6 cells in each well by cell counting every second day.

3.5. Estimation of the Average Cloning Efficiency and Mutant Frequency

1. Mix 2×10^5 cells from each subculture.
2. Make a limited (stepwise) dilution of cells.
3. Seed on two microplates two "mixed" test cells and 2×10^4 irradiated feeder cells per well without TG.
4. Inoculate 10 selection plates with 2×10^4 "mixed" test cells and 1×10^4 feeder cells per well.
5. Wrap the plates in plastic foil to avoid evaporation and incubate at 37°C in 5% CO_2 and 95% humidity for 2 wk without medium change.
6. Score all plates visually using an inverted microscope.
7. Calculate the CE in plates with and without TG from the proportion of negative wells (P_0) assuming a Poisson distribution: CE = $-\ln P_0$/number of cells seeded per well.
8. Obtain the MF by dividing the cloning efficiency in the presence of TG by that in the absence of TG.

3.6. Mutant Selection for Molecular Analysis

1. Prepare for mutant selection of each subculture on a half 96-well plate.
2. Seed in each microwell 2×10^4 test cells and 1×10^4 feeder cells in GM supplemented with TG (2 µg/mL).
3. Incubate for 2 wk.
4. To avoid sibling mutants in the mutational spectrum, only one TG-resistant clone is to be collected from each microplate (subculture) for molecular analysis.

4. Notes

1. The growth-supporting potency of the CM is usually highest when it is used at 15–20% in GM. The CM should produce consistently high CE, but only when combined with human serum *(5)*. The addition of 5% HS together with 5% FCS in GM has been shown to give a remarkable increase in CE *(5)*. Total replacement of FCS, i.e., use of 10% HS, did not give any further increase, nor did addition of IL-2 (Boehringer Mannheim Biochemical, Mannheim, Germany; 10–20 U/mL) to GM *(5)*.
2. In the present protocol, cells are primed with PHA for 20 h before treatment for up to 24 h. This 44 h of incubation before plating of T cells should not allow any cell division, which may give rise to sibling clones.
3. Cell counting may affect the plating efficiency, since differently experienced technicians may count cells in different ways. In particular, counting only the large stimulated cells may introduce an overestimation of CE. However, theoretically, this should not affect the calculated MF, since the CE in the selection plates is affected to the same extent.

4. Inclusion of feeder cells in selection plates promotes the growth of TG-resistant cells. Use of lethally irradiated RJK853 lymphoblastoid cells originated from a Lesch-Nyhan patient with a total deletion of the *HPRT* gene as feeder cells excludes any cross-contamination of mutant *HPRT* DNA by the remaining *HPRT* sequence from feeder cells in the molecular analysis of *HPRT* mutation. Lethally irradiated lymphoblastoid TK6-derived 36X4 cells with a total deletion of the *HPRT* gene can also be used as feeder cells in both nonselection and selection plates.

5. Donor genotypes for enzymes involved in activation and detoxification of mutagenic agents may affect both background and induced MF and thereby the overall mutagenic potency as judged from the dose–response relationship. Knowledge of the metabolic pathways of the chemical agent and relevant genotypes of the blood donors should thus be taken into consideration. Use of cell mixtures made from buffy coats of several different donors or repeated experiments using cells from different donors may be necessary.

References

1. Morley, A. A., Trainor, K. J., Seshadri, R., and Ryall, R. G. (1983) Measurement of in vivo mutations in human lymphocytes. *Nature* **302**, 155–156.
2. Cariello, N. F., Douglas, G. R., Dycaico, M. J., Gorelick, N. J., Provost, G. S., and Soussi, T. (1997) Databases and software for the analysis of mutations in the human *p53* gene, the human *hprt* gene and both the *lacI* and *lacZ* gene in transgenic rodents. *Nucleic Acids Res.* **25**, 136–137.
3. Hou, S. M. (2000) Somatic mutations and aging: methods for molecular analysis of *HPRT* mutations, in *Aging: Methods and Protocols* (Barnett, Y. A. and Barnett, C. R., eds.), Humana, Totowa, NJ, pp. 189–197.
4. Cole, J. and Skopek, T. R. (1994) Somatic mutant frequency, mutation rates and mutational spectra in the human population in vivo. *Mutat. Res.* **304**, 33–105.
5. Hou, S. M., Falt, S., and Steen, A. M. (1995) *Hprt* mutant frequency and GSTM1 genotype in non-smoking healthy individuals. *Environ. Mol. Mutagen.* **25**, 97–105.
6. Andersson, B., Falt, S., and Lambert, B. (1992) Strand specificity for mutations induced by (+)-anti BPDE in the *hprt* gene in human T-lymphocytes. *Mutat. Res.* **269**, 129–140.
7. Bastlova, T. and Podlutsky, A. (1996) Molecular analysis of styrene oxide-induced hprt mutation in human T-lymphocytes. *Mutagenesis* **11**, 581–591.
8. McGregor, W. G., Maher, V. M., and McCormick, J. J. (1994) Kinds and locations of mutations induced in the hypoxanthine-guanine phosphoribosyltransferase gene of human T-lymphocytes by 1-nitrosopyrene, including those caused by V(D)J recombinase. *Cancer Res.* **54**, 4207–4213.
9. Noori, P. and Hou, S. M. (2001) Mutational spectrum induced by acetaldehyde in the *HPRT* gene of human T lymphocytes resembles that in the *p53* gene of esophageal cancers. *Carcinogenesis* **22**, 1825–1830.
10. Hou, S. M., Van Dam, F. J., de Zwart, F., et al. (1999) Validation of the human T-lymphocyte cloning assay—ring test report from the EU concerted action on *HPRT* mutation (EUCAHM). *Mutat. Res.* **431**, 211–221.
11. Norimura, T., Maher, V. M., and McCormick, J. J. (1990) A quantitative assay for measuring the induction of mutations in human peripheral blood T-lymphocytes. *Mutat. Res.* **230**, 101–109.

16

Molecular Analysis of Mutations in the Human *HPRT* Gene

Phouthone Keohavong, Liqiang Xi, and Stephen G. Grant

Summary

The *HPRT* assay uses incorporation of toxic nucleotide analogs to select for cells lacking the purine scavenger enzyme hypoxanthine-guanine phosporibosyltransferase. A major advantage of this assay is the ability to isolate mutant cells and determine the molecular basis for their functional deficiency. Many types of analyses have been performed at this locus: the current protocol involves generation of a cDNA and multiplex PCR of each exon, including the intron/exon junctions, followed by direct sequencing of the products. This analysis detects point mutations, small deletions and insertions within the gene, mutations affecting RNA splicing, and the products of illegitimate V(D)J recombination within the gene. Establishment of and comparisons with mutational spectra hold the promise of identifying exposures to mutation-inducing genotoxicants from their distinctive pattern of gene-specific DNA damage at this easily analyzed reporter gene.

Key Words: *HPRT*; mutation; mutational spectra; deletions; recombination; mutational fingerprint.

1. Introduction

The hypoxanthine-guanine phosphoribosyltransferase *(HPRT)* gene and the mutation selection system based on it have played a major role in molecular genetics. Indeed, this system was used to establish that somatic variants arising in cultured somatic cell populations were mutants, and an amplification mutant allowed for early cloning of the *HPRT* gene *(1)*. One of the earliest mutational spectra compiled was that of inherited mutations in *HPRT (2)*, which is responsible for the self-mutilation disorder Lesch-Nyhan syndrome, and, in less severe forms, gout *(3)*. Ongoing expansion of this mutational spectrum has allowed for genotype/phenotype analyses that have helped map the functional regions of the gene and aid in diagnosis *(4)*.

The *HPRT* gene is located on the mammalian X chromosome and is subject to X inactivation; it is therefore either structurally or functionally hemizygous in all mammalian somatic cells. The HPRT enzyme plays a key role in the purine scavenger pathway, which allowed for the early development of selective systems both for and against enzyme activity *(5–7)*. These selective systems have been used extensively to

From: *Methods in Molecular Biology, vol. 291, Molecular Toxicology Protocols*
Edited by: P. Keohavong and S. G. Grant © Humana Press Inc., Totowa, NJ

genetically manipulate somatic cells, including in the construction of hybridoma cell lines for the generation of monoclonal antibodies. *HPRT* mutations can be selected in almost any established mammalian cell line and in T lymphocytes from humans *(8,9)* and a number of animal species *(10–12)*.

The ability to capture and characterize further mutant clones has always been a major advantage of the *HPRT* assay *(13)*. The latest analysis techniques have always been applied to such mutants, beginning with determination of residual enzyme activity *(14)* and immunological detection of inactive protein *(15)*. Karyotypic analyses confirmed that most *HPRT* mutations do not have detectable chromosomal abnormalities *(16)*, unless the mutations were induced by in vitro exposure to ionizing radiation *(17,18)* or isolated from individuals subjected to whole-body radiation *(19)*.

With the advent of molecular biology techniques, it was found that a variable but significant proportion (10–60%) of in vivo derived *HPRT* mutants had undergone structural rearrangement, based on Southern blot analysis *(20–23*; *see* **Note 1**). The proportion of mutants containing such rearrangements was increased by in vitro *(24,25)* or in vivo *(26,27)* exposure to ionizing radiation, consistent with an overall increase in mutation frequency (*see* **Note 2**). The extent of such rearrangements, including gene deletions, was established by analysis of mutant clones with pulsed-field gel electrophoresis *(28,29)* and analysis of flanking markers *(28,30–32)*.

Polymerase chain reaction (PCR) analysis allowed for the direct sequencing of the *HPRT* transcript *(33)*, and multimeric PCR allowed for the concurrent analysis of all nine exons of the *HPRT* gene *(34)*, identifying point mutations and splicing mutations *(35,36)*. This also allowed for the application of heteroduplex screening techniques for the identification of mutants, such as single-strand conformation polymorphisms *(37,38)* and denaturing gradient gel electrophoresis *(39,40)*.

Of course, the ultimate goal of this type of molecular analysis is identification of the causal agents behind mutations in oncogenes like K-*ras* and *p53* *(41,42*; *see* also Chaps. 18–20). Perhaps the best example of this type of analysis remains the demonstration of distinctive mutations in the *p53* gene of hepatocellular carcinomas from a population in Qidong County, China, which identified aflatoxin B1 as the causative agent *(43)*. *HPRT* mutation frequencies were also elevated in this population *(44)*, and a comparative mutational spectrum was generated for this chemical by in vitro exposure *(45)*.

An on-line compendium of such *HPRT* mutational spectra has been established, which also provides software for pattern analysis and comparison *(46,47)*. The same site contains tumor-derived mutation spectra at the *p53* gene (*see* Chap. 18), as well as spectra based on transgenic systems, such as that described in Chapter 13.

2. Materials

2.1. cDNA Synthesis

1. Microcentrifuge (e.g., Eppendorf 5415 D, Fisher Scientific, Pittsburgh, PA).
2. 0.5-mL Biopur microcentrifuge tubes (Brinkmann Instruments, Westbury, NY).
3. Aerosol Barrier Pipette tips (30, 200, and 1000 µL; Fisher).
4. 20-, 200-, and 1000-µL micropipetors (Rainin, Woburn, MA).

5. RNase- and DNase-free water (Sigma, St. Louis, MO).
6. Phosphate-buffered saline (PBS; Gibco, Gaithersburg, MD).
7. 1.0 *M* Tris-HCl, pH 8.3.
8. 2.5 *M* KCl.
9. 100 m*M* MgCl$_2$.
10. 15 m*M* dithithreitol (DTT).
11. 25 m*M* dNTPs (Promega, Madison, WI).
12. IGEPAL ([octylphenoxyl]polyethoxyethanol; Sigma).
13. 2.8 µg/mL Bovine serum albumin (BSA).
14. 40 U/µL RNAse inhibitors (Invitrogen, Carlsbad, CA).
15. 200 ng/µL Oligo dT (Invitrogen).
16. Super Script II Rnase H$^-$ reverse transcriptase (SSRT; Invitrogen).
17. cDNA synthesis buffer and reagents: 50 m*M* Tris-HCl, 75 m*M* KCl, 3 m*M* MgCl$_2$, pH 8.3, 10 m*M* DTT, 0.1 ng/µL BSA, 500 µ*M* dNTPs, 0.1 ng/µL Rnase inhibitors, 10 ng/µL IGPEAL, 10 ng/mL oligo (dT); 2.5 U/µL SSRT enzyme.

To make 100 mL cDNA synthesis buffer:

Reagent	Stock concentration	Final concentration	Volume added (µL)
KCL	2.5 *M*	75 m*M*	3
MgCL$_2$	0.1 *M*	3 m*M*	3
Tris-HCL	1 *M*	50 m*M*	5
DTT	15 m*M*	10 m*M*	10
dNTPs	15 m*M*	0.5 m*M*	3.3
BSA	2.8 µg/mL	0.1 ng/mL	3.57
RNAase	40 U/µL	1 U/µL	2.5
Oligo dT	200 ng/µL	10 ng/µL	5
IGEPAL			2.5
SSRT			10
Water			52.13
Total			100

18. 42°C heating block or water bath.
19. Vortex mixer.
20. DNA thermocycler (e.g., Perkin Elmer 480, Wellesley, MA).

2.2. PCR Amplification of the HPRT cDNA

1. 0.5-mL Microcentrifuge tubes.
2. 5 U/µL Taq DNA polymerase (Promega).
3. 10X PCR buffer: 500 m*M* KCl, 100 m*M* Tris-HCl, pH 9.0, at 25°C, 15 m*M* MgCl$_2$, 0.1% Triton X-100 (supplied with enzyme).
4. 25 m*M* dNTPs.
5. RNase- and DNase-free water.
6. PCR primers (Midland Certified Reagent, Midland, TX. Each primer is prepared as a 10 µ*M* stock solution in RNase- and DNase-free water and stored at –20°C.
   a. P1: 5'-CTGCTCCGCCACCGGCTTCC-3' (corresponding to bases 1617–1636 of the human *HPRT* gene).

    b. P2: 5'-GATAATTTTACTGGCGATGT-3' (bases 41,565–41,546).

    c. P3: 5'-CCTGAGCAGTCAGCCCGCGC-3' (bases 1641–1660).

    d. P4: 5'-CAATAGGACTCCAGATGTTT-3' (bases 41,545–41,526).

7. 1:37.5 *bis*/acrylamide stock solution: dissolve 1.0 g *bis* and 37.5 g acrylamide (Bio-Rad, Hercules, CA) in a final 100 mL vol with deionized water.

8. 1:19 *bis*/acrylamide stock solution: dissolve 1.0 g *bis* and 19.0 g acrylamide in a final 100 mL vol with deionized water.

9. Vertical gel electrophoresis apparatus: gel boxes, plates, and accessories for a 20-cm wide × 16-cm high gel (Gibco-BRL).

10. Power source (e.g., Pharmacia LKB ECPS 3000/150, Amersham BioSciences, Piscataway, NJ).

11. ABI automated sequencing machine (i.e., University of Pittsburgh DNA Sequencing Facility, Pittsburgh, PA).

2.3. HPRT *Gene Multi-Exon Analysis*

1. Microcentrifuge.

2. PBS.

3. 20-, 200-, and 1000-µL micropipetors and appropriate pipet tips.

4. 0.5-mL Microcentrifuge tubes.

5. Lysis buffer: 6.7 mM MgCl$_2$, 16.6 mM (NH$_4$)$_2$SO$_4$, 6.8 µM EDTA, 67 mM Tris-HCl, pH 8.8, 5 mM 2-mercaptoethanol, 0.45% IGEPAL, 0.45% Tween-20, and 100 µg/mL proteinase K.

6. 56°C heating block or water bath.

7. DNA thermocycler.

8. PCR primers. Each primer is prepared as a 10 µM stock solution in RNase- and DNase-free water and stored at –20°C.

    a. Exon 2:   P796: 5'-TGGGATTACACGTGTGAACCAACC-3'.
                        P797: 5'-GACTCTGGCTAGAGTTCCTTCTTC-3'.

    b. Exon 3:   P983: 5'-CCTTATGAAACATGAGGGCAAAGG-3'.
                        P969: 5'-TGTGACACAGGCAGACTGTGGATC-3'.

    c. Exon 4:   P1147: 5'-TAGCTAGCTAACTTCTCAAATCTTCTAG-3'.
                        P1011: 5'-ATTAACCTAGACTGCTTCCAAGGG-3'.

    d. Exon 5:   P885: 5'-CAGGCTTCCAAATCCCAGCAGATG-3'.
                        P1174: 5'-GGGAACCACATTTTGAGAACCACT-3'.

    e. Exon 6:   P1012: 5'-GACAGTATTGCAGTTATACATGGGG-3'.
                        P1013: 5'-CCAAAATCCTCTGCCATGCTATTC-3'.

    f. Exons 7/8:   P483: 5'-GATCGCTAGAGCCCAAGAAGTCAAG-3'.
                        P854: 5'-TATGAGGTGCTGGAAGGAGAAAAC-3'.

    g. Exon 9:   P1015: 5'-GAGGCAGAAGTCCCATGGATGTGT-3'.
                        P365: 5'-CCGCCCAAAGGGAACTGATAGTC-3'.

    h. Exon 1: this exon is amplified separately, using the following primers:
                pE1: 5'-AGCTTCAGGCGGCTGCGACGAGCCCTCAGG-3',
                (corresponding to bases 1530–1559 of the human *HPRT* gene).
                pE2: 5'-CGGCCGCCCGAGCCCGCACTGCGGATCCCG-3'
                (corresponding to bases 1804–1775).

9. Primer mix preparation (*see* **Note 3**). Primer pairs corresponding to exons 2–9 are premixed as a 10X mixed primer stock solution containing 1 µM each of the exon 2 and 9

primers, 1.5 µ*M* each of the primers for exons 4 and 6, and 2 µ*M* each of the primers for exons 3, 5, and 7/8. Exon 1 is amplified separately, requiring a separate primer stock solution of 10 µ*M* each for primers pE1 and pE2.

10. FailSafe PCR2X Premix A (FSP995A, Epicentre Technologies, Madison, WI).
11. Failsafe PCR Enzyme mix (containing Taq polymerase at 2.5 U/µL; FS99250, Epicentre).
12. 1:37.5 *bis*/acrylamide stock solution.
13. 1:19 *bis*/acrylamide stock solution.
14. Vertical gel electrophoresis apparatus.
15. Power source.

3. Methods

3.1. cDNA Synthesis

1. If beginning with frozen aliquots of cells from a –80°C freezer, thaw the cells on ice in an ice bucket for 30 min. Remove one aliquot of each clone (consisting of 2×10^4 cells in serum-free medium containing 10% dimethyl sulfoxide (DMSO) in a microcentrifuge tube).
2. Microcentrifuge at 8900*g* (microcentrifuge placed inside a 4°C standing refrigerator or a cold room) for 5 min. Remove and discard medium containing DMSO.
3. Wash pellet gently with 50 µL cold PBS, and microcentrifuge at 8900*g* for 2 min.
4. Remove PBS completely, add 5 µL of cDNA synthesis buffer, and incubate at 42°C for 60 min.
5. Heat at 95°C for 5 min in a thermocycler to inactivate reverse transcriptase enzyme and denature the cDNA–mRNA duplex. Cool down to 22°C and microcentrifuge at high speed for 2 s.

3.2. Nested PCR Amplification of the HPRT cDNA

1. For each cDNA, prepare a 0.5-mL PCR tube with 2.5 µL 10X PCR buffer, 0.5 µL 25 m*M* dNTPs, 0.5 µL each of primers P1 and P2 (final concentration 0.2 µ*M*), 0.3 µL Taq enzyme (1.5 U), and 18.2 µL RNase- and DNase-free water.
2. To each tube add 2.5 µL of the appropriate cDNA from **Subheading 3.1.** and mix. Microcentrifuge each tube for 2 s at high speed and cover each PCR solution with mineral oil.
3. Amplify the samples in a thermocycler using a temperature profile of (94°C/1 min + 55°C/45 s + 72°C/2 min) for 25 cycles and then extend at 72°C for 7 min.
4. For the second round of amplification, for each cDNA, prepare a 0.5-mL PCR tube with 2.5 µL 10X PCR buffer, 0.5 µL 25 m*M* dNTPs, 0. 5 µL each of primers P3 and P4 (final concentration 2 µ*M*), 0.3 µL Taq enzyme (1.5 U), and 19.7 µL RNase- and DNase-free water.
5. To each tube add 1 µL of the appropriate first-round PCR product from **Subheading 3.2., step 3**. Mix and microcentrifuge each tube for 2 s at high speed. Cover each reaction with mineral oil.
6. Amplify the samples in a thermocycler using a temperature profile of (94°C/1 min + 55°C/45 s + 72°C/2 min) for 25 cycles, and then extend at 72°C for 7 min.
7. Check the product in a 6% polyacrylamide gel run at 300 V for 1.5 h.
   Possible results:

   a. No product. Indicative of deletion, transcription mutation, or splicing mutation resulting in unstable mRNA.
   b. Full-length product. (~780 bp). Indicative of point mutations, small insertion/deletion (1–10 bases).

   c. Reduced size product. Indicative of intragenic deletion, splicing mutation (specific exon skipping), or frameshift mutation resulting in premature termination.

   d. In rare cases, increased size product, indicative of insertion.

8. Purify the amplified cDNA products by separation on a 6% polyacrylamide gel electrophoresis and DNA fragment isolation from the gel.

9. Sequence with primers P3 and/or P4, using an ABI automated sequencing machine.

3.3. HPRT *Gene Multi-Exon Analysis*

Clones with results from the cDNA analysis consistent with genomic deletion (absence of an amplified cDNA or presence of a shorter than expected cDNA) can be further characterized to potentially identify the deleted genomic sequence, using a multi-exon PCR.

1. If beginning with frozen aliquots of cells, remove one aliquot of each clone (consisting of 10^4 cells in serum-free medium containing 10% DMSO in a microcentrifuge tube) from a –80°C freezer and thaw on ice.

2. Microcentrifuge at 8900g for 5 min. Remove and discard medium containing DMSO.

3. Wash pellet gently with cold 50 µL PBS, and microcentrifuge at 8900g for 2 min.

4. Remove PBS, add 50 µL of lysis buffer, and incubate at 56°C for at least 1 h.

5. Heat at 96°C for 10 min in a thermocycler to inactivate proteinase K and cool down to 22°C. Spin for 2 s (microcentrifuge).

6. For each sample, prepare a PCR tube with 2.5 µL primers mix, 12.5 µL FailSafe PCR 2X Premix A and 7.0 µL RNase- and DNase-free water.

7. Add 2.5 µL crude DNA preparation (from **step 5**).

8. Add 0.5 µL Failsafe PCR Enzyme mix to each tube.

9. Amplify the samples in a thermocycler using a temperature profile of (94°C/4 min) × 1 + (94°C/30 s + 61°C/50 s + 68°C/2 min) × 35 cycles, and then extend at 68°C for 7 min.

10. Analyze 5 µL of each amplified product on a 6–8% polyacrylmide gel.

11. Amplify exon 1 in a separate reaction, using the protocol described in **steps 1–10** above, except that 0.5 µM each of primers pE1 and pE2 are used in **step 6** (*see* **Note 3**).

12. Interpret gel (*see* **Note 4**).

4. Notes

1. A specific type of intragenic deletion involving loss of exons 2 and 3 has been shown to occur through the action of the V(D)J recombinase enzyme at cryptic sites in the second and fourth introns of the *HPRT* gene *(48,49)* (*see* Chap. 17). Although these mutations can be traced to a specific mechanism, "illegitimate" recombination, this mechanism only occurs during the development of the immune system, so it is restricted to T and B cells. If the *HPRT* gene is being used as a surrogate for mutation in another tissue, these recombination-generated mutations are not only irrelevant, they are misleading, because they artificially inflate the mutation frequency (although they should be relevant to leukemia and lymphoma, in which much of the carcinogenic process occurs via this mechanism *[50]*). These recombination-derived deletions can now be enumerated directly *(51)* (*see* Chap. 17*)* and should be accounted for in the compilation of any *HPRT* mutational spectrum generated in T lymphocytes.

2. Another way in which molecular analysis can affect the mutation frequency is by determining how many times a single mutant clone is represented in a sample population (in general, such duplication is a negligible contributor to mutation frequency *[21,52]*, al-

though in rare cases it can have an important effect *[53]*). Because each rearrangement of the T-cell receptor locus is unique, molecular analysis of this locus can identify multiple mutants derived from the same initial event *(54,55)*.

3. The concentrations of primers in the 10X mixed primers stock are those that allowed simultaneous PCR amplification of fragments corresponding to each of exons 2–9, under the reaction mixture and conditions provided, as revealed by the detection of these fragments by polyacrylamide gel electrophoresis analysis. The source of primers, the preparation of each primer stock and of mixed primer stock, and the PCR mixture and reaction conditions have been found to affect the efficiency of amplification of some fragments. Therefore, the concentration of primers in the mixed primers stock may need to be readjusted for some exons to obtain an efficient amplification. Exon 1 is very rich in G/C bases, and it proves very difficult to amplify it by the multi-exon PCR method. This exon is thus amplified separately from the other exons.

4. A shortened cDNA corresponding to specific loss of exons 2 and 3 and/or inability to amplify only these two exons is highly indicative of a mutation caused by illegitimate V(D)J recombination (*see* **Note 1**). A protocol for confirming this mechanism of specific deletion by direct PCR amplification through the characteristic deletion breakpoint is given in Chapter 17.

References

1. Brennand, J., Chinault, A. C., Konecki, D. S., Melton, D. W., and Caskey, C. T. (1982) Cloned cDNA sequences of the hypoxanthine/guanine phosphoribosyltransferase gene from a mouse neuroblastoma cell line found to have amplified genomic sequences. *Proc. Natl. Acad. Sci. USA* **79,** 1950–1954.

2. Patel, P. I., Yang, T. P., Stout, J. T., Konecki, D. S., Chinault, A. C., and Caskey, C. T. (1986) Mutational diversity at the human HPRT locus. *Prog. Clin. Biol. Res.* **209A,** 457–463.

3. Stout, J. T. and Caskey, C. T. (1988) The Lesch-Nyhan syndrome: clinical, molecular and genetic aspects. *Trends Genet.* **4,** 175–178.

4. Jinnah, H. A., De Gregorio, L., Harris, J. C., Nyhan, W. L, and O'Neill, J. P. (2000) The spectrum of inherited mutations causing HPRT deficiency: 75 new cases and a review of 196 previously reported cases. *Mutat. Res.* **463,** 309–326.

5. Szybalski, W. (1959) Genetics of human cell lines. II. Methods or determination of mutation rates to drug resistance. *Exp. Cell Res.* **18,** 588–591.

6. Szybalski, W., Szybalski, E. H., and Ragni, G. (1962) Genetic studies with human cell lines. *Natl. Cancer Inst. Monogr.* **7,** 75–78.

7. Chu, E. H. Y. and Malling, H. V. (1968) Mammalian cell genetics. II. Chemical induction of specific locus mutations in Chinese hamster cells *in vitro*. *Proc. Natl. Acad. Sci. USA* **61,** 1306–1312.

8. Albertini, R. J., Castle, K. L., and Borcherding, W. R. (1982) T-cell cloning to detect the mutant 6-thioguanine-resistant lymphocytes present in human peripheral blood. *Proc. Natl. Acad. Sci. USA* **79,** 6617–6621.

9. Morley, A. A., Cox, S., Wigmore, D., Seshadri, R., and Dempsey, J. L. (1982) Enumeration of thioguanine-resistant lymphocytes using autoradiography. *Mutat. Res.* **95,** 363–375.

10. Jones, I. M., Burkhart-Schultz, K., and Carrano, A. V. (1985) A method to quantify spontaneous and *in vivo* induced thioguanine-resistant mouse lymphocytes. *Mutat. Res.* **147,** 97–105.

11. Zimmer, D. M., Aaron, C. S., O'Neill, J. P., and Albertini, R. J. (1991) Enumeration of 6-thioguanine-resistant T-lymphocytes in the peripheral blood of nonhuman primates (*Cynomolgus* monkeys). *Environ. Mol. Mutagen.* **18,** 161–167.

12. Aidoo, A., Morris, S. M., and Casciano, D. A. (1997) Development and utilization of the rat lymphocyte *hprt* mutation assay. *Mutat. Res.* **387,** 69–88.
13. Grant, S. G. and Jensen, R. H. (1993) Use of hematopoietic cells and markers for the detection and quantitation of human *in vivo* somatic mutation, in *Immunobiology of Transfusion Medicine* (Garratty, G., ed.), Marcel Dekker, New York, pp. 299–323.
14. Clements, G. B. (1975) Selection of biochemically variant, in some cases mutant, mammalian cells in culture. *Adv. Cancer Res.* **21,** 273–390.
15. Epstein, J., Ghangas, G. S., Leyva, A., Milman, G., and Littlefield, J. W. (1979) Analysis of HGPRT⁻ CRM⁺ human lymphoblast mutants. *Somatic Cell Genet.* **5,** 809–820.
16. Muir, P., Osborne, Y., Morley, A. A., and Turner, D. R. (1988) Karyotypic abnormality of the X chromosome is rare in mutant HPRT⁻ lymphocyte clones. *Mutat. Res.* **197,** 157–160.
17. Thacker, J. (1981) The chromosomes of a V79 Chinese hamster line and a mutant subline lacking HPRT activity. *Cytogenet. Cell Genet.* **29,** 16–25.
18. Fuscoe, J. C., Zimmerman, L. J., Fekete, A., Setzer, R.W., and Rossiter, B. J. (1992) Analysis of X-ray-induced HPRT mutations in CHO cells: insertion and deletions. *Mutat. Res.* **269,** 171–183.
19. Kodama, Y., Hakoda, M., Shimba, H., Awa, A. A., and Akiyama, M. (1989) A chromosome study of 6-thioguanine-resistant mutants in T lymphocytes of Hiroshima atomic bomb survivors. *Mutat. Res.* **227,** 31–38.
20. Turner, D. R., Morley, A. A., Haliandros, M., Kutlaca, R., and Sanderson, B. J. (1985) *In vivo* somatic mutations in human lymphocytes frequently result from major gene alterations. *Nature* **315,** 343–345.
21. Albertini, R. J., O'Neill, J. P., Nicklas, J. A., Heintz, N. H., and Kelleher, P. C. (1985) Alterations of the *hprt* gene in human *in vivo*-derived 6-thioguanine-resistant T lymphocytes. *Nature* **316,** 369–371.
22. Nicklas, J. A., Hunter, T. C., Sullivan, L. M., Berman, J. K., O'Neill, J. P., and Albertini, R. J. (1987) Molecular analyses of *in vivo hprt* mutations in human T-lymphocytes. I. Studies of low frequency, 'spontaneous' mutants by Southern blots. *Mutagenesis* **2,** 341–347.
23. Bradley, W. E. C., Gareau, J. L., Seifert, A. M., and Messing, K. (1987) Molecular characterization of 15 rearrangements among 90 human *in vivo* somatic mutants shows that deletions predominate. *Mol. Cell. Biol.* **7,** 956–960.
24. Skulimowski, A. W., Turner, D. R., Morley, A. A., Sanderson, B. J. S., and Haliandros, M. (1986) Molecular basis of X-ray-induced mutation at the *HPRT* locus in human lymphocytes. *Mutat. Res.* **162,** 105–112.
25. O'Neill, J. P., Hunter, T. C., Sullivan, L. M., Nicklas, J. A., and Albertini, R. J. (1990) Southern-blot analyses of human T-lymphocyte mutants induced *in vitro* by γ-irradiation. *Mutat. Res.* **240,** 143–149.
26. Hakoda, M., Hirai, Y., Kyoizumi, S., and Akiyama, M. (1989) Molecular analyses of *in vivo hprt* mutant T cells from atomic bomb survivors. *Environ. Mol. Mutagen.* **13,** 25–33.
27. Nicklas, J. A., O'Neill, J. P., Hunter, T. C., et al. (1991) *In vivo* ionizing irradiations produce deletions in the *hprt* gene of human T-lymphocytes. *Mutat. Res.* **250,** 383–396.
28. Nicklas, J. A., Lippert, M. J., Hunter, T. C., O'Neill, J. P., and Albertini, R. J. (1991) Analysis of human *HPRT* deletion mutations with X-linked probes and pulsed field gel electrophoresis. *Environ. Mol. Mutagen.* **18,** 270–273.
29. Lippert, M. J., Nicklas, J. A., Hunter, T. C., and Albertini, R. J. (1995) Pulsed field analysis of *hprt* T-cell large deletions: telomeric region breakpoint spectrum. *Mutat. Res.* **326,** 51–64.

30. Fuscoe, J. C., Zimmerman, L. J., Harrington-Brock, K., and Moore, M. M. (1992) Large deletions are tolerated at the *hprt* locus of *in vivo* derived human T-lymphocytes. *Mutat. Res.* **283,** 255–262.

31. Fuscoe, J. C., Nelsen, A. J., and Pilia, G. (1994) Detection of deletion mutations extending beyond the HPRT gene by multiplex PCR analysis. *Somat. Cell Mol. Genet.* **20,** 39–46.

32. Nelson, S. L., Jones, I. M., Fuscoe, J. C., Burkhart-Schultz, K., and Grosovsky, A. J. (1995) Mapping the end points of large deletions affecting the *hprt* locus in human peripheral blood cells and cell lines. *Radiat. Res.* **141,** 2–10.

33. Recio, L., Cochrane, J., Simpson, D., et al. (1990) DNA sequence analysis of *in vivo hprt* mutation in human T lymphocytes. *Mutagenesis* **5,** 505–510.

34. Gibbs R. A., Nguyen, P. N., Edwards, A., Civitello, A. B., and Caskey, C. T. (1990) Multiplex DNA deletion detection and exon sequencing of the hypoxanthine phosphoribosyltransferase gene in Lesch-Nyhan families. *Genomics* **7,** 235–244.

35. Rossi, A. M., Tates, A. D., van Zeeland, A. A., and Vrieling, H. (1992) Molecular analysis of mutations affecting *hprt* mRNA splicing in human T-lymphocytes *in vivo*. *Environ. Mol. Mutagen.* **19,** 7–13.

36. Steingrimsdottir, H., Rowley, G., Dorado, G., Cole, J., and Lehmann, A. R. (1992) Mutations which alter splicing in the human hypoxanthine-guanine phosphoribosyltransferase gene. *Nucleic Acids Res.* **20,** 1201–1208.

37. Caggana, M., Benjamin, M. B., Little, J. B., Liber, H. L., and Kelsey, K. T. (1991) Single-strand conformation polymorphisms can be used to detect T cell receptor gene rearrangements: an application to the *in vivo hprt* mutation assay. *Mutagenesis* **6,** 375–379.

38. Fuscoe, J. C., Zimmerman, L. J., Harrington-Brock, K., and Moore, M. M. (1994) Multiplex PCR analysis of *in vivo*-arising deletion mutations in the *hprt* gene of human T-lymphocytes. *Environ. Mol. Mutagen.* **23,** 89–95.

39. Keohavong, P. and Thilly, W. G. (1992) Determination of the point mutational spectra of benzo[*a*]pyrene-diol epoxide in human cells. *Environ. Health Perspect.* **98,** 215–219.

40. Cariello, N. F. and Skopek, T. R. (1993) Mutational analysis using denaturing gel electrophoresis and PCR. *Mutat. Res.* **288,** 103–112.

41. Keohavong, P. and Thilly, W. G. (1992) Mutational spectrometry: a general approach for hot spot point mutations in selectable genes. *Proc. Natl. Acad. Sci. USA* **89,** 4623–4627.

42. Molholt, B. and Finette, B. A. (2000) Distinguishing potential sources of genotoxic exposure via HPRT mutations. *Radiat. Biol. Radioecol.* **40,** 529–534.

43. Hsu, I. C., Metcalf, R. A., Sun, T., Welsh, J. A., Wang, N. J., and Harris, C. C. (1991) Mutational hotspot in the *p53* gene in human hepatocellular carcinomas. *Nature* **350,** 427–428.

44. Wang, S. S., O'Neill, J. P., Qian, G. S., et al. (199) Elevated HPRT mutation frequencies in aflatoxin-exposed residents of daxin, Qidong county, People's Republic of China. *Carcinogenesis* **20,** 2181–2184.

45. Cariello, N. F., Cui, L., and Skopek, T. R. (1994) *In vitro* mutational spectrum of aflatoxin B1 in the human hypoxanthine guanine phosphoribosyltransferase gene. *Cancer Res.* **54,** 4436–4441.

46. Cariello, N. F., Craft, T. R., Vrieling, H., van Zeeland, A. A., Adams, T., and Skopek, T. R. (1992) Human HPRT mutant database: software for data entry and retrieval. *Environ. Mol. Mutagen.* **20,** 81–83.

47. Cariello, N. F., Douglas, G. R., Gorelick, N. J., Hart, D. W., Wilson, J. D., and Soussi, T. (1998) Databases and software for the analysis of mutations in the human *p53* gene, human hprt gene and both the *lacI* and *lacZ* gene in transgenic rodents. *Nucleic Acids Res.* **26,** 198–199.

48. Fuscoe, J. C., Zimmerman, L. J., Lippert, M. J., Nicklas, J. A., O'Neill, J. P., and Albertini, R. J. (1991) V(D)J recombinase-like activity mediates *hprt* gene deletion in human fetal T-lymphocytes. *Cancer Res.* **51,** 6001–6005.
49. Fuscoe, J. C., Zimmerman, L. J., Harrington-Brock, K., et al. (1992) V(D)J recombinase-mediated deletion of the *hprt* gene in T-lymphocytes from adult humans. *Mutat. Res.* **283,** 13–20.
50. Davila, M., Foster, S., Kelsoe, G., and Yang, K. (2001) A role for secondary V(D)J recombination in oncogenic chromosomal translocations? *Adv. Cancer Res.* **81,** 61–92.
51. Fuscoe, J. C., Vira, L. K., Collard, D. D., and Moore, M. M. (1997) Quantification of *hprt* gene deletions mediated by illegitimate V(D)J recombination in peripheral blood cells of humans. *Environ. Mol. Mutagen.* **29,** 28–35.
52. O'Neill, J. P., Nicklas, J. A., Hunter, T. C., et al. (1994) The effect of T-lymphocyte 'clonality' on the calculated *hprt* mutation frequency occurring *in vivo* in humans. *Mutat. Res.* **313,** 215–225.
53. Nicklas, J. A., O'Neill, J. P., Sullivan, L. M., et al. (1988) Molecular analyses of *in vivo* hypoxanthine-guanine phosphoribosyltransferase mutations in human T-lymphocytes: II. Demonstration of a clonal amplification of *hprt* mutant T-lymphocytes *in vivo*. *Environ. Mol. Mutagen.* **12,** 271–284.
54. Nicklas, J. A., O'Neill, J. P., and Albertini, R. J. (1986) Use of T-cell receptor gene probes to quantify the *in vivo hprt* mutations in human T-lymphocytes. *Mutat. Res.* **173,** 67–72.
55. de Boer, J. G., Curry, J. D., and Glickman, B. W. (1993) A fast method to determine the clonal relationship among human T-cell lymphocytes. *Mutat. Res.* **288,** 173–180.

17

Simultaneous Quantification of t(14;18) and *HPRT* Exon 2/3 Deletions in Human Lymphocytes

James C. Fuscoe

Summary

Specific recurring chromosomal translocations and deletions are found in a variety of cancers. In hematopoietic malignancies, many of these chromosomal aberrations result from mistakes involving V(D)J recombination. V(D)J recombination is required for the formation of functional T-cell receptor genes in T cells and antibody genes in B cells. This is an inherently dangerous process, however, because double-strand breaks are introduced into the chromosomes. Molecular evidence indicates that failure of the fidelity of this process results in the activation of proto-oncogenes or the inactivation of tumor suppressor genes. Here we describe sensitive, quantitative PCR assays for the measurement of such events in human lymphocytes. One assay measures the frequency of t(14;18) translocations that result in the dysfunctional regulation of the antiapoptotic gene *BCL-2*. The other assay measures the frequency of a deletion caused by illegitimate V(D)J recombination in the X-linked *HPRT* gene.

Key Words: Translocation; deletion; lymphocytes; V(D)J recombination; illegitimate V(D)J recombination; *HPRT* deletions; t(14;18) translocation; quantitative PCR assay; Poisson statistics; human; cancer; biomarker.

1. Introduction

A t(14;18) chromosomal translocation is found in approx 85% of follicular lymphomas by both cytogenetic and molecular analyses *(1,2)*. This rearrangement deregulates expression of the *BCL-2* oncogene by juxtaposition into the *Ig* heavy chain locus *(3)* and is probably mediated by illegitimate V(D)J recombination. Sensitive polymerase chain reaction (PCR)-based assays have been developed for the detection of this translocation in peripheral blood lymphocytes *(4–10)*. Interestingly, the t(14;18) can be detected at low levels in almost all healthy individuals *(10)*.

A characteristic deletion of exons 2 and 3 of the X-linked hypoxanthine guanine phosphoribosyltransferase *(HPRT)* gene is also mediated by illegitimate V(D)J recombination. This deletion was first discovered in cord blood lymphocytes *(11)* and was subsequently found in adults *(12)*. A quantitative PCR assay was developed to

From: *Methods in Molecular Biology, vol. 291,Molecular Toxicology Protocols*
Edited by: P. Keohavong and S. G. Grant © Humana Press Inc., Totowa, NJ

measure the frequency of this deletion in peripheral blood cells of humans, in which it was found to range from $<1.3 \times 10^{-7}$ to 4.1×10^{-7} *(13)*. We have also shown that this V(D)J recombinase-mediated deletion can be induced in vitro by the chemotherapy drug etoposide *(14)* and that prolonged dosage schedules may reduce the recombinogenic properties of etoposide while maintaining its clinically important cytotoxicity *(15)*. In addition, a human lymphoid leukemia cell line has been isolated as part of these studies that contains a V(D)J recombinase-mediated *HPRT* exon 2/3 deletion *(16)*.

Recently, we have developed a quantitative nested PCR method for simultaneous detection of these two events in human peripheral blood lymphocytes *(17)*. We have used the assay to quantify these mutations in healthy adults and newborns *(18)*, as well as in children treated with etoposide-containing antileukemic therapy *(17)*. Briefly, genomic DNA is purified from peripheral blood lymphocytes, and 2.5 µg (representing approx 4×10^5 cells) are amplified with both translocation-specific primers and deletion-specific primers under conditions in which a single copy of either mutant DNA, if present, will give a detectable PCR product. Multiple replicates are analyzed for each individual, and Poisson statistics are then used to estimate the translocation and deletion mutant frequency. The purpose of this assay, therefore, is to quantify the frequency of lymphocytes containing t(14;18) or deletion of exons 2+3 in the human *HPRT* gene.

2. Materials

2.1. Lymphocyte Isolation

1. Heparinized blood collection tubes (VWR, West Chester, PA).
2. Approximately 50 mL Hanks' phosphate-buffered saline (PBS; Life Technologies, Rockville, MD) or equivalent.
3. 50-mL Centrifuge tubes (e.g., Falcon, BD Biosciences, Franklin Lakes, NJ).
4. 10-mL Pipets.
5. Approximately 60 mL Histopaque-1077 (Sigma, St. Louis, MO) or Ficoll-Paque (Amersham Biosciences, Piscataway, NJ).
6. Benchtop centrifuge (e.g., Thermo IEC HN-SII, Fisher Scientific, Pittsburgh, PA).
7. Approximately 250 mL Tris-buffered saline (TBS): 140 m*M* NaCl, 5 m*M* KCl, 25 m*M* Tris-HCl, pH 7.4 (Sigma). Dissolve 8.0 g NaCl, 380 mg KCl, and 3.0 g Tris-base in 800 mL water. Adjust pH with HCl. Bring to 1 L and then autoclave.

2.2. DNA Isolation (see Note 1)

1. Benchtop centrifuge or microcentrifuge (e.g., Eppendorff, Fisher).
2. Hanks' PBS or equivalent (~5 mL).
3. Approximately 1 mL TEN: 10 m*M* Tris-HCl, pH 7.8, 25 m*M* EDTA, 150 m*M* NaCl (Sigma).
4. Approximately 1 mL PSE: 1 mg/mL proteinase K (Life Technologies) in 3% sarcosyl, 50 m*M* EDTA, pH 8.0 (Sigma).
5. 21-gage Needle and syringe.
6. 55°C Water bath or incubator.
7. RNase (Sigma): 10 mg/mL (<1 mL).
8. Proteinase K: 20 mg/mL (<1 mL).

9. Approximately 5 mL Phenol/chloroform/isoamyl alcohol, 25:24:1 (PCI; Ameresco, Solon, OH).
10. Dialysis tubing.
11. Approximately 7 L TE: 10 mM Tris-HCl, pH 8.0, 1 mM EDTA (Sigma).

2.3. PCR Assay (see Note 2)

1. 10X PCR buffer: 100 mM Tris-HCl, pH 8.3, 500 mM KCl, 15 mM MgCl$_2$, 0.01% gelatin (all molecular biology grade from Sigma).
2. dNTPs: 25 mM dATP, 25 mM dCTP, 25 mM dGTP, 25 mM dTTP (Promega, Madison, WI).
3. Primers:

   a. Primer A262: 5'-AGAAGTGACATCTTCAGCAAATAAAC-3' (*BCL-2* gene) *(9)*.
   b. Primer A263: 5'-ACCTGAGGAGACGGTGACC-3' (IgH J-region consensus primer *[9]*).
   c. Primer A277: 5'-CCGAGGGCAGATTCGGGAATG-3' (human *HPRT* intron 1, nucleotides 2013–2033; GenBank accession number M26434 *[19]*).
   d. Primer A279: 5'-CTACTGCCCTCTTACATGAGACAC-3' (human *HPRT* intron 3, nucleotides 22,718–22,741; GenBank accession number M26434 *[19]*).

4. Master Mix I: 1X PCR buffer, 0.2 µM primer A277, 0.2 µM primer A279, 0.2 µM primer A262, 0.2 µM primer A263, 0.2 mM dNTPs.
5. PCR tubes (*see* **Note 3**).
6. Placental DNA (500 µg/mL; Sigma).
7. LRD2401-1 plasmid cleaved with *Bam*HI (plasmid containing a cloned *HPRT* exon 2+3 deletion junction for use as a positive control; one molecule/µL; available from Dr. James C. Fuscoe, National Center for Toxicological Research, HFT-130, Jefferson, AR 72079).
8. 10 pg/µL SU-DHL-4 DNA: human cell line that contains the t(14;18) chromosome (Oncogene Science). Extract DNA as above or by any standardized protocol.
9. Thermocycler (e.g., PTC-100 thermal cycler, MJ Research, Waltham, MA).
10. Taq polymerase (Promega, Applied Biosystems, Foster City, CA).
11. Primers:

    a. Primer A276: 5'-TCGGGAGAGGCCCTTCCCTGG-3' (internal human *HPRT* intron 1, nucleotides 2064–2084; GenBank accession number M26434 *[19]*).
    b. Primer A278: 5'-CTATGTGAGTTGAGGGATACG-3' (internal human *HPRT* intron 3 primer, nucleotides 22,492–22,512; GenBank accession number M26434 *[19]*).
    c. Primer A264: 5'-ACATTGATGGAATAACTCTGTGG-3' (internal *BCL-2 [9]*).
    d. Primer A265: 5'-CAGGGTCCCTTGGCCCCAG-3' (internal IgH J-region consensus primer *[8]*).

12. 10X Gel loading dye: 25% Ficoll (molecular weight approx 400,000; Sigma), 0.05% xylene cyanole FF (Sigma; *see* **Note 4**).
13. Master Mix II: 1X PCR buffer, 2 mM MgCl$_2$, 0.02 µM primer A276, 0.2 µM primer A278, 0.2 µM primer A264, 0.2 µM primer A265, 1X gel loading dye, 0.2 mM dNTPs, 50 U/mL Taq polymerase. The total MgCl$_2$ concentration is 3.5 mM.
14. 10X TBE: 0.89 M Tris-borate, 0.02 M EDTA, pH 8.3, prepared by dissolving 108 g Tris-base and 55 g boric acid in 900 mL water; add 40 mL 0.5 M EDTA pH 8.0, and then bring to 1 L with water. Autoclave and store at room temperature.
15. Agarose (Bio-Rad, Hercules, CA, or BRL, Life Technologies).
16. Gel electrophoresis equipment (e.g., Mini-sub GT electrophoresis cell, Bio-Rad).

3. Methods

3.1. Lymphocyte Isolation (see Note 5)

1. Collect 48 mL of blood in heparinized tubes.
2. Dilute blood up to 2X with Hanks' PBS to get a multiple of 24 mL (e.g., 96 mL if starting with 48 mL blood). Mix well by inversion.
3. Put 18 mL of Histopaque or Ficoll-Paque into each of four 50-mL centrifuge tubes.
4. Invert blood mixture again and very slowly pipet 24 mL onto Histopaque so that it does not mix with the Histopaque layer.
5. Centrifuge at 350g in tabletop centrifuge at room temperature for 30 min.
6. Remove and discard top serum layer down to lymphocyte layer using a 10-mL pipet.
7. Remove lymphocyte layers and put each into a separate 50-mL centrifuge tube. Fill each tube to 50 mL with TBS.
8. Centrifuge tubes at 350g in a tabletop centrifuge at room temperature for 30 min.
9. Discard supernatant.
10. Suspend cell pellets in 2 mL TBS and combine into one 50-mL tube.
11. Centrifuge tubes at 350g in tabletop centrifuge at room temperature for 30 min.
12. Resuspend cell pellet in 1 mL TBS.

3.2. DNA Isolation

1. Pellet cells in a centrifuge (200g rpm, 10 min in tabletop centrifuge or 10 s in microcentrifuge) and then discard supernatant.
2. Wash cells with 1–2 mL Hanks' PBS or equivalent (resuspend by swirling, and pellet as above).
3. For cells isolated from 48 mL of blood, resuspend cells in 400 μL TEN (scale down for smaller starting volumes). Add 400 μL of PSE and incubate at 55°C overnight (*see* **Note 6**).
4. Shear DNA through 21-gage needle 5 times.
5. Add RNase to 150 μg/mL (12 μL of 10 mg/mL stock). Incubate at 55°C for > 1 h.
6. Add proteinase K to 250 μg/mL (10 μL of 20 mg/mL stock). Incubate at 55°C for > 1 h.
7. Extract with equal volume PCI for 1 h at room temperature.
8. Centrifuge for 10 min in tabletop centrifuge.
9. Remove upper aqueous layer to a new tube.
10. Repeat extraction (**steps 8–10**) two more times.
11. Dialyze overnight against 3.5 L TE, changing the dialysis buffer once.

3.3. PCR Assay (see Note 7)

1. Set up the following primary PCR reactions: 15 μL Master Mix I, 2.5 μg lymphocyte DNA, and water to 47.5 μL in PCR tubes (*see* **Notes 8** and **9**).
2. Set up the following controls:

   a. Negative control: 15 μL Master Mix I, 5 μL placental DNA (500 μg/mL), and water to 47.5 μL.
   b. Positive control: 15 μL Master Mix I, 5 μL placental DNA (500 μg/mL), 5 μL LRD240-1 linearized with *Bam*HI (one molecule/mL), 3 μL SU-DHL-4 DNA (10 pg/μL), and water to 47.5 mL (*see* **Note 10**).

3. Place samples in a PCR thermocycler equipped with a heated lid. Incubate at 80°C for >3 min, and then add 2.5 μL Taq polymerase to the tube without removing it from the thermocycler. (Taq polymerase is diluted to 1 U/μL with sterile water, mixed vigorously, and centrifuged in a microcentrifuge at top speed for 10 s immediately prior to use.)

4. Incubate at 94°C for 4 min.
5. Cycle 40 times at 94°C for 1 min, 60°C for 1 min, and 72°C for 1 min.
6. At completion of cycling, incubate for 5 min at 72°C.
7. Set up the following secondary PCR reactions: 48.5 μL Master Mix II and 0.5 μL Taq polymerase (5 U/μL). Scale up the volume of this mixture for the desired number of reactions and then aliquot 49 μL into prelabeled PCR tubes (*see* **Note 11**).
8. Add 1 μL of primary PCR reaction product to the reaction tubes.
9. Use the following temperature profile, add tubes to the PCR thermocycler *after the instrument reaches 94°C* (hot start): 94°C for 4 min; 20X (94°C for 1 min, 60°C for 1 min, 72°C for 1 min); 72°C for 5 min.
10. Electrophorese 20 μL of secondary PCR product on either a 2% agarose (Bio-Rad Molecular Biology Grade) or a 1.7% agarose (BRL)/0.5X TBE gel. PCR fragments (typically 300–1000 bp) indicate the presence of the t(14;18) junction fragment or *HPRT* exon 2/3 deletion junctions.

3.4. Confirmation of t(14;18) or HPRT Exon 2/3 Deletion

1. For each PCR that produced a fragment, set up a pair of new PCRs for determining whether the fragments are truly representative of the t(14;18) or *HPRT* exon 2/3 deletions.
2. t(14;18) confirmation PCR: 1X PCR buffer, 0.2 μ*M* primer A264, 0.2 μ*M* primer A265, 2 m*M* MgCl$_2$, 0.2 m*M* dNTPs, 1X gel loading dye, 2.5 U Taq polymerase, and 1 μL of primary PCR product.
3. *HPRT* exon 2/3 deletion confirmation PCR: 1X PCR buffer, 0.02 μ*M* primer A276, 0.2 μ*M* primer A278, 2 μ*M* MgCl$_2$, 0.2 m*M* dNTPs, 1X gel loading dye, 2.5 U Taq polymerase, and 1 μL of primary PCR product.
4. Use the following temperature profile and add tubes to the PCR thermocycler *after the instrument reaches 94°C*: 94°C for 4 min; 20X (94°C for 1 min, 60°C for 1 min, 72°C for 1 min) 20; 72°C for 5 min.
5. Electrophorese 20 μL of secondary PCR product on 2% agarose (Bio-Rad Molecular Biology Grade) or 1.7% agarose (BRL)/0.5X TBE gels. A fragment in the t(14;18) confirmation reaction indicates the original sample contained a t(14;18). A fragment in the *HPRT* exon 2/3-deletion confirmation reaction indicates that the original sample contains an *HPRT* exon 2/3 deletion.
6. Calculate the frequency of lymphocytes containing t(14;18) or *HPRT* exon 2/3 deletion (*see* **Note 12**).

4. Notes

1. PSE, 10 mg/mL RNase, and 20 mg/mL proteinase K can be stored at –20°C for at least 1 yr with no significant loss of activity. All water used in this protocol should be of the highest quality (i.e., deionized, sterile, and DNase-free).
2. 10X PCR buffer, gel loading buffer, and genomic DNAs can be stored at 4°C for at least 1 yr. Primers, dNTPs, and Master Mix I and II can be stored at –20°C for at least 2 yr without significant degradation. The LRD240-1 plasmid DNA can be purified with the Qiagen Plasmid Purification Kit (or equivalent) and then cleaved with *Bam*HI under the supplier's recommended conditions. The cleaved plasmid is then quantified by absorbance at 260 nm (1 A$_{260}$ absorbance unit through a 1-cm cuvet is a DNA concentration of 50 μg/mL). The DNA is diluted in TE containing 1 ng/μL placental DNA to a final concentration of one molecule per μL. The diluted LRD240-1 DNA is stored at –80°C. It is stable under these conditions for at least 1 yr. The dilute plasmid will degrade if stored in

sterile water or in TE without the small amount of carrier DNA present, even when stored at –80°C. The LRD240-1 plasmid is composed of the pCRII cloning vector (Invitrogen, Carlsbad, CA) containing an amplified *HPRT* exon 2/3 deletion region isolated from newborn MM30M9 *(11)* in the TA cloning site. The recombinant plasmid (LRD240-1) is 4802 base pairs and has a molecular weight of 3.05×10^6 Daltons.

3. Most of our experience has been with 0.5-mL PCR tubes, but 0.2-mL tubes and 96-well plates work as well.

4. Xylene cyanole FF purchased from another manufacturer inhibited the PCR reactions.

5. Other standard lymphocyte isolation procedures will also work. After resuspension of the combined cell pellet, the cells can be preserved for later processing of DNA by adding DMSO to 8%, mixing well, and then placing at –80°C. The DNA is stable under these conditions for at least 1 yr.

6. At this point, the DNA from the lysed cells is stabilized and can be stored at room temperature for at least a week. It is also a convenient form in which to ship the samples to another site for later processing and analysis, if required.

7. The biggest potential problem in this assay is cross-contamination of the primary PCRs (or the reaction components, including the sample lymphocyte DNAs) with amplified t(14;18)-containing or *HPRT* exon 2/3-containing DNA. The assay is designed to detect a single molecule, so it is imperative to take extraordinary precautions to prevent possible contamination. The threat of contamination is evident when one considers that after the secondary amplification reaction, there are greater than 10^{11} molecules in the reaction tube. Even the act of opening the reaction tube may create enough of an aerosol to be a significant source of contamination. For this reason, it is important to physically isolate all preamplification materials (including racks, pipets, lab coats, gloves, and other materials) from the assembly of the secondary reactions and the subsequent gel analysis. Separate pipets and pipet tips with barrier filters should be used for setting up all primary and secondary PCRs.

8. Under these conditions, the maximum amount of DNA in the primary PCR should be no greater than 2.5 μg, which represents 4×10^5 cells. Greater amounts of DNA have given unreliable results.

9. Scale up for the number of desired reactions and place 47.5 μL into prelabeled PCR tubes. Forming master mixes of common reaction components will aid in the reproducibility of the assay.

10. It is important to include multiple negative controls in each experiment to guard against contamination with t(14;18) and *HPRT* exon 2/3 deletion DNA. The negative control should include all reaction components with placental DNA substituted for the purified genomic DNA. It is also important to verify that all sample DNAs will support the PCR reactions and do not contain an inhibitor. A PCR should be set up with each new sample as follows: 2.5 μg sample DNA, 15 μL Master Mix I, 5 μL LRD240-1 cleaved with *Bam*HI (one molecule per μL), 3 μL SU-DHL-4 DNA (10 pg/μL), and water to 47.5 μL as described in **Subheading 3.3., steps 1–6**. The secondary PCR should be set up as described in **Subheading 3.3., steps 7–10**. The t(14;18) forms a 286-bp primary PCR product, and the *HPRT* exon 2/3 deletion forms a 396-bp product.

11. To help keep track of primary and secondary PCRs, it is convenient to label primary PCRs numerically (e.g., 1–32), and then label secondary PCRs A1–A32.

12. t(14;18) frequency is calculated by use of the Poisson relationship, $P_0 = e^{-x}$, where P_0 is the fraction of PCR reactions without t(14;18) chromosomes and x is the average number of cells (represented by purified DNA) per PCR reaction. Thus, the t(14;18) frequency =

$-\ln P_0/x$. There are approx 6 pg of DNA per human cell, so 2.5 µg human DNA = 400,000 cells. For example, 31 PCR reactions were set up with each containing 2.5 µg (400,000 cells) of lymphocyte DNA. Four of the reactions contained t(14;18) chromosomes. Therefore, 27 reactions (31 − 4) did not contain t(14;18) chromosomes. The frequency of t(14;18)-containing cells is then calculated as $-\ln (27/31)/400,000 = 3.5 \times 10^{-7}$.

References

1. Lipford, E., Wright, J. J., Urba, W., et al. (1987) Refinement of lymphoma cytogenetics by the chromosome 18q21 major breakpoint region. *Blood* **70,** 1816–1823.
2. Yunis, J. J., Oken, M. M., Kaplan, M. E., Ensrud, K. E., Howe, R. R., and Theologides, A. (1982) Distinctive chromosomal abnormalities in histologic subtypes of non-Hodgkin's lymphomas. *N. Engl. J. Med.* **307,** 1231–1236.
3. Hockenbery, D., Nunez, G., Milliman, C., Schreiber, R. D., and Korsmeyer, S. J. (1990) Bcl-2 is an inner mitochondrial membrane protein that blocks programmed cell death. *Nature* **348,** 334–336.
4. Crescenzi, M., Seto, M., Herzig, G. P., Weiss, P. D., Griffith, R. C., and Korsmeyer, S. J. (1988) Thermostable DNA polymerase chain reaction amplification of t(14;18) chromosome breakpoints and detection of minimal residual disease. *Proc. Natl. Acad. Sci. USA* **85,** 4869–4873.
5. Ngan, B. Y., Nourse, J., and Cleary, M. L. (1989) Detection of chromosomal translocation t(14;18) within the minor cluster region of bcl-2 by polymerase chain reaction and direct genomic sequencing of the enzymatically amplified DNA in follicular lymphomas. *Blood* **73,** 1759–1762.
6. Cotter, F., Price, C., Zucca, E., and Young, B. D. (1990) Direct sequence analysis of the 14q+ and 18q- chromosome junctions in follicular lymphoma. *Blood* **76,** 131–135.
7. Eick, S., Krieger, G., Bolz, I., and Kneba, M. (1990) Sequence analysis of amplified t(14;18) chromosomal breakpoints in B-cell lymphomas. *J. Pathol.* **162,** 127–133.
8. Liu, Y., Hernandez, A. M., Shibata, D., and Cortopassi, G. A. (1994) *BCL2* translocation frequency rises with age in humans. *Proc. Natl. Acad. Sci. USA* **91,** 8910–8914.
9. Zhang, X. Y. and Ehrlich, M. (1994) Detection and quantitation of low numbers of chromosomes containing bcl-2 oncogene translocations using semi-nested PCR. *Biotechniques* **16,** 502–507.
10. Fuscoe, J. C., Setzer, R. W., Collard, D. D., and Moore, M. M. (1996) Quantification of t(14;18) in the lymphocytes of healthy adult humans as a possible biomarker for environmental exposures to carcinogens. *Carcinogenesis* **17,** 1013–1020.
11. Fuscoe, J. C., Zimmerman, L. J., Lippert, M. J., Nicklas, J. A., O'Neill, J. P., and Albertini, R. J. (1991) V(D)J recombinase-like activity mediates *hprt* gene deletion in human fetal T-lymphocytes. *Cancer Res.* **51,** 6001–6005.
12. Fuscoe, J. C., Zimmerman, L. J., Harrington-Brock, K., et al. (1992) V(D)J recombinase-mediated deletion of the *hprt* gene in T-lymphocytes from adult humans. *Mutat. Res.* **283,** 13–20.
13. Fuscoe, J. C., Vira, L. K., Collard, D. D., and Moore, M. M. (1997) Quantification of *hprt* gene deletions mediated by illegitimate V(D)J recombination in peripheral blood cells of humans. *Environ. Mol. Mutagen.* **29,** 28–35.
14. Chen, C. L., Fuscoe, J. C., Liu, Q., and Relling, M. V. (1996) Etoposide causes illegitimate V(D)J recombination in human lymphoid leukemic cells. *Blood* **88,** 2210–2218.
15. Chen, C. L., Fuscoe, J. C., Liu, Q., Pui, C. H., Mahmoud, H. H., and Relling, M. V. (1996) Relationship between cytotoxicity and site-specific DNA recombination after in vitro exposure of leukemia cells to etoposide. *J. Natl. Cancer Inst.* **88,** 1840–1847.

16. Chen, C. L., Woo, M. H., Neale, G. A., et al. (1998) A human lymphoid leukemia cell line with a V(D)J recombinase-mediated deletion of hprt. *Mutat. Res.* **403,** 113–125.
17. Fuscoe, J. C., Knapp, G. W., Hanley, N. M., et al. (1998) The frequency of illegitimate V(D)J recombinase-mediated mutations in children treated with etoposide-containing antileukemic therapy. *Mutat. Res.* **419,** 107–121.
18. Scheerer, J. B., Xi, L., Knapp, G. W., Setzer, R. W., Bigbee, W. L., and Fuscoe, J. C. (1999) Quantification of illegitimate V(D)J recombinase-mediated mutations in lymphocytes of newborns and adults. *Mutat. Res.* **431,** 291–303.
19. Edwards, A., Voss, H., Rice, P., et al. (1990) Automated DNA sequencing of the human *HPRT* locus. *Genomics* **6,** 593–608.

18

The *GPA* In Vivo Somatic Mutation Assay

Stephen G. Grant

Summary

The glycophorin A (*GPA*) assay concurrently detects and quantifies two types of erythrocytes with variant phenotypes at the autosomal locus responsible for the polymorphic MN blood group. It uses a pair of allele-specific monoclonal antibodies and flow cytometry to analyze a standard population of 5 million cells efficiently. The two phenotypes detected are simple allele loss and allele loss followed by reduplication of the remaining allele; both are consistent with the mechanisms underlying "loss of heterozygosity" at tumor suppressor genes. The assay is an intermediate biomarker of biological effect, meaning that it integrates both exposure and biological response. It has been applied to populations with a known or suspected genotoxic exposure, to patients with hereditary syndromes causing predisposition to cancer (in which the assay has begun to be moved from validation mode to application), and to patients manifesting a disease endpoint, i.e., cancer.

Key Words: Genotoxicity; carcinogenesis; environmental exposure; DNA repair deficiencies; biomonitoring; mechanisms of mutagenesis; gene inactivation.

1. Introduction

The glycophorin A (*GPA*)-based somatic mutation assay was developed at the Lawrence Livermore National Laboratory (LLNL) in the late 1980s as a potential means of monitoring the exposure of Department of Energy employees to ionizing radiation and other genotoxic agents. Its design took into consideration several factors. First, since mutation is a rare event, the prospective assay had to be able to evaluate literally millions of cells in a cost-effective manner; this looked like a possible application for the flow cytometric technology under development at LLNL at the time. Second, because the assay was to be used as a population screen, it had to be performed on a readily available cell type, and blood, although it required the use of a minimally invasive procedure to obtain, was considered a good source of such tissue samples. Third, because the mutations detected should have pre-existed in vivo, there should be little to no opportunity for mutation to occur ex vivo during the performance of the assay. Although this decision had some disadvantages, erythrocytes, the

From: *Methods in Molecular Biology, vol. 291, Molecular Toxicology Protocols*
Edited by: P. Keohavong and S. G. Grant © Humana Press Inc., Totowa, NJ

most common cell type in the blood, but one that had normally extruded its nucleus in humans, was chosen as the basis of the assay. Finally, because mutation is such a rare event, the assay had to be designed in such a way as to detect mutational outcomes with "single-hit" kinetics, i.e., each mutational event should lead to a detectable and quantifiable change in phenotype.

The detection of potentially recessive mutations is an old problem in genetic toxicology when it comes to dealing with dizygous organisms, such as humans. Traditionally, there have been three ways of designing such a system: detection of a dominant mutation, targeting of a locus in a hemizygous region of the genome (such as the X chromosome), or development of a heterozygous system in which the two alleles can be distinguished unambiguously. Two loci were ultimately targeted, both because of their high expression in erythrocytes and the wealth of data existing on their genetics, which provided a choice of allele-specific monoclonal antibodies to use for detection at the protein level.

The first locus targeted was that of β-hemoglobin, and the assay was designed to detect somatic mutation to the distinctive variant found in sickle cell hemoglobinopathy (1). Although this assay eventually found some limited application (2), several problems were clear: (1) the detectable event required such a specific molecular change that the frequency of variants was very low, and (2) it was difficult to deliver the monoclonal antibody to the target molecule inside the cells without destroying their integrity to the point that their analysis by flow cytometry was compromised. (Indeed, in application this assay was shifted to a computer-assisted slide-based microscopic detection system.) Wishing to retain the advantages of working on the flow cytometer with red blood cells (and therefore with the knowledge and reagents available from clinicians and scientists working on blood groups), a second reporter locus was targeted: GPA.

GPA is the most prevalent protein on the surface of human red cells, and its two common polymorphic forms are the basis of the MN blood group (3,4). Antisera derived against these protein isoforms allowed for the distinctive labeling of the products of each allele in heterozygotes. This, in turn, allowed for the scoring of "inactivation" mutations (actually the true phenotype was loss of antibody binding) at a single allele of this autosomal locus and thus events with single-hit kinetics. Several versions of the basic assay have been published: the 1W1 assay was designed for the unique dual-beam sorter constructed at LLNL (5), the BR6 assay was designed for transfer of the technology to outside users through the use of a commercially available platform (6,7) (see Note 1), and the name of the current DB6 assay refers to the direct conjugation of fluorophors to the allele-specific monoclonal antibodies (8).

The original intent of the GPA assay was to detect and quantitate erythrocytes with "allele-loss" phenotypes, presumably occurring through classical mutation events such as those observed in the HPRT assay (see Chaps. 13 and 15–17). Several in vitro systems had been developed to study "mutation" at heterozygous autosomal loci, however, and it was clear that allele loss could occur by a variety of mechanisms (9). If we define a "classical" mutation as one affecting only the locus under consideration, this includes point mutations in the coding and regulatory regions of the gene (keeping in mind that some regulatory regions affect multiple genes), small intragenic deletions and insertions, and some translocations. In these types of mutants the phenotype is determined only by the differences in activity or expression of the target gene itself. Slightly larger deletions, including or only affecting adjacent genes, may have qualities such as increased inviability that are based more on the effect on those adjacent genes than on the target gene itself, meaning that the genetic context of the target gene plays a role in determining what types of mutants will occur and what types of mutants will be viable enough to be actually detected.

Such distinctions were found to be critical at the thymidine kinase (*Tk*) locus in mouse L5178Y cells, possibly because of its linkage to the *p53* oncogene (*10*). Thus, large deletions, including cytogenetically detectable deletions, would also confer the selected allele-loss phenotype, if they were viable despite the reduction in gene dosage for all loci in the affected region. Indeed, whole chromosome loss would also confer this selected genotype, although it affects the gene dosage of the entire complement of genes on the chromosome. Chromosome loss was frequently observed in somatic cell systems (*11,12*), but this was dismissed as an artifactual mechanism of variation until it was later observed in human carcinogenesis (*13*). Finally, gene inactivation by *de novo* DNA methylation may also produce the allele-loss phenotype and may also affect a region of the genome larger than a single gene (*14*). This epigenetic mechanism really blurs the definition of "mutation" although it is quasistable in the propagation of somatic cells, and it has also been found to play a major role in molecular carcinogenesis (*15,16*). These potential mechanisms of allele loss at the autosomal *GPA* locus are summarized in **Fig. 1**. Chromosome loss is represented as occurring by mitotic nondisjunction, which would produce equal numbers of monosomic and trisomic daughter cells.

With the first application of the *GPA* assay to an exposed population (*17*), it became evident that there was a second class of variant cells that had not only lost one allelic form of the GPA protein, but were also exhibiting twice as much of the other isoform on their cell surface (**Fig. 2**). Once again, such "loss and duplication" phenotypes had previously been observed in vitro. One mechanism shown to account for these variants was mitotic recombination occurring between the centromere and the reporter gene (*18*), although it was a very rare event (*19*). The more localized mechanism of gene conversion would occur at even lower frequency, because it requires either two recombinational events or the transduction of the breakpoint of a single recombinational event through the reporter gene prior to strand resolution. Indeed, the major mechanism of this type of allelic loss and duplication appeared to be the concurrent loss and duplication of homologous chromosomes (*20,21*). Similar chromosomal events are known as *malsegregation* in fungi (*22*), and the actual mechanism remains unknown (*23*) (including such questions as whether chromosome loss and duplication are secondary to an initial chromosome loss). These potential mechanisms of allelic loss and duplication at the *GPA* locus are summarized in **Fig. 3**. Note that mitotic recombination and chromosomal loss and duplication both generate a pair of reciprocal daughter cells homozygous for each of the two parental homologues, whereas gene conversion produces only a single variant daughter cell. Typical flow histograms for the *GPA* assay are given in **Fig. 2**.

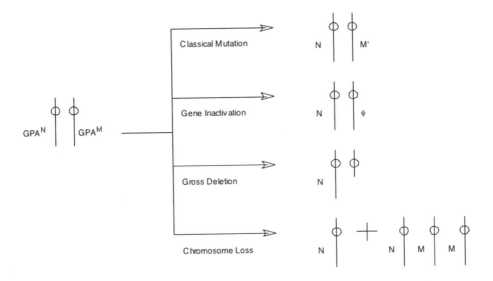

Fig. 1. Possible mechanisms of development of the allele loss phenotype at the *GPA* locus in erythroid bone marrow progenitor cells. Classical mutations refer to any that affect only the target gene, including point mutations, small insertions and deletions, and (potentially) translocations disrupting the integrity of the *GPA* gene. Deletion and chromosome loss define the extremes of events resulting in loss of genetic material including the target locus and any other closely linked gene. Chromosome loss is depicted as occurring by nondisjunction at mitosis, which would result in a second aberrant daughter cell trisomic for chromosome 4, but this is only one possible means of achieving such chromosome loss. This category would also include translocations in the vicinity of the *GPA* locus involving loss of genetic material at the breakpoint(s). Finally, epigenetic gene inactivation by *de novo* DNA hypermethylation would also confer the allele loss phenotype if it occurred at one allele of *GPA*; however, such gene inactivation also has the potential to affect surrounding loci, such as occurs via a position effect in some chromosomal translocations.

The vast majority of studies using the *GPA* assay report these two endpoints separately. Because loss of heterozygosity can occur by either mechanism, however, if the intent of the analysis is linked in any way to carcinogenesis, the frequencies of the two classes of variants can be amalgamated to yield a better idea of overall genotoxic effect. Indeed, the frequency of allele loss and duplication variants has only been affected by one type of exposure, benzene *(24)*, and is only obviously increased in one hereditary cancer-prone disease, Bloom's syndrome *(25)*, although it does seem to have a greater increase with age than simple allele loss *(26)*. Although these separable phenotypes do provide some characterization of the underlying mutations, the fact that allele loss can occur by such diverse mechanisms as point mutation, epigenetic inactivation, or chromosome loss suggests that there is limited specificity in these two classes of variants.

We have previously discussed the three types of mutations involved in multistep carcinogenesis at some length *(26,27)*. These include activation of an oncogene,

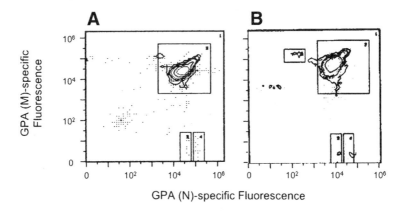

Fig. 2. Flow histograms of 1 million labeled erythrocytes from a normal individual (**A**) and an individual with the premature aging disease Werner's syndrome (**B**). Both individuals were heterozygous for the MN blood groups and exhibit a main peak of cells with approximately equal labeling for both fluorophors. The two windows on the abscissa represent the areas where variant cells with an M-allele loss phenotype would fall (left) and where variant cells with loss of the M allele and duplication of the N allele would fall. (These windows are side by side because the axis is logarithmic.) The higher frequencies of both types of variants observed in the Werner's syndrome patient allow a clear resolution of the two peaks of variants. An N-allele loss window has also been drawn on the histogram of the Werner's syndrome patient demonstrating the occurrence of reciprocal molecular events causing loss or inactivation of the other allele.

through a specific gain (or at least maintenance) of function mutation, inactivation of a tumor suppressor gene (which can involve a broader set of mechanisms), and *segregation* of the remaining wild-type allele of the tumor suppressor gene, also called *loss of heterozygosity*, which can occur by an even greater array of mechanisms *(9,14)*. There are three type of mutation assays that can be used as biomarkers for these processes: dominant mutational assays such a development of resistance to ouabain, inactivation assays at monozygous loci, such as *HPRT*, and inactivation assays at dizygous loci, such as *GPA* and *Tk*. In general, the ability of an assay to represent these types of events is hierarchical; dominant mutation assays, which often involve changes at specific codons or even bases (such as the hemoglobin assay discussed earlier) have little application for inactivation, since there are so many more contributing mechanisms. (This type of mutation is very hard to model because it is so specific; a point mutation that has the potential to activate *K-ras*, for example, may not do the same for *myc*.) Likewise, there are chromosomal mechanisms active in somatic segregation that are not possible at an X-linked locus. Just because a mechanism is theoretically possible in an assay, however, does not mean that it will occur, be easily detectable, or be particularly sensitive to genetic and environmental factors affecting that mechanism (*see* **Note 2**).

In its application, the *GPA* assay is second only to the long-standing *HPRT* assay. However, the *GPA* assay is faster, cheaper, and, at least potentially, responsive to more types of genetic and epigenetic effects. On the other hand, owing to its genetic

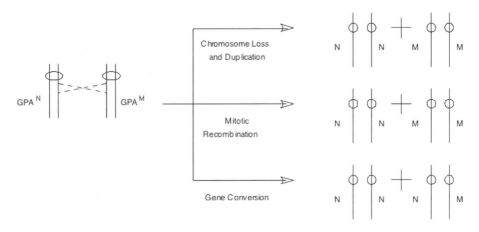

Fig. 3. Possible mechanisms of development of the allele loss and duplication phenotype at the *GPA* locus in erythroid bone marrow progenitor cells. Mitotic recombination results in homozygosity for all markers distal to the site of crossover and the generation of a reciprocal daughter cell at the next mitosis. Chromosome loss and duplication could occur in two steps with successive nondisjunctions (with the second event rescuing a cell of low viability from the first) or by a concerted aberrant disjunction that would accomplish both chromosomal missegregations simultaneously. In the former case there should be an association between the frequency of chromosome loss events contributing to the allele loss endpoint (**Fig. 1**) and the frequency of these variants. In the case of the latter mechanism, this may or may not occur. Gene conversion is probably a low-frequency event associated with mitotic recombination.

basis, the *GPA* assay is applicable to only half the population (those heterozygous for the MN blood group), and, because human erythrocytes have no nucleus, there is no opportunity for molecular analysis *(29)*. We have recently demonstrated, however, that in populations in which the allele loss frequency is expected to be elevated (about threefold), such as in cancer patients undergoing genotoxic chemotherapy or in certain genetic syndromes, the requirement for MN heterozygosity no longer applies *(30)*.

The *GPA* assay has been applied in a large number of studies of accidental, medical, environmental, and occupational exposure to ionizing radiation and genotoxic chemicals *(31)*. Because it requires a biological response, i.e., generation of a viable phenotypic variant, the assay is a biomarker of genotoxic effect rather than simply exposure (meaning that it also integrates individual variation in response) *(32)*. The great majority of these studies have been performed as validation or characterization of either the assay or the population; there does not seem to be an intent to develop this or other molecular toxicological assays into true clinical or public health tools. In addition, several studies have attempted to utilize the *GPA* assay directly as a biomarker of exposure, and these authors have concluded that it was not "sensitive" enough for their application *(33–35)*. The *GPA* assay is a biomarker of biological, and therefore health, effects; it was not designed to detect events that have no biological consequence; in fact, it was designed to discriminate an exposure or level of exposure that might require intervention. DNA adducts might well be a better biomarker of exposure, although the exposure signal does go through some attenuation when you require the adduct to occur in your tissue of choice; however, if these adducts would not have gone on to generate viable, yet deleterious, mutations or other biological effects, then detecting them has no utility. Likewise, chromosomal damage that is lethal to its resident cell may well be indicative of persistent effects in other cells that could have consequences for the health of the individual or population, or the impending cell death may deal with the problem once and for all. The utility of a tool depends on the appropriateness of the tasks to which it is applied.

The *GPA* assay has also documented elevated frequencies of uninduced somatic mutation in a number of hereditary disorders associated with defects in DNA repair, and it is here that we have attempted to move the use of the assay away from validation and into application. We have shown that the *GPA* assay can be used to diagnose ataxia telangiectasia and Fanconi's anemia *(30,36)*, based on their elevated mutation frequencies. Applying the paradigm of Hsu *(37)*, that variability in genetic instability in the human population will have health consequences, resulting in "common" diseases, we *(32)* and others *(38)* have demonstrated similar but more subtle elevations in sporadic cancer patients. Thus, uninduced mutation frequency, representing individual somatic mutational burden, could be measured and considered in cancer risk analyses. These and other applications of the *GPA* assay have been proposed *(7,39)*, and it is our intention to implement them.

2. Materials

2.1. Sample Acquisition and Processing for Storage or Shipment

1. Equipment for blood draw: 21-gage needles, plastic needle holder, tourniquet, alcohol or Betadine swabs, and so on (Daigger, Vernon Hills, IL). Alternate methods, such as use of a syringe or drawing from an IV line are acceptable; refer to relevant guidelines for blood draw in your area.
2. 3-mL Vacutainer tubes with sodium heparin, sodium citrate, or EDTA as anticoagulant (Fisher Scientific, Pittsburgh, PA).
3. Means of keeping samples cold (between 1 and 4°C) for storage or shipping.

2.2. MN Blood Group Typing

1. Anti-M and anti-N blood typing sera (Johnson & Johnson Ortho Clinical Diagnostics, Raritan, NJ).
2. Glass slides (one per sample).
3. 20-µL Micropipetor (Rainin, Woburn, MA) and appropriate pipet tips (Fisher).
4. Wooden applicator sticks (Fisher).

2.3. Sample Processing I: Isovolumetric "Sphering"

1. 1.5-mL Microcentrifuge tubes (two per sample; Brinkmann, Westbury, NY).
2. 15-mL Conical tubes (one per sample; BD Falcon, BD Biosciences, Bedford, MA).
3. 1-, 5-, and 10-mL Serological pipets.
4. 20-, 200-, and 1-mL Pipetors and appropriate tips.
5. Isolyte S (Braun Medical, Irvine, CA, cat. no. L7030).
6. Sodium dodecyl sulphate (SDS; stock 5 mg/mL).

7. Phosphate-buffered saline (PBS; made up as sheath fluid, from **Subheading 2.6., item 3**): add 0.5 g BSA to 10 mL; keep in refrigerator, discard if particulates form or it becomes contaminated.
8. Bovine serum albumin (BSA; Sigma, St. Louis, MO).
9. (Octylphenoxyl)polyethoxyethanol (IGEPAL; Sigma).
10. Formaldehyde (37% solution; Fisher).
11. Plastic transfer pipets (Fisher).
12. Benchtop centrifuge (e.g., Multi with rotor 8947 and 17.5-cm adaptors, Thermo IEC, Needham Heights, MA).
13. Vortex mixer.
14. Staining buffer (amounts for 1 L): 13.6 mM Na$_2$HPO$_4$ (1.93 g), 2.75 mM NaH$_2$PO$_4$ (0.38 g), 0.15 M NaCl (8.5 g), 0.15 mM NaN$_3$ (0.01 g), 0.5% BSA (5.0 g), 0.01% (v/v) IGEPAL (100 μL), distilled water (to 1 L).
15. Microcentrifuge (e.g., Multi with rotor 8848, Thermo IEC).

2.4. Sample Processing II: Antibody Staining

1. 15-mL Conical tubes (one per sample).
2. Staining buffer (*see* **Subheading 2.3., item 14**).
3. Vortex mixer.
4. Microcentrifuge.
5. Labeled, titrated phycoerythrin-conjugated GPA(M)-specific MAb 6A7 and fluorescein-conjugated GPA(N)-specific MAb BRIC157 (International Blood Group Reference Laboratory, Bristol, UK; *see* **Note 3**).
6. Rocker or orbital shaker (e.g., Red Rotor, Hoefer Scientific Instruments, San Francisco, CA).
7. Aluminum foil.
8. Propidium iodide (PI; Sigma P4170). Stock solution is 5 mg/mL. Working solution is 1 mg/mL in staining buffer.

2.5. Preparation of Control Samples

1. Fixed form-spheres from known donors with GPA(M/M), GPA(M/N), and GPA(N/N) phenotypes.
2. Five 1.5-mL microcentrifuge tubes.
3. Staining buffer.
4. Vortex mixer.
5. Microcentrifuge.
6. Labeled, titrated GPA(M)- and GPA(N)-specific antibodies.
7. Rocker or orbital shaker.
8. Aluminum foil.
9. PI.

2.6. Flow Cytometry

1. Flow cytometer, with analysis software (e.g., FACScan with Consort C30 software, BD Biosciences, San Jose, CA; *see* **Note 1**).
2. Nylon mesh filters (Fisher, cat. no. 08-670-202).
3. Sheath fluid (PBS; amounts for 20 L): 13.6 mM Na$_2$HPO$_4$ (38.6 g), 2.75 mM NaH$_2$PO$_4$ (7.6 g), 0.15 M NaCl (170 g), deionized water (to 20 L).
4. Sample tubes (Fisher; 5-mL round-bottomed polystyrene snap cap tubes).

3. Methods

3.1. Sample Acquisition

1. Draw 1–3 mL blood into standard 3-mL Vacutainer tubes (*see* **Notes 4** and **5**).
2. Blood samples should be kept cold (~2°C) prior to fixation. Do not freeze (*see* **Notes 6** and **7**).

3.2. MN Blood Group Typing (see Note 8)

1. Place 1 drop each of anti-M and anti-N typing sera, well-separated, on a microscope slide.
2. Using separate pipet tips, add 20 µL of sample blood to each drop of sera.
3. Mix the blood and sera together with applicator sticks. (Use a fresh stick for each spot.)
4. Lift the slide and swirl it, watching for agglutination in the two blood/sera pools (*see* **Note 9**).

3.3. Sample Processing I: Isovolumetric "Sphering" (see Note 10)

1. Prepare one 1.5-mL microcentrifuge tube for each sample, and, if necessary, M/M, M/N, and N/N controls (*see* **Note 11**). Label each tube and add 1 mL of Isolyte S, 10 µL of 5 mg/mL SDS, and 20 µL of PBS containing 5% BSA. Mix by inversion.
2. Prepare one 15-mL conical tube for each sample, and controls, if necessary. Label each tube and add 9.6 mL Isolyte S, 20 µL of 5 mg/mL SDS, and 300 µL of formaldehyde solution. Mix by inversion.
3. Add 100 µL of well-mixed whole blood to each microcentrifuge tube, and mix by trituration. Let stand 1 min at room temperature.
4. Using a plastic transfer pipet, transfer suspension from microcentrifuge tube to similarly labeled 15-mL conical tube, and immediately mix twice by inversion. Let stand for 90 min at room temperature.
5. Resuspend the cell pellet by gentle shaking and inversion, add 800 µL formaldehyde solution, and immediately mix by inversion. Let stand overnight at room temperature in a fume hood.
6. Resuspend the cell pellet by gentle shaking and inversion. Centrifuge at 1750g (3000 rpm on suggested centrifuge) for 5 min. Pour off supernatant and resuspend by vortexing in 10 mL staining buffer. Incubate for 5 min at room temperature.
7. Resuspend the cell pellet by gentle shaking and inversion. Centrifuge at 1750g for 5 min. Pour off supernatant, add 1 mL staining buffer, mix by trituration, and then transfer the suspension to a labeled 1.5-mL microcentrifuge tube.
8. Centrifuge at 2700g (5000 rpm on suggested centrifuge) for 1 min in a microcentrifuge. Pour off supernatant and resuspend pellet by vortexing in 1 mL staining buffer. Refrigerate until further processing (*see* **Notes 11** and **12**).

3.4. Sample Processing II: Antibody Staining (see Note 13)

Because the antibody-conjugated dyes and the PI are light-sensitive, it is best to perform the following procedure under subdued lighting.

1. Label one 15-mL conical tube for each sample and one for the normal control, a known sample of the same phenotype as the experimental samples (usually M/N; *see* **Note 14**). Add 3 mL of staining buffer to each tube.
2. Add 100 µL of well-mixed fixed spheres to each microcentrifuge tube, and vortex to mix (*see* **Notes 15** and **16**).

3. Centrifuge antibody preparations for 10–15 min at 10,000g in a microcentrifuge. (This step may not be necessary, depending on the purity of your antibody preparation.)

4. Add the required amount of BRIC157 antibody to each tube (determined as described in **Note 3**). Vortex immediately. Add the required amount of 6A7 antibody to each tube. Vortex immediately.

5. Wrap tubes in aluminum foil and incubate for 60 min at room temperature on a rocking platform.

6. Wash each sample twice with 3 mL staining buffer by centrifugation at 1750g for 5 min, followed by resuspension by vortexing. Final resuspension should be in only 2 mL of staining buffer.

7. Add 20 µL of 1 mg/mL PI, mix, and refrigerate overnight. Stained samples should be analyzed within 4 d of staining.

3.5. Preparation of Control Samples

Besides running a known control with each group of experimental samples, it is also necessary to prepare samples with mixtures of the common cell phenotypes M/M, M/N, and N/N in order to set the gains on the flow cytometer. These control samples may be drawn fresh for each run from laboratory volunteers, but we have found it useful to stockpile aliquots of M/M and N/N fixed cells for this purpose (*see* **Note 11**). M/N cells can be taken from the analysis control. Although stained cells may also be kept in the refrigerator for later analysis, because the cytometer will be set by fluorescence measurements based on these controls, we believe it is important to stain the controls and experimental samples at the same time, with the same reagents.

1. Label five 1.5-mL microcentrifuge tubes (1–5), and add 1 mL of staining buffer to each.

2. Add 50 µL of MN fixed cells to each of the first four tubes.

3. Add 17 µL each of the MM, MN, and NN fixed cells to the fifth tube.

4. Microcentrifuge all samples at 1000g for 2 min.

5. Decant supernatant and resuspend pellet in 1 mL staining buffer by vortexing.

6. Add the BRIC157 antibody to tubes 2, 4, and 5. Vortex immediately. Add the 6A7 antibody to tubes 3, 4, and 5. Vortex immediately. Use the same amounts as in **Subheading 3.4., step 4** (as determined in **Note 3**).

7. Wrap tubes in alminum foil and incubate for 60 min at room temperature on a rocking platform.

8. Wash each sample twice with 1 mL staining buffer by microcentrifugation at 1000g for 5 min, followed by resuspension by vortexing. Final resuspension should also be in 1 mL of staining buffer.

9. Add 10 µL of 1 mg/mL PI, mix, and refrigerate overnight. Stained samples should be analyzed within 4 d of staining.

3.6. Flow Cytometry I: Setting Windows With Control Samples

1. Turn on flow cytometer and run water through the sample delivery system to remove bubbles.

2. Turn on computer and start analysis software (C30).

3. Load a 500-µL sample of the M/N control (either the analysis control or tube 4 from **Subheading 3.5.**). Using a low flow rate, use this sample to set a scatter gate around live cells. Try to remove dead cells, cell fragments, nonsphered cells, and cell doublets.

4. Adjust FL1 and FL2 voltages to a mode of channel 45 (in log acquisition mode) in both.

5. Prepare a four-cell sample by adding 100 μL from each of microcentrifuge tubes 1–4 from **Subheading 3.5.** to a fresh sample tube, and mixing by vortexing.

6. Run this sample, and use it to adjust compensation percentages to optimize the orthonogality of the four peaks: unlabeled, M-only, N-only, and M/N (**Fig. 4**; *see* **Note 17**).

7. Run the three-cell sample (tube 5 from **Subheading 3.5.**; **Fig. 4**). Draw three data windows, as follows (*see* **Note 18**):

   a. M/N window: channels 33–57 in both directions.
   b. N/∅; window: channels 43–48, FL1 (abscissa) channels 0–14, FL2 (ordinate).
   c. N/N window: channels 49–54, FL1 (abscissa) channels 0–14, FL2 (ordinate).

8. The M/N window should be centered on the M/N peak and include virtually all cells. The N/∅ window should be centered on the N-only peak but may not contain all such cells. If these conditions are not true, return to the four-cell controls and readjust.

3.7. Flow Cytometry II: Sample Analysis

1. Begin analyzing samples with the known M/N control. Acquire the maximum number of events (1,000,000) within the live gate. A complete standard assay consists of five such runs.

2. Run fresh water through the machine for at least 30 s between samples or until counts have stabilized at a low level. Check the live gate and the FL1/FL2 output for each sample and adjust, if necessary (*see* **Note 19**).

3. After acquiring data, check that the modal channel for the M/N peak in every run is 45. If it is not, adjust the N/∅; and N/N windows to compensate.

4. The variant cell frequencies for total, allele loss, and loss and duplication phenotypes is the average of the number of events in the appropriate windows over the five runs per million total cells (*see* **Notes 20 and 21**).

4. Notes

1. Unfortunately, the FACScan and its C30 software have long been obsolete, and their replacements are not as well suited to the very rare event detection necessary for the *GPA* assay. In designing later generation commercial flow cytometers companies have concentrated on the clinical market, with "rare" defined as a 1% proportion of the lymphocyte population, for example. Later flow cytometers from Becton Dickinson could only collect data in "list mode," meaning that you could not choose what data to store. In the initial machines, this limited a single run to 100,000 events, requiring that data from 50 runs be pooled by hand to perform a single *GPA* assay (the FACScan software allowed accumulation of up to 1 million events). Thus, besides requiring an inordinate (and unnecessary) amount of data storage space, running the *GPA* assay on these machines required a full-time technician to turn the machine back on every 2 min or so. With advances in data storage, there is no longer a definite limit on the length of a "list" of data that can be accumulated, and we have performed runs of 1 million events; however, the data file is still prohibitively large (~40 Mbytes).

   A second problem involves the graphical representation of the data. We have shown that the pattern of the flow distribution, as shown in **Fig. 2**, is an important element in the application of the *GPA* assay *(30,36)*. These data are collected in logarithmic mode, and the representation is simplified by providing contour lines linking areas with successive threefold increases in incidence. This allows us to display single events, such as those in the variant windows, simultaneously with the main M/N peak, with close to 1 million events, in a form that illustrates its distribution. Although the allele loss events should fall

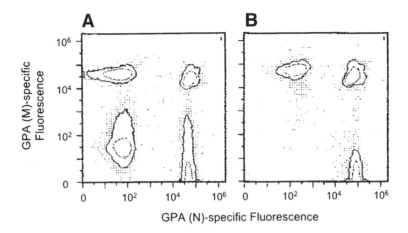

Fig. 4. Examples of the four-cell (**A**) and three-cell (**B**) controls used to set the flow cytometer and software for the *GPA* assay. These labeling controls are used to make sure the two allelic forms of the protein yield equivalent signals and to ensure that variant cells will occur on the abscissa with less than 1% of the labeling of the main peak, directly beneath (allele loss) and to the right (loss and duplication) of the main MN peak.

directly beneath the M/N peak, it is important to know where the true center of this peak lies, which can vary with the donor and condition of the sample. Because they were restricted to capturing only 100,000 events at a time, next-generation software for the flow cytometers subsequent to the FACScan could display only individual events, meaning there was no resolution of the main peak, or of any other peaks (from high-frequency mutations or contaminants such as lymphocytes or transfused blood). Again, this has been addressed to some degree in the more than 10 yr since the FACScan was discontinued; current software has the ability to draw contour lines on the log scale, one-third the resolution of the original machine.

2. Just because a number of molecular mechanisms can potentially contribute to an endpoint doesn't mean that the assay system will really be sensitive to them all. For example, in one in vitro system based on the *APRT* gene, allele loss by gene deletion appeared to be the major mechanism of variation *(40)*, whereas in an in vivo system based on *HLA* polymorphisms, the major mechanism of variation was allele loss and duplication by mitotic recombination *(41)*. In another in vitro system, allele loss occurred primarily by gene inactivation, whereas loss and duplication occurred by chromosome segregation *(14)*. We have argued that the evidence suggests a single mechanism for so-called small-colony mutants in the mouse lymphoma L5178Y *Tk* assay *(42)*, and we have also pointed out that assays with endpoints that have many possible contributing mechanisms are differentially sensitive to those mechanisms with the highest background frequency.

3. Each lot of antibody must be titered upon delivery in order to determine how much is necessary for a standard *GPA* assay. Titering is performed on a sample from a known M/N control individual, by staining, according to the protocol given in **Subheading 3.4.** with 50, 20, 10, 5, 2, and 1 μL of antibody preparation and analysis of staining intensity on the flow cytometer. The amount of antibody necessary to produce 90% of maximum staining intensity is used in the standard assay.

4. Leukoprep tubes (BD Biosciences, Boston, MA) may also be used, but a small amount of serum (~100–200 μL) should be transferred with the red cells to aid in fixation.

5. If very little blood is drawn, or if the sample is to be allocated for several uses, it is best to transfer approx 500 μL for the *GPA* assay to a microcentrifuge tube. Too little blood left in the initial tube will clot or dry onto the side of the tube.

6. If kept cold, samples can be accumulated for up to 2 wk prior to processing.

7. Shipping of samples should be done within 24–48 h of draw, using refrigerated, but not frozen, ice packs and overnight delivery with refrigeration. Shipping early in the week allows time to find lost samples before they are left without refrigeration for the weekend.

8. In its original form, the *GPA* assay requires a heterozygous M/N phenotype to be informative, allowing for quantitation of somatic mutation with single-hit kinetics. We have found, however, that the assay can be informative regardless of donor genotype when the expected mutation frequency exceeds approx 30 allele loss variants per million. (Loss and duplication variants cannot be detected or quantitated under these circumstances, however.)

9. In our experience, the anti-N sera reacts fastest. We therefore watch the anti-M sera while swirling. If the anti-M side agglutinates first, the sample is M/M. If the anti-N side agglutinates first, continue to swirl for about a minute before making a final determination on the anti-M side. (If the anti-M side has agglutinated, the sample is M/N; if the anti-M has not agglutinated, the sample is N/N.)

10. Because the erythrocytes are shaped like biconcave flattened disks, they do not all offer the same surface to the laser during flow cytometry, resulting in excessive light scatter. Expanding them into spheres optimizes their scatter profile, allowing for their discrimination from other blood cells, primarily based on size.

11. Although naive blood samples cannot be frozen for *GPA* analysis, fixed "form spheres," either stained or unstained, may be frozen, allowing for stockpiling of control samples. In practice, we generally only use this for M/M and N/N controls, since the M/N sample will also be analyzed fully, not merely used to set gains and gates on the flow cytometer. (This approach must be adapted if sets of non-M/N samples are to be analyzed; *see* **Note 8.**)

12. If the fixed spheres are not to be stained immediately, they may be kept in the refrigerator (after their overnight incubation) for up to a month with little effect on the performance of the *GPA* assay (although the extra wash described in **Note 16** is recommended if the samples are not processed immediately). Alternatively, these spheres may be frozen for later processing, for stockpiling of samples, or for shipment. To freeze, samples from **Subheading 3.3.** are centrifuged at 450g (2000 rpm on suggested centrifuge) for 1 min, and the supernatant is removed by aspiration. The fixed cells are then resuspended by vortexing in 1 mL of freeze media (RPMI-1640 [Invitrogen, Carlsbad, CA] containing 10% dimethyl sulfoxide [DMSO; Sigma]), separated into 200 μL aliquots in microcentrifuge tubes or cryovials (250-μL tubes; Bio-Rad, Hercules, CA), and frozen at –80°C.

13. Staining of the experimental samples (*see* **Subheading 3.4.**) and the controls (*see* **Subheading 3.5.**) should be done in parallel, if the differences in sample volumes are not too confusing.

14. Because it is essentially useless to run experimental samples if the control is not performed, we often prepare the control in duplicate in case one is dropped or misprocessed.

15. Not all blood samples have the same concentration of red blood cells. Too few cells result in excessively long or incomplete assays, whereas too many cells result in too many cell doublets or even agglutination, which can clog the flow cytometer. We usually compare

the cloudy orange color of this suspension (after mixing) with that of the control, which should represent a sample that is known to run well, and adjust red cell number by adding blood or removing volume (making it up again with staining buffer).

16. An optional wash of the fixed cells can be performed at this stage by centrifuging again at 1750*g* for 5 min, pouring off the supernatant, and resuspending the pellet in 3 mL staining buffer with vortexing. This step is recommended if the form spheres have been in the refrigerator overnight or longer, or if they were frozen.

17. Ideally, the four-cell control should form a perfect square, but it is deformed into a tall rectangle because of crossreaction of the N-specific antibody with another abundant red cell surface protein, glycophorin B, a member of the same gene family as *GPA (3,4)*. The box may be further distorted by overlap of the two fluorophors, causing cells with both alleles to exhibit artifactually high fluorescence for both markers. This causes the angle of the corner of the box marked by the M/N cells to become acute and interferes with the correct positioning of the windows for the variant cells. Likewise, overcompensation causes an obtuse angle at M/N and, again, the mispositioning of the windows for the phenotypic variants.

18. Because the GPB protein is about one-third as abundant on the red cell surface as the GPA protein, a cell expressing a single M allele (an alternate allele loss phenotype) still exhibits one-third of the GPA(N)-specific fluorescence of a parental M/N cell, rather than less than 1% of GPA(M)-specific fluorescence, as does as a cell that has lost an M allele. Although N-allele loss (or loss and duplication) is just as valid a genetic endpoint as M-allele loss, this technical difference in the their detection has led us to consider only M-allele loss variants. (It would be informative to see when the frequencies of mutation are similar at both alleles, and when they are not.) Other groups have established their own versions of the *GPA* assay that include quantitation of N-allele loss variants, however *(43)*, and we quantitate a combined N-allele loss/loss and duplication window when a sample exhibits an unusually high mutation frequency at the M allele (*see* **Note 20**).

19. The M/N peak has a tendency to "drift" toward the ordinate over time.

20. Some adjusting may be necessary owing to changes in denominator if there are obviously scored events that are not possible progenitors of phenotypic variants, such as unusually high number of lymphocytes (in the DB6 assay these appear above and to the left of the main peak) or cells from a recent transfusion *(30)*.

21. When the number of variant cells increases, it may become evident that not all events are contained within the variant windows as originally set. Although the background in this area of the flow histogram is essentially zero (based on analysis of M/M samples that can also manifest an M-allele loss phenotype), we have avoided expanding the windows to accommodate all events, rather, we have simply adjusted the location of the windows so they are centered on the variant cell peak. This avoids the situation in which events from one window overlap the second, producing an artifactual increase in both.

As shown in **Figs. 1** and **3**, in some cases further characterization of the mutational events can be provided by determining whether there are reciprocal products, i.e., a high incidence of N-allele loss in samples in which there are abnormally high frequencies of M-allele loss. In these cases, we simply set a window for variants affecting the N allele empirically, with no attempt to discriminate allele loss from loss and duplication. This is done for all "outliers," samples with frequencies in either phenotypic variant window of 3×10^{-5}, or more or 5×10^{-5} or more in the two windows combined *(30,44)*. We have found that populations generated from these reciprocal events are only evident in the event of a recent or ongoing exposure; when the exposure is distant in time, as in the Hiroshima survivors, there is often no clear association between the M- and N-allele loss populations. We attribute this difference to the differences in cell types contributing to the variant cell populations: when the exposure is recent, most of the mutations are occurring in the highly proliferative, differentiating cell population, and the reciprocal daughter cells contribute equally to the peripheral blood. When a variant peak is caused by an exposure that occurred long ago, it must have affected a stem cell, and the reciprocal event occurred in a daughter cell that may have long since terminally differentiated and disappeared.

All "outlier" samples should be rerun for confirmation of the abnormal phenotype, as well as those rare samples (<1%) in which no variant cells are observed in a standard assay (after ensuring that the sample is not really M/M).

Acknowledgments

The author would like to acknowledge his former colleagues at LLNL who originally conceptualized (Elbert W. Branscomb and William L. Bigbee) and developed (Ronald H. Jensen and Richard G. Langlois) the *GPA* assay, as well as the students (Penelope J. Quintana, Barbara Henry, Reagan K. McLoughlin, and Heather Gordish) and technicians (Barbara A. Nisbet, Ann E. Gorvad, Lynn Biedler, Manda K. Welsh, Britt M. Luccy, Jennifer Adair, Julie A. Conte, and Christian M. Cerceo) who have applied and refined it over the years. He would also like to acknowledge the support of the U.S. Army Breast Cancer Research Program through grants DAMD17-00-1-0409 and DAMD17-01-1-060.

References

1. Mendelsohn, M. L., Bigbee, W. L., Branscomb, E. W., and Stamatoyannopoulos, G. (1980) The detection and sorting of rare sickle-hemoglobin containing cells in normal human blood, in *Flow Cytometry IV* (Laerum, O. D., Lindmo, T., and Thorud, E., eds.), Universitetsforlaget, Oslo, pp. 311–313.
2. Tates, A. D., Bernini, L. F., Natarajan, A. T., et al. (1989) Detection of somatic mutants in man: *HPRT* mutations in lymphocytes and hemoglobin mutations in erythrocytes. *Mutat. Res.* **213,** 73–82.
3. Cartron, J. P. and Rahuel, C. (1995) MNSs and major glycophorins of human erythrocytes. *Transfus. Clin. Biol.* **2,** 251–258.
4. Blumenfeld, O. O. and Huang, C. H. (1997) Molecular genetics of glycophorin MNS variants. *Transfus. Clin. Biol.* **4,** 357–365.
5. Langlois, R. G., Bigbee, W. L., and Jensen, R. H. (1986) Measurements of the frequency of human erythrocytes with gene expression loss phenotypes at the glycophorin A locus. *Hum. Genet.* **74,** 353–362.
6. Langlois, R. G., Nisbet, B. A., Bigbee, W. L., Ridinger, D. N., and Jensen, R. H. (1990) An improved flow cytometric assay for somatic mutations at the glycophorin A locus in humans. *Cytometry* **11,** 513–521.
7. Grant, S. G., Bigbee, W. L., Langlois, R. G., and Jensen, R. H. (1991) Allele loss at the human *GPA* locus: a model for recessive oncogenesis with potential clinical application. *Clin. Biotechnol.* **3,** 177–185.
8. Jensen, R. H. and Bigbee, W. L. (1996) Direct immunofluorescence labeling provides an improved method for the glycophorin A somatic mutation assay. *Cytometry* **23,** 337–343.
9. Worton, R. G. and Grant, S. G. (1985) Segregation-like events in Chinese hamster cells, in *Molecular Cell Genetics* (Gottesman, M. M., ed.), John Wiley & Sons, New York, pp. 831–867.

10. Mitchell, A. D. (1997) Alternate hypothesis for the bimodal size distribution of mutant colonies of L5178Y mouse lymphoma cells. *Environ. Mol. Mutagen.* **29,** 431–433.

11. Farrell, S. A. and Worton, R. G. (1977) Chromosome loss is responsible for segregation at the *HPRT* locus in Chinese hamster cell hybrids. *Somatic Cell Genet.* **3,** 539–551.

12. Eves, E. M. and Farber, R. A. (1981) Chromosome segregation is frequently associated with the expression of recessive mutations in mouse cells. *Proc. Natl. Acad. Sci. USA* **78,** 1768–1772.

13. Gallie, B. L. and Worton, R. G. (1986) Somatic events unmask recessive cancer genes to initiate malignancy. *J. Cell. Biochem.* **32,** 215–222.

14. Grant, S. G., Campbell, C. E., Duff, C., Toth, S. L., and Worton, R. G. (1989) Gene inactivation as a mechanism for the expression of recessive phenotypes. *Am. J. Hum. Genet.* **45,** 619–634.

15. Frost, P. and Kerbel, R. S. (1983) On a possible epigenetic mechanism(s) of tumor cell heterogeneity. The role of DNA methylation. *Cancer Metastasis Rev.* **2,** 375–378.

16. Herman, J. G. and Baylin, S. B. (2003) Gene silencing in cancer in association with promoter hypermethylation. *N. Engl. J. Med.* **349,** 2042–2054.

17. Langlois, R. G., Bigbee, W. L., Kyoizumi, S. K., et al. (1987) Evidence for increased somatic cell mutations at the glycophorin A locus in atomic bomb survivors. *Science* **236,** 445–448.

18. Wasmuth, J. J. and Hall, L. V. (1984) Genetic demonstration of mitotic recombination in cultured Chinese hamster cell hybrids. *Cell* **36,** 697–707.

19. Rosenstraus, M. J. and Chasin, L. A. (1978) Separation of linked markers in Chinese hamster cell hybrids: mitotic recombination is not involved. *Genetics* **90,** 735–760.

20. Campbell, C. E. and Worton, R. G. (1981) Segregation of recessive phenotypes in somatic cell hybrids: role of mitotic recombination, gene inactivation, and chromosome nondisjunction. *Mol. Cell. Biol.* **1,** 336–346.

21. Eves, E. M. and Farber, R. A. (1983) Expression of recessive *Aprt⁻* mutations in mouse CAK cells resulting from chromosome loss and duplication. *Somatic Cell Genet.* **9,** 771–778.

22. Albertini, S. and Zimmermann, F. K. (1991) The detection of chemically induced chromosomal malsegregation in *Saccharomyces cerevisiae* D61.M: a literature survey (1984–1990). *Mutat. Res.* **258,** 237–258.

23. Liu, M., Grant, S. G., Macina, O. T., Klopman, G., and Rosenkranz, H. S. (1997) Structural and mechanistic bases for the induction of mitotic chromosomal loss and duplication ('malsegregation') in the yeast *Saccharomyces cerevisiae*: relevance to human carcinogenesis and developmental toxicology. *Mutat. Res.* **374,** 209–231.

24. Rothman, N., Haas, R., Hayes, R.B., et al. (1995) Benzene induces gene-duplicating but not gene-inactivating mutations at the glycophorin A locus in exposed humans. *Proc. Natl. Acad. Sci. USA* **92,** 4069–4073.

25. Langlois, R. G., Bigbee, W. L., Jensen, R. H., and German, J. (1989) Evidence for elevated *in vivo* mutations and somatic recombination in Bloom's syndrome. *Proc. Natl. Acad. Sci. USA* **86,** 670–674.

26. Compton-Quintana, P. J. E., Jensen, R. H., Bigbee, W. L., et al. (1993) Use of the glycophorin A human mutation assay to study workers exposed to styrene. *Environ. Health Perspect.* **99,** 297–301.

27. Grant, S.G. (1992) Mutation, segregation, and childhood cancer, in *Late Effects of Treatment for Childhood Cancer* (Green, D. M. and D'Angio, G. J., eds.), Wiley-Liss, New York, pp. 121–132.

28. Henry, B., Grant, S. G., Klopman, G., and Rosenkranz, H. S. (1998) Induction of forward mutations at the thymidine kinase locus of mouse lymphoma cells: evidence for electrophilic and non-electrophilic mechanisms. *Mutat. Res.* **397,** 313–335.

29. Grant, S. G. and Jensen, R. H. (1993) Use of hematopoietic cells and markers for the detection and quantitation of human *in vivo* somatic mutation, in *Immunobiology of Transfusion Medicine* (Garratty, G., ed.), Marcel Dekker, New York, pp. 299–323.

30. Evdokimova, V. E., McLoughlin, R. K., Wenger, S. L., and Grant, S. G. Use of the glycophorin A bone marrow somatic mutation assay for rapid, unambiguous identification of Fanconi anemia homozygotes regardless of *GPA* genotype. *Am. J. Med. Genet.*, in press.

31. Grant, S. G. and Bigbee, W. L. (1993) *In vivo* somatic mutation and segregation at the human glycophorin A *(GPA)* locus: phenotypic variation encompassing both gene-specific and chromosomal mechanisms. *Mutat. Res.* **288**, 163–172.

32. Grant, S. G. (2001) Molecular epidemiology of human cancer: biomarkers of genotoxic exposure and susceptibility. *J. Environ. Pathol. Toxicol. Oncol.* **20**, 245–261.

33. Perera, F. P., Tang, D. L., O'Neill, J. P., et al. (1993) HPRT and glycophorin A mutations in foundry workers: relationship to PAH exposure and to PAH-DNA adducts. *Carcinogenesis* **14**, 969–973.

34. Jones, I. M., Galick, H., Kato, P., et al. (2002) Three somatic genetic biomarkers and covariates in radiation-exposed Russian cleanup workers of the chernobyl nuclear reactor 6–13 years after exposure. *Radiat. Res.* **158**, 424–442.

35. Saenko, A. S., Zamulaeva, I. A., Smirnova, S. G., et al. Determination of somatic mutant frequencies at glycophorin A and T-cell receptor loci for biodosimetry of prolonged irradiation. *Int. J. Radiat. Biol.* **73**, 613–618.

36. Grant, S. G., Reeger, W., and Wenger, S. L. (1998) Diagnosis of ataxia telangiectasia with the glycophorin A somatic mutation assay. *Genet. Testing* **1**, 261–267.

37. Hsu, T. C. (1983) Genetic instability in the human population: a working hypothesis. *Hereditas* **98**, 1–9.

38. Okada, S., Ishii, H., Nose, H., et al. (1997) Evidence for increased somatic cell mutations in patients with hepatocellular carcinoma. *Carcinogenesis* **18**, 445–449.

39. Grant, S. G., Bigbee, W. L., Langlois, R. G., and Jensen, R. H. (1991) Methods for the detection of mutational and segregational events: relevance to the monitoring of survivors of childhood cancer, in *Late Effects of Treatment for Childhood Cancer* (Green, D. M. and D'Angio, G. J., ed.), Wiley-Liss, New York, pp. 133–150.

40. Simon, A. E. and Taylor, M. W. (1983) High-frequency mutation at the adenine phosphoribosyltransferase locus in Chinese hamster ovary cells due to deletion of the gene. *Proc. Natl. Acad. Sci. USA* **80**, 810–814.

41. Morley, A. A., Grist, S. A., Turner, D. R., Kutlaca, A., and Bennett, G. (1990) Molecular nature of in vivo mutations in human cells at the autosomal HLA-A locus. *Cancer Res.* **50**, 4584–4587.

42. Grant, S. G., Zhang, Y. P., Klopman, G., and Rosenkranz, H. S. (2000) Modeling the mouse lymphoma forward mutational assay: the Gene-Tox program database. *Mutat. Res.* **465**, 201–229.

43. Kyoizumi, S., Nakamura, N., Hakoda, M., et al. (1989) Detection of somatic mutations at the glycophorin A locus in erythrocytes of atomic bomb survivors using a single beam flow sorter. *Cancer Res.* **49**, 581–588.

44. Bigbee, W. L., Fuscoe, J. C., Grant, S. G., et al. (1998) Human in vivo somatic mutation measured at two loci: individuals with stably elevated background erythrocyte glycophorin A *(gpa)* variant frequencies exhibit normal T-lymphocyte *hprt* mutant frequencies. *Mutat. Res.* **397**, 119–136.

19

Flow Cytometric Measurement of Mutant T Cells With Altered Expression of *TCR*

Detecting Somatic Mutations in Humans and Mice

Seishi Kyoizumi, Yoichiro Kusunoki, and Tomonori Hayashi

Summary

Spontaneously generated mutant T cells defective in T-cell receptor (*TCR*) gene expression are detectable at the frequency of 10^{-4} in vivo, and the mutant fractions are dose-dependently increased by exposure to genotoxic substances such as ionizing radiation. Mutant cells with altered expression of TCR-α or -β among CD4+ T cells can be detected as CD3−/CD4+ cells by two-color flow cytometry using anti-CD3 and anti-CD4 monoclonal antibodies labeled with different fluorescent dyes, because an incomplete TCR$\alpha\beta$/CD3 complex cannot be transported to the cellular membrane. This flow cytometric mutation assay can be applied to CD4+ T cells from human peripheral blood and mouse spleen. Methods for both preparation of target cells and detection of the mutant cells are described.

Key Words: Somatic mutation; flow cytometry; T-cell receptor (TCR), CD4+ T cell; human peripheral blood; mouse spleen.

1. Introduction

Monitoring of somatic mutation in vivo is useful for evaluating cancer risk from exposure to environmental genotoxic substances, including ionizing radiation and chemicals. Assays of in vivo somatic mutations have been established for various target genes *(1)*. The flow cytometric T-cell receptor (*TCR*) mutation assay allows reproducible measurement of mutant fractions (Mfs) at the *TCR-α* (*TCRA*) and *TCR-β* (*TCRB*) genes of peripheral mature CD4+ T cells in individual humans *(2)* and mice *(3)*.

The TCR-α and -β proteins are expressed on the cell surface of normal peripheral CD4− and CD8+ T cells. In most of these T-cell populations, only one of the two alleles of each *TCR* chain gene is actively expressed, although it has been reported that a minor T-cell subpopulation coexpresses dual α or β chains *(4,5)*. The second allele of these loci remains unexpressed owing to nonfunctional recombination or epigenetic inactivation resulting in allelic exclusion *(6)*. Thus, mutants that do not express TCR can be

From: *Methods in Molecular Biology, vol. 291, Molecular Toxicology Protocols*
Edited by: P. Keohavong and S. G. Grant © Humana Press Inc., Totowa, NJ

generated in the majority of the T-cell population by a single inactivation event, even though the *TCR* genes are autosomally located. Further, TCR-α and β chains can be expressed on the cell surface only after formation of large molecular complexes with CD3-γ, -δ, -ϵ, -ζ, and -η chains. If either of the *TCR*-α or β chain genes are not expressed, the TCR$\alpha\beta$/CD3 complex cannot be transported to the cellular membrane, and defective complexes accumulate in the cytoplasm *(2,7)*. Thus, inactivating mutations in the *TCRA* or *TCRB* genes among CD4$^+$ T cells can be detected as CD3$^-$ CD4$^+$ mutant cells by two-color flow cytometry using monoclonal antibodies against the CD3 and CD4 molecules. Specifically, the fraction of CD3$^-$ cells in a population of mature CD4$^+$ T cells is considered to be the total Mf for both the *TCRA* and *TCRB* genes in CD4$^+$ T cells. The background Mf of CD3$^-$ cells in populations of human and mouse mature CD4$^+$ T cells increases significantly with age *(2,8)* but is about 2×10^{-4} *(2,3,9–11)*. *TCR* mutants were found to be dose-dependently induced in normal CD4$^+$ T cells and in a lymphoma cell line by in vitro exposure to ionizing radiation *(12–14)* or chemicals *(12)*.

The *TCR* mutation assay can be used to monitor human exposure to environmental mutagens. For example, it has been applied to lymphocytes from cancer patients who had recently received radiotherapy *(9,14,15)* or chemotherapy *(16)*, from patients who had been treated during the 1930s and 1940s with Thorotrast, a colloidal preparation of radioactive thorium-232 used as a radiological contrast medium *(9,17)*, from a person who was heavily exposed to radiation during the 1986 Chernobyl accident *(9)*, from clean-up workers in the Chernobyl accident *(10)*, and from the residents in a radioactively contaminated area near Chelyabinsk in Russia *(18)*. Although statistically significant dose-dependent increases in *TCR* Mf were found in these individuals, no significant elevation was detected in atomic bomb survivors who were exposed to radiation many years ago *(9)*. This is consistent with the observation that elevated Mfs in radiotherapy patients decline gradually to background levels within about 10 yr after exposure (half-life: about 2 yr) *(15,19)*. Although expression of a *TCR* mutant phenotype can require as long as several months in vivo, we have improved the assay to shorten the expression time of the *TCR* mutant phenotype by using growth stimulation of lymphocytes in culture *(14)*. The Mf of *TCR* was found to be elevated in patients with autosomal recessive inherited diseases with defective DNA repair and premature aging, such as ataxia telangiectasia *(2,11)*, Fanconi's anemia *(2)*, Werner's syndrome *(20)*, and Bloom's syndrome *(20,21)*.

We have used a mouse model to demonstrate the in vivo kinetics and dose response of radiation-induced *TCR* mutations *(3)*. In this system, expression of the *TCR* mutant phenotype reached a peak about 2 wk after whole-body irradiation. The Mf then decreased, with a half-life of about 2 wk. We have also reported on the influence of the genetic background on both spontaneous and radiation-induced mutagenesis *(3)*. Using mutant mice, including bioengineered transgenic knockout mice, we have analyzed the role of the *p53* gene in *TCR* mutagenesis *(22)*.

Both human peripheral blood mononuclear cells and mouse T-cell-enriched splenocytes have been used as the target cells for the *TCR* mutation assay. This chapter gives precise methods for the preparation of these target cells and for the flow cytometric procedures used to detect and quantify CD3$^-$ cell fractions among CD4$^+$ T-cell populations.

2. Materials

2.1. Preparation of Human Peripheral Blood Mononuclear Cells

1. Heparinized peripheral blood (3–5 mL).
2. Ficoll-Hypaque solution (specific density 1.077; e.g., Lymphocyte Separation Medium ICN Biomedicals, Aurora, OH).
3. 15-mL polypropylene centrifuge tube.
4. Phosphate-buffered saline (PBS; e.g., Sigma, St. Louis, MO).
5. PBS containing 2.5% fetal calf serum (FCS; Gibco-BRL, Grand Island, NY); heat-inactivated for 30 min at 56°C; PBS-S.
6. Hemacytometer (e.g., Becton Dickinson Primary Care Diagnostics, Sparks, MD).
7. Turk's solution (e.g., Merck, Darmstadt, Germany).
8. 0.4% Trypan blue stain (e.g., Gibco-BRL).

2.2. Preparation of T-Cell-Enriched Mouse Splenocytes

1. 60 × 15-mm Plastic Petri dish (e.g., Becton Dickinson Labware, Franklin Lakes, NJ).
2. Iris scissors and forceps.
3. Frosted glass slides.
4. RPMI-1640 (e.g., Sigma) containing 10% heat-inactivated FCS, 2 mM L-glutamine, 100 U/mL penicillin, and 100 µg/mL streptomycin (complete RPMI).
5. 15-mL Polypropylene centrifuge tube.
6. 200-µm Mesh nylon screen.
7. Hemacytometer.
8. 0.4% Trypan blue stain.
9. Nylon wool (e.g., Polysciences, Warrington, PA).
10. 5-mL Disposable syringe.
11. Three-way disposable stopcock.
12. 19- and 23-gage Needles.
13. Cell culture incubator.
14. Parafilm (or Saran Wrap).

2.3. Immunofluorescence Staining

1. Fluorescein isothiocyanate (FITC)-labeled antihuman CD4 monoclonal antibody (Leu-3 antibody, BD Biosciences, San Jose, CA).
2. Phycoerythrin (PE)-labeled antihuman CD3ε monoclonal antibody (Leu-4 antibody, BD Biosciences).
3. FITC-labeled antimouse CD4 monoclonal antibody (CT-CD3 antibody, Caltag Laboratories, Burlingame, CA).
4. PE-labeled antimouse CD3ε monoclonal antibody (145-2C11 antibody, BD Pharmingen Biosciences, San Diego, CA).
5. PBS containing 0.01% NaN$_3$ and 1% FCS (PBS-NS).
6. PBS-NS containing 10 µg/mL propidium iodide.
7. 1.5-mL Eppendorf tube.
8. 5-mL Polystyrene round-bottomed tube (Becton Dickinson Labware).

2.4. Flow Cytometry

1. Flow cytometer (e.g., FACScan, BD Biosciences) installed with computer software for data acquisition and analysis (e.g., CELLQuest, BD Biosciences).

3. Methods

3.1. Preparation of Human Peripheral Blood Mononuclear Cells (see Note 1)

1. Place heparinized blood (3–5 mL) into a 15-mL centrifuge tube.
2. Add an equal volume of PBS at room temperature and mix well.
3. Slowly layer the Ficoll-Hypaque solution underneath the blood/PBS mixture by placing the tip of the pipet containing the Ficoll-Hypaque at the bottom of the sample tube. Use 3 mL Ficoll-Hypaque per 10 mL blood/PBS mixture.
4. Centrifuge for a total of 30 min at 400g at room temperature with no brake. (Slowly raise the centrifuge speed to 400g.)
5. Using a pipet, remove the upper layer containing the plasma and platelets. Using another pipet, transfer the mononuclear cell layer (interface between the upper and Ficoll-Hypaque layers) to a new 15-mL centrifuge tube.
6. Wash cells by adding excess PBS-S (about three times the volume of the mononuclear cell layer) at room temperature and centrifuging for 10 min at 510g.
7. Discard supernatant, resuspend cells in 10 mL PBS-S, and centrifuge for 10 min at 240g.
8. Repeat **step 7**.
9. Discard supernatant and resuspend cells in 1 mL PBS-S.
10. Count mononuclear cells in Turk's solution using a hemacytometer and calculate cell yield. Use trypan blue exclusion to determine cell viability. Average yield is about 1×10^6 viable mononuclear cells from 1 mL blood.

3.2. Preparation of T-Cell-Enriched Mouse Splenocytes

1. Sacrifice mice in a humane manner. Make a 1.5-cm incision at the left of the peritoneal wall with scissors. Gently pull the spleen free of the peritoneum, tearing the connective tissue behind the spleen.
2. Place the spleen in a 60 × 15-mm plastic Petri dish containing 3 mL complete RPMI. With scissors, cut the spleen into several pieces.
3. By rubbing between the frosted faces of two glass slides, mash the spleen pieces until mostly fibrous tissue remains.
4. Expel cell suspension into a 15-mL plastic centrifuge tube through a 200-μm-mesh nylon screen. Wash Petri dish with about 4 mL complete RPMI.
5. Centrifuge cell suspension at 240g for 10 min. Resuspend cell pellet in 10 mL complete RPMI and count cells with trypan blue exclusion using a hemacytometer for determining cell yield and viability. The viable cell yield per normal spleen is $5–20 \times 10^7$, depending on the mouse strain and age.
6. Centrifuge again and resuspend in 0.5 mL complete RPMI.
7. Prepare a nylon wool column by packing 0.3 g nylon wool in a 5-mL disposable syringe (*see* **Note 2**). Insert the plunger, and press firmly to compact the nylon wool.
8. Clamp the sterilized nylon wool column to a ring stand. Attach both to a three-way stopcock in an open position and a 19-gage needle.
9. Equilibrate the column by running 10 mL of 37°C warmed complete RPMI through the column. Remove trapped air bubbles by firmly tapping on the sides of the column until no dry areas are visible. Finally, tamp down the nylon wool with a pipet to compact the nylon and extrude any additional trapped air.
10. Close the stopcock and cover the nylon wool with 1–2 mL warmed complete RPMI to prevent drying. Incubate the column in an upright position for 45 min at 37°C, 5% CO_2 in a humidified incubator.
11. Warm cell suspension at 37°C.

12. Open the stopcock and allow the medium to drain completely. Using a Pasteur pipet, add dropwise 0.5 mL warmed cell suspension onto the nylon wool and again allow to drain completely. Close the stopcock, and cover the top of the column with plastic (Parafilm or Saran Wrap).
13. Incubate the column for 1 h in an upright position in a 37°C, 5% CO_2 humidified incubator.
14. Remove the column from the incubator, and clamp to the ring stand. Replace the 19-gage needle with a 23-gage needle.
15. Open the stopcock and elute the column with 10 mL total warmed complete RPMI. Collect the effluent (nonadherent) cells in a 15-mL centrifuge tube.
16. Centrifuge harvested cells at 240g, 4°C for 10 min.
17. Discard supernatant and resuspend cells in 10 mL complete RPMI.
18. Count cells with trypan blue exclusion using a hemacytometer for determining cell yield and viability. Average yield is about $2–3 \times 10^7$ T-cell–enriched cells from a spleen (*see* **Notes 3** and **4**).

3.3. Immunofluorescence Staining

1. Transfer 2×10^6 human peripheral blood mononuclear cells or mouse T-cell-enriched splenocytes suspended in PBS-NS to a 1.5-mL Eppendorf tube, and centrifuge at 340g, 4°C for 2 min.
2. Discard supernatant, and add 2 μg each of FITC-labeled antihuman or -mouse CD4 and PE-labeled antihuman or -mouse CD3 antibodies to the cell pellet, mix well, and incubate for 30 min on ice.
3. Wash cells by adding 0.75 mL PBS-NS and centrifuging at 340g, 4°C for 2 min.
4. Discard supernatant and resuspend cells in 0.5 mL PBS-NS containing propidium iodide to stain dead cells. Transfer cell suspension to a 5-mL polystyrene tube for flow cytometry.

3.4. Flow Cytometry (see Note 5)

1. *TCR* mutant CD4+ T cells (CD3-/CD4+) can be measured using a FACScan installed with the operation and analysis software CELLQuest. Set up the FACScan and CELLQuest, and optimize settings according to the manufacturer's instructions (*see* **Note 6**).
2. First, run a small number of the stained lymphocytes (about 1000 events) through the FACScan. Set a gate for the lymphocyte fraction using the forward and side light scatter (FSC and SSC) profile (**Fig. 1A** and **B**).
3. Acquire and store FL1 (CD4 FITC fluorescence) and FL2 (CD3 PE fluorescence) data for a minimum of 500,000 lymphocyte-gated events (*see* **Note 7**).
4. Display acquired data on the screen in histograms of FL1 (CD4) and FL2 (CD3) and in density plots of FL1 vs. FL2 (**Fig. 1B, C, E,** and **F**). Obtain the peak fluorescence intensities (channel number) of the FL1 (CD4) and FL2 (CD3) of normal CD3+/CD4+ cell population in the histograms by gating this population in the density plot. (Gate out propidium iodide-stained dead cells from the population; **Fig. 1B, C, E,** and **F**).
5. Set a mutant window on the region for CD3-/CD4+ in the density plot as follows. Set the left and right limits of FL1 at the half and two times values of the peak intensity of FL1 (CD4) for normal CD3+/CD4+ cells, respectively. Set the upper limit of the FL2 for the mutant window at the 1/25 value of the peak intensity of CD3 for normal CD3+/CD4+ cells as mentioned above, and set the lower limit at 10^0 (*see* **Note 8**).
6. Calculate the Mf as the number of events in the mutant window (**Fig. 1B, C, E,** and **F**) divided by the total number of events corresponding to CD4+ cells.

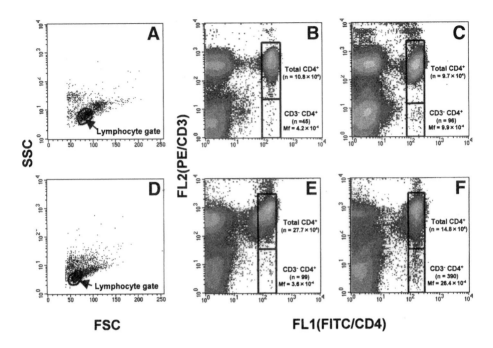

FSC   **FL1(FITC/CD4)**

Fig. 1. Representative flow cytograms of human peripheral blood mononuclear cells (**A–C**) and nylon-wool-passed mouse splenocytes (**D–F**) stained with FITC-labeled anti-CD4 (FL1) and PE-labeled anti-CD3 (FL2) monoclonal antibodies. (**A and D**) Gates for lymphocytes on forward and side light scatter (FSC and SSC) profiles (dot plot). (**B, C, E, and F**) Windows for total CD4$^+$ and mutant CD3$^-$/CD4$^+$ T cells on fluorescence profiles (density plot). The number of events in each window is shown in each panel. The mutant fraction (Mf) was calculated as the number of events in the mutant window divided by the number of events in the total CD4$^+$ T cells. Events representing the highest FL2 fluorescence (nearly 10^4) are dead cells stained with propidium iodide. (**A and B**) Laboratory control (48-yr-old male). (**C**) A patient who had received Thorotrast. (**D and E**) C57BL/6 mouse (4-mo-old female). (**F**) C57BL/6 mouse irradiated with 2.5 Gy X-rays (2 wk after whole-body irradiation).

4. Notes

1. Tubes for one-step mononuclear cell separation from whole blood are commercially available (e.g., BD Vacutainer CPT tube, Becton Dickinson Primary Care Diagnostics). These tubes contain anticoagulant (sodium heparin or sodium citrate) and the cell separation medium, which is composed of a polyester gel and a density gradient liquid.
2. Prepacked nylon wool fiber columns are also commercially available (e.g., Polysciences).
3. Generally, effluent cells are 80–90% T cells and 10–20% B cells and macrophages. Viable cell yield after nylon column passage is generally 15–20% of the initial number of cells loaded on the column.
4. T-cell-enriched mouse splenocytes can also be prepared using a magnetic cell sorting system (MACS) for the *TCR* mutation assay. A pan-T-cell isolation kit containing cock-

tail of magnetic beads for depleting non-T cells is commercially available (e.g., Miltenyi Biotec, Bergish-Gladbach, Germany).

5. The general principles of methodological flow cytometry have been described elsewhere *(23)*.

6. Setup procedures for flow cytometry using the FACScan are described elsewhere *(24)*.

7. Data correlated by four parameters (FSC, SSC, FL1, and FL2) can be acquired and stored if disk storage space is large enough. The lymphocyte gate should be set on the light scatter profile for the mutant analyses of the stored four-parameter data.

8. The mutant window may be set by other reasonable rules. For example, the upper limit of the mutant window can be set at the value of the mean plus 3 standard deviations of PE fluorescence intensity (FL2) of CD3⁻/CD4⁻ cells *(10)*.

Acknowledgments

The authors would like to acknowledge M. Yamaoka and K. Koyama for excellent technical help and C. A. Waldren for valuable suggestions.

References

1. Cole, J. and Skopek, T. R. (1994) Somatic mutant frequency, mutation rates and mutational spectra in the human population in vivo. *Mutat. Res.* **304**, 33–105.

2. Kyoizumi, S., Akiyama, M., Hirai, Y., Kusunoki, Y., Tanabe, K., and Umeki, S. (1990) Spontaneous loss and alteration of antigen receptor expression in mature CD4+ T cells. *J. Exp. Med.* **171**, 1981–1999.

3. Umeki, S., Suzuki, T., Kusunoki, Y., Seyama, T., Fujita, S., and Kyoizumi, S. (1997) Development of a mouse model for studying in vivo T-cell receptor mutations. *Mutat. Res.* **393**, 37–46.

4. Davodeau, F., Peyrat, M. A., Romagne, F., et al. (1995) Dual T cell receptor beta chain expression on human T lymphocytes. *J. Exp. Med.* **181**, 1391–1398.

5. Padovan, E., Casorati, G., Dellabona, P., Meyer, S., Brockhaus, M., and Lanzavecchia, A. (1993) Expression of two T cell receptor alpha chains: dual receptor T cells. *Science* **262**, 422–424.

6. Malissen, M., Trucy, J., Jouvin-Marche, E., Cazenave, P. A., Scollay, R., and Malissen, B. (1992) Regulation of TCR alpha and beta gene allelic exclusion during T-cell development. *Immunol. Today* **13**, 315–322.

7. Clevers, H., Alarcon, B., Wileman, T., and Terhorst, C. (1988) The T cell receptor/CD3 complex: a dynamic protein ensemble. *Annu. Rev. Immunol.* **6**, 629–662.

8. Akiyama, M., Kyoizumi, S., Hirai, Y., Kusunoki, Y., Iwamoto, K. S., and Nakamura, N. (1995). Mutation frequency in human blood cells increases with age. *Mutat. Res.* **338**, 141–149.

9. Kyoizumi, S., Umeki, S., Akiyama, M., et al. (1992) Frequency of mutant T lymphocytes defective in the expression of the T-cell antigen receptor gene among radiation-exposed people. *Mutat. Res.* **265**, 173–180.

10. Saenko, A. S., Zamulaeva, I. A., Smirnova, S. G., et al. (1998) Determination of somatic mutant frequencies at glycophorin A and T-cell receptor loci for biodosimetry of prolonged irradiation. *Int. J. Radiat. Biol.* **73**, 613–618.

11. Lantelme, E., Mantovani, S., Palermo, B., et al. (2000) Increased frequency of RAG-expressing, CD4(+)CD3(low) peripheral T lymphocytes in patients with defective responses to DNA damage. *Eur. J. Immunol.* **30**, 1520–1525.

12. Mei, N., Kunugita, N., Nomoto, S., and Norimura, T. (1996) Comparison of the frequency of T-cell receptor mutants and thioguanine resistance induced by X-rays and ethylnitrosourea in cultured human blood T-lymphocytes. *Mutat. Res.* **357,** 191–197.

13. Iwamoto, K. S., Mizuno, T., Ito, T., Tsuyama, N., Kyoizumi, S., and Seyama, T. (1996) Gain-of-function *p53* mutations enhance alteration of the T-cell receptor following X-irradiation, independently of the cell cycle and cell survival. *Cancer Res.* **56,** 3862–3865.

14. Ishioka, N., Umeki, S., Hirai, Y., et al. (1997) Stimulated rapid expression in vitro for early detection of in vivo T-cell receptor mutations induced by radiation exposure. *Mutat. Res.* **390,** 269–282.

15. Iwamoto, K. S., Hirai, Y., Umeki, S., et al. (1994) A positive correlation between T-cell-receptor mutant frequencies and dicentric chromosome frequencies in lymphocytes from radiotherapy patients. *J. Radiat. Res.* **35,** 92–103.

16. Hirota, H., Kubota, M., Adachi, S., et al. (1994) Somatic mutations at T-cell antigen receptor and glycophorin A loci in pediatric leukemia patients following chemotherapy: comparison with HPRT locus mutation. *Mutat. Res.* **315,** 95–103.

17. Umeki, S., Kyoizumi, S., Kusunoki, Y., et al. (1991) Flow cytometric measurements of somatic cell mutations in Thorotrast patients. *Jpn. J. Cancer Res.* **82,** 1349–1353.

18. Akleyev, A. V., Kossenko, M. M., Silkina, L. A., et al. (1995). Health effects of radiation incidents in the southern Urals. *Stem Cells* **13(suppl. 1),** 58–68.

19. Umeki, S., Kusunoki, Y., Cologne, J. B., et al. (1998). Lifespan of human memory T-cells in the absence of T-cell receptor expression. *Immunol. Lett.* **62,** 99–104.

20. Kyoizumi, S., Kusunoki, Y., Seyama, T., Hatamochi, A., and Goto, M. (1998) In vivo somatic mutations in Werner's syndrome. *Hum. Genet.* **103,** 405–410.

21. Kusunoki, Y., Hayashi, T., Hirai, Y., et al. (1994) Increased rate of spontaneous mitotic recombination in T lymphocytes from a Bloom's syndrome patient using a flow-cytometric assay at HLA-A locus. *Jpn. J. Cancer Res.* **85,** 610–618.

22. Suzuki, T., Kusunoki, Y., Tsuyama, N., Ohnishi, H., Seyama, T., and Kyoizumi, S. (2001) Elevated in vivo frequencies of mutant T cells with altered functional expression of the T-cell receptor or hypoxanthine phosphoribosyltransferase genes in *p53*-deficient mice. *Mutat. Res.* **483,** 13–17.

23. Shallow, S. O. (1999) Overview of flow cytometry, in *Current Protocols in Immunology* (Coligan, J. E., Kruisbreek, A. M., Margulies, D. H., Shevach, E. M., and Strober, W., eds.), John Wiley & Sons, New York, Units 5.1 and 5.2.

24. Otten, G., Yokoyama, W. M., and Holmes, K. L. (1999) Flow cytometry analysis using the Becton Dickinson FACScan, in *Current Protocols in Immunology* (Coligan, J. E., Kruisbreek, A. M., Margulies, D. H., Shevach, E. M., and Stroer, W., eds.), John Wiley & Sons, New York, Unit 5.4.

IV

DETECTION AND CHARACTERIZATION OF CANCER GENE MUTATION

20

Mutation Screening of the *TP53* Gene by Temporal Temperature Gradient Gel Electrophoresis

Therese Sørlie, Hilde Johnsen, Phuong Vu, Guro Elisabeth Lind, Ragnhild Lothe, and Anne-Lise Børresen-Dale

Summary

A protocol for detection of mutations in the *TP53* gene using temporal temperature gradient gel electrophoresis (TTGE) is described. TTGE is a mutation detection technique that separates DNA fragments differing by single base pairs according to their melting properties in a denaturing gel. It is based on constant denaturing conditions in the gel combined with a temperature gradient during the electrophoretic run. This method combines some of the advantages of the related techniques denaturing gradient gel electrophoresis (DGGE) and constant denaturant gel electrophoresis (CDGE) and eliminates some of the problems. The result is a rapid and sensitive screening technique that is robust and easily set up in smaller laboratory environments.

Key Words: *TP53*; TTGE; DGGE; CDGE; mutation screening.

1. Introduction

The tumor suppressor protein TP53 is a central regulator of the cell cycle, and mutations in the *TP53* gene are found in almost all types of human cancer with a frequency ranging from 20 to 60% (http://www.iarc.fr/P53/) *(1)*. Our increasing knowledge about how different *TP53* mutations have arisen, and how they impair the function of the protein and alter the many p53 pathways *(2)*, makes it a suitable molecular marker for (1) exposure to various DNA insults; (2) prognosis evaluation; (3) prediction of response to therapy; and (4) molecular targeting for therapy *(3–6)*. Reported frequencies of mutations have been dependent on several factors, such as population differences in exposure risks and susceptibility and type and stage of the tumors analyzed, as well as the sensitivity and specificity of the method used for detection of mutations. Although most *TP53* mutations are located in the most conserved region of the gene, exons 5–8, sequence alterations, especially small deletions and insertions, are found outside this region. A precise knowledge of the complete *TP53*

From: *Methods in Molecular Biology, vol. 291, Molecular Toxicology Protocols*
Edited by: P. Keohavong and S. G. Grant © Humana Press Inc., Totowa, NJ

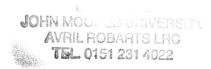

mutation spectrum, including the nature and location of the different sequence changes, can provide insight into the different processes (exogenous and endogenous factors) that cause these mutations *(4)*. This information is essential if it is to be used in the evaluation of tumor aggressiveness and therapeutic response *(7–11)*.

In addition to direct sequencing, a variety of screening methods are currently in use to detect mutations in the *TP53* gene. Major techniques include single-stranded conformation polymorphism analysis (SSCP) *(12,13)*, denaturing gradient gel electrophoresis (DGGE) *(14)*, constant denaturant gel electrophoresis (CDGE) *(15,16)*, constant denaturant capillary electrophoresis (CDCE) *(17,18)*, and dideoxy fingerprinting (ddF) *(19)*. These gene scanning techniques are followed by sequencing of the region of interest to determine the exact nature of the mutation.

Temporal temperature gradient gel electrophoresis (TTGE) is an improved mutation screening technique that combines the maximized separation achieved by the calculated constant denaturant in CDGE with a temporal temperature gradient *(20,21)*. DNA fragments melt in a sequence-specific manner under denaturing conditions during polyacrylamide gel electrophoresis, resulting in abrupt stepwise decreases in mobility. By using a constant denaturant corresponding to the specific melting domains, the fragments migrate with a consistently different mobility through the gel. In TTGE, the separation of fragments differing by as little as 1 bp is enhanced by the addition of a second denaturing condition provided by the temperature gradient. The temperature is gradually and uniformly increased during electrophoresis, resulting in a linear temperature gradient over time *(22,23)*. This provides TTGE with an advantage over CDGE for fragments with a short time interval for the transition from double-stranded DNA to complete denaturation to single-stranded structures. In TTGE, the denaturing conditions span a wider range, making this system more flexible than CDGE and DGGE with respect to time and denaturing conditions. Consequently, this allows fragments with different melting profiles to be analyzed on the same gel (*see* **Note 1**). TTGE also shows an increased sensitivity for the detection of mutant cells in a wild-type background (*see* **Note 2**). In this chapter, we present a protocol for mutation screening of the *TP53* gene using TTGE. This protocol should be adaptable to the mutational screening of other human genes whose sequence is known.

2. Materials
2.1. Primer Design and Optimizing Melting Profiles

1. Oligo primer analysis program (National Biosciences, Plymouth, MN).
2. MacMelt or WinMelt program (MedProbe, Oslo, Norway).

2.2. PCR

1. 5 U/µL AmpliTaq DNA polymerase (PE Biosystems, Foster City, CA).
2. 10X Polymerase chain reaction (PCR) buffer: 500 mM KCl, 100 mM Tris-HCl, pH 8.3 (supplied with AmpliTaq enzyme).
3. 25 mM MgCl$_2$ (supplied with the enzyme).
4. 10 mM dNTPs.
5. 100–200 ng/µL Genomic DNA (*see* **Note 3**).
6. Primers (prepared as a stock solution in distilled water and stored at –20°C).

7. Distilled water.
8. Thin-walled 0.2-mL PCR tubes.
9. Mastercycler (Eppendorf, Hamburg, Germany).

2.3. Preparation of Polyacrylamide Gels

1. 40% Polyacrylamide/*bis*-acrylamide 37.5:1 (Bio-Rad, Hercules, CA).
2. 1.25X and 1.75X TAE, both prepared from a 50X stock solution (2 *M* Tris-acetate, 50 m*M* EDTA, pH 8.0).
3. Urea.
4. Formamide.
5. Ammonium persulfate (APS).
6. *N,N,N,N*-tetramethyl-ethylenediamine (TEMED; Bio-Rad).

2.4. Sample Loading, Electrophoresis, and Visualization of Bands

1. DCode™ Universal Mutation Detection System (Bio-Rad).
2. 16 × 16-cm Glass plates, with 1-mm spacers.
3. Loading buffer: 0.1% bromophenol blue, 20% Ficoll 400, 1X TAE.
7. 1X, 1.25X, and 1.75X TAE, freshly prepared from 50X stock (*see* **Subheading 2.3.**, **item 2**).
8. SYBR Green I (FMC BioProducts, Rockland, ME).
9. UV transilluminator (e.g., Fotodyne, Hartland, WI).

3. Methods

3.1. Optimizing Melting Profiles and Primer Design

1. Design primers with minimal secondary structures and minimal ability to form dimers (*see* **Note 4**). The sequences of a set of optimized primers for analysis of the *TP53* gene are given in **Table 1**.
2. Calculate theoretical melting profiles for each DNA fragment to be analyzed using the MacMelt or WinMelt programs (based on the melting algorithm from the Melt87 program developed by Lerman and Silverstein *[24]*) (*see* **Note 4** and **Fig. 1**).

3.2. PCR

1. Amplify the 12 different DNA fragments representing exons 2–11 according to the optimized conditions presented in **Table 2**. Mix the components to the following final concentrations in a total volume of 25 µL: 50 m*M* KCl, 10 m*M* Tris-HCl, pH 8.3, 800 µ*M* dNTPs, 0.65 U AmpliTaq DNA polymerase, approx 50 ng of genomic DNA, and 15 pmol of each primer. The concentration of $MgCl_2$ is given in **Table 2**.
2. Incubate samples in a thermal cycler for 35 cycles at the temperatures specified in **Table 2**. Initiate all PCR programs with a 5-min denaturation step at 94°C and terminate with an 8-min extension step at 72°C. Generate heteroduplexes by denaturing the completed PCR products at 94°C for 30 s followed by a 30-min incubation at 65°C (*see* **Note 5**).
3. PCR products should be seen as high-quality single bands in each lane when analyzed by gel electrophoresis (*see* **Note 6**).

3.3. Preparation of Polyacrylamide Gels

1. Prepare stock solutions of 10% polyacrylamide/*bis*-acrylamide with 70% denaturant (147 g urea, 140 mL formamide, and 500 mL 1.25X TAE) or with 7 *M* urea (210 g urea to 500 mL 1.75X TAE; *see* **Note 7** for fragment 4B).
2. Fill the electrophoresis chamber with 1.25X TAE buffer, and preheat to the appropriate temperature.

Table 1
Primers for Amplification of the *TP53* Gene[a]

Fragment	5' Primer sequence[b]	3' Primer sequence[b]	Fragment length (bp)
2	gatcccacttctc	GC$_{cl1}$-cctgcccttccaatgga	191
3	GC$_{cl1}$-catgggactgacttctgctc	ccccagcctccaggt	135
4A	GC$_{cl1}$-gctgggggctgaggacc	gccgccggtg**aaaa**taggagctg	246
4B	ctcccgg**aaaaa**tggcccctgc	GC$_{cl1}$-gatacggccaggcattgaagtc	260
5A	ctctgtccttcctctt	GC$_{cl1}$-tgtgactgcttgtagatg	190
5B	GC$_{cl1}$-ttccacacccccgcccg	gccctgcgtctctcca	181
6	GC$_{cl1}$-tctgattcctcactgatt	tcccagagacccagttg	207
7	GC$_{cl1}$-gcctgtgttatcctcta	cagggtggcaagtggct	191
8	cctctgcttctctttc	GC$_{cl1}$-ccaccgcttcttgtcctg	240
9	acctttccttgcctctt	GC$_{cl1}$-tgataagaggtcccaaga	163
10	GC$_{cl2}$-tgtatatacttactttctcccctcc	aggggagtagggccaggaagg	212
11	ctccctgcttcgtctcc	GC$_{cl1}$-tcagtggggaacaagaag	172

[a]One of the primers in each pair has a GC clamp attached, as indicated. Stretches of "a" in bold represent nucleotides added to the primers to lower the melting temperature of the corresponding fragment.

[b]GC$_{cl1}$ = cgcccgccgcccgccgccccgccccgccgcccgcccccgcccg (40-mer).

GC$_{cl2}$ = ccccgccgcccgccgcccgccgcccgccgcccgcccgccgcccgtccccgccccgccgccccgcccg (56-mer).

3. Prepare 30-mL gel solution with the appropriate denaturant concentration according to **Table 2** (*see* **Note 8** for fragment 4B).
4. Add 116 μL APS and 48 μL TEMED per 30 mL of gel solution.
5. Pour the gel according to the manual provided with the DCode system (Bio-Rad) and polymerize for about 60 min at room temperature.
   or:
6. Fill the electrophoresis chamber with 1.75X TAE buffer, and preheat to the appropriate temperature.
7. Add 116 μL ammonium persulfate and 48 μL TEMED to 30 mL of gel solution containing 7 *M* urea.
8. Pour the gel and let polymerize for about 60 min.

3.4. Sample Loading, Electrophoresis, and Visualization of Bands

1. Prerun the gel for about 15 min in the warm buffer at 130 V.
2. Mix 5 μL of the PCR product with 3 μL of loading buffer, and load into the wells on the gel (*see* **Note 1**).
3. Run electrophoreses at 130 V in the appropriate buffer (1.25X or 1.75X TAE) and with the temperature range indicated in **Table 2** (*see* also **Notes 9** and **10**).
4. Stain gels in 1.25X TAE or 1.75X TAE containing 2 μL SYBR Green I for 3–5 min, and visualize the banding pattern on a UV transilluminator.

4. Notes

1. Fragments with similar melting profiles can be analyzed simultaneously, which is most useful in a diagnostic setting. For example, fragments 2, 5A, 5B, 6, 7, 8, 9, and 11 can all be analyzed on the same gel containing 7 *M* urea. The separation achieved as the fragments migrate through the gel is not lost with time, and the focusing of the bands seems to be less time-dependent.
2. The sensitivity in detecting mutations present in only a small fraction of the sample is around 10% at the homoduplex level and 1–3% at the heteroduplex level (*25*), which is considerably better than can be achieved by direct sequencing (**Fig. 2**).
3. High-quality genomic DNA is extracted from fresh frozen tissue or leukocytes using the phenol–chloroform extraction protocol on a 340A Nucleic Acid Extractor (Applied Biosystems, Foster City, CA) or similar technique. Extraction of DNA from formalin-fixed and paraffin-embedded tissue requires a manual phenol–chloroform extraction procedure to achieve good-quality DNA with high purity (*26*); in general, a higher concentration of template is required in the PCR reaction (100–200 ng).
4. Primers should be designed to achieve fragments in which the region to be screened resides in the lower melting domain. A GC clamp is usually attached to one end of each fragment to ensure one high-melting domain, thereby preventing complete strand dissociation (*27*). The increased robustness of TTGE enables fragments containing more than one melting domain to be consistently analyzed, provided that the different domains are descending in order starting with the melting domain generated by the GC clamp (**Fig. 1**). All *TP53* primers were selected from intron sequences to cover the exon–intron boundaries in the analysis and were designed using the OLIGO primer analysis program. Primer sequences are listed in **Table 1**. Note that stretches of adenines have been added to the primer sequences for exon 4 in order to lower the melting temperature for the fragments (*28*). The exact sequences of the GC clamps are given in the footnote to **Table 1**. Primers should be ordered already purified by high-performance liquid chromatography.

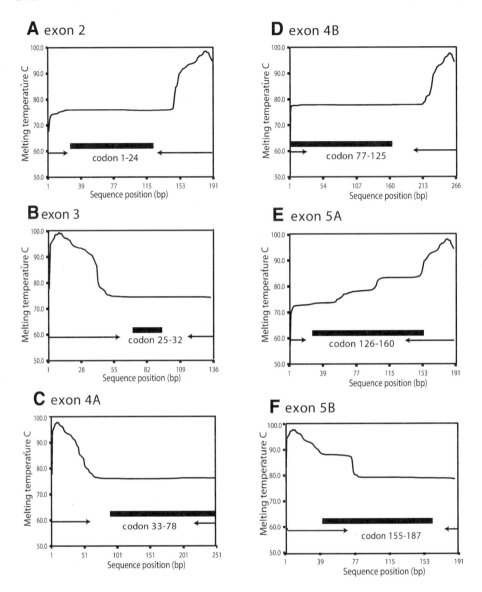

Fig. 1. Fifty percent melting probability curves for the 12 different *TP53* fragments analyzed by TTGE. Thick black bars indicate the positions of the exons; arrows indicate the locations of the primers.

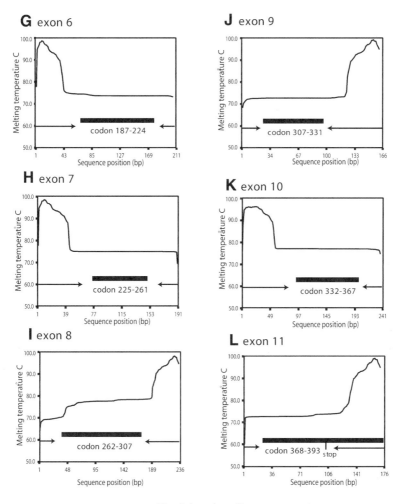

G exon 6

H exon 7

I exon 8

J exon 9

K exon 10

L exon 11

Fig. 1 (continued)

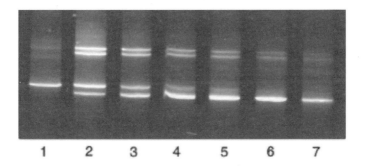

Fig. 2. Sensitivity of TTGE. DNA from a *TP53* mutant sample (G to A in codon 285, exon 8) mixed with wild-type in different concentrations and analyzed by TTGE. The mutant present in 100, 50, 25, 10, 5, 3 and 1% is shown in lanes 1–7, respectively.

Table 2
PCR and TTGE Conditions for the Various *TP53* Fragments

	PCR conditions[a]		TTGE conditions	
TP53 Fragment (exon)	MgCl$_2$ (m*M*)	Annealing temp. (°C)	Denaturant concentration[b] (%)	Temperature range (°C)[c]
2	1.5	57	45 (7 *M*)	60–65 (58–70)
3	1.0	59	45	60–65
4A	1.5	66	48	60–65
4B[d]	1.5	66	20–80	60
5A	1.5	58	45 (7 *M*)	60–65 (58–70)
5B	0.8	53	53 (7 *M*)	60–65 (58–70)
6	1.5	56	40 (7 *M*)	60–65 (58–70)
7	1.0	59	45 (7 *M*)	60–65 (58–70)
8	1.5	56	40 (7 *M*)	60–65 (58–70)
9	1.5	56	40 (7 *M*)	60–65 (58–70)
10	0.8	56	48	60–65
11	1.5	57	40 (7 *M*)	60–65 (58–70)

[a]PCR programs: 94°C for 5 min, 35 cycles of 94°C for 30 s, annealing for 30 s, 72°C for 30 s, followed by an extension for 8 min at 72°C.

[b]One hundred percent denaturant corresponds to 7 *M* urea and 40% formamide.

[c]Temperature range in parentheses is used for 7 *M* urea gels (*see* **Note 10**).

[d]Fragment 4B was analyzed in a 6% acrylamide DGGE (20–80% denaturant) at 60°C for 4 h (*see* **Note 8**).

5. When DNA from formalin-fixed and paraffin-embedded tissue is used as template, a slightly different PCR protocol is required. We have experienced good results by increasing the incubation times to 1.5 min for denaturation, 1.5 min for primer annealing, and 2 min for elongation. Furthermore, the number of cycles can be increased up to 40, and the specific annealing temperatures may need to be decreased 2–4°C. Generation of heteroduplexes will increase the possibility of detecting mutations because the difference in migration between mutated and wild-type fragments may be minimal, whereas the decreased stability of the heteroduplexes results in considerably less migration.

6. If the PCR products do not meet the quality criteria, i.e., no nonspecific products, the PCR conditions should be further optimized, or, alternatively, the specific product can be excised from the gel and purified before further analysis.

7. All gels contain 10% polyacrylamide/*bis*-acrylamide, except for that used for fragment 4B, which is analyzed in 6% gels.

8. Fragment 4B is very GC-rich and consequently its melting probability profile shows a high melting temperature (**Fig. 1D**). The best results for this fragment are obtained by analysis in a gel containing a denaturing gradient from 20 to 80% in 1.25X TAE and with a constant temperature of 60°C during the run. The gradient is poured using the gradient wheel provided with the DCode system.

9. In TTGE, urea and formamide, or only urea, form the constant denaturant in the acrylamide gels. Formamide as a second denaturant in the gel may improve the focusing of the bands for some fragments. The optimal constant denaturant can easily be deter-

mined from a perpendicular DGGE gel by subtracting approx 10 U from the % denaturant that corresponds to the steepest part of the S-shaped curve *(23)*. Fragments 2, 3, 4A, 4B, and 10 of the *TP53* gene are best analyzed in gels containing 1.25X TAE and varying concentrations of urea and formamide. The concentrations for each individual fragment are shown in **Table 2**. Gels are run submerged in 1.25X TAE with a temperature ramp of 1.7°C/h from 60 to 65°C for a total of 3 h. This is the preferred method of analysis for large series of samples.

10. The temperature range in the buffer and the denaturant concentration for a particular fragment in TTGE can also be determined from the theoretical melting curve of the DNA sequence (**Fig. 1**). Using urea (7 *M*) as the sole denaturant in the gel, the theoretical melting temperature of DNA is lowered 14°C (approx 2°C for every mole/liter of urea) *(29)*. Hence, the resulting temperature range in the buffer during the TTGE run is determined from the temperature range of the non-GC–clamped portion of the theoretical profile and corrected for urea denaturant. Fragments 2, 5A, 5B, 6, 7, 8, 9, and 11 can be analyzed in gels containing 7 *M* urea and 1.75X TAE. Gels are run submerged in 1.75X TAE for a total of 4 h, simultaneously increasing the temperature from 58 to 70°C with a ramp rate of 3°C/h.

References

1. Hernandez-Boussard, T., Montesano, R., and Hainaut, P. (1999) Sources of bias in the detection and reporting of *p53* mutations in human cancer: analysis of the IARC *p53* mutation database. *Genet. Anal.* **14,** 229–233.

2. Hollstein, M., Rice, K., Greenblatt, M. S., et al. (1994) Database of *p53* gene somatic mutations in human tumors and cell lines. *Nucleic Acids Res.* **22,** 3551–3555.

3. Hussain, S. P., Hofseth, L. J., and Harris, C. C. (2001) Tumor suppressor genes: at the crossroads of molecular carcinogenesis, molecular epidemiology and human risk assessment. *Lung Cancer* **34(suppl. 2),** S7–S15.

4. Martin, A. C., Facchiano, A. M., Cuff, A. L., et al. (2002) Integrating mutation data and structural analysis of the TP53 tumor-suppressor protein. *Hum. Mutat.* **19,** 149–164.

5. Soussi, T. and Beroud, C. (2002) Assessing TP53 status in human tumours to evaluate clinical outcome. *Nat. Rev. Cancer* **1,** 233–240.

6. Tyner, S. D., Venkatachalam, S., Choi, J., et al. (2002) *p53* mutant mice that display early ageing-associated phenotypes. *Nature* **415,** 45–53.

7. Aas, T., Børresen, A.-L., Geisler, S., et al. (1996) Specific *p53* mutations are associated with de novo resistance to doxorubicin in breast cancer patients. *Nat. Med.* **2,** 811–814.

8. Børresen-Dale, A.-L., Lothe, R. A., Meling, G. I., Hainaut, P., Rognum, T. O., and Skovlund, E. (1998) TP53 and long-term prognosis in colorectal cancer: mutations in the L3 zinc-binding domain predict poor survival. *Clin. Cancer Res.* **4,** 203–210.

9. Geisler, S., Lønning, P. E., Aas, T., et al. (2001) Influence of TP53 gene alterations and c-erbB2 expression on the response to treatment with doxorubicin in locally advanced breast cancer. *Cancer Res.* **61,** 2505–2512.

10. Wallace-Brodeur, R. R. and Lowe, S. W. (1999) Clinical implications of *p53* mutations. *Cell. Mol. Life Sci.* **55,** 64–75.

11. Wattel, E., Preudhomme, C., Hecquet, B., et al. (1994) *p53* mutations are associated with resistance to chemotherapy and short survival in hematologic malignancies. *Blood* **84,** 3148–3157.

12. Orita, M., Iwahana, H., Kanazawa, H., Hayashi, K., and Sekiya, T. (1989) Detection of polymorphisms of human DNA by gel electrophoresis as single-strand conformation polymorphisms. *Proc. Natl. Acad. Sci. USA* **86,** 2766–2770.

13. Orita, M., Suzuki, Y., Sekiya, T., and Hayashi, K. (1989) Rapid and sensitive detection of point mutations and DNA polymorphisms using the polymerase chain reaction. *Genomics* **5,** 874–879.

14. Fischer, S. G. and Lerman, L. S. (1983) DNA fragments differing by single base-pair substitutions are separated in denaturing gradient gels: correspondence with melting theory. *Proc. Natl. Acad. Sci. USA* **80,** 1579–1583.

15. Børresen, A.-L., Hovig, E., Smith-Sorensen, B., et al. (1991) Constant denaturant gel electrophoresis as a rapid screening technique for *p53* mutations. *Proc. Natl. Acad. Sci. USA* **88,** 8405–8409.

16. Hovig, E., Smith-Sorensen, B., Brogger, A., and Børresen, A.-L. (1991) Constant denaturant gel electrophoresis, a modification of denaturing gradient gel electrophoresis, in mutation detection. *Mutat. Res.* **262,** 63–71 [Published erratum: *Mutat. Res.* **263,** 61].

17. Bjorheim, J., Gaudernack, G., and Ekstrom, P. O. (2001) Mutation analysis of TP53 exons 5-8 by automated constant denaturant capillary electrophoresis. *Tumour Biol.* **22,** 323–327.

18. Khrapko, K., Hanekamp, J. S., Thilly, W. G., Belenkii, A., Foret, F., and Karger, B. L. (1994) Constant denaturant capillary electrophoresis (CDCE): a high resolution approach to mutational analysis. *Nucleic Acids Res.* **22,** 364–369.

19. Sarkar, G., Yoon, H. S., and Sommer, S. S. (1992) Dideoxy fingerprinting (ddF): a rapid and efficient screen for the presence of mutations. *Genomics* **13,** 441–443.

20. Gelfi, C., Cremonesi, L., Ferrari, M., and Righetti, P. G. (1996) Temperature-programmed capillary electrophoresis for detection of DNA point mutations. *BioTechniques* **21,** 926–928, 930, 932.

21. Riesner, D., Steger, G., Zimmat, R., et al. (1989). Temperature-gradient gel electrophoresis of nucleic acids: analysis of conformational transitions, sequence variations, and protein-nucleic acid interactions. *Electrophoresis* **10,** 377–389.

22. Børresen-Dale, A.-L., Lystad, S., and Langeroed, A. (1997) Temporal temperature gradient electrophoresis on the DCode system. *Biorad Bull.* **2133**.

23. Zoller, P., Redila-Flores, T., Chu, D., and Patel, A. (1998) Temporal temperature gradient electrophoresis—a powerful mutation screening technique. *Biomed. Prod.* **9**.

24. Lerman, L. S. and Silverstein, K. (1987) Computational simulation of DNA melting and its application to denaturing gradient gel electrophoresis. *Methods Enzymol.* **155,** 482–501.

25. Børresen, A.-L. (1996) Constant denaturant gel electrophoresis (CDGE) in mutation screening, in *Technologies for Detection of DNA Damage and Mutation* (Pfeifer, G. P., ed.), Plenum, New York, pp. 267–279.

26. Kraggerud, S. M., Szymanska, J., Abeler, V. M., et al. (2000) DNA copy number changes in malignant ovarian germ cell tumors. *Cancer Res.* **60,** 3025–3030.

27. Sheffield, V. C., Cox, D. R., Lerman, L. S., and Myers, R. M. (1989) Attachment of a 40-base-pair G + C-rich sequence (GC-clamp) to genomic DNA fragments by the polymerase chain reaction results in improved detection of single-base changes. *Proc. Natl. Acad. Sci. USA* **86,** 232–236.

28. Guldberg, P., Nedergaard, T., Nielsen, H. J., Olsen, A. C., Ahrenkiel, V., and Zeuthen, J. (1997) Single-step DGGE-based mutation scanning of the *p53* gene: application to genetic diagnosis of colorectal cancer. *Hum. Mutat.* **9,** 348–355.

29. Steger, G. (1994) Thermal denaturation of double-stranded nucleic acids: prediction of temperatures critical for gradient gel electrophoresis and polymerase chain reaction. *Nucleic Acids Res.* **22,** 2760–2768.

21

Analysis of K-*RAS* and *P53* Mutations in Sputum Samples

Weimin Gao and Phouthone Keohavong

Summary

Mutations in the *P53* tumor suppressor gene and the K-*RAS* oncogene have frequently been found in sputum and bronchoalveolar lavage (BAL) samples of lung cancer patients, and also in samples from patients prior to presenting clinical symptoms of lung cancer, suggesting they may provide useful biomarkers for early lung cancer diagnosis. However, the detection of these mutations has been complicated by the fact that they often occur in only a small fraction of epithelial cells among sputum cells, and, in the case of the *P53* gene, inactivating mutations may occur at many codons. This chapter describes methods to identify *P53* and K-*RAS* mutations present in low fractions of epithelial cells among the excess of other cell types in sputum samples from lung cancer patients.

Key Words: Lung cancer; sputum; laser capture microdissection; K-*RAS* and *P53* mutations.

1. Introduction

Lung cancer remains the most common cause of death from cancer, both in the United States and worldwide *(1,2)*. One goal of lung cancer research has been to develop assays that facilitate early detection and treatment of this disease and thus decrease the mortality *(3–5)*.

Lung cancer, like other cancers, results from the accumulation of genetic alterations in genes involved in the control of cell growth and differentiation *(6,7)*. Mutations in two of these genes, the K-*RAS* oncogene and the *P53* tumor suppressor gene, have frequently been found in lung tumors and are implicated in the development of lung cancer. K-*RAS* mutations occur in 20–50% of adenocarcinoma and undifferentiated large cell carcinoma of the lung, and, to a lesser extent, in squamous cell carcinoma *(8–12)*. More than 90% of the mutations detected in the K-*RAS* oncogene is in codon 12 *(12)*. Therefore, these mutations can be specifically targeted and are easily detected using sufficiently sensitive methods. Mutations in the *P53* gene have been detected in 30–50% of lung tumors and lung tumor-derived cell lines *(13–19)*. Contrary to the specificity of K-*RAS* mutations, cancer-associated *P53* mutations have

From: *Methods in Molecular Biology, vol. 291, Molecular Toxicology Protocols*
Edited by: P. Keohavong and S. G. Grant © Humana Press Inc., Totowa, NJ

been documented at more than 100 sites in the gene. In lung cancer, some of these mutations are found clustered at hot spots in codons 158, 175, 245, 248, 249, 273, and 282 within exons 5–8, where the four evolutionarily conserved domains of the *P53* gene are located *(20–23)*. The high prevalence of mutations in both the K-*RAS* and *P53* genes in lung cancer should make these mutations useful biomarkers for this disease.

To evaluate the roles of K-*RAS* and *P53* mutations in lung carcinogenesis and establish their significance as early-detection biomarkers, sufficiently sensitive methods are necessary to facilitate the determination of a complete spectrum of mutations in these genes. Moreover, the technique must be able to discriminate a small population of mutant cells within a larger population of normal cells in sputum and/or bronchoalveolar (BAL) samples. Several molecular approaches have been applied to enhance the detection of point mutations in cultured cells, tissue, or sputum samples *(24–33)*. A specific and sensitive method has been developed for K-*RAS* mutation detection that is a significant improvement upon existing methodology. Through a combination of polymerase chain reaction (PCR), mutant allele enrichment (MAE), nested amplification, and denaturing gradient gel electrophoresis (DGGE), a sensitivity of detection of one mutated cell in 10^4–10^5 normal cells can be attained *(34)*. This method has been applied to analyze K-*RAS* codon 12 mutations in sputum samples of lung cancer patients *(35)*. All of these methods are adaptable for the detection of mutations at specific codons of other oncogenes. However, more than half the mutations in the *P53* tumor suppressor gene in lung cancer occur outside the hot spot codons and are thus not detectable by most existing sensitive methods that target mutations at specific codons.

We have designed two methods for the molecular analysis of low fraction K-*RAS* and *P53* mutations in sputum samples. In the first case, cancer cells carrying mutations are isolated from the vast majority of normal cells by laser capture microdissection (LCM). With this fairly pure sample of mutant cells, it is possible to analyze the complete spectrum of mutations that might occur at the K-*RAS* and *P53* genes, using PCR and DGGE or single-stranded conformational polymorphism (SSCP). If laser capture microscopy is not available, molecular analysis of mutations in these oncogenes is still possible from DNA extracted directly from whole sputum samples via repeated steps of MAE, by using codon-specific restriction enzyme digestion; however, this type of analysis is more limited and may only be used to detect mutations within known hot spots.

We therefore set out to design a method to detect the complete spectrum of low-frequency *P53* and K-*RAS* mutations in sputum samples of lung cancer patients. We combined sputum cytocentrifugation with LCM microscopy to isolate epithelial cells from sputum samples. We then screened for K-*RAS* and *P53* mutations in these isolated cells using DGGE and SSCP, respectively (*see* **Subheading 3.1.**). This mutation detection method was then compared with existing methods that used MAE by restriction enzyme digestion of bulk PCR products at codons of interest, before analysis of mutant sequences by DGGE, for K-*RAS* mutants, or polyacrylamide gel electrophoresis (PAGE), for *P53* mutants (*see* **Subheading 3.2.** and **Table 1**).

2. Materials

2.1. Epithelial Cell Isolation From Sputum Samples

1. Obtain sputum samples (each containing about 2×10^4 cells in 1 mL) from lung cancer patients. Prior to analysis they are stored in 1 mL saccomanno fluid (International Medical Equipment, San Marcos, CA) in 1.5-mL microcentrifuge tubes at $-20°C$ (e.g., freezer model 525F, Fisher Scientific, Pittsburgh, PA).
2. 1.5-mL Microcentrifuge tubes (Brinkmann, Westbury, NY).
3. Phosphate-buffered saline (PBS; Gibco-BRL, Gaithersburgh, MD).
4. 20-, 200-, and 1000-µL pipetors (Rainin, Woburn, MA) and appropriate tips (Fisher).
5. Centrifugable 1-mL specimen chamber and chamber holder with membrane filter (Sakura Finetek, Torrance, CA).
6. Cyto-Tex centrifuge (VWR, Bridgeport, NJ).
7. Hematoxylin (Sigma, St. Louis, MO).
8. Eosin (Sigma).
9. LCM microscope (e.g., Pix Cell II LCM, Arcturius Engineering, Mountain View, CA).
10. CapSure™ LCM caps (Arcturius Engineering).

2.2. DNA Extraction From Sputum and Laser-Captured Cells (see Note 1)

1. Stock buffers and solutions for DNA extraction (all chemicals purchased from Sigma): 10% (w/v) sodium dodecyl sulfate (SDS), 5 M NaCl, 0.5 M EDTA, 1 M Tris-HCl, pH 7.4, 1 M Tris-HCl, pH 8.0, and 1.0 M Tris-base.
2. Lysis solution: 40 mM Tris-HCl, 1 mM EDTA, pH 8.0, 0.5% Tween-20 (Sigma), 0.5 µg/µL proteinase K (Gibco-BRL).
3. Sputum cell lysis buffer: 0.5% (w/v) SDS, 150 mM NaCl, 100 mM EDTA, 10 mM Tris-HCl, pH 7.4.
4. Proteinase K: 20 mg/mL stock (Gibco-BRL)
5. Saturated phenol, pH 7.8 (Gibco-BRL). For 100 mL: 60 mL phenol, 39 mL distilled water, 0.8 mL 1.0 M Tris-base, 0.1% (w/v) 8-hydroxyquinoline (Sigma; *see* **Note 2**).
6. Chloroform (Sigma).
7. Chloroform/isoamyl alcohol (22:1, v/v; Fisher).
8. Ammonium acetate (Sigma): 7.5 M stock solution.
9. 100% and 70% Ethanol (Fisher), both solutions kept at $+4°C$.
10. TE buffer: 10 mM Tris-HCl, 1 mM EDTA, pH 7.5.
11. Microcentrifuge and microcentrifuge tubes.
12. Pipetors and pipet tips.

2.3. DNA Amplification by PCR

1. DNA Thermocyclers (e.g., Perkin Elmer 480, Shelton, CT).
2. Gold AmpliTaq DNA polymerase, 5 U/µL (Perkin Elmer).
3. 10X PCR buffer: 500 mM KCl, 100 mM Tris-HCl, pH 8.3 (supplied with enzyme).
4. 25 mM MgCl$_2$ (supplied with enzyme).
5. 10 mM dNTP (Sigma).
6. $[\alpha^{32}P]$-dATP (3000 Ci/mmol, Perkin Elmer).

7. Primers (Midland Certified Reagent, Midland, TX; each primer is prepared as a 10 μ*M* stock solution in distilled water and stored at −20°C).

   a. Primers for mutations at codon 12/13 of the K-*RAS* gene (*see* **Note 3**):

      i. KI1-1 (sense):   5'-TATTATAAGGCCTGCTGAAA-3'.
      ii. PK12/13 (antisense): 5'-GTCAAGGCACTCTTGCCTAC-3'.
      iii. PKB (antisense):   5'-AGGCACTCTTGCCTACGGCA-3'.
      iv. PKGC(sense):   5'-GCCGCCTGCAGCCCGCGCCCCCGTGCC
      CCCGCCCCGCCGCCGGCCCGGCGCCTATAA
      GGCCTGCTGAAAATG-3'.

   b. Primers for sensitive analysis of specific hot spot *P53* mutations:

      i. Exon 5: pE5 sense: 5'-TTCCTCTTCCTACAGTACTC-3'.
                 pE5 antisense: 5'-CGCTATCTGAGCAGCGCCCA-3'.
      ii. Exon 7: pE7 sense: 5'-GTAACAGTTCCTGCATGAGC-3'.
                 pE7 antisense: 5'-TCTTCCAGTGTGATGATGGTGAGGATA
      GG-3'.
      iii. Exon 8: pE8 sense: 5'-GACGGAACAGCTTTGAGGCG-3'.
                 pE8 antisense: 5'-GGTGAGGCTCCCCTTTCTTG-3'.

   c. Primers for SSCP analysis of *P53* mutations:

      i. Exon 5-6: pE5-5':   5'-AACTCTGTCTCCTTCCTCTT-3'.
                  pE6-3':   5'-GGAGGGCCACTGACAACCA-3'.
      ii. Exon 7: pE7-5':   5'-GTGTTATCTCCTAGGTTGGC-3'.
                 pE7-3':   5'-GTGTGCAGGGTGGCAAGTGG-3'.
      iii. Exon 8: pE8-5':   5'-AGGACCTGATTTCCTTACTG-3'.
                 pE8-3':   5'-TCCACCGCTTCTTGTCCTGCT-3'.

8. Distilled water.
9. 0.5-mL Microcentrifuge tubes (Brinkmann).
10. Microcentrifuge.
11. Pipetors and pipet tips.
12. Mineral oil (Sigma).

2.4. Restriction Enzyme Digestion

For K-*RAS* codon 12 mutations:

1. *Ban*I enzyme stock, 20 U/μL (New England Biolabs, Beverly, MA).
2. 10X digestion buffer: 0.5 *M* potassium acetate, 0.2 *M* Tris-acetate, 0.1 *M* magnesium-acetate, 0.01 *M* dithiothreitol (DTT); supplied with enzyme.
3. 37°C Incubator or water bath (e.g., Fisher).
4. Distilled water.
5. 0.5-mL Microcentrifuge tubes.

For *P53* hotspot codon mutations:

1. 10 U/μL stock *Aci*I, 10 U/μL *Bsr*BI, 10 U/mL *Bst*UI, 20 U/μL *Msp*I, 10 U/μL *Nco*I, and 10 U/μL *Stu*I (all from New England Biolabs).
2. 10X digestion buffers supplied with the enzymes: 0.5 *M* NaCl, 0.1 *M* Tris-HCl, pH 7.9, at 25°C, 0.1 *M* MgCl$_2$, 0.01 *M* DTT, and an incubation at 37°C for *Bsr*BI, *Msp*I, and *Stu*I,

and at 60°C for *Bst*UI. The same buffer is used for *Aci*I, except that NaCl is adjusted to 1.0 *M* and Tris-HCl, pH 7.9, to 0.5 *M*. For *Nco*I, the same buffer and digestion conditions as for *Ban*I are used.

3. Distilled water.
4. 0.5-mL Microcentrifuge tubes.
5. 37°C Water bath (e.g., from Fisher).

2.5. Polyacrylamide Gel Electrophoresis

1. Vertical gel electrophoresis apparatus: gel boxes, plates, and accessories for a 20-cm-wide × 16-cm-high gel (Gibco-BRL).
2. Power sources, i.e., Pharmacia LKB ECPS 3000/150 (Amersham BioSiences, Piscataway, NJ).
3. (1:37.5)% *bis*/acrylamide stock solution: dissolve 1.0 g *bis* and 37.5 g acrylamide (Bio-Rad, Hercules, CA) in a final 100 mL vol with distilled water.
4. (1:19)% *bis*/acrylamide stock solution: dissolve 1.0 g *bis* and 19.0 g acrylamide in a final 100 mL vol with distilled water.
5. 20X TBE buffer: dissolve 216 g Trizma base (Sigma), 110 g boric acid (Fisher), 80 mL 0.5 *M* EDTA, and complete to 1 L with distilled water. Aliquot the solution in 500-mL bottles and autoclave.
6. *N,N,N,N*-tetramethyl-ethylenediamine (TEMED; Bio-Rad).
7. 10% (w/v) Ammonium persulfate (APS) in distilled water, stored at 4°C (Bio-Rad).
8. 6X PAGE stock loading solution: 30% glycerol (Mallinckrodt, Paris, KY), 0.6% SDS, 0.06% bromphenol blue-xylene cyanole (Sigma). The solution is kept at 4°C.
9. DNA elution buffer: 10 m*M* Tris-HCl, pH 7.4, 1 m*M* EDTA, 200 m*M* NaCl, 0.05% SDS.

2.6. Denaturing Gradient Gel Electrophoresis (DGGE)

1. Vertical gel DGGE apparatus: glass plates, gel boxes, buffer tank, buffer heater, circulating system, and accessories for a 20-cm-wide × 16-cm-high gel (Bio-Rad).
2. Gradient gel maker (Bio-Rad).
3. Power sources, i.e., Pharmacia LKB ECPS 3000/150 (Amersham BioSiences).
4. (1:37.5)% *bis*/acrylamide stock solution (*see* **Subheading 2.5.**, **item 3**).
5. 50X TAE buffer (for 1 L): dissolve 230 g Trizma base, 14.9 g Tris-HCl, and 37.25 g EDTA in 0.8 L of distilled water. In a fume hood and wearing eye protection glasses, add carefully, and in small volumes, 171.3 mL of glacial acetic acid (J.T. Baker, Phillipsburg, NJ), and then adjust to a final volume of 1 L with distilled water. Aliquot the solution in 500-mL bottles and autoclave.
6. Stock 50% denaturant solution (for 200 mL): mix 4 mL 50X TAE, 66 mL (1:37.5)% *bis*/acrylamide solution, 40 g urea (Sigma), 40 mL formamide (Boehringer Mannheim), adjust to 200 mL with distilled water, and store at 4°C (*see* **Note 4**).
7. Stock 0% denaturant solution (for 200 mL): mix 4 mL 50X TAE, 66 mL (1:37.5)% *bis*/acrylamide solution, complete to 200 mL with distilled water, and store at 4°C.
8. DGGE 6X loading solution: 40% glycerol, 0.6% SDS, 0.06% bromphenol blue-xylene cyanole. The solution is kept at +4°C.

2.7. Single-Stranded Conformational Polymorphism (SSCP)

1. Sequencing gel electrophoresis apparatus, glass plates, gel box, and accessories (Gibco-BRL).
2. MDE™ gel solution (2X concentrate; BioWhittaker Molecular Applications, Rockland, ME).
3. Glycerol (Sigma).
4. 20X TBE buffer.

A   **B**   **C**   **D**

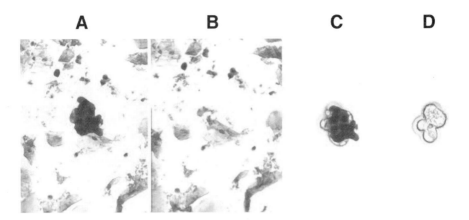

Fig. 1. An example of laser capture of epithelial cells from a sputum sample. A group of malignant cells collected on a filter membrane by cytocentrifugation of a sputum sample obtained from one of the patients before (**A**) and after (**B**) laser capture. Collected cells were stained with H&E then analyzed histopathologically. Malignant epithelial cells appeared as a group of dark-stained cells. Sputum cells consisted of a mixture of mostly leucocytes, buccal cells, and malignant and/or atypical epithelial cells. About 10% of sputum cells from this patient corresponded to malignant and atypical epithelial cells. Approximately 100 malignant cells in each sputum sample were laser-captured on a cap and molecularly analyzed. The cells captured on a cap (**C**) were then lysed to release the cell content used for mutation analysis. The captured cells after treatment with proteinase K are shown in (**D**).

5. Power source.
6. SSCP loading solution: 95% formamide, 10 m*M* NaOH, 0.25% xylene cyanol, and 0.25% bromophenol blue.

3. Methods

Mutations can be analyzed either in epithelial cells isolated from sputum by LCM (*see* **Subheading 3.1.**) or in DNA extracted directly from whole sputum cells (*see* **Subheading 3.2.**, and **Note 1**).

3.1. Analysis of Mutations in Laser-Captured Epithelial Cells

3.1.1. Epithelial Cell Isolation From Sputum Samples

Ideally, this work is performed by a pathologist with appropriate experience in sputum cytology using an LCM microscope and is not described in great detail in this chapter. Briefly, the following steps are used to isolate epithelial cells from sputum:

1. Remove sputum samples from the freezer and leave on ice for 15 min.
2. Dilute an aliquot of each sputum sample (equivalent to 5000 total cells or 250 μL saccomanno fluid) in 1 mL of PBS in a 1.5-mL microcentrifuge tube.
3. Transfer the cell solution to a specimen chamber fixed onto a chamber holder equipped with a membrane filter.

4. Centrifuge the specimen chamber at 62g (Cyto-Tex centrifuge) for 5 min to collect sputum cells on the filter.
5. Remove the filter from the chamber and air-dry on a lab bench for 15–30 min.
6. Stain the cells retained on the filter with H&E and examine histopathologically.
7. Capture 100–150 epithelial cells from each sputum sample on an LCM cap, by LCM (*see* **Fig. 1**).

3.1.2. DNA Extraction From Laser-Captured Cells

1. Add 20 µL of lysis solution directly on top of the cells captured on each LCM cap.
2. Enclose the LCM cap with a 0.5-mL microcentrifuge tube on top (in an upside-down position), and incubate at room temperature for 36 h with occasional gentle horizontal shaking manually (*see* **Note 5**).
3. To recover the cell lysate, put the microcentrifuge tube back into the "up" position with the LCM cap on top, and spin at 750g for 1 s in an Eppendorf microcentrifuge.
4. Remove the LCM cap and close the microcentrifuge tube containing the cell lysate. Heat the cell lysate at 95°C for 5 min to inactivate the proteinase K, and then spin at 750g for 1 s in a microcentrifuge. The cell lysate is then kept at –20°C until use.

3.1.3. Analysis of K-RAS Exon 1 Mutations by PCR and DGGE

3.1.3.1. FIRST-ROUND PCR

1. Use an aliquot of cell lysate (corresponding to 10–20 epithelial cells laser-captured from sputum) as a template for PCR amplification of a 79-bp fragment corresponding to the 5' half of exon 1 of the K-*RAS* gene, which includes codons 12 and 13. PCR is carried out in a 50 µL reaction mixture in a 0.5-µL PCR tube containing 10 mM Tris-HCl, pH 8.3, 1.5 mM MgCl$_2$, 50 mM KCl, 100 µM each dNTP, 0.5 µM each primer (KI1-1 and PK12/13), and 2.5 U Gold AmpliTaq DNA polymerase.
2. Cover the mixture with mineral oil, place in a thermocycler heated at 95°C for 9 min, and subject it to 12 PCR cycles of 94°C/1 min, 53°C/1 min, 72°C/2 min.

3.1.3.2. SECOND-ROUND PCR

1. Dilute 1 µL of the first-round PCR product into a final 25-µL reaction mixture containing the same buffer composition as in the first round, except that 0.25 µL of [α^{32}P]dATP is added and primer KI1-1 is replaced by primer PKGC.
2. Heat the mixture at 95°C for 9 min and subject it to 35 PCR cycles of 94°C/1 min, 60°C/1 min, 72°C/2 min.
3. Take 10 µL from each of the second-round PCR products, add 2 µL of 6X dye, and load onto the PAGE gel.

3.1.3.3. PAGE PURIFICATION OF PCR PRODUCTS

1. Prepare 25 mL of 8% polyacrylamide gel solution containing 5.2 mL of the (1:37.5)% *bis*/acrylamide, 1.25 mL 20X TBE, 18.5 mL distilled water, 250 µL 10% APS, and 25 µL TEMED, and mix.
2. Pour the solution into a preassembled 0.5-mm-thick × 20-cm-wide × 16-cm-high set of gel plates. Insert a 20-well comb. The gel polymerizes within 30 min.
3. Place the gel onto the gel box with 1X TBE buffer. Remove the comb, and rinse the wells with the buffer. Load each sample onto the gel well, and electrophorese the DNA at 250 constant V for 90 min.
4. Remove one glass plate from the gel. Cover the gel while still on top of the second glass plate with Saran Wrap. In a dark room, take a sheet of X-ray film, and tape it on top of the

gel. Use a marker to draw a thin line surrounding the edge of the film on the gel. Expose the gel for 30–45 min, and develop the film.

5. Superimpose the autoradiogram on the gel to locate the position of the DNA in the gel. Mark the position of the band of DNA in the gel. Excise the appropriate band containing the expected-size DNA fragment (in this case 129 bp) from the gel.

6. Place the gel slice in a 1.5-mL microcentrifuge tube, crush the gel using a pipet tip, add 300 μL of elution buffer, and incubate the solution at 60°C in a water bath for 30 min. Shake the tube vigorously for 1 min every 10 min.

7. Centrifuge each tube at 9800*g* (microcentrifuge) for 1 min.

8. Recover the elution solution in a new 1.5-mL microcentrifuge tube, add 2 vol of 100% cold ethanol, close the tube, mix, and precipitate the DNA at –20°C for 1 h.

9. Recover the DNA by centrifugation at 9800*g* (microcentrifuge) for 15 min. Remove the ethanol, add 500 μL 70% cold ethanol, and centrifuge at 9800*g* for 5 min. Remove the ethanol completely.

10. Dry the DNA pellet at room temperature for 15 min, dissolved in 15 μL of 1X DGGE loading solution.

3.1.3.4. DGGE Separation of K-*RAS* Mutant DNA

1. Prepare a 1-mm-thick × 20-cm-wide × 16-cm-high gel containing a denaturant gradient from 50% (bottom of the gel) to 35% (top of the gel). Use two gel solutions, one containing a 50% denaturant (13.5 mL of the 50% denaturant stock solution) and the other containing a 35% denaturant (9.45 mL of the 50% denaturant stock solution mixed with 4.05 mL of the 0% denaturant stock).

2. Add 75 μL 10% APS and 7.5 μL TEMED to each of the solutions and mix.

3. Transfer the 50% and 35% denaturant solutions into their respective chambers of a gradient mixer (Bio-Rad) and pour them into preassembled gel plates as described in the manual provided by Bio-Rad for DGGE. Insert a 20-well comb, and let the gel polymerize for 1–2 h at room temperature.

4. Place the polymerized gel into the gel box submerged under 1X TAE buffer in a buffer tank heated at 60°C. Prerun the gel at 100 constant V for 30 min.

5. Remove the comb from the gel and immediately rinse the wells using a syringe and the 1X TAE buffer from the tank. Load the above 15-μL gel-purified DNA sample in 1X dye solution.

6. Run the gel at 100 V at 60°C for 12–15 h.

7. Dry and autoradiograph the gel (*see* **Fig. 2**).

8. Isolate mutant DNA from the denaturing gradient gel by following a procedure similar to that described in **Subheading 3.1.3.**, **steps 4** and **5**.

9. Transfer each dried gel slice excised from the gel into a 0.5-μL microcentrifuge tube, and soak and wash in 50 μL of distilled water once for 5 min. Discard the water and break the gel slice by squeezing it against the inner wall of the tube using the end of a 200-μL pipet tip. Add 50 μL of distilled water, mix, and heat at 98°C for 10 min in a thermocycler. After a 10–15 min cooling down period at room temperature, spin the tube quickly for 2 s (microcentrifuge).

10. Use a 5-μL aliquot of the eluted DNA as a template for further PCR amplification, using the 25-μL reaction mixture, primers of the second-round PCR, buffer composition, and PCR cycling conditions as described above in **Subheading 3.1.3.**, **step 2**, except that only an equivalence of 0.01 μL of [α^{32}P]dATP is added per reaction.

11. PAGE-purify the PCR product as described in **Subheading 3.1.3.**, **step 3**. Analyze an aliquot of each DNA sample on PAGE (8% polyacrylamide gel, 1:37.5% = *bis*/acrylamide) against known amount of marker DNA to estimate the amount of DNA isolated.

12. Characterize the eluted mutant DNA using an automated sequencer.

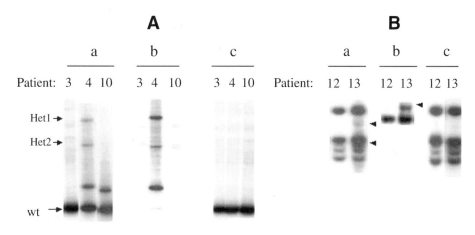

Fig. 2. Molecular analysis of sputum samples of lung cancer patients. Example of mutation analysis **(A)** by DGGE of exon 1 of the K-*RAS* gene for three patients (patients 3, 4, and 10) and **(B)** by SSCP and PAGE in exons 5–8 of the *P53* gene for two patients (patients 12 and 13). For each patient, mutations were analyzed by three approaches. **(A)** Analysis was performed using cells taken from sputum and the PCR + DGGE method *(a)*, or DNA extracted from sputum and the PCR + MAE + DGGE method *(b)*, or the PCR + DGGE method *(c)*. wt indicates the position of the wild-type K-*RAS* exon 1 allele in the gel. DGGE analysis showed that patient 4 had K-*RAS* codon exon 1 mutant sequences in the laser-captured cells (indicated by Het1 and Het2 in lane a4, corresponding to the two respective mutant/wild-type heteroduplexes and the mutant homoduplex focusing between the wt and Het2). This mutant corresponded to a GGT to TGT in codon 12 of the K-*RAS* gene. This same mutation was also detected in DNA isolated from sputum cells of this patient by the PCR + MAE + DGGE method (lane b4), but not by the PCR + DGGE method (lane c4). For comparison, patient 10 did not reveal any mutant sequence pattern when DNA extracted from sputum cells was analyzed using either the PCR + DGGE (lane c10) or the PCR + MAE + DGGE (lane b10) method. However, when cells isolated from this patient's sputum were analyzed by the PCR + DGGE method, a mutant sequence corresponding to a GGC to TGC in codon 13 of the K-*RAS* gene was detected (lane a10). As expected, this mutation was not detected using the PCR+MAE+DGGE method because it targeted only codon 12 mutations (lane b10). For comparison, patient 3 showed no mutations in either the cells isolated from sputum (lane a3) or DNA extracted from sputum cells by using both the PCR+MAE+DGGE (lane b3) or PCR+DGGE (lane c3) method. **(B)** *P53* mutations were analyzed using, **(a)** cells isolated from sputum and the PCR+SSCP method, or DNA extracted from sputum and the PCR+SSCP method **(c)**, or the PCR+MAE+PAGE method **(b)**. Patient 13 showed a *P53* mutant in cells captured from sputum (arrowheads in lane a13). This mutant corresponded to a CGG to CAG mutation at codon 248 of the *P53* gene. The identical mutation was detected in DNA extracted from sputum by using the PCR+MAE+PAGE method (arrowhead in lane b13), but not by using directly the less sensitive PCR+SSCP method (lane c13).

3.1.4. Analysis of P53 Mutations in Laser-Captured Cells by PCR and SSCP

1. The first-round PCR is used to amplify three fragments corresponding to exons 5-6, 7, and 8, simultaneously in a single reaction. PCR is carried out in a 50-µL reaction mixture containing cell lysate (corresponding to 10–20 laser-captured epithelial cells) and the

same reagents as those described in **Subheading 3.1.3., step 1** for the first-round PCR for K-*RAS* exon 1, except that: (1) 0.25 µ*M* of each of the six primers is used; and (2) the PCR reaction mixture is heated at 95°C for 9 min and subjected to 12 cycles of 94°C/1 min, 60°C/2 min, and 72°C/2 min.

2. For the second-round PCR, 1 µL of the above first-round PCR product is subjected to further amplification of each fragment containing exons 5-6, 7, and 8, in a separate reaction mixture. PCR is performed in a final 25-µL reaction mixture containing the same buffer composition as those used above, except that: (1) only one pair of appropriate primers (0.5 µ*M* each) is used, i.e., pE5-5'+ pE6-3' (for exons 5-6 fragment), or pE7-5'+ pE7-3' (for exon 7), or pE8-5'+ pE8-3' (for exon 8); (2) 0.25 µL of [α³²P]dATP is added; and (3) the mixture is heated at 95°C for 9 min and subjected to 35 PCR cycles of 94°C/1 min, 60°C/2 min, and 72°C/2 min.

3. Add 1 µL of each PCR product above to 9 µL of SSCP loading solution in a 0.5 µL microcentrifuge tube, heat at 98°C for 2 min, and then immediately chill on ice for 5 min before analysis by SSCP.

4. Assemble glass plates for a 0.8-mm-thick × 33.5-cm-wide × 39.5-cm-high SSCP gel. Prepare 125 mL of SSCP solution containing 0.5X MDE (31.25 mL of the 2X MDE gel solution), 5% glycerol (6.25 mL glycerol stock), 0.6X TBE buffer (3.75 mL 20X TBE), and 83.75 mL distilled water. Add 750 µL 10% APS and 75 µL TEMED and mix.

5. Pour the solution onto the preassembled SSCP plates. Insert a 38-well comb, and let the gel polymerize for 2 h at room temperature.

6. Remove the comb and rinse the gel wells immediately with 0.6X TBE buffer. Place the gel on the gel box containing 0.6X TBE buffer in the top and bottom tanks. Load the 10 µL denatured PCR product.

7. Run the gel at 7 constant W for 18–24 h at room temperature (*see* **Note 6**).

8. Dry and autoradiograph the gel.

9. Isolate mutant alleles from the gel by following the steps described in **Subheading 3.1.3., step 3**.

10. Transfer each dried gel slice excised from the gel into a 0.5-mL microcentrifuge tube, and elute the DNA as described in **Subheading 3.1.3., step 9**.

11. Use a 5-µL aliquot of the eluted DNA as a template for further PCR amplification, using the 25-µL reaction mixture and the appropriate pair of primers, buffer composition, and PCR cycling conditions as described above in **Subheading 3.1.4., step 2**, for each specific exon, except that only an equivalence of 0.01 µL of [α³²P]dATP is added per reaction.

12. The PCR product is PAGE-purified as described in **Subheading 3.1.3., step 3**, and quantified as described in **Subheading 3.1.3., step 11**. An aliquot of the purified DNA is used for mutation determination by automated sequencer.

3.2. Analysis of Mutations From DNA Extracted From Whole Sputum Cells

*3.2.1. DNA Extraction From Sputum Samples (see **Note 7**)*

1. Remove sputum samples from the freezer, and leave the tubes on ice in an ice bucket for 30 min. Take an aliquot (an equivalence of 10^4 cells or 500 µL of saccomanno solution) of each sample, transfer it into a 1.5-mL microcentrifuge tube, and centrifuge at 7500*g* for 5 min (microcentrifuge) at 4°C. Discard the saccommanno solution and wash the pellet once with 500 µL cold PBS.

2. Add 250 µL lysis buffer containing 50 µg of proteinase K to the pellet, mix gently for 1 min, and incubate the solution at 37°C for 2 h with occasional manual shaking.

3. Spin down each tube in an microcentrifuge for 1 s. In a fume hood and wearing eye protection, open the tube and add 250 μL saturated phenol, close the tube, and shake vigorously for 1 min. Quickly spin down for 1 s before opening the tube and adding 250 μL chloroform. Close the tube and shake vigorously for 30 s.

4. Centrifuge at 3000*g* for 5 min.

5. Transfer the top (aqueous) layer to a new 1.5-mL microcentrifuge tube, and add 500 μL chloroform/isoamylic alcohol (22:1). Mix vigorously for 1 min, and centrifuge at 3000*g* for 1 min.

6. Repeat the chloroform/isoamylic alcohol extraction (**step 5**) once more.

7. Transfer the aqueous layer into a new 1.5-mL microcentrifuge tube, add 1/2 vol of 7.5 *M* ammonium acetate, and mix gently.

8. Add 2.5 vol of cold 100% ethanol, close the tube, mix, and place the tube at –20°C for at least 2 h.

9. Centrifuge the precipitated DNA at 9800*g* for 15 min.

10. Carefully discard the ethanol, then wash the tube with 500 μL cold 70% ethanol, and centrifuge at 9800*g* for 5 min.

11. Discard the 70% ethanol.

12. Spin down for 1 s in an Eppendorf centrifuge, carefully discard the remainder of the 70% ethanol using a thin gel loading tip, and dry the pellet at room temperature for 15 min.

13. Dissolve each DNA pellet in 20 μL distilled water and store at –20°C until use.

3.2.2. Analysis of K-RAS Mutations by PCR + MAE + DGGE

Enrichment for K-*RAS* codon 12 mutant alleles:

1. The same procedure described above in **Subheading 3.1.**, **step 3**, is used here, with the following modifications:

   a. Genomic DNA extracted from whole sputum cells is used as the template for PCR.

   b. Antisense primer PKB is used instead of PK12/13 to generate the *Ban*I restriction site.

   c. Two steps of *Ban*I restriction enzyme digestion of the PCR products to enrich for codon 12 mutant alleles are added, with the first step being used to digest the first-round PCR product, which is then used as template for a second-round PCR, and the second step to digest the second-round PCR product.

   d. Only the digestion-resistant fragment is PAGE-purified and analyzed by DGGE. These steps are performed as follows: an aliquot of the genomic DNA extracted from whole sputum cells (equivalent to 10^3 cells) is used as template for the first-round PCR, using the same reagents and concentrations, and PCR reaction conditions and cycle number are as described in **Subheading 3.1.3.**, **step 1**; the set of primers used includes KI1-1 and PKB to amplify a 75-bp fragment.

2. Dilute 1 μL of the first-round PCR product to a final 5-μL mixture containing 1X *Ban*I restriction enzyme buffer and 3 U of *Ban*I restriction enzyme in a 0.5-mL microcentrifuge tube.

3. Incubate the mixture at 37°C for 2 h.

4. Dilute the digested product to a final 25-μL PCR mixture containing the same reagents, isotope, and respective concentrations as those described in **Subheading 3.1.3.**, **step 2**; the primers used are PKGC and PKB to amplify a 125-bp fragment.

5. Subject the mixture to a second-round PCR for 35 cycles as described in **Subheading 3.1.3.**, **step 2**.

6. Digest 10 mL of the second-round PCR product in a final 50-μL mixture containing 1X *Ban*I restriction enzyme buffer and 30 U of *Ban*I enzyme at 37°C for 2 h (*see* **Note 8**).

7. Spin down for 1 s in a microcentrifuge, and add 1/2 vol (25 μL) of 7.5 *M* ammonium acetate. Mix and add 2.5 vol (187.5 μL) of cold 100% ethanol.

8. Mix and chill the tube at –20°C for 1 h.

9. Centrifuge the tube at 9800*g* for 15 min in a microcentrifuge.

10. Discard the ethanol, add 250 μL of 70% cold ethanol, centrifuge at 9800*g* for 3 min, discard the ethanol completely, and dry the DNA pellet at room temperature for 15 min.

11. Dissolve each pellet in 15 μL of 1X PAGE loading solution, and separate the DNA by PAGE.

12. PAGE purification of restriction enzyme digestion-resistant fragments. The procedure described in **Subheading 3.1.3., step 3** is used here to prepare the gel, separate the DNA, and purify the wanted DNA fragment from the gel for analysis by DGGE, with the following modifications to increase the resolution of fragment separation: Prepare a 10% polyacrylamide gel, using the (1:19)% (*bis*/acrylamide) stock solution (for 25 mL, add 12.5 mL *bis*/acrylamide solution, 1.25 mL 20X TBE, 11.25 mL distilled water, 250 μL 10% AP, and 25 μL TEMED. The gel polymerizes within 30 min (*see* **Note 9**).

13. Load and electrophorese the above 15-μL DNA sample in 1X loading solution at 250 constant V for 3 h.

14. Autoradiograph the gel, purify, and sequence-analyze the 125-bp wanted fragment as described in **Subheading 3.1.3., step 3** and **3.1.3., step 4**.

3.2.3. Analysis of P53 Mutations by PCR + MAE + PAGE

For a sensitive analysis of *P53* mutations occurring at hot spot codons 158, 175/176, 245, 248, 249, 273, or 282, PCR+MAE+PAGE is used. These codons are located in exons 5, 7, and 8 of the *P53* gene. The screening for mutations at each of these codons is carried out using a procedure similar to that used for K-*RAS* mutation detection. To simplify the screening for mutations at each of these codons, the three exons are first amplified simultaneously in a single reaction mixture during the first-round PCR. Aliquots of the amplified DNA are then used for screening for mutations at each specific codon individually. These steps include the digestion of the first-round PCR product with an appropriate restriction enzyme, followed by a second-round PCR and a second restriction enzyme digestion, before PAGE purification of the digestion-resistant fragment and sequencing analysis of mutations.

1. Carry out the first-round PCR in a 50-μL reaction mixture containing genomic DNA extracted from whole sputum cells (an equivalence of 1000 sputum cells), 10 m*M* Tris-HCl , pH 8.0, 2.5 m*M* MgCl2, 50 m*M* KCl, 100 μ*M* each dNTP, 0.25 μ*M* of each of the three pairs of the *P53* gene primers, and 1 U of Gold AmpliTaq DNA polymerase. Heat the mixture at 95°C for 9 min and then subject it to 12 PCR cycles of 94°C/1 min, 65°C/2 min, and 72°C/2 min.

2. The stock template, obtained from the first round of amplification, contains:
   a. A *P53* gene exon 5 segment of 196 bp with hot spot codons 158 and 175/176, which correspond to *Aci*I and *Nco*I restriction enzyme sites, respectively.
   b. A *P53* gene exon 7 segment of 64 bp with hot spot codons 245, 248, and 249, which correspond to *Bsr*BI, *Msp*I and *Stu*I sites, respectively.

   c. A *P53* gene exon 8 segment of 93 bp with hot spot codons 273 and 282, which correspond to *Bst*UI and *Msp*I sites, respectively.

3. Dilute 1 µL of the first-round PCR stock template to a final 4-µL reaction mixture in a 0.5-mL microcentrifuge tube containing 1X the appropriate buffer and 3 U of the appropriate enzyme, and incubate for 2 h at 37°C (or 60°C for *Bst*UI). Heat the digestion mixture at 85°C for 5 min and then dilute to a final 25-µL PCR reaction mixture containing the same PCR reagents as shown above, except that only one pair of the appropriate primers (0.5 µ*M* each) is used, and 0.25-µL [α^{32}P]dATP is added. Carry out the amplification using 2 U of Gold AmpliTaq DNA polymerase, heated at 95°C/9 min for 30 cycles of 94°C/1 min, 60°C/2 min, and 72°C/2 min.

4. Dilute a 10-µL aliquot into a final 50 µL vol in a 0.5-mL microcentrifuge tube containing 5 µL of the appropriate 10X buffer, 1–2 µL (20 U) of each appropriate enzyme, and distilled water to make 50 µL. Incubate the mixture for 2 h at 37°C (or 60°C for *Bst*UI).

5. Precipitate the digested material by adding into each tube 25 µL 7.5 *M* ammonium acetate and 187.5 µL cold 100% ethanol, and place at –20°C for 1 h. Centrifuge each tube at 9800*g* in an Eppendorf centrifuge for 15 min. Discard the ethanol, and wash each pellet with 250 µL cold 70% ethanol. Centrifuge at 9800*g* for 5 min, discard the ethanol completely, and dry the pellet at room temperature for 10–15 min. Dissolve each pellet in 15 µL 1X PAGE loading solution.

6. Separate the DNA by PAGE, using a 10% polyacrylamide gel solution prepared from (1:19)% *bis*/acrylamide. The preparation of gel, loading of sample onto the gel, gel electrophoresis, isolation of the restriction enzyme-resistant fragment from the gel, and sequencing determination of mutations are carried out as described in **Subheading 3.2.2.**, **steps 12–14** for K-*RAS* exon 12 mutants.

4. Notes

1. Most sputum samples obtained from lung cancer patients contain between 5 and 10% epithelial cells. Most other cell types are inflammatory cells, buccal epithelial cells, macrophages, and neutrophils.

2. 8-Hydroxyquinoline is an oxidization indicator in the saturated phenol. If the color goes from yellow to red, it means that the phenol is oxidized and it cannot be used any more.

3. The codon 12 sequence of the human K-*RAS* gene, 5'-GGT-3', and its flanking codons do not correspond naturally to the site for any restriction enzyme. However, the sequence formed between codons 12-13, 5'-GGT GGC-3', closely resembles the restriction enzyme site for *Ban*I, 5'-GGT GCC-3'. We used a mismatch-primer, PKB: 5'-AGGCACTCTTGCCTACG<u>G</u>CA-3', to substitute the second G of codon 13 with a C to create the site for the restriction enzyme *Ban*I in the first-round PCR. Meanwhile, antisense primer PK12/13 can be used to detect K-*RAS* mutations in codons 12 and 13.

4. Both the 50% and 0% denaturant stock solutions should be kept at 4°C for no more than 2 mo.

5. Microscopic examination of the cap after an incubation of laser-captured cells with the lysis solution at room temperature for 36 h shows that 98–100% of the cells are emptied of their contents, i.e., completely lyzed. A similar rate of cell lysis can be achieved by carrying out the incubation at 37°C or 42°C overnight (~12–16 h). However, incubation at these temperatures leads to a leak of the lysis solution from the cap in approx 15–20% of the cases.

6. The electrophoresis power is based on the size of the fragment with 6 W at 150–200 bp and 7–8 W at more than 200 bp. Running the gel in a 4°C cold room for more than 24 h provides a better separation.

Table 1
Summary of *P53* and *K-RAS* Mutations of 15 Lung Cancer Patients from XuanWei, China[a]

Patient	P53		K-RAS	
	Mutations	Amino acid changes	Mutations	Amino acid changes
1				
2[b]	E5cod.136 CAA to CAG	Gln to Gln		
3				
4[c]			Cod.12 GGT to TGT	Gly to Cys
5				
6				
7[b]	E5cod.151 CCC to TCC	Pro to Ser		
8[b]	E7cod.244 GGC to TGC	Gly to Cys		
9				
10[b]	E5cod.139 AAG to TAG	Lys to Stop	Cod.13 GGC to TGC	Gly to Cys
11				
12				
13[c]	E7cod.248 CGG to CAG	Arg to Gln		
14[b]	E7cod.244 GGC to GTC	Gly to Val		
15				

[a]Summary of the mutations detected using three approaches in sputum samples of 7 (46.6%) of the 15 patients investigated. Five patients each had a *P53* mutation, including patient 2 (with a silent CAA to CAG transition at codon 136 in exon 5), patient 7 (with a CCC to TCC transition at codon 151 in exon 5), patient 8 (with a GGC to TGC transversions at codon 244 in exon 7), patient 13 (with a CGG to CAG transition at codon 248 in exon 7), and patient 14 (with a GGC to GTC transversion at codon 244 in exon 7). Patient 4 had a GGT to TGT transversion in codon 12 of the K-*RAS* gene. Patient 10 had a GGC to TGC transversion at codon 13 of the K-*RAS* gene and an AAG to TAG transversion at codon 139 in exon 5 of the *P53* gene. None of these mutations were detected in the matched nonmalignant epithelial cells or the matched buccal cells taken from sputum of these patients (data not shown). Therefore, two mutations were detected in DNA extracted directly from sputum of two patients, including a K-*RAS* codon 12 mutation (patient 4) and a *P53* mutation at codon 248 (patient 13), by using sensitive methods. Both of these mutations and six additional mutations, including a K-*RAS* codon 13 mutation and five *P53* mutations, were detected when epithelial cells isolated by LCM from sputum were analyzed using less sensitive but less laborious methods.

[b]Mutations detected only in tumor cells isolated from sputum by the laser capture/mutation analysis method.

[c]Mutations detected by both the PCR+MAE+PAGE (for *P53*) or PCR+MAE+DGGE (for K-*RAS*) method in DNA extracted from sputum cells, and by the laser capture/mutation analysis method in tumor cells isolated from sputum.

7. Because the DNA extraction is carried out from only 10^4 cells, there is no need for treatment with RNase to eliminate cellular RNA. On the other hand, treatment with proteinase (50 mg) is needed, since each sputum sample contains mucus. If protein is still present at the interface between the phenol and aqueous phase, one additional step of phenol extraction is needed before the chloroform/isoamyl alcohol extraction.

8. The digestion is performed with 10–50 U *Ban*I for 1–6 h at 37°C. A complete digestion of the 10-µL PCR product can be achieved with 30 U of the enzymes for 2 h. A longer incubation time (6–12 h) with 10–50 U *Ban*I leads to nonspecific digestion of a fraction of some of the mutant/wild-type heteroduplex fragment, as revealed by their respective band intensity after separation by DGGE (unpublished data).

9. The use of PAGE made of the (1:37.5)% *bis*/acrylamide solution does not allow a satisfactory separation of the undigested (codon 12 mutant alleles) from the digested fragments (nonmutant alleles).

Acknowledgments

This work was supported by grants from the American Cancer Society (RPG-99-61-01-CNE and RSG-99-161-04-CNE).

References

1. Pisani, P., Parkin, D. M., Bray, F., and Ferlay, J. (1999) Estimates of the worldwide mortality from 25 major cancers in 1990. *Int. J. Cancer* **83,** 18–29.
2. *Cancer Facts and Figures—2002.* American Cancer Society, Atlanta, GA.
3. Fontana, R. S. (1977) Early diagnosis of lung cancer. *Am. Rev. Respir. Dis.* **116,** 399–402.
4. Birrer, M. J. and Brown, P. H. (1992) Application of molecular genetics to the early diagnosis and screening of lung cancer. *Cancer Res.* **52,** 2658s–2664s.
5. Szabo, E., Birrer, M. J., and Mulshire, J. L. (1993) Early detection of lung cancer. *Semin. Oncol.* **20,** 374–382.
6. Vogelstein, B. and Kinzler, K. W. (1992) p53 function and disfunction. *Cell* **70,** 523–526.
7. Khosravi-Far, R. and Der, C. J. (1994) The ras signal transduction pathway. *Cancer Metastasis Rev.* **13,** 67–89.
8. Suzuki, Y., Orita, M., Shiraishi, M., Hayashi, K., and Sekiya, T. (1990) Detection of *ras* gene mutations in human lung cancers by single-strand conformation polymorphism analysis of polymerase chain reaction products. *Oncogene* **5,** 1037–1043.
9. Sugio, K., Ishida, T., Yokoyama, H., Inoue, T., Sugimachi, and K., Sasazuki, T. (1992) *ras* gene mutation as a prognostic marker in adenocarcinoma of the human lung without lymph node metastasis. *Cancer Res.* **52,** 2903–2906.
10. Rodenhuis, S. and Slebos, R. J. (1992) Clinical significance of ras oncogene activation in human lung cancer. *Cancer Res.* **52,** 2665s–2669s.
11. Husgafvel-Pursianen, K., Hackman, P., Ridanpaa, M., et al. (1993) K-*ras* mutations in human adenocarcinoma of the lung: association with smoking and occupational exposure to asbestos. *Int. J. Cancer* **53,** 250-256.
12. Keohavong, P., DeMichele, M. A., Melacrinos, A. C., Landreneau, R. J., Weyant, R. J., and Siegfried, J. M. (1996) Detection of K-*RAS* mutations in lung carcinomas: relationship to prognosis. *Clin. Cancer Res.* **2,** 411–418.
13. Hollstein, M., Sidransky, D., Vogelstein, B., and Harris, C. C. (1991) *p53* mutations in human cancers. *Science* **253,** 49–53.
14. Greenblatt, M. S., Bennett, W. P., Hollstein, M., and Harris, C. C. (1994) Mutations in the *p53* tumor suppressor gene: clues to cancer etiology and molecular pathogenesis. *Cancer Res.* **54,** 4855–4878.

15. Yokota, J., Wada, M., Shimosato, Y., Terada, M., and Sugimura, T. (1987) Loss of heterozygosity on chromosomes 3, 13, and 17 in small-cell carcinoma and on chromosome 3 in adenocarcinoma of the lung. *Proc. Natl. Acad. Sci. USA* **84**, 9252–9256.

16. Chiba, I., Takahashi, T., Nau, M. M., et al. (1990) Mutations in the *p53* gene are frequent in primary, resected non-small cell lung cancer. *Oncogene* **5**, 1603–1610.

17. Kishimoto, Y., Murakami, Y., Shiraishi, M., Hayashi, K., and Sekiya, T. (1992) Aberrations of the p53 tumor suppressor gene in human non-small cell carcinomas of the lung. *Cancer Res.* **52**, 4799–4804.

18. Takahashi, T., Nau, M. M., Chiba, I., et al. (1989) p53: a frequent target for genetic abnormalities in lung cancer. *Science* **246**, 491–494.

19. Cho, Y., Gorina, S., Jeffrey, P. D., and Pavletich, N. P. (1994) Crystal structure of a *p53* tumor suppressor-DNA complex: understanding tumorigenic mutations. *Science* **265**, 346–355.

20. Hainaut, P. and Hollstein, M. (2000) *p53* and human cancer: the first ten thousand mutations. *Adv. Cancer Res.* **77**, 81–137.

21. Jassem, E., Niklinski, J., Rosell, R., et al. (2001) Types and localisation of p53 gene mutations: a report on 332 non-small cell lung cancer patients. *Lung Cancer* **34**, 47s–51s.

22. Caron de Fromentel, C. and Soussi, T. (1992) TP53 tumor suppressor gene: a model for investigating human mutagenesis. *Genes Chromosomes Cancer* **4**, 1–15.

23. de Anta, J. M., Jassem, E., Rosell, R., et al. (1997) TP53 mutational pattern in Spanish and Polish non-small cell lung cancer patients: null mutations are associated with poor prognosis. *Oncogene* **15**, 2951–2958.

24. Cha, R. S., Zarbl, H., Keohavong, P., and Thilly, W. G. (1992) Mismatch amplification mutation assay (MAMA): application to the c-H-*ras* gene. *PCR Methods Appl.* **2**, 14–20.

25. Mitsudomi, T., Viallet, J., Mulshine, J. L., Linnoila, R. I., Minna, J. D., and Gazdar, A. F. (1991) Mutations of *ras* genes distinguish a subset of non-small-cell lung cancer cell lines from small-cell lung cancer cell lines. *Oncogene* **6**, 1353–1362.

26. Jiang, W., Kahn, S. M., Guillem, J. G., Lu, S. H., and Weinstein, I. B. (1989) Rapid detection of ras oncogenes in human tumors: application to colon, esophageal, and gastric cancer. *Oncogene* **4**, 923–928.

27. Kumar, R. and Dunn, L. L. (1989) Designed diagnostic restriction fragment length polymorphism for the detection of point mutations in ras oncogenes. *Oncogene Res.* **1**, 235–241.

28. Levi, S., Urbano-Ispizua, A., Gill, R., et al. (1991) Multiple K-*ras* 12 mutations in cholangiocarcinomas demonstrated with a sensitive polymerase chain reaction technique. *Cancer Res.* **51**, 3497–3502.

29. Kahn, S. M., Jiang, W., Culbertson, T. A., et al. (1991) Rapid and sensitive non-radioactive detection of mutant K-*ras* genes via enriched PCR amplification. *Oncogene* **6**, 1079–1083.

30. Yakubovskaya, M. S., Spiegelman, V., Luo, F. C., et al. (1995) High frequency of K-*ras* mutations in normal appearing lung tissues and sputum of patients with lung cancer. *Int. J. Cancer* **63**, 810–814.

31. Mills, N. E., Fishman, C. L., Scholes, J., Anderson, S. E., Rom, W. N., and Jacobson, D. R. (1995) Detection of K-*ras* oncogene mutations in bronchoalveolar lavage fluid for lung cancer diagnosis. *J. Natl. Cancer Inst.* **87**, 1056–1060.

32. Mao, L., Hruban, R. H., Boyle, J. O., Tockman, M., and Sidransky, D. (1994) Detection of oncogene mutations in sputum precedes diagnosis of lung cancer. *Cancer Res.* **54**, 1634–1637.

33. Scott, F. M., Modali, R., Lehman, T. A., et al. (1997) High frequency of K-*RAS* codon 12 mutations in bronchoalveolar lavage fluid of patients at high risk for second primary lung cancer. *Clin. Cancer Res.* **3**, 479–482.

34. Keohavong, P., Zhu, D., Whiteside, T. L., et al. (1997) Detection of infrequent and multiple K-*ras* mutations in human tumors and tumor-adjacent tissues. *Anal. Biochem.* **247,** 394–403.

35. Zhang, L. F., Gao, W. M., Gealy, R., et al. (2003) Comparison of K-*ras* gene mutations in tumor and sputum DNA of patients with lung cancer. *Biomarkers* **8,** 156–161.

22

Allele-Specific Competitive Blocker–PCR Detection of Rare Base Substitution

Barbara L. Parsons, Page B. McKinzie, and Robert H. Heflich

Summary

Methods that detect rare base substitutions within populations of DNA molecules are valuable tools for studying the DNA-damaging effects of chemicals and for pool screening for single-nucleotide polymorphisms. Allele-specific competitive blocker–polymerase chain reaction (ACB–PCR) uses a mutant-specific PCR primer with more 3'-terminal mismatches to an abundant or wild-type sequence than to a rare or mutant sequence in order to amplify specifically an allele that differs from the wild-type by a single base pair. ACB–PCR reactions include a blocker primer to reduce the amount of background signal generated from the abundant wild-type template. The nonextendable blocker primer preferentially anneals to the wild-type DNA sequence, thereby excluding the annealing of the extendable mutant-specific primer to the wild-type sequence. Inclusion of single-strand DNA binding protein in the ACB–PCR reaction and use of the Stoffel fragment of *Taq* DNA polymerase both significantly increase allele discrimination. The concurrent analysis of mutant fraction standards and equivalent PCR products amplified from genomic DNA samples makes ACB–PCR a quantitative method that can detect a base pair substitution in the presence of a 10^5-fold excess of wild-type DNA. Methods for the ACB–PCR measurement of the mouse H-*ras* codon 61 CAA $\rightarrow$ AAA mutation are presented.

Key Words: ACB–PCR; point mutation; allele-specific amplification; mutation detection; base substitution; H-*ras*; PCR; single-strand DNA binding protein; single nucleotide polymorphism; SNP.

1. Introduction

There are two main classes of DNA-based methods for the detection of point mutation: scanning methods that detect unknown mutations within a given length of DNA sequence and diagnostic methods that detect only one or a few specific point mutations *(1)*. Because sequence specificity is incorporated into diagnostic mutation detection methods, they are generally more sensitive than scanning methods. Unfortunately, the sequence specificity also makes diagnostic mutation detection methods more difficult to adapt to new mutational targets. Allele-specific amplification (ASA) is one

From: *Methods in Molecular Biology, vol. 291, Molecular Toxicology Protocols*
Edited by: P. Keohavong and S. G. Grant © Humana Press Inc., Totowa, NJ

approach for the diagnostic detection of specific point mutations *(2)*. Many different variations of ASA have been reported, all of which use a mutant-specific primer (MSP) to amplify preferentially a rare, "mutant" DNA sequence in a polymerase chain reaction (PCR). With a sensitivity of 10^{-5}, allele-specific competitive blocker (ACB)–PCR is among the most sensitive allele-specific amplification methods *(2–4)*. Application of ACB–PCR to the detection of several different point mutations has defined a relatively narrow range of ACB–PCR reaction conditions that now can be used to develop the ACB–PCR detection of new mutational targets.

ACB–PCR sensitivity is derived from the use of two different allele-discriminating primers *(3–5)*. In ACB–PCR, the MSP is designed with a mismatch in the 3'-penultimate position with respect to both the mutant and wild-type alleles (**Fig. 1**). The 3'-terminal base of the MSP is complementary to the base substitution being detected. This design results in a single 3'-terminal mismatch between the mutant-specific primer and the mutant template, but a double, 3'-terminal mismatch between the mutant-specific primer and the wild-type template. It has been shown that greater allele selectivity is achieved when mutant allele-specific amplification is based on extension of a singly vs doubly mismatched primer than when allele discrimination is based on amplification of a perfectly matched vs a singly mismatched primer *(2,3)*.

The second allele-selecting primer used in ACB–PCR is the blocker primer (BP). The BP carries a 3'-terminal dideoxynucleotide and thus cannot be extended. Like the mutant-specific primer, this primer is designed with a 3'-penultimate mismatch. The 3'-terminal base of this primer is complementary to the wild-type template. The BP, therefore, has a single, 3'-penultimate mismatch relative to the wild-type template but a double, 3'-terminal mismatch relative to the mutant template (**Fig. 1**). This causes the nonextendable BP to anneal selectively to the wild-type allele, thereby reducing the availability of this priming site for the mutant-specific primer. Ultimately, the use of a BP in the ACB–PCR reaction reduces the background level of PCR product that is synthesized from the abundant wild-type allele. Because at low mutant fractions a signal must be generated from relatively few mutant template molecules, the lower the amplification of wild-type molecules, the greater the sensitivity of the assay.

Other aspects of the ACB–PCR reaction that contribute to mutation detection sensitivity are the use of the Stoffel fragment of *Taq* DNA polymerase, Perfect Match PCR enhancer, and a "hot start." The Stoffel fragment of *Taq* DNA polymerase is a less processive enzyme that shows greater allele selectivity than the holoenzyme *(6)*. Perfect Match PCR enhancer is a commercial composition that includes single-strand DNA binding protein (SSB). SSB lowers the melting temperature of DNA, but it lowers the melting temperature of mismatched DNA to a greater extent than perfectly matched DNA and magnifies the discrimination between singly and doubly mismatched primer/template pairs *(7–9)*.

ACB–PCR is a quantitative assay in which mutant fraction standards are analyzed in parallel with unknown samples *(10)*. Cloned mutant and wild-type DNAs can be used as templates to generate PCR products. Once purified and quantified, the mutant and wild-type PCR products can be mixed in known proportions to construct mutant fraction standards. Mutant fraction standards are exceedingly valuable for monitoring

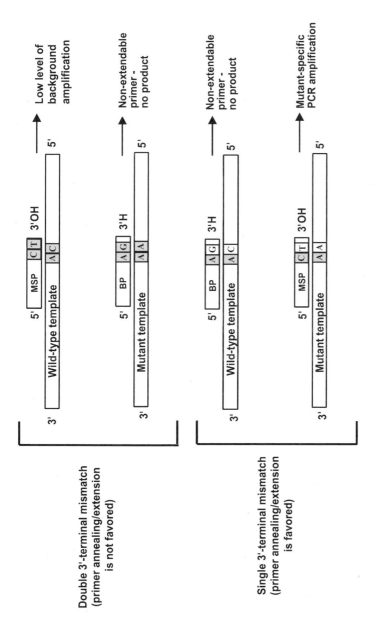

Fig. 1. Significance of mutant-specific primer (MSP) and blocker primer (BP) design in ACB–PCR amplification. The four potential primer/template pairs that may occur between the mutant-specific and blocker primers, and the mutant and wild-type templates are depicted (mismatched basepairs are shaded). The result of each pairing in the ACB–PCR reaction is indicated. The depicted ACB–PCR primer design is used to detect mouse H-*ras* codon 61 CAA → AAA mutation (*3,10*).

assay performance and sensitivity. PCR products that are equivalent in sequence are amplified from the genomic DNA samples to be analyzed for mutation. These products are also purified and quantified. Finally, 10^8 copies of each mutant fraction standard and PCR product generated from the genomic "test" DNAs are analyzed in parallel by ACB–PCR. Samples of the ACB–PCR reactions are run on polyacrylamide gels, whereby the diagnostic products are detected and quantified (**Fig. 2**). A standard curve is constructed based on the signal from the mutant fraction standards, and the mutant fractions of the test DNAs are calculated using this standard curve.

ACB–PCR has been used to detect three of the six possible base pair substitution mutations known to activate the *ras* gene, including the three most common point mutations (G:C → T:A, G:C → A:T, and T:A → A:T) *(4)*. Somewhat different conditions are needed to detect these different point mutations. However, the optimal ACB–PCR reaction conditions established for the detection of G:C → T:A mutation in two different mutational targets (mouse H-*ras* codon 61 and human K-*ras* codon 12) are identical, suggesting that they may be broadly applicable to the detection of this point mutation *(3,4)*. The ACB–PCR methods presented below specifically describe the detection of the mouse H-*ras* codon 61 CAA → AAA point mutation, but ranges of reaction conditions that should be optimized in the detection of other point mutations are also provided *(4)*.

2. Materials

2.1. Preparation of Mutant and Wild-Type Standard DNAs and First-Round PCR Products From Genomic DNA Samples (see Note 1)

1. All H_2O used is Ultra Pure Reagent Grade Water (New England Reagent Laboratory, East Providence, RI).
2. The wild-type plasmid, p94 (codon 61, CAA) has all of mouse H-*ras* exon 1, intron 1, and part of exon 2, cloned into the TA cloning vector PCR II (Invitrogen, Carlsbad, CA) *(11)*. The mutant plasmid p91 (codon 61, AAA) is similarly constructed.
3. Cloned *Pfu* DNA polymerase and 10X reaction buffer: 100 m*M* KCl, 100 m*M* $(NH_4)_2SO_4$, 200 m*M* Tris-HCl (pH 8.75), 20 m*M* $MgSO_4$, 1% Triton X-100, 1 mg/mL bovine serum albumin (BSA; Stratagene, La Jolla, CA).
4. GeneAmp dNTPs, 10 m*M* stocks (Applied Biosystems, Foster City, CA).
5. PCR primers (Sigma Genosys, The Woodlands, TX): reconstituted with H_2O at 100 μ*M*.

   a. TR3 (5'-TTCTGTGGATTCTCTGGT-3').
   b. H2 (5'-GTGCGCATGTACTGGTCCCG-3').

6. 0.5-mL Thin-walled PCR tubes.
7. Single-use aliquots of 1 mL mineral oil (Sigma, St. Louis, MO).
8. 6X Loading dye: 0.25% bromophenol blue, 0.25% xylene cyanole FF, 15% Ficoll (type 400); all purchased from Sigma.
9. 0.7% TAE agarose gels: agarose (Invitrogen Life Technologies, Carlsbad, CA), 1X TAE (40 m*M* Tris-base, 50 m*M* sodium acetate, 10 m*M* Na_2EDTA, pH 7.9; reagents purchased from Sigma).
10. 10 mg/mL Ethidium bromide stock solution (Sigma).
11. UV source (transilluminator or hand-held).

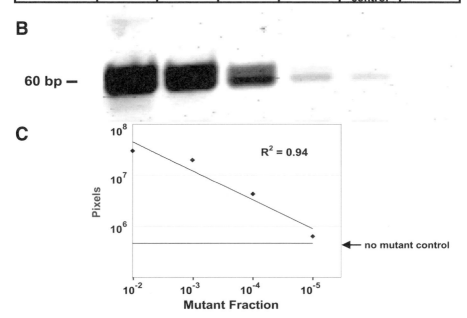

Fig. 2. ACB–PCR detection of mouse H-*ras* codon 61 CAA → AAA mutation. (**A**) Composition of mutant fraction standards. (**B**) Fluorescent detection of ACB–PCR products generated from the mutant fraction standards (with lanes aligned beneath mutant fraction labels). (**C**) Construction of a standard curve from the fluorescent data.

12. Razor blade or scalpel.
13. Geneclean Spin Kit (BIO 101, Vista, CA).
14. 0.5X TE: 5 mM Tris-HCl, 0.5 mM Na$_2$EDTA, pH 8.0.
15. Barrier pipet tips (LabSource, Chicago, IL, or equivalent).
16. 0.5-mL Microcentrifuge tubes.

2.2. Quantification of Standard DNAs and First-Round PCR Products

1. Low DNA Mass Ladder (Invitrogen).
2. 1X TE: 10 mM Tris-HCl, 1.0 mM Na$_2$EDTA, pH 8.0.
3. 0.5-mL Microcentrifuge tubes.
4. Vertical slab gel electrophoresis system (CBS Scientific, Del Mar, CA).
5. 8% Polyacrylamide gels (20 cm × 20 cm × 0.75 mm): 40 mL of acrylamide solution are prepared using 27 mL of H$_2$O, 4 mL of 10X TAE buffer, 8 mL of 40% acrylamide/

bis-acrylamide solution (37.5:1), 1 mL of 10% ammonium persulfate, and 60 µL of TEMED. Acrylamide, ammonium persulfate, and TEMED purchased from Bio-Rad (Hercules, CA).

6. Vistra Green (Amersham Biosciences, Piscataway, NJ).
7. FluorImager SI with ImageQuaNT (Molecular Dynamics, Sunnyvale, CA).
8. Excel (Microsoft, Redmond, WA).

2.3. Preparation of ACB–PCR Reaction Mix, Mutant Fraction Standards, and ACB–PCR Reactions

1. Primers: primer stocks are reconstituted with H_2O at 100 µ*M*, and working solutions of 10 µ*M* are prepared as needed.

   a. MSP: TR10 5'-ATGGCACTATACTCTTGTCT-3'.
   b. BP: TR27 5'-ATGGCACTATACTCTTCTAddG-3' (synthesized with a 3'-deoxy G chain terminator).
   After synthesis, both these primers are gel-purified (Sigma Genosys).
   c. Upstream ACB–PCR primer: TR31 5'-TGGGGAGACATGTCTACTG -3'.

2. AmpliTaq DNA polymerase Stoffel fragment (10 U/mL), 10X Stoffel buffer (100 m*M* KCl, 100 m*M* Tris-HCl, pH 8.3) and 25 m*M* $MgCl_2$ solution (Applied Biosystems).
3. 0.5-mL Microcentrifuge tubes.
4. Single-use aliquots of 100 µL 10 m*M* sequencing grade dNTPs (Amersham Biosciences) are apportioned and can be stored at –20°C for at least 2 yr. A 1.25 m*M* dNTP working solution is prepared by adding 50 µL of each of the four 10 m*M* dNTP stocks to 200 µL of H_2O.
5. Perfect Match PCR Enhancer, 1 U/µL (Stratagene).
6. A working solution of 1% Triton X-100 (Sigma) is apportioned into 150-µL single-use aliquots.
7. A 20 mg/mL stock solution of gelatin (Sigma) can be stored at 4°C for up to 2 yr. This stock is diluted to the working concentration of 1 mg/mL and apportioned into 150-µL single-use aliquots.
8. Single-use aliquots of gel-purified wild-type and mutant standard DNAs (from **Subheading 3.1., steps 3** and **6**).
9. First-round PCR products prepared from genomic DNAs (from **Subheading 3.1., step 5**).
10. 0.5-mL Thin-walled PCR tubes.
11. Single-use aliquots of 1 mL mineral oil (Sigma).

2.4. Hot Start ACB–PCR Reactions

1. A microcentrifuge that can be pulsed and from which the samples can be removed quickly (e.g., Costar Variable Speed Microcentrifuge, Daigger, Vernon Hills, IL).
2. Two Perkin Elmer 480 thermocyclers (Boston, MA; or the equivalent) positioned side by side.

2.5. Sample and Data Analysis

1. 0.5-mL Microcentrifuge tubes.
2. 6X Loading dye.
3. Vertical slab gel electrophoresis system.
4. 8% Polyacrylamide gel.
5. 50-bp DNA Ladder (Gibco-BRL).

6. Vistra Green.
7. FluorImager SI with ImageQuaNT.
8. Microsoft Excel.

3. Methods

3.1. Preparation of Mutant and Wild-Type Standard DNAs and First-Round PCR Products From Genomic DNA Samples

1. Using 3.75 ng of wild-type plasmid DNA as template (*see* **Note 2**), set up a 100 μL PCR reaction containing: 10 μL 10X *Pfu* reaction buffer, 7.5 μL of each 10 m*M* dNTP, 1.5 μL of 100 μ*M* primer TR3, 1.5 μL of 100 μ*M* primer H2, and 1.5 μL (3.75 U) *Pfu* DNA polymerase. Overlay with 100 μL of mineral oil. Amplify using a single cycle of 1 min at 94°C, 5 min at 48°C, and 1 min at 72°C, followed by 28 cycles of 1 min at 94°C, 1 min at 48°C, and 2 min at 72°C.
2. Add 20 μL of 6X loading dye and run the PCR reaction on a preparative 0.7% TAE agarose gel.
3. Use a razor blade to cut out the 189-bp H-*ras* PCR product (*see* **Note 3**) and recover the DNA from the gel slice using two Geneclean Spin Kit columns (≤300 mg agarose per column, per the manufacturer's instructions). Each column is eluted with 25 μL of 0.5X TE, and the two samples are pooled. All pipeting is performed using barrier pipet tips. Because little DNA standard is needed for each ACB–PCR (picograms) and to reduce the potential for cross-contamination, many single-use aliquots (5–15 ng) of the purified PCR product are prepared from a single DNA isolation. These aliquots are stable for approx 1 yr when DNAs at 0.5–5 ng/μL are stored at –80°C.
4. Set up and run 100 μL PCR reactions identical to those described in **Subheading 3.1.**, **step 1** to synthesize first-round H-*ras* PCR products from the genomic DNA samples, using 1.5 μg of each genomic DNA (4.5×10^5 copies of a single-copy nuclear gene) as template.
5. Purify the PCR products amplified from the genomic DNAs from agarose gels. Apportion the gel-purified DNAs into single-use aliquots (5–15 ng).
6. Using 3.75 ng of mutant plasmid DNA as template, set up and run a 100-μL PCR reaction as described above, and then purify and aliquot the standard in single-use aliquots (5–15 ng; *see* **Note 4**).

3.2. Quantification of Standard DNAs and First-Round PCR Products

1. Prepare 10 μL samples of 1:10 and 1:100 dilutions of the DNA Mass Ladder in 1X TE buffer.
2. Set up DNA mass standards, each sample containing 1 μL of 6X loading buffer; 1, 2, or 4 μL of either the 1:100 or 1:10 dilution of the DNA Mass Ladder; and H_2O to bring the volume of each to 6 μL. These standards will contain 0.05, 0.1, 0.2. 0.5, 1, and 2 ng of a 200-bp DNA, respectively.
3. Prepare 6-μL samples of all standard DNAs (wild-type and mutant) and first-round PCR products containing: 1 μL of 6X loading buffer, 4 μL of H_2O, and 1 μL DNA (*see* **Note 5**).
4. Load samples on 8% polyacrylamide gels (run at ~200 V, for 2 h at 4°C).
5. Stain the gel with Vistra Green per the manufacturer's instructions. Scan the gel using a Molecular Dynamics FluorImager SI or the equivalent. Quantify the fluorescence of the 189-bp PCR products and the 200-bp DNA mass standards using ImageQuaNT software.
6. Import the ImageQuaNT data into Microsoft Excel and construct a standard curve of pixels vs nanograms of DNA (using the linear function). Use the equation of this line to calculate the mass of the 189-bp DNA per volume loaded for each unknown (*see* **Note 6**).

3.3. Preparation of Mutant Fraction Standards and First-Round PCR Products for ACB–PCR (see Note 7)

1. Using the conversion 19.4 pg of 189-bp H-*ras* DNA = 10^8 copies, dilute the wild-type PCR product to 2.5×10^7 copies per µL in H_2O.
2. Label 0.5-mL tubes in which to set up the mutant fraction standard and the no-mutant control DNA mixes, as shown in **Table 1**.
3. Add H_2O and wild-type DNA to the tubes, as shown in **Table 1**.
4. Dilute the unknown samples to 2.0×10^7 copies per µL in H_2O.
5. Dilute mutant DNA to 1×10^8 copies per µL in H_2O, and then make five 10-fold serial dilutions of the mutant DNA (1×10^7 to 1×10^3 copies per µL).
6. Add mutant DNA standard to the mixes as shown in **Table 1**.

3.4. Preparation of ACB–PCR Reaction Mix and ACB–PCR Reactions (see Note 8)

1. The following reagent volumes are combined (on ice) to prepare 1 mL of ACB–PCR reaction mix (enough for 20 50-µL reactions): 408 µL of H_2O, 100 µL of 10X Stoffel buffer, 100 µL of 1 mg/mL gelatin, 100 µL of 1% Triton X-100, 32 µL of 1.25 m*M* dNTPs, 60 µL of 25 m*M* $MgCl_2$, 40 µL of 10 µ*M* TR10 (MSP), 33 µL of 10 µ*M* TR31 (upstream primer), and 20 µL of 10 µ*M* TR27 (BP) for a total of 893 µL. Template DNA (20 reactions × 5 µL/reaction = 100 µL) and enzyme/Perfect Match (~7 µL) are added later and bring the total volume to 1 mL. Vortex and briefly centrifuge the ACB–PCR reaction mix several times to ensure homogeneity.
2. Remove 100 µL of ACB-PCR reaction mix and transfer to a separate tube. Add to this aliquot 6 µL of *Taq* DNA polymerase Stoffel fragment (60 U) and 1.3 µL of Perfect Match PCR Enhancer (1.3 U). Mix and briefly centrifuge to ensure homogeneity, and then distribute into three tubes (36 µL each).
3. Place 40 µL of ACB–PCR reaction mix into labeled, 0.5-mL thin-walled PCR tubes (one tube per sample, including mutant fraction standards, the "no mutant" [i.e., wild-type] control, a "no DNA" control, and unknowns; up to 18 samples).
4. Add 5 µL of H_2O to the "no DNA" control tube. Then add 5 µL of each mutant fraction standard, "no mutant" control, or first-round PCR product to the ACB–PCR reaction mix in each labeled tube (*see* **Note 9**).
5. Mix and briefly centrifuge the samples twice, overlay the samples with 45 µL of mineral oil, and briefly centrifuge once more.

3.5. Hot Start ACB–PCR Reactions

1. With two thermocyclers (A and B) side by side, set up and save the following step-cycle program: 30 s at 94°C, 45 s at 46°C, 1 min at 72°C, for 37 cycles on thermocycler A.
2. Preheat both thermocyclers to 94°C (94°C soak cycle). Place a set of five or six ACB–PCR reactions (from **Subheading 3.4., step 5**) into thermocycler B (*see* **Note 10**). Hit stop twice and start once so the thermocycler begins to time from 0. After 1 min 40 s, place one of the tubes of enzyme mix into thermocycler B. After an additional 20 s (timer now reads 2 min), transfer 5 µL of the enzyme mix (from **Subheading 3.4., step 2**) into each ACB–PCR reaction. Specifically, remove the enzyme mix from the block, open the tube, and position it so you can hold it and another tube in the same hand. Remove a sample from the block, place it in the same hand, open it, transfer the enzyme, close the sample tube, and return the sample tube to the block before picking up the next sample and repeating the procedure.

Table 1
Preparation of Mutant Fraction Standard DNAs

Mutant fraction standard	Wild-Type DNA	Mutant DNA	H_2O
10^{-1}	18 μL @ 2.5×10^7 copies/μL	5 μL @ 1×10^7 copies/μL	2 μL
10^{-2}	20 μL @ 2.5×10^7 copies/μL	5 μL @ 1×10^6 copies/μL	—
10^{-3}	20 μL @ 2.5×10^7 copies/μL	5 μL @ 1×10^5 copies/μL	—
10^{-4}	20 μL @ 2.5×10^7 copies/μL	5 μL @ 1×10^4 copies/μL	—
10^{-5}	20 μL @ 2.5×10^7 copies/μL	5 μL @ 1×10^3 copies/μL	—
No mutant control	20 μL @ 2.5×10^7 copies/μL	—	5 μL

3. After enzyme has been added to each tube, quickly vortex and spin the set of five or six samples.
4. Quickly transfer the tubes to thermocycler A and start cycling.
5. After the 94°C incubation of the first cycle has finished, wait 15 s, and then place the second set of five or six samples into thermocycler B. Press stop twice and start to begin timing and repeat the hot start for the second set of samples. The samples should be vortexed and spun in time to transfer them to thermocycler A just as the second cycle (94°C incubation) is starting (*see* **Note 10**).
6. Repeat this procedure to start the third set of samples.
7. Because each set of samples is offset by one cycle, the thermocycler is programmed for 37 cycles, but each set of samples is subject to only 35 cycles. Remove the first set of samples before the last two cycles, the second set before the last cycle, and the third set at the end of the last cycle. As the samples are removed, transfer them to ice.

3.6. Sample and Data Analysis

1. Add 10 μL of 6X loading dye to each ACB–PCR reaction and then mix and spin.
2. Load 12 μL of each ACB–PCR sample and a marker on an 8% polyacrylamide gel and run as described in **Subheading 3.2., step 4**.
3. Stain the gel with Vistra Green and scan the gel to collect a fluorescent image (*see* **Subheading 3.2., step 5,** and **Note 11**). Determine the fluorescence in pixels of the diagnostic 60-bp H-*ras*-specific ACB-PCR product for each sample using ImageQuaNT software.
4. Export ImageQuaNT data to Excel and construct a standard curve of pixels vs mutant fraction. Derive the best-fit equation for the data (use the Excel exponential function). Then use that equation to calculate the mutant fractions of the unknown samples from their pixel intensities (**Fig. 2**).

4. Notes

1. Two different preparatory laboratory spaces (each with microfuge and pipetor sets) should be used for this procedure, one to dilute wild-type, mutant, and test DNAs and prepare mutant fraction standards, and the other to set up PCR reactions.
2. A 428-bp *Pvu*II to *Hin*dIII fragment (3.75 ng) purified from wild-type plasmid p94 was used as template to amplify the wild-type standard (**Fig. 2**) *(10)*. However, an equimolar amount of uncut plasmid DNA could be used directly for the same purpose. Plasmid DNA is considered the best source of template for generating the standard DNAs because it should contain an insignificant level of mutation. (The error rate for in vivo bacterial DNA replication is $\sim10^{-8}$/bp.) Also, *Pfu* DNA polymerase is used to generate the first-

round PCR products because its error rate is below the level of ACB–PCR detection *(2,9)*. Similarly, 3.75 ng of a 428-bp *Pvu*II to *Hin*dIII fragment purified from mutant plasmid p91 was used as template to amplify the mutant standard.

3. Amplified bands can be visualized by intercalation with ethidium bromide at 0.5 µg/mL in both the agarose gel and the running buffer. Alternatively, to minimize ethidium bromide exposure, the gel can be rocked gently for 10 min in a staining pan containing approx 100 mL of a 0.5 µg/mL ethidium bromide solution (enough to submerge the gel), followed by one or more "destains" with distilled water. The DNA bands can then be seen on a UV transilluminator or with a hand-held UV source.

4. It is necessary to amplify and purify the wild-type and mutant DNAs separately (on different days) to avoid cross-contamination of the samples. Isolating the wild-type standard and first-round PCR products from the unknown samples first reduces the risk of contaminating them with the mutant.

5. Remove one DNA aliquot from the freezer at a time and discard after use.

6. Ideally, only the DNA standards closest in length to the unknowns should be used to generate the standard curve and calculate the DNA concentrations of the unknowns. Initially, some of the DNAs to be quantified may not fall within the range of the DNA mass standards. If this is the case, use the initial quantitation to adjust the volumes of DNA loaded so they will fall within the range of the standards on subsequent gels. The more accurate the DNA concentration determination for the DNA standards and the first-round PCR products, the more accurate the ACB–PCR measurement will be. Obtaining three separate DNA concentration measurements that vary by $\leq 10\%$ from the average determination is recommended.

7. All DNAs should be kept on ice during dilution and mutant fraction standard construction. ACB–PCR has been performed successfully using both 10^8 and 4.6×10^8 total H-*ras* copies. ACB–PCR using 10^8 total H-*ras* copies is described here.

8. Final ACB-PCR reaction conditions are: 10^8 copies of template, 1X Stoffel buffer (10 m*M* KCl, 10 m*M* Tris-HCl, pH 8.3), 0.1 mg/mL gelatin, 0.1% Triton X-100, 40 µ*M* dNTPs, 1.5 m*M* MgCl$_2$, 0.4 µ*M* TR10 (the MSP), 0.33 µ*M* TR31 (the upstream primer), 0.2 µ*M* TR27 (the BP), 3 U of Stoffel fragment, and 0.06 U of Perfect Match PCR Enhancer (for 50-µL reactions). The ranges of final reaction conditions that should be tested (in the order listed) to optimize the ACB–PCR detection of other (non-G $\rightarrow$ T) point mutations are: 0.06–0.006 U of Perfect Match PCR enhancer per 50 µL sample, 41–51°C annealing temperatures, 0.4–0.57 µ*M* MSP, 0.2–0.57 µ*M* BP, and 40–60 µ*M* dNTPs *(4)*.

9. When working with the mutant fraction standards, always work from control and low mutant fractions to high mutant fractions, changing gloves after working with the high mutant fraction DNAs.

10. Hot start together the "no mutant" control and one of each mutant fraction standard, working from low to high mutant fraction and changing gloves between starting the different sets. Ideally, standards should be analyzed in duplicate (two sets). Larger volumes of ACB–PCR reaction mix can be prepared and additional sets of five or six samples added as needed, depending on the number of unknowns to be analyzed. (Simply add one PCR cycle to the program for every additional set of samples to be started.) Getting a set of samples ready just as the previous set begins a new cycle requires some precision and will depend on how quickly the pipeting is performed. A dry run may be useful to determine the exact point in the cycle (on thermocycler A) at which the hot start procedure for the next set should be initiated. If two thermocyclers are not available, a 94°C heating block and timer can be used instead of thermocycler B.

11. A fluorescein label at the 5'-end of the MSP or the upstream primer can be used for fluorescent imaging in place of Vistra Green staining. (Such images often have less background than Vistra Green-stained images.) Imaging based on a fluorescein label, however, should be followed by Vistra Green staining and reimaging, so that the length of the diagnostic band can be confirmed relative to the DNA length marker.

References

1. Cotton, R. G. (1993) Current methods of mutation detection. *Mutat. Res.* **285,** 125–144.
2. Parsons, B. L. and Heflich, R. H. (1997) Genotypic selection methods for the direct analysis of point mutations. *Mutat. Res.* **387,** 97–121.
3. Parsons, B. L. and Heflich, R. H. (1998) Detection of a mouse H-*ras* codon 61 mutation using a modified allele-specific competitive blocker PCR genotypic selection method. *Mutagenesis* **13,** 581–588.
4. McKinzie, P. B. and Parsons, B. L. (2002) Detection of rare K-*ras* codon 12 mutants using allele-specific competitive blocker PCR. *Mutat. Res.* **517,** 209–220.
5. Orou, A., Fechner, B., Utermann, G., and Menzel, H. J. (1995) Allele-specific competitive blocker PCR: a one-step method with applicability to pool screening. *Hum. Mutat.* **6,** 163–169.
6. Lawyer, F. C., Stoffel, S., Saiki, R. K., et al. (1993) High-level expression, purification, and enzymatic characterication of full-length *Thermus aquaticus* DNA polymerase and a truncated form deficient in 5' to 3' exonuclease activity. *PCR Methods Appl.* **2,** 275–287.
7. Weiner, J. H., Bertsch, L. L., and Kornberg, A. (1975) The deoxyribonucleotide acid unwinding protein of *Escherichia coli. J. Biol. Chem.* **250,** 1972–1980.
8. De Milito, A., Catuccie, M., Iannelli, F., Romano, L., Zazzi, M. and Valensin, P. E. (1995) Increased reliability of selective PCR by using additionally mutated primers and a commercial Taq DNA polymerase enhancer. *Mol. Biotech.* **3,** 166–169.
9. Parsons, B. L. and Heflich, R. H. (1998) Detection of basepair substitution mutation at a frequency of 1×10^{-7} by combining two genotypic selection methods, MutEx enrichment and allele-specific competitive blocker PCR. *Environ. Mol. Mutagen.* **32,** 200–211.
10. Parsons, B. L., Culp, S. J., Manjanatha, M. G., and Heflich, R. H. (2002) Occurrence of H-*ras* codon 61 CAA to AAA mutation during mouse liver tumor progression. *Carcinogenesis* **23,** 943–948.
11. Parsons, B. L. and Heflich, R. H. (1997) Evaluation of MutS as a tool for direct measurement of point mutations in genomic DNA. *Mutat. Res.* **374,** 277–285.

23

Gel-Based Nonradioactive Single-Strand Conformational Polymorphism and Mutation Detection

Limitations and Solutions

Vibhuti Gupta, Reetakshi Arora, Anand Ranjan, Narendra K. Bairwa, Dheeraj K. Malhotra, P. T. Udhayasuriyan, Anjana Saha, and Ramesh Bamezai

Summary

Single-strand conformation polymorphism (SSCP) for screening mutations/single-nucleotide polymorphisms (SNPs) is a simple, cost-effective technique, saving an expensive exercise of sequencing each and every PCR reaction product and assisting in choosing only the amplicons of interest with expected mutation. The principle of detection of small changes in DNA sequences is based on the changes in single-strand DNA conformations. The changes in electrophoretic mobility that SSCP detects are sequence-dependent. The limitations faced in SSCP range from the routine polyacrylamide gel electrophoresis (PAGE) problems to the problems of resolving mutant DNA bands. Both these problems could be solved by controlling PAGE conditions and by varying physical and environmental conditions such as pH, temperature, voltage, gel type and percentage, addition of additives or denaturants, and others. Despite much upgrading of the technology for mutation detection, SSCP continues to remain the method of choice to analyze mutations and SNPs in order to understand genomic variations, spontaneous and induced, and the genetic basis of diseases.

Key Words: SSCP (single-strand conformation polymorphism); PCR (polymerase chain reaction); PCR-SSCP; PAGE (polyacrylamide gel electrophoresis); polymorphism; chemical mutagenesis; SNP (single-nucleotide polymorphism); mutation detection.

1. Introduction
1.1. What is SSCP?

The study of genomic variations has become important in understanding human history and disease susceptibility. A variety of techniques are described in the literature that can detect single base mutations, insertions, and deletions, and all of these have one or the other advantage. In recent years, high-throughput methods like solid

From: *Methods in Molecular Biology, vol. 291, Molecular Toxicology Protocols*
Edited by: P. Keohavong and S. G. Grant © Humana Press Inc., Totowa, NJ

phase minisequencing, detection of dissimilarly sized extension fragments by matrix-assisted laser description ionization-time of flight mass spectroscopy (MALDI-MS), mismatch cleavage detection, oligoarray hybridization, molecular beacon signaling, fluorescence monitoring of polymerase chain reaction (PCR), electronic dot-blot assay, and denaturation high-performance liquid chromatography are already in use (for review, *see* **ref.** *1*). Nevertheless, one of the commonest, simplest, and also reasonably sensitive methods for rapid detection of gene mutations is that of single-strand conformation polymorphism (SSCP). It has been useful in finding associations with a number of diseases ranging from hemophilia A *(2)*, Parkinson's disease *(3)*, hereditary spastic paraplegia *(4)* to schizophrenia *(5)* and cancer *(6)*. Also, the technique has been useful in detecting induction of mutations in DNA/cDNA in toxicology studies. Chemically induced mutagenesis has been studied using the SSCP technique in rats *(7–10)*, humans *(11–13)*, and cell lines *(14)*.

SSCP relies on the ability of a single (or multiple) nucleotide change(s) to alter the electrophoretic mobility of a single-strand DNA molecule under native (nondenaturing) conditions. Under nondenaturing conditions, most single-stranded DNA molecules assume one or more stable 3D conformations that depend on the nucleotide sequence. This change in a single nucleotide leads to a conformational change that is reflected in the electrophoretic mobility of the polymorphic sequence in comparison with the more common "wild-type" sequence (**Figs. 1** and **2**).

Mutations/polymorphisms occur within many different regions of a gene (promoter, 5' untranslated region [5' UTR], exons, introns, exon–intron junctions, 3' UTR, and others), and are screened by the following steps: (1) designing primers complementary to the region flanking the specified region; (2) subjecting the amplicons produced by PCR to SSCP analysis; (3) eluting the variant bands for characterization through sequencing; and (4) using these bands (DNA) for comparison in further analysis. A large number of samples can be prescreened for mutation(s) and single-nuleotide polymorphisms (SNPs).

The basic protocol of SSCP described by Orita in 1989 was based on PCR *(15)* or restriction fragment length polymorphism *(16)* -based detection of mutations in radiolabeled fragments on a sequencing apparatus. This basic protocol has undergone drastic changes since then, and nonradiolabeled *(17)* and fluorescence-based detection *(18)* has subsequently been used for SSCP analysis.

The advantages of the SSCP technique are that it is easy and cost-effective and requires low technical input. It can be used as a basic tool to identify variations before sequencing. If properly standardized, it can also be applied to find loss of heterozygosity (LOH) and microsatellite instability (MIS). Another advantage is the ease of separation, direct elution, and cloning of the variant band in both heterozygous and homozygous mutant situations. However, among its disadvantages are that it is at times difficult to standardize. SSCP results may be misleading if nonspecific bands are seen in some gels, a problem that can be overcome by repeating and obtaining reproducible results. Some mutations may not be resolved at all using SSCP. Also, it is a low-throughput technique: at the most, a worker can analyze 30–40 samples in a day.

In the literature, a variety of parameters have been found to improve the efficiency of the SSCP technique. Additives (such as sucrose, glycerol *[19]*, urea *[20,21]*, formamide *[20]*, and *[22]* polyethylene glycol *[23]*), use of shorter length fragments for analysis *(24)*, varying acrylamide percentage *(25)* and acrylamide to *bis*-acrylamide ratio *(20)*, optimization of PCR conditions *(26)*, use of acrylamide substitutes (such as the mutation detection enhancer [MDE] *[27]*, PHAST SYSTEM *[28,29]*, and agarose *[30]*), varying pH, current, and voltage *(31)*, use of multitemperature SSCP *(32)*, use of cold SSCPs *(33)*, and use of combined SSCP/duplex analysis by capillary electrophoresis *(34)* have all been proposed to improve the resolution of single strands of the denatured double-stranded DNA

1.2. Standardizing SSCP

It is important to remember that the optimum SSCP conditions for a particular fragment are determined by sequence, i.e., the length, base composition, and type of mutation to be studied. At least 90% of single-base pair substitutions can be detected if the fragment length is within the optimal size range of 130–320 bp. Also, 80% of single base pair substitutions can be detected if the PCR products are kept under 400 bp in length *(35)*. Low pH greatly increases the sensitivity of the mutation detection and allows the screening of fragments of 800 bp in length *(20)*, although in our experience, amplicon length remains a limiting factor.

Factors important for standardization are:

1. *Gel temperature:* temperature is an important factor as it affects the stable DNA conformation as well as the mobility. As the temperature increases, the mobility also increases, and the total run time decreases. Low temperature is maintained either by running the gel in a cold room or by circulating cold running buffer in the gel apparatus. Running the same sample at different temperatures maximizes the chances of detecting mutations, as the variations missed under one temperature may be picked up at another. The same sequence can show two absolutely different profiles at two different temperatures. Temperature is one of the most important factors affecting the resolution of the single-strand DNA bands in the gels. The temperature range of 4°C (cold room) to 25–30°C (room temperature) shows the best differentiation of the single-stranded (ss)DNA bands. Migration of the bands is directly related to the increase in temperature.

2. *Gel pH:* generally, SSCP gels are run in 1X TBE solution, pH 8.3. However, TBE concentrations can be varied from 0.089 *M* to 134 *M* TBE. pH can also be lowered by adding 5–10% glycerol. Low pH can enhance sensitivity for longer fragments *(20)*. pH can also be varied by the addition of sucrose, formamide, polyethylene glycol (PEG), and so on. Running buffer pH can also be lowered to 6.8.

3. *Voltage:* high voltage increases mobility and hence lowers the run time. However, the heat produced at higher voltage can lead to uneven heating of the gel matrix, which can result in band smiling or frowning, if the heat dissipation system is not effective.

4. *Gel matrix:* bands move more slowly and resolve better at higher acrylamide concentrations. The gel % is mainly determined according to the size of the sequence to be analyzed. Sometimes the use of alternative matrixes like MDE, gene amp, Hydrolinks, agarose, or PHAST can also increase the possibility of finding a mutation.

5. *Additives:* sucrose (10%), urea, glycerol (5–10%), PEG, ethylene glycol, or formamide may be added to gel. It has also been suggested that 5–10% glycerol stabilizes the 3D DNA conformations, especially at higher temperature, although in our experiments we have not found any difference in resolution of bands. Glycerol enhances the mutation

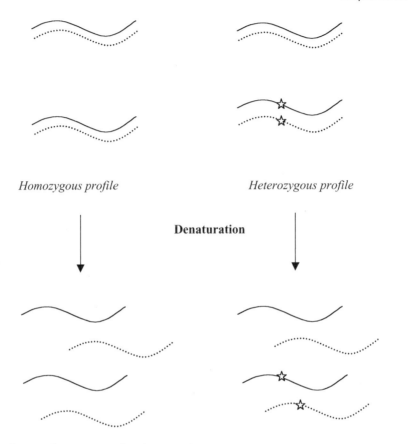

Single strand separation after denaturation

(Continued next page)

Fig. 1. Schematic representation of hypothetical conformation differences adopted by the mutation-bearing ssDNA molecules (☆) in comparison with the wild-type (nonmutant) ssDNA molecule, thus resulting in the mobility shifts of the two strands of DNA. The heterozygous profile in some cases may only resolve into three bands instead of four.

    detection and interpretation of bands, as it reduces deformer formation and is known to affect pH in the TBE buffer system *(19)*.

6. Another option is to label both strands. Using different colors for each strand allows the detection of the residual double-stranded molecules remaining after denaturation and also overlapping peaks in the two colors may confirm the presence of unresolved bands in the three-band situation. Dedicating a color to each fragment allows one to confirm the origin of extra peaks.

It is difficult to predict optimum conditions for a particular fragment even if its complete sequence is known. Optimum conditions have to be standardized by trial-

Snap chilling and gel analysis

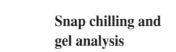

22

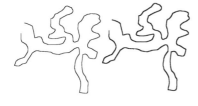

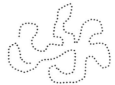

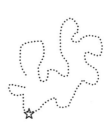

Homozygous profile

(two DNA bands)

Heterozygous profile

(four DNA bands)

Fig. 1 (Continued)

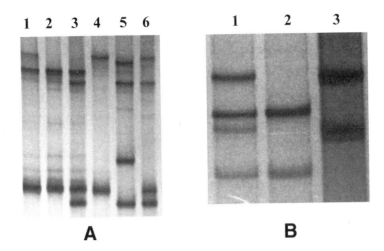

Fig. 2. SSCP profile seen for two different amplicons. The conditions are: 15% acrylamide, 160 V, 1X TBE. The gels were run at room temperature for 22 h. (**A**) A 231-bp-long fragment of TGF-β1 5' UTR showing variations in all the lanes. Lane 1, a three-band pattern heterozygous profile; lanes 3, 5, and 6, four-band pattern heterozygous profiles; lanes 2 and 4, homozygous profiles. (**B**) A different region, a 231-bp fragment for the TGF-β1 promoter. Lane 1, a four-band heterozygous profile; lanes 2 and 3, homozygous profiles.

and-error methods, trying out various permutations and combinations of the parameters influencing the outcome.

To start with, 200–325-bp DNA fragments can be run in 12–15% gels at 160–200 V. The total run time increases as the gel percentage and fragment size increases, and it decreases as the temperature and voltage decrease. Sometimes increasing the run time can also resolve some bands not resolved in less time. A major percentage of the fragments can be resolved this way. For the rest, various additives and different physical conditions (as already discussed) can be varied.

2. Materials

2.1. Genomic DNA Isolation

1. Lysis buffer: 0.32 M sucrose (autoclaved), 5 mM MgCl$_2$, 0.01 M Tris-HCl, pH 8.0, 1% Triton X-100 (e.g., Sigma, St. Louis, MO, or Qualigen, Mumbai, India). Store at room temperature.
2. Digestion buffer: 100 mM NaCl, 25 mM EDTA, 0.5% sodium dodecyl sulfate (SDS), 10 mM Tris-HCl, pH 8.0.
3. 20 mg/mL Proteinase K in solution.
4. Tris-HCl–saturated phenol, pH 8.0 (store at 4°C) and chloroform.
5. TE buffer: 10 mM Tris-HCl, pH 8.0, 1 mM EDTA, pH 8.0.
6. Gel loading dye: 0.25% bromophenol blue, 0.25% xylene cyanol, and 30% glycerol (use gloves and store at 4°C).

7. TBE buffer: 80 m*M* Tris-base, 40 m*M* boric acid, 2 m*M* EDTA. Make as 10X stock solution and store at room temperature.
8. Ethidium bromide: 10 mg/mL stock solution in autoclaved distilled water (use gloves and protect from direct light; store at 4°C).
9. 1% Agarose in 1X TBE buffer.

2.2. Polymerase Chain Reactions

Use gloves to handle.

1. Sterile 0.5-mL PCR tubes and microtips.
2. PCR kit (reaction buffer, enzyme, dNTP mix; store at –20°C).
3. Primers for the region to be studied (store at –20°C until use and after).
4. Mineral oil (store at room temperature).
5. Thermal Cycler (e.g., MJ Research, Miami, FL).

2.3. Polyacrylamide Gel Preparation and Gel Eletrophoresis

1. Autoclaved distilled water.
2. Glass plates of 20 × 18 cm, spacers, and combs of 1-mm thickness each, with a well size of 3.5 mm.
3. Gel electrophoresis system.
4. Acrylamide: *bis*-acrylamide stock (29:1); store at 4°C.
5. 10% APS solution and TEMED.
6. TBE running buffer: *see* **Subheading 2.1., item 7**.
7. SSCP dye: 0.15 g Ficoll, 0.0025 g bromophenol blue, 0.0025 g xylene cyanol, 950 μL formamide, and 50 μL 1X TBE.
8. Power pack (e.g., Bio-Rad PAC 3000, Hercules, CA).

2.4. Silver Staining of SSCP Gel

1. Fixative: 10% ethanol and 1% acetic acid solution.
2. Staining solution: 0.1% silver nitrate solution.
3. Developing solution: 1.5% NaOH solution.
4. 0.75% Sodium carbonate and *X*% acetic acid solution.

2.5. PAGE Elution of DNA

1. Elution buffer preparation (for 25 mL): add 0.9365 g ammonium acetate and 0.0536 g magnesium acetate to 10 mL water and autoclave. Add to this 125 μL 0.2 *M* EDTA and 250 μL of 10% SDS and make up the volume to 25 mL.

2.6. Agarose Purification of DNA Bands

1. Agarose (molecular biology grade; e.g., Sigma or Pronadisa, Rehovat, Israel).
2. Tris-HCl–saturated phenol, pH 8.0 (store at 4°C).
3. 3 *M* Sodium acetate, pH 5.2 (store at room temperature).
4. Absolute ethanol (e.g., Merck, Mumbia, India).

2.7. Ligation of DNA Bands for Sequencing

1. PCR product ligation kit (e.g., Promega, Madison, WI).
2. Insert DNA.

2.8. Transformation of Ligated Product and Screening of Positive Clones

1. Competent bacterial cells (e.g., DH5α).
2. Sterile culture plates.
3. Luria broth medium (e.g., Himedia, Mumbai, India).
4. Ampicillin (store at –20°C).

3. Methods (*see* Note 1)

3.1. Preparation of Template

1. Incubate blood (5 mL) with 4.5 mL lysis buffer for 30 min on ice. Break the clumps or clots with the help of a Pasteur pipet.
2. Centrifuge at 4°C for 20 min at 1100*g*.
3. Resuspend the pellet gently in 4.5 mL of digestion buffer.
4. Add Proteinase K solution to the homogenous cell suspension at a final concentration of 100 ng/mL.
5. Incubate the suspension at 65°C for 1 h, followed by overnight incubation at 37°C with gentle shaking.
6. Next day, deproteinate the cell suspension by extracting twice with an equal volume of phenol/choloroform and twice with chloroform, centrifuging at 2200–3500*g* for 20 min at room temperature.
7. Precipitate by adding 1/10th vol of 3 *M* sodium acetate and 2 vol of ethanol.
8. Spool DNA by binding on a glass rod or pick DNA in a broad-mouthed Pasteur pipet and wash with chilled 70% ethanol.
9. Dry the DNA and dissolve in TE.
10. Mix the genomic DNA with 1/6th vol of gel loading dye and load into wells of a 0.8% agarose gel. Run at low voltage of 40–45 volts. Visualize on a UV transilluminator. The high-quality genomic DNA should be seen as a band without shearing.
11. Quantitate by taking the optical density (OD) at 260 nm. Also compare the ratio of OD at 260 nm with that at 280 nm to check the quality; DNA samples having OD ratios > 1.5 are considered to have low protein contamination. Dilute the samples to the concentration of 25 ng/μL in autoclaved distilled water, and store at –20°C until analysis.

3.2. Polymerase Chain Reaction for Amplification of the Region to Be Studied

1. A 12.5 μL vol of PCR reaction for each sample includes: 6.25 pmol of each primer, 10 ng target DNA, 100 n*M* dNTPs, 1X PCR reaction buffer, 0.5 U *Taq* polymerase (e.g., Promega PCR kit).
2. PCR reaction is done for 30 cycles (denaturation at 94°C for 2 min, annealing at 55–65°C for 1 min, and extension at 72°C for 1 min) and final extension at 72°C for 10 min.
3. PCR products are checked by loading in 0.8% agarose gel at 120 V.

3.3. Preparation of Nondenaturing Polyacrylamide Gel (12–15%) for SSCP Analysis (see Notes 3–6, 8–10)

1. Clean the gel plates with detergent and rinse well with distilled water.
2. Wipe the plates with absolute ethanol.
3. Clean the spacers with absolute ethanol and place securely on the bottom plate. Secure the plates properly with clamps.

4. Clean the combs with absolute ethanol and keep it ready to be inserted between the two plates after pouring the gel mix.
5. Prepare the gel mix (12–15%) by adding a premade solution of acrylamide and *bis*-acrylamide at a ratio of 29:1, adding 10X TBE to make final concentration of 1X, 200 μL of 10% APS, and 50 μL of TEMED.
6. Mix all the constituents properly and pour between the two plates (*see* **Notes 3–5**).
7. Leave the assembly undisturbed until the gel becomes polymerized.
8. Prepare the samples for loading by taking 5 μL of PCR product, adding 4.5 μL 1X TBE, and 0.5 μL of loading dye.
9. Denature samples at 95°C for 5 min and chill immediately on ice for 5 min prior to loading.
10. Load all of the sample prepared into the appropriate wells of the non-denaturing gel, and electrophorese at a constant voltage at room temperature or at 4°C. (*See* **Note 6**.)

3.4. Silver Staining of SSCP Gel

1. After completion of the gel run, fix the gel in fixative for about 30 min.
2. Stain the gel in 0.1% silver nitrate solution for 15 min.
3. Wash the gel three times with autoclaved water.
4. Develop by adding 1.5% NaOH solution and wait till the bands appear.
5. Throw away the previous solution and add 0.75% sodium carbonate solution.
6. Photograph/scan the gels for record purposes.
7. For long-term storage: dry the gels in a gel dryer or store in a 1% acetic acid solution. (*See* **Note 7**.)

3.5. PAGE Elution of Bands Showing Variation (see Notes 2 and 3)

1. Cut out the band showing variation, and mince it well with the help of a microtip in an Eppendorf tube.
2. Add 400 μL of PAGE elution buffer and incubate at 37°C overnight with shaking.
3. Centifuge at 16,000*g* 4°C for 1 min.
4. Take the supernatant and add 1/10th vol of sodium acetate, pH 5.2, followed by 1 mL ethanol.
5. Keep at –80°C for 1 h.
6. Centrifuge at 16,000*g* 4°C for 20 min.
7. Wash twice with 70% ethanol, followed by centrifugation at 16,000*g*, 4°C for 10 min.
8. Air-dry DNA and dissolve in 10 μL autoclaved and double-distilled water.
9. PCR-amplify the eluted fragment DNA.

3.6. Agarose Purification of DNA Bands

1. Run the PCR product to be eluted in a 0.8% agarose gel.
2. Excise the PCR-amplified product from the agarose gel and put it in a 1.5-mL Eppendorf tube.
3. Add 1 mL of saturated phenol, pH 8.0 into the tube, and freeze it at –80°C. Take out the frozen tube, and thaw it completely. Freeze-thaw the tube three times.
4. In the final step, take out the frozen tube and centrifuge at a high speed of 13,000*g* for 20 min at room temperature.
5. Take out the aqueous phase and transfer to a fresh tube. Add an equal volume of chloroform into the tube, mix, and centrifuge again at 13,000*g* for 10 min.
6. Transfer the aqueous phase and add 1/10th vol of 3 *M* sodium acetate, pH 5.2, and make up to1 mL vol by absolute ethanol. Allow the DNA to precipitate for 30–45 min at –80°C.
7. Centrifuge at 16,000*g* at 4°C for 20 min for precipitating DNA.

8. Wash the DNA pellet with chilled 70% ethanol for 10 min at 4°C.
9. Dry the pellet and finally dissolve it in 10 µL of autoclaved distilled water.
10. Check the quality of DNA by running in an agarose gel and quantitate the amount for cloning.

3.7. Ligation of Gel-Eluted Product for Determination of Allele Sequence

1. Mix 2X reaction buffer, T-tailed vector (e.g., pGEM-T Promega ligation kit), enzyme (ligase), and DNA insert (gel-eluted product) in a 0.5-mL Eppendorf tube. Mix well and make up the volume to 10 µL (per instructions given in, e.g., the Promega PCR ligation kit).
2. Incubate at 16°C for 4–6 h, followed by an overnight incubation at 4°C.

3.8. Transformation of Ligated Product and Screening of Positive Clones

1. Carry out the transformation using competent cells (e.g., *E.coli* strains DH5α, XL-1).
2. Rescreen for positive clones through colony PCR using the same set of primers as was used for amplifying genomic DNA and at the same PCR conditions.
3. Sequence the resulting PCR product manually, or by an automated sequencer.

3.9. Recombinant Plasmid Isolation From Positive Clone for Further Use as Control in SSCP Gels (see Note 3d)

1. Inoculate 5 mL of fresh LB medium with a single colony and grow it at 37°C overnight with high-speed shaking.
2. Isolate the plasmid as in the instructions of a plasmid isolation kit (e.g., Sigma or Promega plasmid isolation kit).
3. PCR-amplify the plasmid and run it for all subsequent gels of the same amplicon.

4. Notes

1. General considerations while doing PCR-SSCP:

   a. Prepare and store the chemicals as mentioned, and handle with care.
   b. While isolating genomic DNA, handle with care to minimize the shearing of DNA.
   c. DNA is better purified with phenol/chloroform.
   d. For PCR reaction, use fresh sterile tips, tubes, and aseptic bench area.
   e. Filter the gel mix before adding APS and TEMED. APS should be freshly prepared.
   f. Any indecision in band shifts can be removed by repeating the PCR either fresh or by reamplifying the eluted variant band.

2. False bands seen: sometimes SSCP results may be misleading, and false bands may appear:

   a. At times, deformer bands appear in some lanes. Therefore, during sample preparation, ensure an equal quantity of DNA and uniform treatment of all samples. In order to confirm that the extra bands appearing in some lanes are the variant bands, these should be cut out, eluted, amplified, and run again in an SSCP gel (*see* **Note 3**).
   b. The presence of repetitive sequences causes primer slippage and hence the generation of extra bands during PCR amplification, a possible cause of false bands. To avoid this, try to keep PCR conditions as stringent as possible.
   c. The *Taq* polymerase used for PCR amplification can also introduce mutations. It is preferable to use high-proofreading-activity polymerase rather than other polymerases with high fidelity. PCR-SSCP should be repeated for all the samples showing variations, and their profiles should be confirmed before they are sequenced.

3. Appearance of extra bands in all the lanes: sometimes all the lanes show a number of bands, which makes the analysis difficult, as these may be confused with the mutant bands:

   a. Nonspecific bands generated during PCR, which could be owing to nonstringent conditions or primer dimers. This can be controlled by maintaining stringent PCR conditions by reducing target or salt concentration, or keeping annealing temperature high. Also, the primer concentration should be kept low. It is suggested to always check the PCR standardization results on acrylamide gel along with marker. An agarose gel is not sensitive enough to discriminate bands differing by only a few base pairs.

   b. Loading of high amounts of PCR products can also make visible the otherwise faint bands. Therefore, it would be good to optimize the amount of PCR sample to be used for loading depending on the PCR amplification, gel thickness, and well size. Sometimes reducing the PCR amount can also reduce the intensity of the extra bands.

   c. The PCR fragment adopts more than a single conformation or deformer. Adoption of more than one stable form is sequence-dependent, but varying physical conditions like pH, temperature, voltage, and so on may reduce the appearance of extra bands. This can also occur during temperature fluctuations. It is important to check for temperature fluctuations during the run. A deformer is less intense than the original band. Bands can be PAGE-eluted and PCR-amplified. Reamplified products should be electrophoresed along with the genomic control samples. A similar multiple band profile as earlier indicates the band is a deformer.

   d. Double-stranded DNA, as seen in gels of higher concentration: run two to three control samples for which the profile is known with the samples to be analyzed. Also, run a sample that has not been denatured to determine the location of double strands in the gel.

   e. Partially denatured double-stranded DNA takes a different conformation than single-stranded DNA and fully double-stranded DNA: denature the samples for at least 5 min, chill immediately, and load immediately.

4. Gel polymerization problems: sometimes the gel does not polymerize well:

   a. This could be caused by dirty plates or the use of chemicals of poor quality. It can be avoided by proper cleaning of plates using detergent, rinsing with autoclaved water followed by ethanol, wiping, and air-drying. Also, the gel solution should be made fresh and filtered, TEMED and APS should be of good quality, APS should be made fresh, and its concentration should be checked; this can also be increased (under the optimal range).

   b. Gel polymerization may take longer at low room temperatures. A table lamp or a heat convector should be used in such conditions.

5. Difficulty in resolving variant bands: sometimes variant bands do not resolve at all from the normal bands:

   a. At times, three bands appear under heterozygous conditions instead of the expected four-band profile, in which two bands take a similar conformation and hence show an identical mobility. In such cases, it is not important to resolve the three-band profile into a four-band profile.

   b. Sometimes the variant strand may not resolve from the normal band under a particular set of conditions, as both of them may have same mobility. In such cases, SSCP has to be standardized, as mentioned in **Subheading 1.2.**

   c. An inadequate run of the sample also may not resolve the variant bands completely.

6. Problems in sample loading: sometimes improper loading leads to formation of a diffused band pattern:

    a. The presence of mineral oil may interfere with loading. Try using no mineral oil while loading.

    b. The sample may not settle in the well; use Ficoll or glycerol in the denaturing dye.

7. Silver staining problems: sometimes the gel may not stain well, or ghost bands may appear in the middle section of the gel; instead of staining black, it remains clear and without stain:

    a. Improper fixing and improper staining. Gels should be fixed properly, and freshly made silver nitrate and developer should be used.

    b. Bands are not clearly visible after staining if the amplification during PCR is low. Therefore, PCR conditions and the amount loaded should be standardized by checking the efficiency of PCR amplification and its signal on agarose gel.

    c. If the signal is good enough to be detected on PAGE, then the problem is in the staining step. Reduce the number of intermediate washings. Shake the gel well, and mix all the solution with the gel for uniform staining.

8. Sample forms large streaks back toward the well:

    a. This may be owing to the dry run of the gel. Try to avoid the dry run, which might allow evaporation of the buffer or some leakage. Seal the space between the plates and the tank to avoid leakage from the upper tank to the lower tank.

    b. Try changing the gel percentage; an inappropriate percentage might lead to streak formation.

9. Uneven band patterns: sometimes bands are U-shaped, smeary, or diffused; they may show smiling or frowning:

    a. The bottom of the well may not be flat. This could be owing to improper polymerization of the gel. Take care during polymerization, as discussed in **Note 1**. Also, take out the combs only after the gel is properly polymerized. Always flush the well with buffer or water before loading in order to remove the residual gel solution, which might polymerize in the wells and lead to an uneven well bottom.

    b. Uneven thickness of the gels owing to a lack of compatibility between combs and spacers causes film formation in the wells and hence improper loading and band pattern. Therefore, spacers and combs should be of identical thickness to avoid uneven polymerization and film formation.

    c. At times the appearance of bubbles in the gel matrix or at the interface of the gel and the buffer interfere with the current flow and affect the quality of the run. The lanes which show the presence of air bubbles within the matrix could be avoided when running precious samples, and the bubbles at the interface could be removed by flushing with the help of a syringe and a needle.

    d. This pattern may occur because the temperature is higher at the center than at the edges as joule heating effects are more easily dissipated at the edges of the gel; since electrophoretic mobilities vary inversely with the viscosity of the solvent, DNA samples in the center of the gel migrate faster than sample near the edges. Therefore, it is important to maintain the temperature of the matrix.

10. Gel-to-gel variations are seen even under similar running conditions: sometimes two gels run at different times but in the similar conditions show varying profiles. Minor variations in gel percentage, temperature, buffer concentration, pH, and so on can give a dif-

ferent profile for the same amplicon in two different gels. The parameters influencing the outcome should be maintained as constant as possible. The following important points should be taken into account:

a. Genomic DNA should be quantitated carefully, and the amount used for PCR should be optimal.
b. The pH of the running buffer should not increase. The running buffer should not be reused again and again, although it can be used at least twice.
c. Try to maintain a constant temperature, voltage, and running time of the samples.

References

1. Graber, J. H., O'Donnell, M. J., Smith, C. L., and Cantor, C. R. (1998) Advances in DNA diagnostics. *Curr. Opin. Biotechnol.* **9**, 14–18.
2. Lin, S. W., Lin, S. R., and Shen, M. C. (1993) Characterization of genetic defects of hemophilia A in patients of Chinese origin. *Genomics* **18**, 496–504.
3. Pastor, P., Munoz, E., Ezquerra, M., et al. (2001) Analysis of the coding and the 5' flanking regions of the α-synuclein gene in patients with Parkinson's disease. *Mov. Disord.* **16**, 1115–1119.
4. Higgins, J. J., Loveless, J. M., Goswami, S., et al. (2001) An atypical intronic deletion widens the spectrum of mutations in hereditary spastic paraplegia. *Neurology* **56**, 1482–1485.
5. Chiavetto, L. B., Boin, F., Zanardini, R., et al. (2002) Association between promoter polymorphic haplotypes of interleukin-10 gene and schizophrenia. *Biol. Psych.* **51**, 480–484.
6. Strippoli, P., Sarchielli, S., Santucci, R., Bagnara, G. N., Brandi, G., and Biasco, G. (2001) Cold single-strand conformation polymorphism analysis: optimization for detection of APC gene mutations in patients with familial adenomatous polyposis. *Int. J. Mol. Med.* **8**, 567–572.
7. Suzui, M., Sugie, S., Mori, H., Okuno, M., Tanaka, T., and Moriwaki, H. (2001) Different mutation status of the β-catenin gene in carcinogen-induced colon, brain, and oral tumors in rats. *Mol. Carcinogen.* **32**, 206–212.
8. French, J. E., Lacks, G. D., Trempus, C., et al. (2001) Loss of heterozygosity frequency at the Trp53 locus in p53-deficient (+/–) mouse tumors is carcinogen-and tissue-dependent. *Carcinogenesis* **22**, 99–106 [Erratum in *Carcinogenesis* **23**, 373 (2002)].
9. Yamamoto, S., Tatematsu, M., Yamamoto, M., Fukami, H., and Fukushima, S. (1998) Clonal analysis of urothelial carcinomas in C3H/HeN↔BALB/c chimeric mice treated with N-butyl-N-(4-hydroxybutyl)nitrosamine. *Carcinogenesis* **19**, 855–860.
10. Devereux, T. R., Anna, C. H., Foley, J. F., White, C. M., Sills, R. C., and Barrett, J. C. (1999) Mutation of β-catenin is an early event in chemically induced mouse hepatocellular carcinogenesis. *Oncogene* **18**, 4726-4733.
11. Wanner, R., Zober, A., Abraham, K., Kleffe, J., Henz, B. M., and Wittig, B. (1999) Polymorphism at codon 554 of the human Ah receptor: different allelic frequencies in Caucasians and Japanese and no correlation with severity of TCDD induced chloracne in chemical workers. *Pharmacogenetics* **9**, 777–780.
12. Hsu, C. H., Yang, S. A., Wang, J. Y., Yu, H. S., and Lin, S. R. (1999) Mutational spectrum of p53 gene in arsenic-related skin cancers from the blackfoot disease endemic area of Taiwan. *Br. J. Cancer* **80**, 1080–1086.
13. Sarkar, F. H., Li, Y., and Vallyathan, V. (2001) Molecular analysis of p53 and K-ras in lung carcinomas of coal miners. *Int. J. Mol. Med.* **8**, 453–459.
14. Nohturfft, A., Hua, X., Brown, M. S., and Goldstein, J. L. (1996) Recurrent G-to-A substi-

tution in a single codon of SREBP cleavage-activating protein causes sterol resistance in three mutant Chinese hamster ovary cell lines. *Proc. Natl. Acad. Sci. USA* **93,** 13709–13714.

15. Orita, M., Iwahana, H., Kanazawa, H., Hayashi, K., and Sekiya, T. (1989) Detection of polymorphisms of human DNA by gel electrophoresis as single-strand conformation polymorphisms. *Proc. Natl. Acad. Sci. USA* **86,** 2766–2770.

16. Orita, M., Suzuki, Y., Sekiya, T., and Hayashi, K. (1989) Rapid and sensitive detection of point mutations and DNA polymorphisms using the polymerase chain reaction. *Genomics* **5,** 874–879.

17. Oto, M., Miyake, S., and Yuasa, Y. (1993) Optimization of nonradioisotopic single strand conformation polymorphism analysis with a conventional minislab gel electrophoresis apparatus. *Anal. Biochem.* **213,** 19–22.

18. Iwahana, H., Yoshimoto, K., Mizusawa, N., Kudo, E., and Itakura, M. (1999) Multiple fluorescence-based PCR-SSCP analysis. *BioTechniques* **27,** 20–22, 24.

19. Kukita, Y., Tahira, T., Sommer, S. S., and Hayashi, K. (1997) SSCP analysis of long DNA fragments in low pH gel. *Hum. Mutat.* **10,** 400–407.

20. Glavac, D. and Dean, M. (1993) Optimization of the single-strand conformation polymorphism (SSCP) technique for detection of point mutations. *Hum. Mutat.* **2,** 404–414.

21. Yip, S. P., Hopkinson, D. A., and Whitehouse, D. B. (1999) Improvement of SSCP analysis by use of denaturants. *BioTechniques* **27,** 20–22, 24.

22. Xie, T., Ho, S. L., and Ma, O. C. (1997) High resolution single strand conformation polymorphism analysis using formamide and ethidium bromide staining. *Mol. Pathol.* **50,** 276–278.

23. Markoff, A., Savoa, A., Vladimirov, V., Bogdanova, N., Kremensky, I., and Ganev, V. (1997) Optimization of single-strand conformation polymorphism analysis in the presence of polyethylene glycol. *Clin. Chem.* **43,** 30–33.

24. Ushijima, T., Hosoya, Y., Suzuki, T., Sofuni, T., Sugimura, T., and Nagao, M. (1994) A rapid method for detection of mutations in the lacI gene using PCR-single strand conformation polymorphism analysis: demonstration of its high sensitivity. *Nucleic Acids Res.* **22,** 2155–2157.

25. Savov, A., Angelicheva, D., Jordanova, A., Eigel, A., and Kalaydjieva, L. (1992) High percentage acrylamide gels improve resolution in SSCP analysis. *Nucleic Acids Res.* **20,** 6741–6742.

26. Lallas, T. A. and Buller, R. E. (1998) Optimization of PCR and electrophoresis conditions enhances mutation analysis of the BRCA1 gene. *Mol. Genet. Metab.* **64,** 173–176.

27. Ravnik-Glavac, M., Glavac, D., and Dean, M. (1994) Sensitivity of single-strand conformation polymorphism and heteroduplex method for mutation detection in the cystic fibrosis gene. *Hum. Mol. Genet.* **3,** 801–807.

28. Vidal-Puig, A. and Moller, D. E. (1994) Comparative sensitivity of alternative single-strand conformation polymorphism (SSCP) methods. *BioTechniques* **17,** 490–492, 494, 496.

29. Mohabeer, A. J., Hiti, A. L., and Martin, W. J. (1991) Non-radioactive single strand conformation polymorphism (SSCP) using the Pharmacia 'PhastSystem. *Nucleic Acids Res.* **19,** 3154.

30. Monckton, D. G. and Jeffreys, A. J. (1994) Minisatellite isoalleles can be distinguished by single-stranded conformational polymorphism analysis in agarose gels. *Nucleic Acids Res.* **22,** 2155–2157.

31. Liu, Q., Li, X., and Sommer, S. S. (1999) pK-matched running buffers for gel electrophoresis. *Anal. Biochem.* **270,** 112–122.

32. Kaczanowski, R., Trzeciak, L., and Kucharczyk, K. (2001) Multitemperature single-strand conformation polymorphism. *Electrophoresis* **22,** 3539–3545.
33. Hongyo, T., Buzard, G. S., Calvert, R. J., and Weghorst, C. M. (1993) 'Cold SSCP': a simple, rapid and non-radioactive method for optimized single-strand conformation polymorphism analyses. *Nucleic Acids Res.* **21,** 3637–3642.
34. Kozlowski, P. and Krzyzosiak, W. J. (2001) Combined SSCP/duplex analysis by capillary electrophoresis for more efficient mutation detection. *Nucleic Acids Res.* **29,** E71.
35. Hayashi, K. (1992) PCR-SSCP: a method for detection of mutations. *Genet. Anal. Tech. Appl.* **9,** 73–79.

24

Detection and Characterization of Oncogene Mutations in Preneoplastic and Early Neoplastic Lesions

Toshinari Minamoto

Summary

Although it has been more than 20 yr since its discovery, the *ras* family of genes has not yet lost its impact on basic and clinical oncology. These genes remain central to the field of molecular oncology as tools for investigating carcinogenesis and oncogenic signaling, as powerful biomarkers for the identification of those who have or are at high risk of developing cancer, and as oncogene targets for the design and development of new chemotherapeutic drugs. Mutational activation of the K-*RAS* proto-oncogene is an early event in the development and progression of the colorectal, pancreatic, and lung cancers that are the major causes of cancer death in the world. The presence of point mutational "hot spots" at sites necessary for the activation of this proto-oncogene has led to the development of a number of highly sensitive PCR-based methods that are feasible for the early detection of K-*RAS* oncogene mutations in the clinical setting. In light of these facts, mutation at the K-*RAS* oncogene has the potential to serve as a useful biomarker in the early diagnosis and risk assessment of cancers with oncogenic *Ras* signaling. This chapter describes a highly sensitive method for detecting mutant K-*RAS*, enriched PCR, and its application to early detection of this oncogene in preneoplastic and early neoplastic lesions of the colon and rectum.

Key Words: Oncogene; K-*RAS*; enriched PCR; molecular diagnosis; risk assessment; biomarker; colorectal cancer; preneoplastic lesion; aberrant crypt foci.

1. Introduction

A detailed scenario of molecular alterations, including epigenetic events, has been identified in the development and progression of human cancers. Multistep genetic alterations are known to affect oncogenes and tumor suppressor genes, including the genes for DNA mismatch and excision repair *(1,2)*. Genetic testing for susceptibility has become part of the standard management of patients with well-defined and uncommon hereditary cancers, in which cancer predisposing mutations occur in the germ line *(3)*. However, a molecular diagnostic approach to sporadic cancers, which comprise the majority of clinically documented malignant tumors, is still under development.

From: *Methods in Molecular Biology, vol. 291, Molecular Toxicology Protocols*
Edited by: P. Keohavong and S. G. Grant © Humana Press Inc., Totowa, NJ

Of the first identified oncogenes, some of the best characterized form the *ras* family of genes (H-*ras*, N-*ras,* and K-*RAS*), the products of which regulate GTP signal transduction. Common to all mutant forms of *ras* genes is a mutation pattern that results in constitutive activation of signaling cascades, including PI3K, PKB/AKT, and MAPK, and the stress kinases *(4)*. Activated *ras* genes efficiently over-ride cellular growth control and attenuate its ability to initiate programmed cell death. Somatic mutational activation of *ras* genes is frequent in various human cancers *(5,6)*. Activation of K-*RAS* is an early event in the development of certain types of cancer, i.e., colorectal, pancreas, and lung cancers, in both humans and experimental animals. Accordingly, this mutation has the potential to serve as a useful biomarker, both in early diagnosis and in susceptibility assessment *(7)*. In clinical samples subjected to molecular diagnosis and risk assessment, the ratio of neoplastic or preneoplastic to normal cells is extremely low and varies in different target organs and among individuals. The fact that K-*RAS* mutations occur exclusively in three hot spots (codons 12,13, and 61) *(5,6)* has led to the development of various polymerase chain reaction (PCR)-based methods that are much more sensitive and feasible for the early detection of cancer *(8,9)* than methods developed for other genes (i.e., *p53*, *APC*), in which mutations are distributed throughout their entire sequences.

Modified PCR protocols have been established to enhance the amplification of mutant, but not wild-type, alleles in nontransformed tissues that appear normal. These modifications include combinations of PCR with restriction fragment length polymorphisms (RFLP) or single-strand conformation polymorphisms (SSCP), mutant-enriched PCR (EPCR), EPCR-SSCP, mutant allele-specific amplification (MASA; *see* Chap. 23), and the mutation–ligation assay *(8,9)*.

The EPCR procedure, as outlined in **Fig. 1A**, consists of a mismatched primer-mediated two-step PCR amplification, with digestion of the wild-type PCR product with a restriction enzyme in between *(10)*. The upstream primer (K5') encodes a G to C substitution at the first position of codon 11, creating a product with a recognition site (CCTGG) specific to the DNA restriction enzymes *Bst*NI or *Mva*I that overlaps the first two nucleotides of the wild-type codon 12. Since this restriction enzyme site is absent in the product amplified from the K-*RAS* gene with a mutant codon 12, RFLP analysis of the PCR products can distinguish wild-type and mutant genes (**Fig. 1B** and **1C**). Of particular importance is the strategic incorporation of a second *Bst*NI or *Mva*I site into the downstream primer (K3'), as an internal control for restriction enzyme activity and fidelity *(11)*.

As shown in **Fig. 1A**, the first exon fragments of K-*RAS* are PCR-amplified with the set of upstream primer K5' and a new downstream primer, K3' wild-type (wt) that lacks an internal copy of the restriction enzyme site. The 157-bp fragment amplified in this first-step PCR is digested with *Bst*NI or *Mva*I, thereby cleaving the wild-type products and rendering them inaccessible for subsequent amplification. The products of the intermediate digestion, enriched in full-length mutant codon 12 sequences, are then amplified by the second-step PCR with primers K5' and K3'. The resultant products are subjected to RFLP analysis by digestion with the same restriction enzyme and native polyacrylamide gel electrophoresis. The 157-bp product of mutant K-*RAS* is

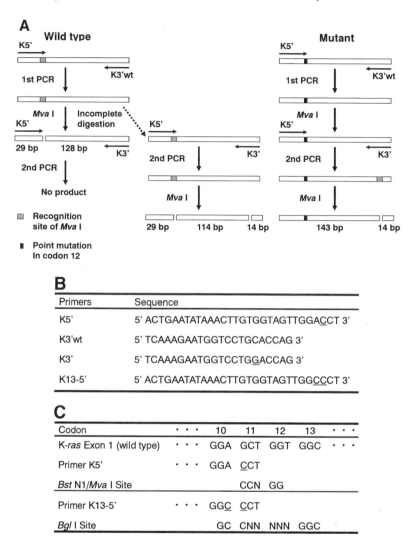

Fig. 1. Schematic representation of the two-step procedure of EPCR amplification of mutant K-*RAS* codon 12 sequences (**A**), the primers used for EPCR (**B**), and comparison of the sequences of wild-type K-*RAS* exon 1, mismatched primers, and restriction sites of *Bst*NI/*Mva*I and *Bgl*I (**C**). In the first step of amplification (1st PCR), a set of primers K5' and K3' wt is used for amplification of 157-bp fragments including codon 12 sequences. The K5' contains a nucleotide substitution at the first position of codon 11, creating a *Bst*NI/*Mva*I restriction site (CCTGG, gray box) that overlaps the first two nucleotides of wild-type codon 12. Intermediate digestion of the first-step PCR product with *Bst*NI or *Mva*I leaves products enriched in mutant codon 12 sequences (black box). An aliquot of the undigested products is subjected to the second-step PCR (2nd PCR) with a set of primers K5' and K3' (containing a control site specific to *Bst*NI/*Mva*I). RFLP analysis with *Bst*NI/*Mva*I distinguishes the mutant fragments of 143 bp from wild-type alleles of 114 bp, as shown in **Fig. 2**.

cleaved only at the control site created by the primer K3', to give fragments of 143 and 14 bp, whereas the wild-type product is cleaved at two sites mediated by the primers K5' and K3', generating fragments of 114, 29, and 14 bp. Elimination of normal alleles from the amplification process has been found to allow detection of one mutant allele of *ras* among 1000–10,000 normal alleles (**Fig. 2**) *(10,12)*. Similarly, the two-step EPCR amplification of a K-*RAS* gene with mutant codon 13 is possible using the upstream primer K5'-13, which encodes substitutions of A to C in the third nucleotide of codon 10, and G to C in the first position of codon 11 (**Fig. 1B**). When the wild-type K-*RAS* codon 13 is amplified with the downstream primer K3'wt, the primer K5'-13 creates a new recognition site (GCCNNNNNGGC) specific to the restriction enzyme *Bgl*I (**Fig. 1C**).

1.1. Detection of K-RAS Oncogene Mutations in Normal-Appearing (Nonneoplastic) Tissues of Colorectal Cancer Patients

Along with early diagnosis of tumors, one of the optimal ways to reduce mortality from (or prevent) colorectal cancer is to identify those who are at increased risk of developing sporadic cancer (by analogy with the known hereditary cancer syndromes *[2,3]*). The precise localization of *ras* oncogene-activating mutations allows for their detection even when they are present in a very small fraction of cells, as is often found in the early stages of tumor development. In fact, mutant *ras* has served as a classic paradigm of the ability to detect mutations in oncogenes in tissues that appear normal at histopathological examination *(7)*. A good representative of this paradigm comes from our experiences in analyzing matched pairs of normal and tumor tissues from colorectal cancer patients, since the molecular foundation of the multistep carcinogenesis process in human colorectal cancer has been established in great detail *(13)*. Many independent studies have been directed toward sensitive detection of mutations in K-*RAS* (reviewed in **refs.** 7 and *14*), which occur in more than 40% of colorectal cancers.

Our recent series of EPCR-based studies has clearly demonstrated activating K-*RAS* mutations in apparently normal tissues taken from surgical specimens of patients who underwent surgery for colorectal cancer *(12,15–17)*. When one sample is taken from the adjoining non-neoplastic mucosa of surgical specimens, mutant K-*RAS* is detected in 5–18% of patients *(12,15)*. As shown in **Fig. 3**, when multiple (three to seven) samples are collected from each patient for EPCR analysis of K-*RAS*, activating mutations are detected in 20% of the patients *(16,17)*. The latter study also shows confined localization of the epithelial cells harboring this mutant gene in the nonneoplastic mucosa. Interestingly, sequencing analysis showed that the specific mutant K-*RAS* allele found in mucosa that appeared to be normal was not always the same as that found in the tumors (**Fig. 3**). We have also demonstrated microsatellite DNA instability in normal-appearing tissues adjacent to the tumor *(18)*, suggesting that colorectal cancer patients with mutant K-*RAS* in apparently normal tissue may harbor genetically unstable mucosa that may predispose to development of second primary tumors. These findings suggest that the mutant K-*RAS* identified in nonneoplastic mucosa may sometimes represent *de novo* mutations and serve as a useful biomarker for identifying persons at higher risk of colorectal cancer. Presupposing either of these speculations

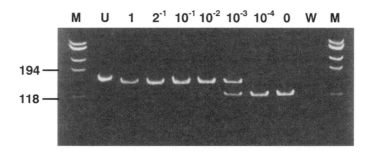

Fig. 2. Sensitivity of EPCR for detecting mutant K-*RAS*. The genomic DNA mixtures with different ratios of mutant DNA (derived from the SW480 colon cancer cell line) to wild-type (human placenta) DNA were amplified by EPCR to determine the sensitivity for detecting mutant K-*RAS* gene sequences (143-bp fragment). Each PCR product was digested with *Mva*I and subjected to electrophoresis on a 10% native polyacrylamide minigel. Ratios of SW480 cell line-derived DNA to human placental DNA in templates for EPCR are shown in the respective sample lanes. An EPCR product from a negative control, containing no DNA, was loaded in the W (distilled water) lane. U, undigested EPCR product from SW480 DNA; M, molecular weight marker DNA (ϕX174 DNA digested with *Hae*III).

in a pilot study, we could detect mutant K-*RAS* by EPCR in colonic lavage fluids (effluents) in persons who are at high risk for development of colorectal cancer *(19)*.

These surprising findings also raise concern as to the biological importance of *ras* mutations and consequently the value of their early detection. It is clear today that *ras* mutation *per se* is not sufficient to yield a transformed phenotype and that cooperation of mutant *ras* with other oncogenes and tumor suppressor genes must take place. For these reasons, it is important to analyze *ras* oncogene mutation in combination with the analysis of other markers known to be associated with tumor development *(7,14,18,20)*.

1.2. Detection of Mutant K-RAS Oncogenes in Aberrant Crypt Foci of Human Colon

Studies on very minute preneoplastic or early neoplastic lesions are essential for understanding the molecular details of the mechanism of colorectal carcinogenesis. Among these lesions are aberrant crypt foci (ACFs), first identified in methylene blue-stained, whole-mount preparations of colon mucosa from carcinogen-treated rodents. An aberrant crypt is two to three times larger than normal crypts in the same field, has a thickened epithelial layer, frequently has a slit-, asteroid-, or oval-shaped lumen, has an increased pericryptal zone separating it from the surrounding normal crypts, and is microscopically elevated above the surrounding mucosa. Multiple aberrant crypts frequently appear together as a cluster, forming a single unit that is referred to as an ACF (**Fig. 4A**) *(21)*. Multiple phenotypic alterations, i.e., decreased hexosaminidase activity, have been identified in ACF. These minute foci are also found in surgical specimens of human colon cancer (**Fig. 4A**) *(22)* and have recently been identified in patients both with and without colorectal tumors by magnifying dye endoscopy *(23)*.

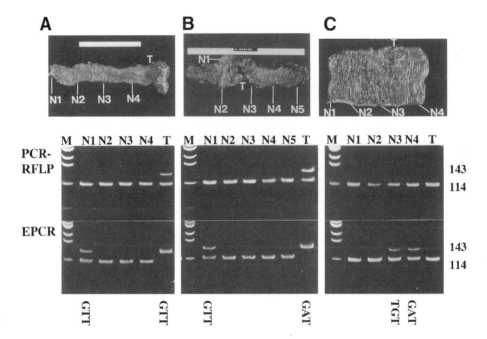

Fig. 3. Representative detection patterns of mutant K-*RAS* in the nonneoplastic mucosa (N) and tumors (T) of the colon and rectum, by conventional polymerase chain reaction-restriction fragment length polymorphism (PCR-RFLP) and mutant-enriched PCR (EPCR). In each case, the sample numbers shown above the lanes of 10% polyacrylamide gel electrophoresis are identical to those depicted in the figures of the corresponding surgical specimen. (**A**) A 59-yr-old woman with rectal cancer. The conventional PCR-RFLP analysis shows mutant K-*RAS* (143 bp) in the tumor. By EPCR, a mutant with a base pair alteration identical to that of the tumor is detected in one (proximal to the tumor) of four non-neoplastic mucosal samples. (**B**) A 65-yr-old woman with ascending colon cancer. The EPCR detects a mutant in a nonneoplastic sample taken from the cecum. The base pair alteration in this sample is different from that in the tumor. (**C**) A 75-yr-old man with sigmoid colon cancer. Two different types of mutants are identified in two of four nonneoplastic samples, by EPCR. The tumor, however, has no mutant allele.

Histological characteristics of ACF include findings of hyperplasia, dysplasia, adenoma, and adenocarcinoma *(24,25)*.

K-*RAS* mutation was the first molecular alteration reported in human ACFs *(26)*. Practically, ACFs are identified and dissected from the methylene blue-stained mucosal strips of formalin-fixed surgical specimens under a stereo microscope (**Fig. 4A** and **B**). Each focus is divided into two pieces, one for histopathological examination and the other for DNA extraction (**Fig. 4B**). By conventional PCR-RFLP and EPCR, K-*RAS* mutations at codon 12 and 13 are detected in 46% and 12% of ACFs, respectively (**Fig. 4C**) *(22)*. Sequencing shows that, in ACFs, GAT mutants are as frequent as GTT mutations in codon 12, whereas the latter type of mutation is predominant in

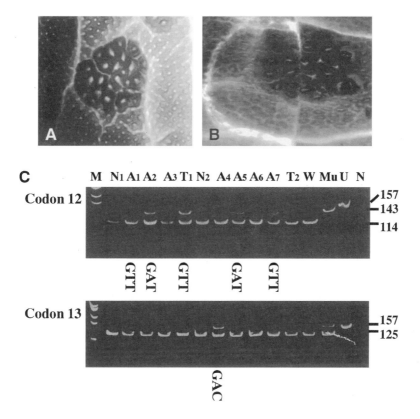

Fig. 4. Detection of mutant K-*RAS* in human colon ACF. (**A**) An ACF, identified in methylene blue-stained grossly normal mucosa, consists of a cluster of aberrant crypts showing thickened epithelial layer, slit-, asteroid-, or oval-shaped lumen, increased pericryptal zone and microscopic elevation above the surrounding normal mucosa. (**B**) Under microscopic observation, an ACF is isolated and divided into two pieces, one for conventional histopathological examinations and the other for DNA extraction. (**C**) EPCR and RFLP analysis of K-*RAS* mutations in codon 12 (upper panel) and codon 13 (lower panel) in ACF, carcinomas and microscopically normal mucosa sampled from the same patients with colorectal cancer. N1 and N2, normal colorectal mucosa; A1–A7, ACF; T1 and T2, colorectal carcinomas (N1, A1–A3, and T1 were taken from a 53-yr-old woman with rectal cancer. N2, A4–A7, and T2 were from a 63-yr-old man with sigmoid colon cancer); W, wild-type DNA derived from human placenta; Mu, mutant DNA controls derived from a colon cancer cell line SW 480 (codon 12) and from an adenocarcinoma known to harbor a heterozygous mutation in codon 13; U, undigested PCR product (157 bp); N, a PCR product from a negative control reaction with no DNA template; M, molecular size marker (φX174 DNA digested with *Hae*III). In the former case, mutation was detected in two ACFs and a carcinoma, and the sequence of one mutant (GAT) in ACF was different from that (GTT) in the carcinoma. In the latter case, K-*RAS* mutations were detected in three of four ACFs: two ACFs showed a mutation in codon 12 and one in codon 13, whereas the carcinoma harbored no mutation.

adenocarcinomas. The high frequency of these oncogene mutations and subsequent demonstration of molecular alterations in these lesions *(27)* support the idea that ACFs are genetically monoclonal in their evolution. Although ACFs are highly heterogeneous biologically and morphologically, and their fate has yet to be determined definitely, these minute foci represent one of the plausible candidates for prenoplastic colorectal epithelial foci mutated at various tumor-related genes, including the K-*RAS* locus.

2. Materials

Chemicals and reagents not specifically sourced may be purchased from local vendors or international suppliers (e.g., Sigma-Aldrich, St. Louis, MO).

2.1. Control DNA for Validation of EPCR

1. Sources of homozygous mutant DNA: human colon cancer cell lines SW480 (codon 12: GGT to GTT) and HCT116 (codon 13: GGC to GAC) (American Type Culture Collection, Rockville, MD).
2. RPMI cell culture medium supplemented with 10% fetal bovine serum (FBS; Gibco, Grand Island, NY).
3. 10-mL Disposable pipets and pipet aid.
4. 10- and 15-cm Tissue culture dishes (Falcon, BD Biosciences, Franklin Lakes, NJ).
5. Cell culture incubator.
6. Trypsin-EDTA solution (Gibco).
7. Phosphate-buffered saline (PBS), pH 7.4: 137 mM NaCl, 2.7 mM KCl, 4.3 mM Na$_2$HPO$_4$ (Gibco).
8. 50-mL Polypropylene conical tubes (Blue Max, BD Biosciences).
9. Cell scraper (e.g., Cell Lifter, Costar, Cambridge, MA).
10. Table top centrifuge with swing rotor (e.g., KN-70, Kubota, Tokyo, Japan).
11. 1.5-mL Polypropylene microcentrifuge tubes (Sarstedt AG, Nümbrecht, Germany).
12. Refrigerated microcentrifuge (e.g., Kubota 1920).
13. 1-mL Micropipetor and appropriate tips.
14. Cell lysis buffer: 10 mM Tris-HCl, pH 7.5, 10 mM EDTA, 15 mM NaCl, 2% sodium dodecyl sulfate (SDS). Ten milliliters is sufficient for 25–50 cell-pellet samples (200–400 μL each in volume) and can be stored at –20°C for over a year.
15. Proteinase K (Beckman, San Ramon, CA): small volume of stock solution (at 20 mg/mL) initially made by dissolving in deionized distilled water. This stock solution is then diluted in cell lysis buffer to a concentration of 100 μg/mL immediately prior to use. Cell lysis buffer (2 mL) with proteinase K should be sufficient for at least 5 samples. Once the proteinase K has been dissolved or added, these solutions must be used or discarded; they cannot be stored.
16. 37°C water bath.
17. Phenol equilibrated with Tris-HCl, pH 8.0 (Wako, Osaka, Japan).
18. Chloroform.
19. Ethanol: 99% (absolute), 95%, 70% solutions.
20. 10 mg/mL RNase A stock solution (Roche Diagnostics, Mannheim, Germany; *see* **Note 1**). Thaw one aliquot per experiment (can include multiple samples), and discard the unused portion.
21. Human placenta DNA (Sigma).

2.2. Preparation of Tissue Samples and DNA Extraction

1. Nonneoplastic mucosa and tumor tissues taken from fresh surgical specimen of patients with colorectal cancer.
2. ACFs of colon dissected from formalin-fixed mucosal strips of a surgical specimen.
3. Frozen storage container.
4. Liquid nitrogen.
5. Mortar and pestle; autoclaved.
6. Tissue lysis buffer: 10 mM Tris-HCl, pH 8.0, 1 mM EDTA, 10 mM NaCl, 0.1% SDS. Ten milliliters of this buffer is sufficient for 25–50 tissue samples and can be stored at –20°C for over a year.
7. Proteinase K (Beckman): small volume of stock solution (at 20 mg/mL) initially made by dissolving in deionized distilled water. This stock solution is then diluted in tissue lysis buffer to a concentration of 100 μg/mL immediately prior to use. Tissue lysis buffer (2 mL) with proteinase K should be sufficient for at least five samples. Once the proteinase K has been dissolved or added, these solutions must be used or discarded; they cannot be stored.
8. 45°C water bath.
9. Phenol equilibrated with Tris-HCl, pH 8.0 (Wako).
10. Chloroform.
11. Ethanol: 99% (absolute), 95%, 70% solutions.
12. Tris-EDTA solution (TE): 10 mM Tris-HCl, pH 8.0, 1 mM EDTA (*see* **Note 2**). This solution is also commercially available from a number of sources.
13. 10 mg/mL RNase A stock solution (Roche; *see* **Note 1**). Thaw one aliquot per experiment (can include multiple samples), and discard the unused portion.
14. Glass slides used for conventional microscopic examination.
15. 0.2% Methylene blue solution—will require 2 mL per a strip of colon mucosa with a size of slide glass for identifying ACF. This solution can be stored indefinitely at 4°C and can be reused. (Filter before returning to storage container.)
16. Light microscope (e.g., Olympus model BX50, Tokyo, Japan).
17. Pasteur pipets.
18. Ampoule cutter (or file).
19. DNA concentrater (e.g., Microcon model 100, Amicon, Beverly, MA).

2.3. Enriched PCR

1. Primers (*see* **Fig. 1B** and **Note 3**):
   K5': 5'-ACTGAATATAAACTTGTGGTAGTTGGA<u>C</u>CT-3'
   K3'wt: 5'-TCAAAGAATGGTCCTGCACCAG-3'
   K3': 5'-TCAAAGAATGGTCCTG<u>G</u>ACCAG-3'
   K5'-13: 5'-ACTGAATATAAACTTGTGGTAGTTGG<u>C</u>CCT-3'
2. *Taq* DNA polymerase (Applied Biosystems, Foster City, CA).
3. 10X PCR buffer containing MgCl$_2$; comes with commercial purchase of *Taq* DNA polymerase (Applied Biosystems): 1X buffer consists of 10 mM Tris-HCl, pH 8.3, 50 mM KCl, 1.5 mM MgCl$_2$, and 0.01% gelatin.
4. dNTPs (Applied Biosystems).
5. AmpliWax PCR Gems 100 (Applied Biosystems).
6. Distilled and sterilized water in ampoules for medical use commercially available from pharmaceutical companies (e.g., Ohtsuka or Kobayashi Seiyaku, Tokyo, Japan).
7. Thin-walled tubes for PCR: GeneAmp Thin-Walled Reaction Tubes with Flat Caps (Applied Biosystems), or Thin-Wall Tube with Flat Cap (MJ Research, Waltham, MA).

8. Thermal cycler: GeneAmp PCR System 9600 (Applied Biosystems), or DNA Engine Peltier Thermal Cycler PTC-200 (MJ Research).
9. Restriction enzymes:
   *Mva*I (Takara, Kyoto, Japan)
   *Bst*NI (New England Biolabs, Beverly, MA)
   *Bgl*I (Toyobo, Osaka, Japan)
10. 4 M NH$_3$COOCH$_3$.

2.4. Polyacrylamide Gel Electrophoresis

1. Acrylamide stock solution: 40% acrylamide/*bis*-acrylamide (ratio 29:1) dissolved in distilled water and filtered through Whatman chromatography paper (3MM Chr, Whatman International, Maidstone, England) or a bottle top filter (Nalgene, Nalge Nunc International, Rochester, NY). Stored in a dark bottle at 4°C, this solution will be stable for more than a year, so it can be prepared in bulk (500 mL). Recently, the same solution has become commercially available (Sigma). A 2.5-mL aliquot of this stock solution is used for preparation of 10 mL of 10% native acrylamide gel solution for a 1.0-mm-thick minigel.
2. 20X TBE buffer: 1 M Tris-base, 1 M boric acid, 0.02 M EDTA (EDTA-2Na-2H$_2$O). Five hundred to 1000 mL of this solution can be prepared at a time, as it is stable for more than a year at room temperature. Precipitate, when it appears after longer storage, can be redissolved with warming. An aliquot of 0.5 mL is used for preparation of a 1.0-mm-thick minigel (10 mL).
3. 10% Ammonium peroxodisulfate (APS; Sigma). APS solid powder is stable when stored in the dark at room temperature. Practically, aliquots of 100 mg (0.1 g) of APS powder are stored in dark-colored, 1.5-mL microcentrifuge tubes at 4°C. Prior to use, an aliquot of the powder is dissolved in 1.0 mL of distilled water to make a 10% solution. It is important to inscribe the date of preparation on the tube, because this solution is stable only for 1 or 2 wk at 4°C. Typically, 100 µL of 10% APS solution is used for preparation of 10 mL acrylamide gel solution for a 1.0-mm-thick minigel.
4. N,N,N',N'-tetramethyl ethylene diamine (TMED; Wako).
5. 6X Gel loading buffer: 0.25% bromophenol blue, 0.25% xylene cyanol FF, 15% Ficoll (type 400, Amersham Biosciences, Piscataway, NJ) dissolved in water. Typically, 10 mL of this solution is prepared, which is stable at room temperature for over a year. Similar solutions are now available commercially.
6. Minislab gel apparatus (Bio-Rad, Hercules, CA, or Hoeffer Pharmacia Biotech, San Francisco, CA) and power supply (Crosspower 500L, ATTO, Tokyo, Japan, or PowerPac 300, Bio-Rad).
7. Ethidium bromide (stock solution, 10 mg/mL) or SYBR Green I nucleic acid stain (Molecular Probes, Eugene, OR). Ten to 100 mL of ethidium bromide stock solution is prepared, depending on the frequency of electrophoresis, size of gels to be stained, and other factors in each laboratory. The stock solution is stable in the dark at 4°C. Similar solutions are now available commercially. For staining minigels, a working solution is prepared by dissolving 10 µL of ethidium bromide stock solution in 100 mL of distilled water. A 1.0-mm-thick 10% acrylamide minigel can be stained in this solution in 5 min. This working solution can be used several times if recovered and stored in the dark.
8. Molecular marker DNA: Bluescript SKII (+) plasmid DNA (Stratagene, La Jolla, CA) digested with *Hpa*II (TaKaRa or Toyobo, Tokyo, Japan; *see* **Note 4**).
9. UV transilluminator (UVP, Upland, CA).
10. Gel photography equipment (e.g., LightCapture Type AE-6960/C/FC, ATTO, Tokyo, Japan).

3. Methods

3.1. Preparation of Mutant DNA Used for Validation of the Sensitivity of EPCR

1. Plate an aliquot of frozen stock of the SW480 and/or the HCT116 human colon adenocarcinoma cell line into a 10-cm tissue culture dish containing 10 mL RPMI supplemented with 10% FBS. When this culture is semiconfluent, it is used to initiate three 15-cm tissue culture dishes.

2. Pelleting:

    a. Grow the three cell cultures to semiconfluent to confluent status, then decant the medium, and gently wash each dish three times with 10 mL ice-cold PBS. (Introduce PBS with a pipet along the inner wall of the dish and swirl gently before decanting.)
    b. Harvest cells in the first dish by scraping in a further 10 mL ice-cold PBS.
    c. Transfer this cell suspension into a second dish and harvest it by scraping; meanwhile wash the first dish with a further 10 mL ice-cold PBS.
    d. Transfer the cell suspension from the second dish to the third and harvest by scraping; transfer the wash solution from the first dish to the second and wash.
    e. Transfer the cell suspension in 10 mL ice-cold PBS from the third dish into a 50-mL polypropylene conical tube, and wash the third dish with the wash solution from the second dish.
    f. Finally, transfer the wash solution to the tube, such that it contains harvested cells from all three dishes in about 30 mL of ice-cold PBS.
    g. Centrifuge this cell suspension at 3000–5000 rpm ($1670g$ +) for 5–10 min to pellet the cells.

3. Centrifugation:

    a. After centrifugation, remove and discard the supernatant by gentle decantation.
    b. Wash the cell pellet three times with 40 mL ice-cold PBS (resuspend by vortexing, pellet, and decant wash as in **step 2**).
    c. Resuspend the cell pellet in 1.0 mL of ice-cold PBS by gentle pipeting, and transfer the suspension into a 1.5-mL polypropylene microcentrifuge tube.
    d. Centrifuge the cell suspension at 10,000 rpm ($9200g$) for 5 min at 4°C to pellet the cells.
    e. After centrifugation, aspirate the supernatant through a 1 mL micropipet tip using a vacuum pump system and discard.

4. Resuspend the cell pellet in 100–200 µL (1 µL per initial mg of wet weight, or 1 µL per 1 µL (=1 mg) of cell pellet volume) cell lysis buffer containing 100 µg/mL proteinase K by pipeting, and incubate for 1–2 h at 37°C in a water bath, with occasional tapping to keep the cells suspended in the lysis buffer.

5. Extract genomic DNA and purify by serial treatment with phenol and chloroform, and then precipitate with 99% ethanol, all according to standardized methodologies *(28–30)*.

6. Serially wash the precipitated DNA with 1 mL of 95% and 70% ethanol (resuspension by gentle mixing or vortexing, followed by microcentrifugation), and then dissolve in distilled water at a concentration of 1 µg/µL. Divide this DNA solution into conveniently sized aliquots (~50 µL) and store at –20°C.

7. To prepare mixtures with different ratios of mutant to wild-type control DNAs, dilute 1 µg/µL of SW480- or HCT116-derived mutant DNA 10-fold with a 1 µg/µL solution of placenta-derived wild-type DNA. Use 0.5 or 1.0 µL of each mixture for validation of EPCR sensitivity.

3.2. DNA Extraction From Fresh Tissue Samples

1. Take 0.1–0.2 g (wet weight) samples of fresh tissue from normal mucosa and colon cancer immediately after removal of surgical specimens (*see* **Note 5**).
2. Snap-freeze samples (*see* **Note 6**) and store at –80°C until use.
3. To begin DNA extraction, homogenize selected frozen tissue samples and powder in a mortar containing liquid nitrogen (*see* **Note 7**).
4. Suspend powdered tissue in 1 or 2 vol (assume 0.1 g wet weight = 100 μL) of tissue lysis buffer containing 100 μg/mL of proteinase K in a microcentrifuge tube, and incubate in a water bath at 45°C for 2–5 h.
5. Extract genomic DNA and purify by serial treatment with phenol and chloroform, precipitating with ethanol, all according to standardized methodologies *(28–30)*.
6. Wash precipitated DNA serially in 95% and 70% ethanol (resuspension by gentle mixing or vortexing, followed by microcentrifugation), then dissolve in 100–200 μL TE (the exact volume is dependent on the amount of input tissue and the efficiency of the extraction), and treat with 25–50 ng/μL of RNase A at 37°C for 30 min.
7. Repurify DNA by treatment with phenol and chloroform, and precipitate with ethanol *(31)*.
8. Wash precipitated DNA again serially in 1 mL 95% and 70% ethanol, then dissolve in distilled and sterilized water or TE at a concentration of 1.0 μg/μL, and store at –20°C. Again, the exact volume of water or TE is dependent on the amount and quality of the original tissue sample and the efficiency of the DNA extraction.

3.3. Extraction of DNA From Formalin-Fixed ACF

1. Strip off the grossly normal mucosal layer from the formalin-fixed surgical specimen of colorectal cancer.
2. Cut mucosal strips into pieces the size of a conventional glass slide used for light microscopic examination.
3. Stain each mucosal piece by overlaying it with 2 mL of 0.2% methylene blue solution for a few minutes, and then wash briefly by immersion in distilled water and gentle shaking. This distilled water may be exchanged several times until no excess dye appears in the wash.
4. Place the stained mucosal strip on a glass slide and overlay it with distilled water, suitable for observation under the microscope at 40-fold magnification.
5. Under microscopic observation, excise ACF showing characteristic morphological findings (**Fig. 4A**) from the mucosal strip using a Pasteur pipet, the tip of which has been precut with an ampoule cutter.
6. Divide each isolated ACF into two pieces (**Fig. 4B**), one for histopathological examination and the other for DNA extraction after removal of as many normal crypts as possible, under microscopic observation.
7. Extract genomic DNA from each individual ACF by serial treatment with proteinase K (100 μg/mL) and RNase A (25–50 ng/μL) in 20–50 μL of tissue lysis buffer, depending on the size of the sample.
8. Purify the extracted DNA and concentrate according to the manufacturer's instructions (Microcon Model 100, Amicon, Beverly, MA). An aliquot of 0.5–1.0 μL of this DNA solution is used for PCR analysis.

3.4. Enriched PCR

1. Prepare the two reaction mixtures for the first-step PCR; divide them into two layers with AmpliWax according to the supplier's instruction: the lower layer should contain 100 ng of primer K5', 70 ng of primer K3'wt (not K3'), and 0.2 mM each of dNTP in a volume of

13.5 μL; the upper layer should contain 7.5 μL of 10X PCR buffer with $MgCl_2$, 1.25 U of *Taq* DNA polymerase, and 0.5–1.0 μg of genomic DNA in a volume of 61.5 μL (*see* **Notes 8–10**).

2. Run the first-step amplification for 20 cycles of 1 min denaturation at 94°C, 1 min annealing at 59°C, and 1 min extension at 72°C, and followed by 10 min extension at 72°C (*see* **Note 11**).
3. Intermediate digestion: digest 1 μL of the first-step PCR products with 10 U of *Mva*I in a final volume of 10 μL at 37°C for more than 2 h (*see* **Note 12**).
4. Prepare the reaction mixtures for the second-step PCR in the presence of AmpliWax. The mixture should contain 140 ng of primer K5', 100 ng of K3' (not K3'wt), 0.2 m*M* each of dNTP, 1.25 U of *Taq* DNA polymerase, and 1 μL of *Mva*I-digested first-step PCR product in a final volume of 75 μL (13.5 μL of lower layer + 61.5 μL of upper layer) of 1X PCR buffer (*see* **Notes 8–10**).
5. Run the second-step amplification for 30 cycles of 1 min denaturation at 94°C, 1 min annealing at 59°C, and 1 min extension at 72°C, followed by 10 min extension at 72°C (*see* **Note 11**).

3.5. Detection of Mutant K-RAS by RFLP Analysis

1. Digest 8 μL of the second-step PCR product with 10 U of *Mva*I in a total volume of 10 μL containing 1 μL of 10X enzyme buffer, at 37°C for 1 h.
2. Add 2 μL of 6X gel loading buffer to the digested PCR product solution.
3. Separate digested products on a 10% native polyacrylamide (29:1) minislab gel at 100 V for 1 h in the presence of 1X TBE buffer (*see* **Note 13**) *(32)*.
4. Stain the gel with 0.5 μg/mL ethidium bromide solution at room temperature for 5–10 min with gentle shaking.
5. Wash the stained gel with distilled water for 1 min with gentle shaking.
6. Detect and photograph the characteristic mutant signal (142 bp) under the UV transilluminator, and save the picture.

3.6. Characterization of Mutant K-RAS Detected by EPCR

1. If a mutant band is detected in a sample, the second-step PCR is repeated in duplicate.
2. Digest 8 μL of PCR product from each tube with *Mva*I and separate on a native polyacrylamide gel (*see* **Subheading 3.5.**, **step 3**), to confirm reproducibility of enrichment of the mutant.
3. Digest the remaining PCR product (about 130 μL in total from two tubes) with 50 U of *Mva*I in 160 μL solution containing 1X enzyme buffer, at 37°C for 1 h.
4. Mix the digested PCR product with an equal amount of 4 *M* NH_3COOCH_3, and precipitate with ethanol at –80°C for 15–30 min.
5. Dissolve the precipitated PCR product in 20 μL of TE, and separate on a 10% native polyacrylamide gel as described previously (*see* **Subheading 3.5.**, **step 3**).
6. Cut out a piece of gel (~5 × 1–2 mm, 1 mm thick) containing the mutant band from the ethidium bromide-stained gel under the UV transilluminator.
7. Elute the mutant PCR product from the cut-out piece of gel in 50 μL of sterilized water in a 1.5-mL microcentrifuge tube by heating at 80°C for 20 min.
8. Analyze this purified product by sequencing using one of the following methods (*see* **Note 14**):

   a. The dideoxy chain-termination method using the Sequenase DNA Sequencing Kit (USB, Cleveland, OH).

b. The dye terminator method using the Dye Primer Cycle Sequencing Kit (Applied Biosystems) after cloning PCR product by blunt-end ligation.

c. Direct sequencing by the dye terminator method.

4. Notes

1. Dissolve 20 mg of RNase A powder in 2 mL of 10 mM Tris-HCl (pH 7.5) buffer containing 15 mM NaCl. Heat the enzyme solution at 100°C for 15 min, and then allow to cool down slowly to room temperature. Aliquot this stock solution (~50 µL), and store at –20°C (should be usable for 1 yr or longer).

2. TE is chemically stable but easily contaminated biologically. Whether small amounts are made fresh or a larger stock solution is kept on hand must be decided by the individual laboratory.

3. As a prerequisite, to maximize the sensitivity of EPCR, all synthesized primers must be gel-purified.

4. Prepare the molecular weight marker DNA as follows: digest 10 µg of Bluescript SKII (+) plasmid DNA with 30 U of HpaII in 30 µL of 1X enzyme buffer at 37°C for 1 h. Add 6 µL of 6X gel loading buffer to this solution. A 1–2-µL aliquot of this marker solution is sufficient for a lane of a gel.

5. When collecting tissue samples, normal tissue should be excised prior to tumor tissue, using different forceps and scissors. Before storage, normal tissue is extensively washed with cold PBS to remove desquamated tumor cells.

6. "Snap" freezing simply implies freezing samples as fast as possible. We use a unique method with equipment of our own design: two special metal plates joined with hinges. This piece of equipment is chilled in liquid nitrogen prior to use. Then each tissue sample is placed in a 8 × 5-cm plastic bag, sealed, frozen by compression between the two plates (this also causes the tissue to be flattened), and stored at –80°C.

7. Pour liquid nitrogen into a mortar just before homogenization of tissue sample to prechill both mortar and pestle.

8. In the original method *(10)*, 10 ng each and 150 ng each of primers were used in the first and second step of PCR amplification, respectively. However, the optimal enrichment of mutant is obtained in the amounts of primers given in this protocol.

9. Concentration of each NTP should be kept at 0.2 mM to obtain optimal amplification.

10. AmpliWax PCR Gem 100 is used to minimize nonspecific amplification.

11. To confirm the validity of the assay and to avoid contamination, placenta DNA (wild-type control), SW 480 cell–derived DNA (mutant control), and sterilized water instead of DNA are amplified in parallel with DNA samples in every PCR run.

12. When a mutant band is detected, the intermediate digestion mixture is stored at –20°C for further use with the sequencing reactions.

13. Detection and separation of a mutant signal is more sensitive and feasible on a 10–15% polyacrylamide gel than on an agarose gel. The method for elution of the target DNA band from the former type of gel is also simpler and more feasible than from the latter type.

14. The exact protocols of the respective sequencing methods are not described here, owing to space limitations. These protocols are available from the suppliers' instructions. The upstream primer K5' is used for sequencing in the forward direction. The sequence of the downstream primer SK3' used for sequencing in the reverse direction is: 5'-CTCTATTGTTGGATCATATTC-3' *(12)*.

References

1. Karp, J. E. and Broder, S. (1995) Molecular foundations of cancer: new targets for intervention. *Nat. Med.* **1**, 309–320.
2. Ponder B. A. J. (2001) Cancer genetics. *Nature* **411**, 336–341.
3. Fearon, E. R. (1997) Human cancer syndromes: clues to the origin and nature of cancer. *Science* **278**, 1043–1050.
4. Blume-Jensen, P. and Hunter, T. (2001) Oncogenic kinase signaling. *Nature* **411**, 355–365.
5. Bos, J. L. (1989) *ras* oncogenes in human cancer: a review. *Cancer Res.* **49**, 4682–4689.
6. Kiaris, H. and Spandidos, D. A. (1995) Mutations of *ras* genes in human tumors. *Int. J. Oncol.* **7**, 413–421.
7. Minamoto, T., Mai, M., and Ronai, Z. (2000) K-*RAS* mutation: early detection in molecular diagnosis and risk assessment of colorectal, pancreas, and lung cancers—a review. *Cancer Detect. Prev.* **4**, 1–12.
8. van Mansfeld, A. D. M. and Bos, J. L. (1992) PCR-based approaches for detection of mutated *ras* genes. *PCR Methods Appl.* **1**, 211–216.
9. Ronai, Z. and Yakubovskaya, M. (1995) PCR in clinical diagnosis. *J. Clin. Lab. Anal.* **9**, 269–283.
10. Kahn, S. M., Jiang, W., Culbertson, T. A., et al. (1991) Rapid and sensitive nonradioactive detection of mutant K-*RAS* genes via 'enriched' PCR amplification. *Oncogene* **6**, 1079–1083.
11. Jiang, W., Kahn, S., Guillem, J., Lu, S., and Weinstein, I. B. (1989) Rapid detection of *ras* oncogenes in human tissues: applications to colon, esophageal, and gastric cancer. *Oncogene* **4**, 923–928.
12. Minamoto, T., Ronai, Z., Yamashita, N., et al. (1994) Detection of Ki-*RAS* mutation in non-neoplastic mucosa of Japanese patients with colorectal cancers. *Int. J. Oncol.* **4**, 397–401.
13. Chung, D. C. (2000) The genetic basis of colorectal cancer: insights into critical pathways of tumorigenesis. *Gastroenterology* **119**, 864–865.
14. Minamoto, T. and Ronai, Z. (2001) Gene mutation as a target for early detection in cancer diagnosis. *Crit. Rev. Oncol. Hematol.* **40**, 195–213.
15. Ronai, Z., Luo, F. C., Gradia, S., Hart, W. J., and Butler, R. (1994) Detection of K-*RAS* mutation in normal and malignant colonic tissues by an enriched PCR method. *Int. J. Oncol.* **4**, 391–396.
16. Minamoto, T., Yamashita, N., Ochiai, A., et al. (1995) Mutant K-*RAS* in apparently normal mucosa of colorectal cancer patients. Its potential as a biomarker of colorectal cancer patients. *Cancer* **75**, 1520–1526.
17. Ronai, Z., Minamoto, T., Butler, R., et al. (1995) Sampling method as a key factor in identifying K-*RAS* oncogene mutations in preneoplastic colorectal lesions. *Cancer Detect. Prev.* **19**, 512–517.
18. Minamoto, T., Esumi, H., Ochiai, A., et al. (1997) Combined analysis of microsatellite instability and K-*RAS* mutation increases detection incidence of normal samples from colorectal cancer patients. *Clin. Cancer Res.* **3**, 1413–1417.
19. Tobi, M., Luo, F.-C., and Ronai, Z. (1994) Detection of K-*RAS* mutation in colonic effluent samples from patients without evidence of colorectal carcinoma. *J. Natl. Cancer Inst.* **86**, 1007–1010.
20. Zhang, B., Ougolkov, A., Yamashita, K., Takahashi, Y., Mai, M., and Minamoto, T. (2003) β-*catenin* and *ras* oncogenes detect most human colorectal cancers. *Clin. Cancer Res.* **3**, 3073–3079.

21. Pretlow, T. P. (1995) Aberrant crypt foci and K-*RAS* mutations: earliest recognized players or innocent bystanders in colon carcinogenesis? *Gastroenterology* **108,** 600–603.
22. Yamashita, N., Minamoto, T., Ochiai, A., Onda, M., and Esumi, H. (1995) Frequent and characteristic K-*RAS* activation and absence of p53 protein accumulation in aberrant crypt foci of the colon. *Gastroenterology* **108,** 434-440.
23. Takayama, T., Katsuki, S., Takahashi, Y., et al. (1998) Aberrant crypt foci of the colon as precursors of adenoma and cancer. *N. Engl. J. Med.* **339,** 1277–1284.
24. Otori, K., Sugiyama, K., Hasebe, T., Fukushima, S., and Esumi, H. (1995) Emergence of adenomatous aberrant crypt foci (ACF) from hyperplastic ACF with concomitant increase in cell proliferation. *Cancer Res.* **55,** 4743–4746.
25. Konstantakos, A. K., Siu, I.-M., Pretlow, T. G., Stellato, T. A., and Pretlow, T. P. (1996) Human aberrant crypt foci with carcinoma in situ from a patient with sporadic colon cancer. *Gastroenterology* **111,** 772–777.
26. Pretlow, T. P., Brasitus, T. A., Fulton, N. C., Cheyer, C., and Kaplan, E. L. (1993) K-*RAS* mutation in putative preneoplastic lesions in human colon. *J. Natl. Cancer Inst.* **85,** 2004–2007.
27. Takayama, T., Ohi, M., Hayashi, T., et al. (2001) Analysis of K-*RAS*, *APC*, and β-*catenin* in aberrant crypt foci in sporadic adenoma, cancer, and familial adenomatous polyposis. *Gastroenterology* **121,** 599–611.
28. Sambrook, J., Fritsch, E. F., and Maniatis, T. (1989) Isolation of high-molecular-weight DNA from mammalian cells, in *Molecular Cloning: A Laboratory Manual,* 2nd ed., Cold Spring Harbor Laboratory Press, Plainview, NY, pp. 9.14–9.23.
29. Moore, D. D. and Strauss, W. M. (1995) Preparation of genomic DNA from mammalian tissue, in *Short Protocols in Molecular Biology,* 3rd ed. (Ausubel, F., Brent, R., Kingston, R. E., et al., eds.), Wiley, Hoboken, NJ, pp. 2–8.
30. Wolff, R. and Gemmill, R. (1997) DNA from mammalian sources, in *Genome Analysis: A Laboratory Manual,* vol. 1 (Birren, B., Green, E. D., Klapholz, S., Myers, R. M., and Roskams, J., eds.), Cold Spring Harbor Laboratory Press, Plainview, NY, pp. 4–16.
31. Sambrook, J., Fritsch, E. F., and Maniatis, T. (1989) Extraction with phenol:chloroform, in *Molecular Cloning: A Laboratory Manual,* 2nd ed., Cold Spring Harbor Laboratory Press, Plainview, NY, pp. E.3–E.4.
32. Sambrook, J., Fritsch, E. F., and Maniatis, T. (1989) Polyacrylamide gel electrophoresis, in *Molecular Cloning: A Laboratory Manual,* 2nd ed., Cold Spring Harbor Laboratory Press, Plainview, NY, pp. 6.36–6.59.

25

Detection of DNA Double-Strand Breaks and Chromosome Translocations Using Ligation-Mediated PCR and Inverse PCR

Michael J. Villalobos, Christopher J. Betti, and Andrew T. M. Vaughan

Summary

Current techniques for examining the global creation and repair of DNA double-strand breaks are restricted in their sensitivity, and such techniques mask any site-dependent variations in breakage and repair rate or fidelity. We present here a system for analyzing the fate of documented DNA breaks, using the *MLL* gene as an example, through application of ligation-mediated PCR. Here, a simple asymmetric double-stranded DNA adapter molecule is ligated to experimentally induced DNA breaks and subjected to seminested PCR using adapter and gene-specific primers. The rate of appearance and loss of specific PCR products allows detection of both the break and its repair. Using the additional technique of inverse PCR, the presence of misrepaired products (translocations) can be detected at the same site, providing information on the fidelity of the ligation reaction in intact cells. Such techniques may be adapted for the analysis of DNA breaks introduced into any identifiable genomic location.

Key Words: LM-PCR; IPCR; translocation; DNA; double-strand break repair; apoptosis; *MLL*.

1. Introduction

Chromosome translocations involving the mixed-lineage leukemia (*MLL*) gene are a frequent finding in infant, adult, and therapy-related leukemias *(1,2)*. Although the mechanism(s) responsible for the formation of a translocation is unknown, two models are beginning to evolve. The two mechanisms, illegitimate V(D)J recombination and apoptosis, share one element in common, in that both involve the presence of DNA double-strand breaks (DSBs) *(3–7)*. DNA DSBs have been shown to be potent inducers of chromosome translocations and can be produced by a multitude of agents, including ionizing radiation, genotoxic chemicals, and cellular processes such as apoptosis *(8,9)*. Traditional Southern blot-based techniques have been used in the past to visualize the presence of DNA breaks in a gene, but such methods have two major drawbacks: they require large amounts of starting material and are rather insensitive.

From: *Methods in Molecular Biology, vol. 291, Molecular Toxicology Protocols*
Edited by: P. Keohavong and S. G. Grant © Humana Press Inc., Totowa, NJ

The technique of ligation-mediated polymerase chain reaction (LM-PCR) coupled with nested PCR allows for greater sensitivity to detect DNA breaks and for the use of small amounts of DNA template.

The detection of chromosome translocations has previously employed both the Southern blot technique and *in situ* hybridization. However, these techniques are only capable of detecting chromosome translocations when both partner genes are known. Inverse PCR (IPCR) is performed using a gene-specific primer set oriented in opposing directions. Therefore, IPCR allows for the detection of chromosome translocations when only one of the translocation partners is known.

1.1. Ligation-Mediated PCR

This technique takes advantage of the extreme sensitivity of seminested PCR coupled with the specificity of LM-PCR to amplify gene fragments produced during apoptosis. LM-PCR has been used to amplify DNA adjacent to internucleosomal breaks induced during apoptosis, as well as breaks introduced during V(D)J recombination *(5,6)*. Although DNA lesions introduced by apoptotic nucleases produce blunt-end double-strand DNA breaks, it is possible to ligate a blunt-end linker molecule to the break site. This allows for the specific amplification of DNA sequences ligated to the linker molecule, using primers to the linker and to the gene of interest. In the second round of PCR, the use of nested primers exponentially increases the sensitivity of the assay to detect DNA breaks.

Prior to PCR amplification, the double-stranded linker molecule must be constructed and ligated to the genomic DNA. The linker is made by incubating two homologous oligonucleotides under a gradually decreasing temperature gradient. This is most easily achieved using the thermocycling file type on a Perkin Elmer 480 thermocycler. After the linker is made, it will have a staggered and a blunt-end terminus (**Fig. 1A**). Next, the linker is ligated to isolated genomic DNA using T4 DNA ligase. Just prior to LM-PCR, the reaction is heated to 72°C, causing the 11-mer oligomer to dissociate from the ligated linker molecule, leaving a 5' 25-mer overhang. The 25-mer remains ligated to the DNA because the genomic DNA contributed its 5' phosphate to the ligation reaction, and the 11-mer dissociates because the ligation lacked a 5' phosphate, resulting in incomplete ligation (**Fig. 1B**). During PCR, *Taq* polymerase elongates the staggered 25-mer end to create the homologous strand. Now the DNA end has a double-stranded 25-mer linker molecule ligated to its terminus. LM-PCR is conducted using the linker-ligated DNA as a template, the 25-mer oligomer as a primer, and a primer specific to the gene or target of interest, in this case *MLL*. Seminested PCR is conducted using the PCR products from the first-round reactions. It is seminested because only the *MLL* primer is nested, whereas the same 25-mer oligomer is used as a primer. The second-round PCR products are analyzed by Southern blot using a 0.75-kb cDNA probe to the *MLL* breakpoint cluster region *(10)*. Amplification of cleaved *MLL* fragments with these primers results in a product of approx 290 bp (**Fig. 2**).

1.2. Inverse PCR

During apoptosis, the *MLL* breakpoint cluster region (bcr) is subjected to cleavage, creating a DNA DSB. One possible consequence of nonhomologous end joining

A
```
5'- GCG GTG ACC CGG GAG ATC TGA ATT C -3'
      3'- C TAG ACT TAA G -5'
```

B

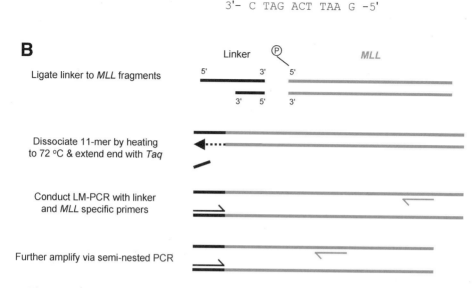

Fig. 1. Ligation-mediated polymerase chain reaction (LM-PCR) amplification of apoptotically cleaved *MLL*. (**A**) Depiction of the double-stranded blunt-end linker molecule used for LM-PCR. (**B**) Schematic of the LM-PCR technique used to amplify apoptotically cleaved *MLL*. The linker and linker-specific primers are black. *MLL* and its primers are in gray.

(NHEJ) repair operating at the *MLL* cleavage site is incorrect repair of the break, leading to the formation of a chromosomal translocation. The identification of such misrepair events within early apoptotic cells would provide specific evidence that a break–rejoining cycle had occurred. To determine whether the apoptotic program is capable of generating a chromosomal translocation, an IPCR strategy was employed (**Fig. 3**). This procedure is able to amplify both the germline *MLL* sequence at the location of the apoptotic cut site and any rearranged fragments that contain a *MLL* translocation.

IPCR was first described by Ochman et al. *(11)* as a means of chromosome walking and identifying bacterial genes that were inactivated by insertional mutagenesis. Since its advent, this technique has been further tailored to identify DNA translocations when the partner gene is unknown *(12,13)*. The template for IPCR is a circularized DNA molecule created by restriction enzyme digestion followed by ligation. A restriction enzyme is chosen such that it has a high probability of cutting the unknown DNA sequence. This is achieved through the use of an enzyme with a short, 4-bp recognition sequence. Statistically, such an enzyme cuts random DNA sequences every 256 bp and thus would be very likely to cut an unknown DNA sequence.

The protocol described here utilizes a second infrequent cutting restriction enzyme with a 6-bp recognition sequence that is predicted to cut a DNA sequence once every 4096 bp. This second restriction enzyme specifically allows for the detection of

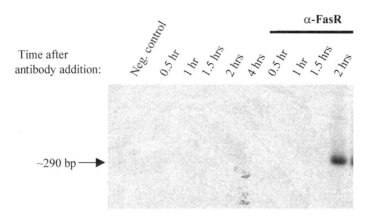

Fig. 2. Detection of *MLL* cleavage by LM-PCR. TK6 cells were induced to apoptosis by treatment with anti-Fas receptor antibody. Cell aliquots were removed at the stated times and DNA prepared. *MLL* cleavage was analyzed by LM-PCR. Control cells were not induced to undergo apoptosis. Negative control contains sfH$_2$O instead of DNA.

a chromosome translocation within a population of germline DNA sequences. The infrequently cutting restriction enzyme is chosen such that it lies on the 3' side of the presumed chromosomal break site. The infrequent cutter also prevents the circularization of germline DNA molecules containing only the known DNA sequence (frequent cutter to frequent cutter) when both restriction enzymes are used. An infrequent restriction site would have a low probability of lying between two frequent cutting restriction enzyme sites. Therefore, circular germline molecules can be removed from the reaction mixture, thereby favoring the PCR amplification of molecules containing a DNA translocation (**Fig. 3**). However, any DNA translocations that contain this infrequent cutter site lying between the two frequent cutter sites will be eliminated from the pool. PCR is conducted from the circular templates using a pair of primers oriented in opposite directions that are specific to the known DNA sequence. This allows the PCR reaction to proceed from the known sequence through the unknown sequence. An example of the IPCR technique's ability to detect *MLL* translocations is shown in **Fig. 4**. Here, DNA from both the TK6 cell line (not containing an *MLL* translocation) and the MM6 cell line (containing an *MLL-AF9* translocation) were both subjected to the IPCR assay.

2. Materials

2.1. Ligation-Mediated PCR

2.1.1. Construction of the Asymmetric Double-Stranded Linker

1. 0.22-μm filtered and autoclaved H$_2$O (sfH$_2$O).
2. Oligonucleotides (MWG Biotech, High Point, NC):

   a. Linker 11 (5'-GAA TTC AGA TC-3').
   b. Linker 25 (5'-GCG GTG ACC CGG GAG ATC TGA ATT C-3').

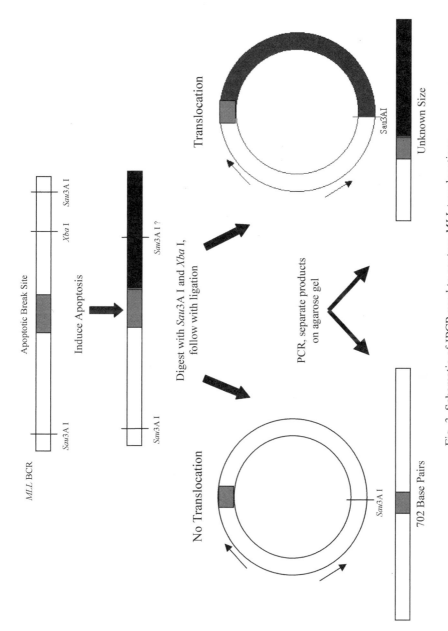

Fig. 3. Schematic of IPCR used to capture *MLL* translocations.

3. Oligonucleotide resuspension buffer: 75 m*M* Tris-HCl, pH 8.8 (Sigma, St. Louis, MO).
4. 1X T4 DNA ligase buffer: dilute from 10X with sfH$_2$0, keep at −20°C (Promega, Madison, WI).

2.1.2. Purification and Preparation of Template DNA

1. Puregene DNA isolation kit (Gentra Systems, Minneapolis, MN).
2. Asymmetric double-stranded linker.
3. 10X T4 DNA ligase buffer (Promega).
4. T4 DNA ligase (Promega).
5. 70°C Heating block.

2.1.3. Seminested PCR Amplification of Linker-Ligated DNA

1. *Taq* DNA polymerase (MBI Fermentas, Hanover, MD).
2. 10X and 1X (NH$_4$)$_2$SO$_4$ buffer: 10X stock comes with *Taq* polymerase; dilute to 1X with sfH$_2$0.
3. 500 μ*M* Oligonucleotides (MWG Biotech).
   a. in12.2F (5'-ATG CCC AAG TCC CTA GAC AAA ATG GTG-3').
   b. Nin12.3F (5'-GTC TGT TCA CAT AGA GTA CAG AGG CAA CTA-3').
4. Oligonucleotide resuspension buffer: 75 m*M* Tris-HCl, pH 8.8.
5. 50 μ*M* stock solutions of Linker 11, Linker 25, in12.2F, and Nin12.3F.
6. 25 m*M* MgCl$_2$ (Sigma).
7. 25 m*M* dNTP stock: equal volumes of 100 m*M* dCTP, dTTP, dATP, and dGTP.
8. Thermocycler (e.g., Perkin Elmer 480, Foster City, CA).

2.1.4. Southern Blot Analysis of PCR-Amplified DNA

1. ZetaProbe GT nylon membrane (Bio-Rad, Hercules, CA).
2. 0.4 *M* NaOH buffer (Sigma).
3. Prime-a-Gene kit (Promega, Madison, WI).
4. 6000 Ci/mmol [α-^{32}P]dCTP (Amersham Pharmacia, Piscataway, NJ).
5. 0.75-kb cDNA fragment to *MLL* exons 8–14.

2.2. Inverse PCR

2.2.1. Preparation and Purification of the DNA Template

1 TK6 cells (American Type Culture Collection [ATCC]; Manassas, VA).
2. 25- and 75-cm^2 Tissue culture flasks (e.g., Corning, Corning, NY).
3. RPMI cell culture medium (e.g., Sigma), or medium appropriate for cells of interest.
4. Fetal bovine serum (FBS; e.g., Biologos, Naperville, IL).
5. Apoptotic stimulus: anti-Fas antibody (Kamiya Biomedical, Seattle, WA), radiation source (e.g., dual-head Cs-137 Gammacell irradiator, Nordion International, Ontario, Canada, or equivalent).
6. Centrifuge (e.g., Jouan, Winchester, VA).
7. Phosphate-buffered saline (PBS; Cambrex BioScience, Walkersville, MD).
8. Nuclei lysis solution (Promega).
9. 10 mg/mL RNase (Sigma).
10. Protein precipitation solution (Promega).
11. 100% Isopropanol (Sigma).
12. Vortex mixer.
13. Ice.

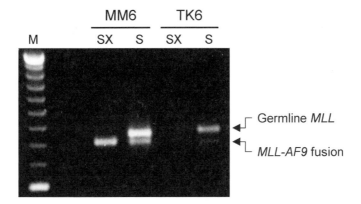

Fig. 4. IPCR detection of native and translocated *MLL*. In an effort to confirm the feasibility of detecting a chromosomal translocation, the IPCR technique was implemented using known positive and negative controls. The TK6 cell line contains one copy of the native (untranslocated) *MLL* gene, and the MM6 cell line is pseudotetraploid with respect to *MLL*, containing two native and two translocated copies of *MLL*. Using DNA cut only with the frequent cutter, a parental 782 bp is seen in both cell lines. Additionally, a 687-bp band is seen under the parental 782-bp band in the MM6 cell line, representing the *MLL-AF9* translocation. Both parental bands disappear when the DNA is digested with both the frequent (*Sau*3A I) and infrequent (*Xba*I) cutting enzymes. However, the 687-bp band under the MM6 parental remains as expected since no *Xba*I site lies within this region of the *MLL-AF9* translocation.

14. 70% Ethanol (Sigma).
15. 0.22-μm Filtered and autoclaved H_2O.

2.2.2. Restriction Enzyme Digestion

1. *Sau*3AI and *Xba*I (Promega).
2. 3 *M* Sodium acetate, pH 5.2 (Sigma).

2.2.3. Ligation Reaction

1. T4 DNA ligase (Promega).
2. 0.1 *M* Spermidine (Sigma).

2.2.4. Inverse PCR

1. For intron 11, use the following primers:
   Forward 1 (5'-ATG TCC ATG ACA TAT CAC TG-3').
   Reverse 1 (5'-TAG GAC TTC ATA TTT GCC A-3').
   Forward 2 (5'-AGC ACA ATC CCA TCT TAG T-3').
   Reverse 2 (5'-TGA GAC GGA GTC TTG CT-3').

   For exon 12, use the following primers:
   Forward 1 (5'-CTT TGT TTA TAC CAC TC-3').
   Reverse 1 (5'-TAT GGG AAT ATA AAG GAG TGG G-3').
   Forward 2 (5'-TTA GGT CAC TTA GCA TGT TCT G-3').
   Reverse 2 (5'-CAG TTG TAA GGT CTG GTT TGT C-3') (Invitrogen, Carlsbad, CA).

2. *Taq* DNA polymerase (MBI Fermentas).
3. Thermocycler (e.g., Perkin Elmer 480).

2.2.5. Cloning and Sequencing of IPCR Products

1. Qiaquick gel extraction kit (Qiagen, Valencia, CA).
2. TOPO TA Cloning® Kit (Invitrogen).
3. Wizard Miniprep kit (Promega).
4. DNA sequencer (e.g., model 377 Prism DNA Sequencer®, Applied Biosystems, Foster City, CA).

2.2.6. Translocation Sequence Analysis

1. Computer with internet access.

3. Methods

3.1. Ligation-Mediated PCR

3.1.1. Construction of the Asymmetric Double-Stranded Linker

1. Resuspend Linker 11 and Linker 25 to 500 μM with oligonucleotide resuspension buffer by vortexing.
2. Mix 500 pmols Linker 11 and 500 pmols Linker 25 by pipeting in the presence of 1X T4 DNA ligase buffer and sfH$_2$O, to a total volume of 5 μL.
3. Incubate the reaction in the thermocycler at 95°C for 5 min, 70°C for 1 s, and then lower the temperature from 70°C to 25°C over 60 min.
4. Continue to incubate the reaction at 25°C for 60 min, and subsequently lower the temperature from 25°C to 4°C over 60 min.
5. Store the double-stranded linker at –20°C.

3.1.2. Purification and Preparation of Template DNA

1. Isolate genomic DNA from approx 1–2 × 10^6 cells using the Puregene DNA isolation kit according to manufacturer's instruction (*see* **Note 1**).
2. To 1.0 µg of genomic DNA, add 100 pmols (1.0 µL) of double-strand linker, 6 µL of 10X T4 DNA ligase buffer, 1.0 µL (3 U) of T4 DNA ligase, and add sfH$_2$O to a final volume of 60 µL (*see* **Note 2**). Flick-mix the tubes.
3. Incubate the reaction at 15°C for 14 h, 70°C for 10 min in a heating block and then at 4°C (*see* **Note 3**).
4. Dilute the reaction to 5 ng/µL and then 0.5 ng/µL with sfH$_2$O (*see* **Note 4**).

3.1.3. Seminested PCR Amplification of Linker-Ligated DNA

1. Dilute *Taq* DNA polymerase 1:1 with 1X (NH$_4$)$_2$SO$_4$ buffer, for a final concentration of 2.5 U/µL.
2. Dilute 5 µL of 500 μM primers to 50 μM with 45 µL of oligonucleotide resuspension buffer.
3. To 2.0 µL (1.0 ng) of linker-ligated DNA add: 5.0 µL of 10X (NH$_4$)$_2$SO$_4$ buffer, 6.0 µL of 25 mM MgCl$_2$, 0.5 µL of 50 μM Linker 25 primer, 0.5 µL of 50 μM in 12.2F primer, 0.5 µL of 25 mM dNTP mix, and 34.5 µL of sfH$_2$O (*see* **Notes 5** and **6**).
4. Incubate the reactions at 72°C for 3 min, and then add 1.0 µL of diluted *Taq* DNA polymerase. Mix the reactions by vortexing and centrifuge briefly (*see* **Note 7**).
5. Process the PCR reactions at 72°C for 5 min, then increase to 95°C for 4 min, then 30 cycles of 95°C for 45 s, 66°C for 60 s, 72°C for 45 s, followed by 72°C for 10 min, and reduce to 4°C until removed from the machine.

6. To 1.0 μL of first-round PCR product add: 2.5 μL of 10X $(NH_4)_2SO_4$ buffer, 3.0 μL of 25 mM $MgCl_2$, 0.25 μL of 50 μM Linker 25 primer, 0.25 μL of 50 μM in 12.3F primer, 0.25 μL of 25 mM dNTP mix, 0.25 μL (1.25 U) of *Taq* polymerase, and 17.5 μL of sfH$_2$O (*see* **Note 6**).

7. Process the reactions at 95°C for 4 min, then 25 cycles at 95°C for 45 s, 66°C for 60 s, 72°C for 45 s, then 72°C for 5 min, and leave at 4°C.

8. Size-fractionate the second-round PCR products on a 2.0% agarose gel, and transfer the DNA to a ZetaProbe GT membrane with 0.4 M NaOH buffer according to the manufacturer's instructions.

9. Construct an *MLL* cDNA probe using the 0.75-kb fragment *(10,14)*, the Prime-a-Gene kit, and [α-^{32}P]dCTP.

10. Perform Southern blot analysis by standard methods using the *MLL* cDNA probe *(14)*.

3.2. Inverse PCR

3.2.1. Preparation and Purification of the DNA Template

1. Resuspend 1×10^7 TK6 cells in 20 mL of fresh RPMI medium supplemented with 10% FBS by vortexing. Treat with anti-Fas antibody (0.5 μg/mL final concentration) or 8 Gy γ-radiation.

2. Remove aliquots containing 3×10^6 cells at 0, 2, 4, 6, 8, and 24 h after addition of the apoptotic stimulus. Pellet cells by centrifugation at 700g for 5 min.

3. Wash cell pellets once in 500 μL of PBS and centrifuge again at 700g.

4. Resuspend pellets in 600 μL nuclei lysis solution, and mix by pipeting to ensure cell lysis.

5. Next, add 3 μL of RNase (stock 10 mg/mL) to each sample, and incubate at 37°C for 30 min.

6. Allow the samples to cool to room temperature.

7. Add 200 μL of protein precipitation solution and vortex on high for 20 s.

8. Allow the protein to precipitate for 5 min on ice.

9. Centrifuge at 14,000g to precipitate the protein.

10. Remove the liquid phase, leaving behind the white protein pellet, and transfer it to a clean microcentrifuge tube containing 600 μL of 100% cold isopropanol.

11. Repeatedly invert the tube until the white thread-like strands of DNA appear.

12. Pellet the DNA by centrifugation at 14,000g for 1 min, wash the pellet in 70% ethanol, and resuspend in 50 μL sfH$_2$O.

3.2.2. Restriction Enzyme Digestion

1. Set up a restriction enzyme digestion in a 1.5-mL microcentrifuge tube containing 6 μg of TK6 DNA (prepared as in **Subheading 3.1.1.**). Digest with 10 U *Sau*3AI or a combination of both *Sau*3AI (10 U) and *Xba*I (10 U) in a reaction volume of 50 μL according to the supplier's instructions with the restriction buffer provided.

2. Incubate the reaction at 37°C for 18 h.

3. Inactivate the restriction enzyme(s) by heating the reaction mixture to 70°C for 15 min.

4. Precipitate the DNA by adding 2 vol of ice-cold 100% ethanol and 1/10 vol of 3 M NaOAc, pH 5.2. Incubate at –80°C for 20 min, and then pellet at 14,000g in a microcentrifuge for 20 min at 4°C. Wash the pellet once in 70% ethanol, dry the pellet, and resuspend it in 172 μL of sfH$_2$O.

3.2.3. Ligation Reaction

1. Ligate cleaved DNA from **Subheading 3.2.2.** with 0.05 U of T4 ligase in a 200 μL vol with the addition of 5 μL of 0.1 M spermadine to a final concentration of 2.5 mM (*see* **Note 8**).

2. Allow reaction to proceed for 48 h at 14°C (e.g., using a water bath).
3. Inactivate T4 ligase by heating to 70°C for 10 min.
4. Precipitate DNA by adding 2 vol of ice-cold 100% ethanol and 1/10 vol of 3 M NaOAc, pH 5.2. Incubate at –80°C for 20 min, then pellet at 14,000g in a microcentrifuge for 20 min at 4°C. Wash the pellet once in 70% ethanol, dry the pellet, and resuspend it in 40 µL of sfH$_2$O (*see* **Note 9**).

3.2.4. Inverse PCR

1. Use 100 ng of the ligated DNA from **Subheading 3.2.3.** as a template for nested PCR analysis of the *MLL* gene. PCR is conducted using a nested set of primers to examine both the intron 11 control region and the exon 12 apoptotic cleavage site. Both sets were used identically for 28 cycles in the first round and 18 cycles in the second round at PCR reaction temperatures of 95°C/55°C/72°C for 1 min/step using reaction conditions stated by Perkin Elmer (*see* **Note 10**).
2. Following PCR, analyze the samples by electrophoresis on a 1.2% agarose gel.

3.2.5. Cloning of Inverse PCR Products

1. Stain agarose gels with ethidium bromide and visualize under UV light. Excise bands present in lanes digested with both *Sau*3AI and *Xba*I, and gel-purify using a kit according to the manufacturer's instructions.
2. Clone gel-purified PCR products into pCR4-TOPO and select on plates containing 50 mg/mL ampicillin, according to the manufacturer's instructions.
3. Select and expand resistant colonies in 5 mL each of liquid LB and purify the cloned PCR product by performing a miniprep according to the manufacturer's protocol.
4. Sequence the cloned PCR product using either the T7 or T3 primers.

3.2.6. Translocation Sequence Analysis

1. Search obtained DNA sequences against the NCBI database (http://www.ncbi.nlm.nih.gov/ BLAST/). Select accession numbers providing a match to the input DNA sequence, and analyze the region of DNA extending beyond the point at which it breaks off at *MLL*.

4. Notes

1. This protocol has been successfully conducted on the lymphoblastoid cell lines TK6 and WIL2-NS and the glioblastoma cell lines M059K and M059J. The genomic DNA must be fully resuspended. This can be achieved by resuspending the DNA with 200–350 µL of DNA hydration buffer and incubating it at 65°C for 2–3 h. During this incubation, flick-mix the tubes frequently.
2. The reaction stated is for one sample. It is best to make a master mix of double-stranded linker, T4 DNA ligase buffer, and T4 DNA ligase that can be added to each sample of DNA diluted in the required amount of sfH$_2$O. The master mix provides for greater accuracy in measuring small volumes and uniformity between samples.
3. The 70°C incubation heat-inactivates the T4 DNA ligase.
4. Vortex the DNA dilutions rigorously to ensure uniform solutions.
5. The amount of linker-ligated DNA used for amplification must be titrated. This is done to minimize the signal produced by basal levels of apoptosis in culture. Titrate the linker-ligated DNA to the point at which the break of interest is undetectable in control cells. A good titration range is 1.0–5.0 ng of linker-ligated DNA as template for LM-PCR.
6. Make a master mix of PCR components to ensure PCR reaction uniformity.

7. Use of *Taq* DNA polymerase from Fermentas eliminates the need to optimize $MgCl_2$ concentrations in PCR reactions.

8. The volume of the ligation reaction should not be less than 200 µL. A large volume is necessary to favor intramolecular ligation kinetically.

9. Use of a master mix for PCR ensures equal concentration of reagents in each reaction.

10. DNA pellets resuspended in water can be incubated in a 50°C water bath to solubilize the DNA more readily.

References

1. Super, H. J., McCabe, N. R., Thirman, M. J., et al. (1993) Rearrangements of the *MLL* gene in therapy-related acute myeloid leukemia in patients previously treated with agents targeting DNA-topoisomerase II. *Blood* **82,** 3705–3711.

2. Rowley, J. D. (1993) Rearrangements involving chromosome band 11q23 in acute leukaemia. *Semin. Cancer Biol.* **4,** 377–385.

3. Aplan, P. D., Lombardi, D. P., Ginsberg, A. M., Cossman, J., Bertness, V. L., and Kirsch, I. R. (1990) Disruption of the human SCL locus by "illegitimate" V-(D)-J recombinase activity. *Science* **250,** 1426–1429.

4. Tycko, B. and Sklar, J. (1990) Chromosomal translocations in lymphoid neoplasia: a reappraisal of the recombinase model. *Cancer Cells* **2,** 1–8.

5. Schlissel, M. S. (1998) Structure of nonhairpin coding-end DNA breaks in cells undergoing V(D)J recombination. *Mol. Cell. Biol.* **18,** 2029–2037.

6. Staley, K., Blaschke, A. J., and Chun, J. (1997) Apoptotic DNA fragmentation is detected by a semi-quantitative ligation-mediated PCR of blunt DNA ends. *Cell Death Differ.* **4,** 66–75.

7. Wyllie, A. H. (1980) Glucocorticoid-induced thymocyte apoptosis is associated with endogenous endonuclease activation. *Nature* **284,** 555–556.

8. Richardson, C. and Jasin, M. (2000) Frequent chromosomal translocations induced by DNA double-strand breaks. *Nature* **405,** 697–700.

9. Vaux, D. L. and Strasser, A. (1996) The molecular biology of apoptosis. *Proc. Natl. Acad. Sci. USA* **93,** 2239–2244.

10. Betti, C. J., Villalobos, M. J., Diaz, M. O., and Vaughan, A. T. (2001) Apoptotic triggers initiate translocations within the *MLL* gene involving the nonhomologous end joining repair system. *Cancer Res.* **61,** 4550–4555.

11. Ochman, H., Gerber, A. S., and Hartl, D. L. (1988) Genetic applications of an inverse polymerase chain reaction. *Genetics* **120,** 621–623.

12. Forrester, H. B., Yeh, R. F., and Dewey, W. C. (1999) A dose response for radiation-induced intrachromosomal DNA rearrangements detected by inverse polymerase chain reaction. *Radiat. Res.* **152,** 232–238.

13. Forrester, H. B. and Radford, I. R. (1998) Detection and sequencing of ionizing radiation-induced DNA rearrangements using the inverse polymerase chain reaction. *Int. J. Radiat. Biol.* **74,** 1–15.

14. Ausubel, F. M., Brent, R., Kingston, R. E., et al. (eds.) (1997) *Short Protocols in Molecular Biology.* John Wiley & Sons, New York.

V

ANALYSIS OF DNA REPAIR MECHANISMS

26

Microsatellite Instability

An Indirect Assay to Detect Defects in the Cellular Mismatch Repair Machinery

Anjana Saha, Narendra K. Bairwa, and Ramesh Bamezai

Summary

The DNA mismatch repair (MMR) pathway plays a prominent role in the correction of errors made during DNA replication and genetic recombination and in the repair of small deletions and loops in DNA. Mismatched nucleotides can occur by replication error, damage to nucleotide precursors, damage to DNA, or during heteroduplex formation between two homologous DNA molecules in the process of genetic recombination. Defects in MMR can precipitate instability in simple sequence repeats (SSRs), also referred to as microsatellite instability (MSI), which appears to be important in certain types of cancers, both spontaneous and hereditary. Variation in the highly polymorphic alleles of specific microsatellite repeats can be identified using PCR with primers derived from the unique flanking sequences. These PCR products are analyzed on denaturing polyacrylamide gels to resolve differences in allele sizes of more than 2 bp. Although $(CA)_n$ repeats are the most abundant class among dinucleotide SSRs, trinucleotide and tetranucleotide repeats are also frequent. These polymorphic repeats have the advantage of producing band patterns that are easy to analyze and can be used as an indication of a possible MMR defect in a cell. The presumed association between such allelic variation and an MMR defect should be confirmed by molecular analysis of the structure and/or expression of MMR genes.

Key Words: Allele sizes; denaturing PAGE; loss of heterozygosity (LOH); microsatellite instability (MSI); microsatellite markers; mismatch repair (MMR) genes; DNA sequencing; simple sequence repeats (SSRs); simple sequence length polymorphism (SSLP).

1. Introduction

DNA repair is present in all organisms as a major defense against damage to cellular DNA. It is involved in processes that minimize cell killing, mutations, replication errors, persistence of DNA damage, and genomic instability. DNA mismatch repair (MMR) has a prominent role in the correction of errors made during DNA replication and genetic recombination. The MMR pathway is responsible for detecting and repair-

From: *Methods in Molecular Biology, vol. 291, Molecular Toxicology Protocols*
Edited by: P. Keohavong and S. G. Grant © Humana Press Inc., Totowa, NJ

ing short segments of mismatched base pairs, such as T opposite G, or an addition of extra nucleotides, resulting in unpaired bases within the DNA. Thus, MMR recognizes normal nucleotides that are either unpaired or paired with a noncomplementary nucleotide. The formation of mismatched nucleotides can occur by polymerase misincorporations (i.e., replication error), damage to nucleotide precursors, damage to DNA, or heteroduplex formation between two homologous DNA molecules during genetic recombination. Rapid repair of replicative errors provides the genome with a protection against mutation and guards the genome by preventing recombination between nonhomologous regions of DNA *(1,2)*.

In *E. coli*, methyl-directed MMR involves the products of the mutator genes *mutS*, *mutL*, *mutH*, and *uvrD*. In vitro, MutS is a DNA mismatch-binding protein, UvrD is a DNA helicase II, and MutH is an endonuclease that incises at the transiently unmethylated DNA strand *(3)*. In eukaryotes, the mismatch repair system is more complex. Genetic studies have demonstrated that the major DNA mismatch repair pathway in *Streptomyces cerevisiae* requires three bacterial MutS homologs, MSH2, MSH3, and MSH6, and two bacterial MutL homologs, MLH1 and PMS1. Human homologs of the yeast mismatch repair genes *hMSH2*, *hMLH1*, and *hPMS2* have been identified and have been shown to be mutated in patients and their kindred with hereditary nonpolyposis colon cancer (HNPCC) *(1,2,4)*.

The first clue that an MMR defect might be responsible for HNPCC came from the observation of a previously unrecognized phenomenon in colon cancer cells from patients with HNPCC. These tumors often exhibited "ladders" of new microsatellite alleles created by insertion and deletion of multiples of the repeat length in tumor DNA compared with nonneoplastic DNA. The addition of novel microsatellite alleles in the tumor was called microsatellite instability (MSI). In HNPCC, MSI was discovered to be the result of germline mutations in the MMR genes.

MSI occurs mainly because of DNA biosynthetic errors that are generated by DNA polymerase and escape the proofreading mechanism *(5)*. Strand slippages result in misaligned intermediates in repetitive sequences, creating the potential for insertion and deletion mutations if they are not corrected prior to replication in the subsequent cell cycle, as in MMR-deficient cells *(6,7)*. Because microsatellite repeats fall into this category, tumors from patients with HNPCC have elevated mutation rates in microsatellite sequences, and monitoring of MSI has become an indirect, semiquantitative tool to characterize MMR. Experiments demonstrating how certain DNA-damaging agents can transiently inactivate the MMR system by saturating its repair capacity, creating a temporary "mutator" phenotype with MSI, have reinforced the ability of MSI to assess the MMR status of a cell *(9)*.

As the list of MMR proteins grows, studies are beginning to identify many ways that these proteins can mix and match to generate distinct complexes with specificities for different substrates involved in meiotic recombination, base mismatch repair, and the repair of small deletions and loops in DNA *(3,8)*. Biochemical studies have demonstrated that mismatch recognition is mediated primarily by a heterodimer of *hMSH2* and *hMSH6*. Interestingly, although mutations in the *hMSH2* gene are shown to segregate frequently with HNPCC *(10,11)*, *hMSH6* has been shown to be mutated to date in only a few atypical HNPCC families, as well as in a few sporadic colon tumors *(12)*.

Moreover, there are significant differences between the mutator phenotypes of cell lines lacking *hMSH2* or *hMSH6*, inasmuch as both are deficient in the correction of base/base mismatches, but only the former is also deficient in the repair of insertion/deletion loops, resulting in MSI *(13)*. The hMSH2/6 heterodimer has been shown to recognize base/base mispairs efficiently, but its affinity for loops of more than one extra helical nucleotide is relatively low, depending on flanking sequence context. In later studies, it was shown that a third MutS homolog, hMSH3, could form a heterodimer with hMSH2 and that this latter complex efficiently recognizes loops of two or more extrahelical nucleotides. Thus, the two MSH heterodimers, hMSH2/6 and hMSH2/3, are functionally complementary in the correction of slippage products in insertion/deletion loops *(14,15)*.

Defective MMR results in abnormalities in the processes of DNA repair that have been implicated in carcinogenesis and aging. It has been suggested that MMR defects are themselves procarcinogenic and may also be involved in the development of resistance to cancer chemotherapy. This chapter describes gel-based radioactive and nonradioactive methods to detect an MMR defect indirectly by analyzing microsatellite sequence variation in matched samples of tumor and nontumor DNA.

2. Materials

2.1. Genomic DNA Isolation

1. Lysis buffer: 0.32 M sucrose (autoclaved), 5 mM MgCl$_2$, 0.01 M Tris-HCl, pH 8.0, 1% Triton X-100. Store at room temperature.
2. Digestion buffer: 100 mM NaCl, 25 mM EDTA, 0.5% sodium dodecyl sulfate (SDS), 10 mM Tris-HCl, pH 8.0.
3. Phenol equilibrated with 0.1 M Tris-HCl, pH 8.0. Use gloves and store at 4°C.
4. Chloroform.
5. Isoamyl alcohol.
6. 3 M Sodium acetate, pH 5.2.
7. Absolute ethanol (Merck, Mumbai, India).
8. TE buffer: 10 mM Tris-HCl, pH 8.0, 1 mM EDTA, pH 8.0.
9. Gel loading dye: 0.25% bromophenol blue, 0.25% xylene cyanol, 0.25% and 30% glycerol. Use gloves and store at 4°C.
10. TBE buffer: 80 mM Tris-base, 40 mM boric acid, 2 mM EDTA. Make as 10X stock solution, and store at room temperature.
11. Ethidium bromide: 10 mg/mL stock solution in autoclaved distilled water. Use gloves, protect from direct light, and store at 4°C.
12. 1% Agarose in 1X TBE buffer.
13. Genomic DNA diluted in autoclaved distilled water from test samples to be analyzed. Store at 4°C.

2.2. Polymerase Chain Reaction

Use gloves to handle.

1. Sterile PCR tubes.
2. PCR kit: reaction buffer, enzyme, dNTP mix, [α^{32}P]dCTP (e.g., Amersham Pharmacia, Piscataway, NJ). Store at –20°C.

3. Primers for microsatellite region. Store at –20°C until use and after.
4. Mineral oil. Store at room temperature.
5. Thermal cycler (e.g., MJ Research, Miami, FL).

2.3. Preparation of Polyacrylamide Gel and Gel Electrophoresis

1. Autoclaved distilled water.
2. Sequencing gel apparatus.
3. Sigmacoat (Sigma). Store at 4°C.
4. 29:1 Acrylamide/*bis*-acrylamide stock. Store at 4°C.
5. Urea.
6. 10X TBE running buffer: 0.8 M Tris-base, 0.4 M boric acid, 20 mM EDTA.
7. Stop buffer or loading dye: 0.25% bromophenol blue, 0.25% xylene cyanole, 1 mM EDTA, 95% formamide, 5% 1X TBE (e.g., Sigma). Store at 4°C.
8. Sequencing gel apparatus (e.g., Bio-Rad, Hercules, CA).
9. Power pack (e.g., Bio-Rad PAC 3000).

2.4. Processing of Denaturing Acrylamide Gel Data for Analysis

1. Phosphorimager (e.g., Shimmazdu) or, alternatively, X-ray film and X-ray film developing solutions. (e.g., Kodak and Sigma).

2.5. Agarose Purification of DNA Bands

1. Agarose, molecular biology grade (e.g., Sigma or Pronadisa, Rehovot, Israel).
2. Tris-saturated phenol, pH 8.0. Store at 4°C.
3. 3 M Sodium acetate, pH 5.2. Store at room temperature.
4. Absolute ethanol.

2.6. Ligation of DNA Bands for Sequencing

1. PCR product ligation kit (e.g., Promega, Madison, WI).
2. Insert DNA.

2.7. Transformation of Ligated Product and Screening of Positive Clones

1. Competent bacterial cells (e.g., DH5α).
2. Sterile culture plates.
3. Luria broth medium.
4. Ampicillin. Store at –20°C.

2.8. Sequencing Reactions for Confirming and Determining Microsatellite Allele Sizes

1. PCR tubes.
2. Primers for sequencing the allele (e.g., Genemed Synthesis, South San Francisco, CA).
3. Sequenase-dye termination kit (e.g., Epicentre, Madison, WI).
4. Mineral oil (e.g., Sigma).
5. Thermal cycler (e.g., MJ Research).

2.9. Preparation of Polyacrylamide Gel for Nonradioactive Microsatellite Marker Analysis

1. Autoclaved distilled water.
2. Acrylamide/*bis*-acrylamide stock (19:1).
3. Ammonium persulfate (APS; 10%) and TEMED.
4. 1X TBE buffer: 80 mM Tris-base, 40 mM boric acid, and 2 mM EDTA. Make as a 10X stock solution.
5. Gel loading dye: 98% formamide, 10 mM EDTA, 0.05% bromophenol blue, 0.05% xylene cyanole.

3. Methods

3.1. Preparation of Template

Set up all reactions on ice.

1. Isolate total genomic DNA from blood samples using a standard genomic DNA isolation protocol (*see* **Notes 1** and **2**).
2. Check the quality of DNA by running an 0.8% agarose gel at a low voltage of 40–50 V. Mix the genomic DNA with 1/6 volume of gel loading dye and load onto the wells. Visualize the high-quality genomic DNA on a UV transilluminator; it should be seen as a single band without shearing.
3. Quantify the DNA by taking the optical density (OD$_{260}$) spectrophotometrically, dilute the samples at a concentration of 25 ng/µL in autoclaved distal water, and store at –20°C until analysis (*see* **Note 3**).

3.2. Polymerase Chain Reaction for Amplification of Microsatellite Markers (see Notes 4 and 5)

1. 12.5 µL vol for polymerase chain reaction (PCR) reaction of each sample includes a microsatellite marker primer set: 6.25 pM of each primer, 10 ng target DNA, 100 nM dNTPs, 1X PCR reaction buffer, 0.5 U *Taq* polymerase (*see* **Note 6**) and [α^{32}P]dCTP.
2. Process the PCR reaction for 25 cycles with denaturation at 94°C for 2 min, annealing at 55–65°C for 30 s, and extension at 72°C for 1 min and a final extension at 72°C for 5 min (*see* **Notes 7** and **8**).
3. Stop the PCR by adding 3 µL of stop buffer containing formamide.

3.3. Preparation of Denaturing Polyacrylamide Gel for Microsatellite Marker Analysis

1. Clean the sequencing gel plates very well with distilled water.
2. Wipe the plates with absolute ethanol.
3. Coat one of the sequencing gel plates with fresh Sigmacoat.
4. Clean spacers with absolute ethanol and place securely on the bottom plate. Secure the plates properly with clamps.
5. Clean the shark-tooth comb with absolute ethanol, and keep it ready to be inserted between the two plates after pouring the gel mix.

6. Prepare the gel mix (8%) by adding 5.7 g of acrylamide, 0.3 g of *bis*-acrylamide, 31.5 g of urea (8 *M*), 7.5 mL of 10X TBE, 300 µL of 10% APS, and 20 µL of TEMED. Mix all the constituents properly, and pour between the two plates (*see* **Notes 9–11**).
7. Leave the assembly undisturbed until the gel is polymerized.
8. Denature the samples at 95°C for 5 min, and chill immediately on ice for 5 min prior to loading.
9. Load around 3 µL vol of each reaction into the appropriate well of the denaturing gel, and electrophorese at a high temperature of 40–45°C at constant watt (45 W) for 2–4 h (*see* **Note 12**).

3.4. Processing of Denaturing Acrylamide Gels for Microsatellite Analysis

1. After completion of the gel run, fix the gel in 10% methanol, 10% acetic acid for 15–20 min, and wash the urea; then carefully transfer it onto a 3MM Whatman sheet and dry in a gel dryer.
2. Use phosphorimager intensifying plates to expose the dried gel, and analyze the results in a phosphorimager. Alternatively, expose the gel to X-ray film and develop. (*See* **Fig. 1** and **Notes 13** and **14**.)

3.5. Agarose Purification of DNA Bands From Samples, Which Differ in Mobility Shift (Depicting MSI) in Denaturing Gel

1. Excise the PCR-amplified product from the agarose gel, and put gel fragment in a 1.5-mL microcentrifuge tube (*see* **Note 14**).
2. Add 1 mL of saturated phenol, pH 8.0, to the tube and freeze it at –80°C. Take out the frozen tube, and thaw it completely.
3. Repeat the freeze-thaw steps three times (**steps 1** and **2**).
4. Take out the frozen tube containing the agarose piece, and centrifuge at a high speed of 16,000g for 20 min at room temperature.
5. Take out the aqueous phase, and transfer to a fresh tube. Add an equal volume of chloroform to the tube, mix, and centrifuge again at 13,500g for 10 min.
6. Transfer the aqueous phase, add 1/10 vol of 3 *M* sodium acetate, pH 5.2, and make up to 1 mL with absolute ethanol. Allow the DNA to precipitate for 30–45 min at –20°C.
7. Centrifuge at 16,000g at 4°C for 20 min to precipitate the DNA.
8. Wash the DNA pellet with chilled 70% ethanol for 10 min at 4°C.
9. Dry the pellet and finally dissolve it in 10 µL of autoclaved distilled water.
10. Check the quality of the DNA by running on an agarose gel, and quantitate concentration (*see* **Subheading 3.1.**, **step 3**).

3.6. Ligation of Gel-Eluted Product for Determination of Allele Size or Repeats

1. Mix 2X reaction buffer, T-tailed Vector (e.g., pGEM-T Promega ligation kit), enzyme (ligase), and DNA insert (gel-eluted product) in a 0.5-mL microcentrifuge tube. Mix well, and make up the volume to 10 µL (per instructions given in, e.g., Promega PCR ligation kit. Determine the quantity of insert required for carrying out ligation according to kit instructions.)
2. Incubate at 16°C for 4–6 h, followed by an overnight incubation at 4°C.

3.7. Transformation of Ligated Product and Screening of Positive Clones

1. Carry out the transformation using competent cells of *E. coli* strain (e.g., DH5α, XL-1).
2. Rescreen for positive clones through colony PCR using the same set of primers as was used for amplifying the genomic DNA, under the same PCR conditions as given in **Subheading 3.2.**

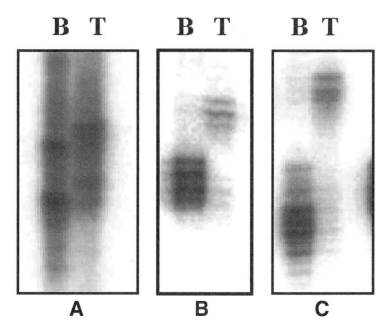

Fig. 1. (**A–C**) Microsatellite instability (MSI) observed with microsatellite markers in breast tumors (lane B, blood DNA; lane T, tumor DNA) by the radioactive method (8% denaturing polyacrylamide gel).

3.8. Recombinant Plasmid Isolation From Positive Clones for Sequencing of Insert (Amplified Microsatellite Region)

1. Grow positive clones overnight in 5 mL of LB medium.
2. Isolate the plasmid as described in the plasmid isolation kit (e.g., Sigma or Promega).

3.9. Sequencing of Plasmid With Microsatellite Insert

1. For each template, label four 0.5-mL PCR tubes "G," "A," "T," and "C," respectively.
2. Aliquot 2 µL each of ddGTP mix, ddATP mix, ddTTP mix, and ddCTP mix into the corresponding microcentrifuge tubes.
3. For each template (containing set of four tubes: G, A, T, C), prepare a master mix consisting of 7.2 µL of 3.5X reaction buffer, template (plasmid with insert DNA), 0.7 µL of 15 pmols/µL sequencing primer, 0.5 µL of labeled dNTP (^{32}P-dCTP/dATP), 1.0 of enzyme (e.g., Epicentre sequencing reaction kit), and water to make up the volume to 17 µL.
4. Gently vortex the mix, then briefly spin down the tube containing the master mix.
5. Dispense 4 µL of the master mix in each of tube containing ddGTP mix, ddATP mix, ddTTP mix, and ddCTP mix. Mix them by pipeting up and down a few times, and finally overlay the reaction mix with mineral oil.
6. Carry out sequencing reactions in a thermal cycler using the following conditions: denaturation at 95°C for 30 s, annealing at 42°C for 30 s, extension at 72°C for 1 min; repeat the cycle 30 times, followed by a final extension for 10 min at 72°C.
7. Stop each reaction by adding 2 µL of stop buffer provided with the sequencing kit.

B   T

GATC GAT C

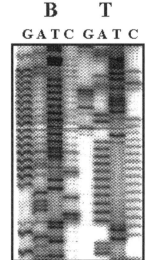

Fig. 2. Partial sequence showed $(CA/GT)_n$ repeats of variant alleles in blood and tumor DNA (8% denaturing polyacrylamide gel). Lane B, blood DNA; lane T, tumor DNA.

3.10. Preparation of Polyacrylamide Gel for Sequencing of Microsatellite Product

1. Prepare and run the gel as described in **Subheading 3.3.**
2. Fix and process the gel as described in **Subheading 3.4.**
3. Develop the gel to read the microsatellite sequence (*see* **Fig. 2**).

3.11. Preparation of Polyacrylamide Gel (10–12%) for Nonradioactive Microsatellite Marker Study

1. Prepare the gel apparatus as described in **Subheading 3.3., steps 1–5**.
2. Prepare (20%) acrylamide stock of 19:1 acrylamide/*bis*-acrylamide, and filter it, and store it at 4°C. Prepare the required gel concentration from the stock solution when required as described in **Subheading 3.3., step 6**.
3. Leave the assembly undisturbed until the gel is polymerized.
4. Prepare the samples by adding appropriate amplicons and 2 µL of dye (98% formamide, 10 m*M* EDTA, 0.05% bromophenol blue, and 0.05% xylene cyanol) in each sample. Make up the volume to 10 µL.
5. Load the full volume of each reaction into the appropriate well of the nondenaturing gel, and electrophorese at room temperature at 120 V for different time periods depending on the length of the amplicon (*see* **Note 12**).

3.12. Processing of Nondenaturing Acrylamide Gels for MSI Analysis

1. After completion of the gel run, stain the gel in ethidium bromide stain and visualize on a UV transilluminator.

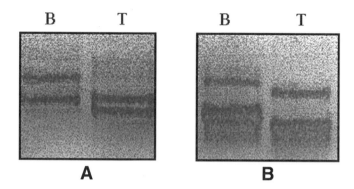

Fig. 3. (**A,B**) Microsatellite instability (MSI) observed with microsatellite markes in breast tumors (lane B, blood DNA; lane T, tumor DNA) by the nonradioactive method (silver-stained nondenurating polyacrylamide gel).

2. For storage of the gels and further processing, fix the gel in 10% ethanol/0.5% acetic acid for 15–20 min.
3. Stain the gel in 0.1% silver nitrate solution for 30 min.
4. Wash the gel properly three times with distilled water.
5. Develop in 1.5% sodium hydroxide solution in the presence of 400 μL of formaldehyde until the bands appear.
6. Finally, when bands start appearing, replace the solution with 0.75% sodium bicarbonate solution until the bands become intense.
7. Stop, and store the gels in 2% acetic acid (*see* **Fig. 3**).

4. Notes

1. While isolating genomic DNA, handle with care to minimize the shearing of DNA.
2. DNA is better purified with phenol/chloroform.
3. Target template should be well-quantified because PCR sensitivity and product amplification are directly correlated.
4. For all PCR reactions, use fresh sterile tips, tubes, and aseptic bench area.
5. The protocol describes the analysis of MSI through simple sequence length polymorphism (SSLP) analysis. The primers used should flank the microsatellite loci of interest and be specific to avoid amplification of any undesirable region in the genome.
6. High-proofreading-activity polymerase is preferred to other polymerases.
7. The PCR conditions should be standardized for each microsatellite marker under study. Optimization or standardization of cycling conditions may be required for specific PCR product apart from other factors, e.g., $MgCl_2$, target concentration, annealing temperature, and so on.
8. For microsatellite PCR primer standardization, three-step touch-down PCR is preferred (three different annealing temperatures to obtain specific product and to avoid short size products).
9. APS should be freshly prepared.
10. Filter the gel mix before adding APS and TEMED.

11. While polymerizing the gel, avoid air bubbles in the gel matrix.
12. Wash the wells properly to remove traces of urea prior to sample loading, using a syringe and a needle; otherwise smiling and distortion of bands may occur.
13. While analyzing the results of microsatellite marker study, the most intense band should be considered the authentic band, as there may be "stutter" bands.
14. Any indecision in band shifts can be removed by repeating the PCR either fresh or by reamplifying the eluted variant band.

References

1. Fishel, R., Acharya, S., Berardini, M., et al. (2000) Signalling mismatch repair: the mechanics of an adenosine-nucleotide molecular switch. *Cold Spring Harbor Symp. Quant. Biol.* **65,** 217–224.
2. Yang, W., Junop, M. S., Ban, C., Obmolova, G., and Hsieh, P. (2000) DNA mismatch repair: from structure to mechanism. *Cold Spring Harbor Symp. Quant. Biol.* **65,** 225–232.
3. Modrich, P. and Lahue, R. (1996) Mismatch repair in replication fidelity, genetic recombination, and cancer biology. *Annu. Rev. Biochem.* **65,** 101–133.
4. Schär, P. and Jiricny, J. (1998) Eukaryotic mismatch repairs, in: *Nucleic Acids and Molecular Biology*, vol. 12 (Eckstein, F. and Lilley, D. M. J., eds.), Springer-Verlag, New York.
5. Minnick, D. T. and Kunkel, T. A. (1996) DNA synthesis errors, mutators and cancer. *Cancer Surv.* **28,** 3–20.
6. Buermeyer, A. B., Deshenes, S. M., Baker, S. M., and Liskey, R. M. (1999) Mammalian DNA mismatch repair. *Annu. Rev. Genet.* **33,** 533–564.
7. Bebenek, K. and Kunkel, T. A. (2000) Streisinger revisited: DNA synthesis errors mediated by substrate misalignments. *Cold Spring Harbor Symp. Quant. Biol.* **65,** 81–91.
8. Jiricny, J. (1998) Replication errors: challenging the genome. *EMBO J.* **17,** 6427–6436.
9. Miller, J. H., Yeung, A., Funchain, P., et al. (2000) Temporary and permanent mutators lacking the mismatch repair system: the enhancement of mutators in cell populations. *Cold Spring Harbor Symp. Quant. Biol.* **65,** 241–252.
10. Kolodner, R. D. (1995) Mismatch repair: mechanisms and relationship to cancer susceptibility. *Trends Biochem. Sci.* **20,** 397–401.
11. Jiricny, J. (1996) Mismatch repair and cancer. *Cancer Surv.* **28,** 47–68.
12. Papadopoulos, N., Nicolaides, N. C., Liu, B., et al. (1995) Mutations of GTBP in genetically unstable cells. *Science* **268,** 1915–1917.
13. Kunkel, T. A. (1993) Nucleotide repeats. Slippery DNA and diseases. *Nature* **365,** 207–208.
14. Palombo, F., Iaccarino, I., Nakajima, E., Ikejima, M., Shimada, T., and Jiricny, J. (1996) hMutb, a heterodimer of hMSH2 and hMSH3, binds to insertion/deletion loops in DNA. *Curr. Biol.* **6,** 1181–1184.
15. Iaccarino, I., Marra, G., Dufner, P., and Jiricny, J. (2000) Mutation in the magnesium-binding site of hMSH6 disables the hMutS-alpha sliding clamp from translocating along DNA. *J. Biol. Chem.* **275,** 2080–2086.

27

Unscheduled DNA Synthesis

A Functional Assay for Global Genomic Nucleotide Excision Repair

Crystal M. Kelly and Jean J. Latimer

Summary

The unscheduled DNA synthesis (UDS) assay measures a cell's ability to perform global genomic nucleotide excision repair (NER). This chapter provides instructions for the application of this technique in living cells by creating 6-4 photoproducts and pyrimidine dimers using UVC irradiation, then allowing for their repair. Repair is quantified by the amount of radioactive thymidine incorporated after this insult, and the length of time allowed for this incorporation is specific for repair of particular lesions. Radioactivity is evaluated by grain counting after autoradiography. The results are used to diagnosis repair-deficient disorders clinically and provide a basis for investigation of repair deficiency in human tissues or tumors. At the present time, no other functional assay is available that directly measures the capacity to perform NER on the entire genome without the use of specific antibodies. Since live cells are required for this assay, explant culture techniques must be previously established. Host cell reactivation, as discussed in Chapter 28, is not an equivalent technique, as it specifically measures transcription-coupled repair at active genes, a subset of total NER.

Key Words: Unscheduled DNA synthesis (UDS); nucleotide excision repair (NER); DNA repair; DNA damage; UV light; pyrimidine dimers; 6-4 photoproducts; global genomic repair (GGR); transcription coupled repair (TCR).

1. Introduction

Long patch, or nucleotide excision repair (NER), is the primary process by which cyclobutane pyrimidine dimers, 6-4 photoproducts, and DNA crosslinks are removed from DNA *(1,2)*. Ultraviolet $(UV)_{254 \text{ nm}}$ light (UVC), as well as UV mimetic drugs, induces DNA lesions that are corrected by this pathway. Damage lesions caused by agents that act as inter- and intrastrand crosslinkers, such as cisplatin *(3)*, covalently bind to DNA, creating "bulky" adducts such as *N*-acetoxyaminoacetylfluorene (AAAF) *(4)* and, perhaps, alkylating agents such as cyclophosphamide *(5,6)* are also remediated by this pathway. NER is a complicated process requiring the protein

From: *Methods in Molecular Biology, vol. 291, Molecular Toxicology Protocols*
Edited by: P. Keohavong and S. G. Grant © Humana Press Inc., Totowa, NJ

products of 25–30 genes *(7)*. NER involves the recognition of a damage lesion causing distortion of the DNA helix, incisions flanking the lesion on the damaged strand, excision of 27–29 bases including the damage lesion, and replication and ligation to replace the excised information and seal the strand breaks at each end of the newly synthesized region *(8–11)*. This pathway can also be recruited for other types of DNA damage lesions that have not been corrected by base excision and other single-stranded DNA repair mechanisms *(12,13)*. In effect, the NER pathway provides redundancy for these other repair systems should they be overwhelmed by a genotoxic exposure *(1)*.

Human cells perform NER at two levels: the rapid and efficient removal of lesions that block ongoing transcription and thus need to be eliminated quickly, also known as transcription-coupled repair (TCR) *(14,15)*, and the slower, less efficient repair of bulk DNA, including the nontranscribed strand of active genes, also referred to as global genomic repair (GGR). In addition, the sense strand of the actively transcribed gene is repaired before the antisense strand.

NER of the overall genome can be measured quantitatively using the unscheduled DNA synthesis assay (UDS). The UDS assay involves the measurement of labeled base incorporation into the DNA after in vitro exposure to UV light or certain chemicals (**Fig. 1**). The UDS assay is a cell-autonomous, functional assay, in that it allows one to look at the complex process of NER as a whole, at least as it is expressed in a particular cell type *(16–18)*. As applied in our laboratory, this assay predominantly quantifies the repair of UV-induced DNA 6-4 photoproducts, and elements of both the GGR as well as the TCR components of NER contribute to the results (*see* **Note 1**).

The autoradiographic UDS assay requires the analysis of living cells. It has previously been applied primarily to skin fibroblasts and peripheral blood lymphocytes (PBLs) for diagnosis of xeroderma pigmentosum (XP) and other DNA repair diseases impacting specifically on the NER pathway. Classical NER deficiency disorders are characterized by UV sensitivity manifesting mainly in the skin and cornea *(1)*.

Studies involving functional assays in general, and specifically functional assays of DNA repair capacity, have been hampered by a technical lack of ability to perform primary explant culture on all cell types. The one notable exception is that of rat hepatocyte primary cultures, which have been used extensively in UDS assays for evaluation of the carcinogenic potential of chemicals *(19,20)*. Although repair assays can be performed on established, transformed cell lines, the generation of cell lines from normal adult tissue has proved to be a technical challenge. In addition, during the process of passaging, established cell lines undergo clonal evolution that may alter or extinguish many of the original characteristics of the cells, including their intrinsic repair capacity *(21,22)*.

Until recently, cell culture techniques have not existed to support primary culture explants of most human tissues. These tissues require attachment to a substratum of some sort of extracellular matrix. Our laboratory has developed methods for primary culture of various cell types *(23,24)*.

The UDS assay was first described by Rassmussen and Painter *(25)*. Its name stems from the fact that the assay evaluates the DNA repair mechanisms of cells in all stages

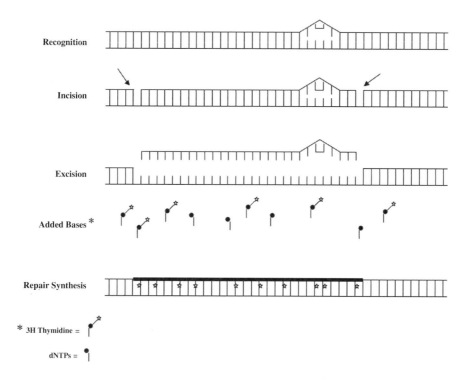

Fig. 1. NER schematic as measured by the UDS assay. The assay involves damaging cells with UVC light, then allowing the cells to repair themselves over a designated period of time. The UV light causes the formation of pyrimidine dimers and 6-4 photoproducts. Over time, the cells utilize the NER pathway to remove a single-stranded DNA molecule containing 23–27 bases including the damage lesion. Resynthesis of the removed strand is then performed in the presence of radioactive thymidine. The amount of repair is therefore correlated with the total incorporation of radioactive thymidine.

of replication except synthesis or S phase, when "scheduled" DNA synthesis of the entire genome takes place. (We know of no technique that will measure NER during S phase.) There are two methods of quantifying data from the assay: autoradiography and scintillation counting. Autoradiography is the preferred method and is described in this chapter. Although it is labor-intensive, software packages have been designed in an attempt to remove the human subjectivity of this aspect of data analysis *(26–28)*. However, our laboratory still performs grain counting with two to three independent counters on each slide, because the current software is still inadequate for appreciating the differences between, for example, darkly stained nucleoli and silver grains in some cases. An additional problem with the automated counting system is the fact that emulsion is more than one focal-length thick; i.e., one has to focus up and down to see all of the silver grains over a nucleus. Finding rare cells can also be difficult without integrating control of an automated stage into the grain counting software program. The greatest strength of software-based grain counting is the evaluation of background, as this is the area in which individual reader subjectivity is greatest.

Scintillation counting is a simplified form of the autoradiographic assay that was popularized in industry for the hepatocyte evaluation of mutagenic chemicals. In order for it to be accurate, all the S-phase cells have to be eliminated. from the analysis, because radiolabel incorporation during replicative synthesis is orders of magnitude greater than during repair synthesis. In an attempt to achieve this, the use of hydrox-yurea was incorporated into the original UDS protocol. However, we have found that up to 40% of S phase cells can still persist in the presence of hydroxyurea, which would significantly affect the results and render them inaccurate. Indeed, because S-phase nuclei incorporate hundreds of times more radioactive label than non-S-phase cells, only a few cells that happen to be in synthesis mode would render these experiments quite inaccurate. We therefore recommend the autoradiographic form of this assay over the scintillation counting form, which probably should only be used to determine rough trends. Autoradiography has the added benefit of allowing the counter to deter-mine different cell types present on each slide and evaluate each type for NER.

Controls for use in combination with this assay can include commercially avail-able, repair-deficient XP cell lines. Our laboratory usually utilizes foreskin fibroblasts (FF) as a positive standard for comparison. These cells can reliably be used as extended explants up to passage 13. Explants beyond 13 passages show a decreasing repair capacity relative to the earliest passages. We have recently demonstrated considerable tissue variation in NER capacity, suggesting that a tissue-matched control should also be used *(23,24)*. For lymphocyte studies, we recommend the lymphoblastoid cell line TK6 *(23)*, although transformed cell lines do not always accurately reflect the NER capacity of their progenitor tissue.

Published doses of UV irradiation utilized for UDS experiments range from 5–50 J/M^2. It is recommended that a dose–response curve be performed to determine the optimal dose of UVC for a given cell type.

2. Materials

2.1. Cell Irradiation, Labeling, and Fixation

1. Viable experimental samples (*see* **Note 2**).
2. Positive (and, if appropriate, negative) controls, including "tester" slides (*see* **Notes 3–5**).
3. Two-chamber chamber slides (made by Nunc, ordered from Fisher Scientific, Pittsburgh, PA), two to four slides per sample; controls, four slides minimum.
4. 10-cm^2 Round cell tissue culture dish (one per chamber slide; made by Corning, ordered from Fisher).
5. Whatman filter paper (3-mm CHR in 35 × 45-cm sheets; Thomas Scientific, Swedesboro, NJ) cut into 2.5 × 5-cm strips, wrapped in tinfoil and autoclaved (one strip per chamber slide).
6. Appropriate growth medium for each type of cell that will be analyzed.
7. Fetal bovine serum (FBS; Hyclone, Logan, UT).
8. Sterile tissue culture hood (class IIA/B3 Biological Safety Cabinet, Forma Scientific, Marietta, OH).
9. Tissue culture incubator with 5% CO_2 (ThermoForma Series II Water Jacketed CO_2 Incu-bator, Forma Scientific).

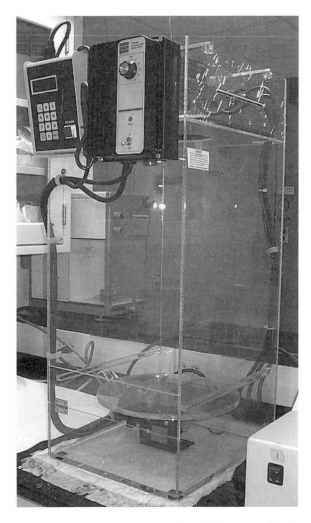

Fig. 2. Specialized UV irradiation device created to deliver a specific damaging dosage of UVC light. The machine consists of three appropriate UV bulbs, a turntable, and a timed shutter, all enclosed by plexiglass. The distance from the bulbs to the sample determines the amount of DNA damage the device can induce over a set time.

10. Vortex mixer.
11. UV delivery device (Design Specialties, Bethel Park, PA; **Fig. 2**) *(29)*.
12. Short-wave UV meter (e.g., Spectroline model DM-254XA, Spectronics, Westbury, NY).
13. 80 Ci/mmol [³H]thymidine (NET 027Z, New England Nuclear, Boston, MA). Thaw and allow to warm to room temperature before use (*see* **Note 6**).
14. Hot thymidine incubation medium: 10 µCi [³H]thymidine label (80 Ci/mmol) per mL of appropriate medium for each cell type, including serum and 1X penicillin-streptomycin (10,000 U/mL penicillin G sodium, 100,000 µg/mL streptomycin sulfate in 85% saline,

Invitrogen [Gibco], Carlsbad, CA). For example, for 20 slides, in a total volume of 20 mL of medium with serum, 200 µL of label are added. Add [^{3}H]thymidine to the medium immediately before use.

15. Cold thymidine chase medium: medium of choice supplemented with 10^{-3} M thymidine nucleoside (Sigma, St. Louis, MO). Add 10% serum just prior to use and filter through a 0.4-µm filter (Nalgene, through Fisher; *see* **Note 7**).
16. 1X Salt sodium citrate (SSC; Sigma).
17. 100 mL 70% Ethanol (made fresh to prevent evaporation; AAPER, Shelbyville, KY).
18. 33% Acetic acid (Fisher) in ethanol (made fresh), total 100 mL.
19. Scalpel.
20. Two hemostats.
21. Vertical glass slide Copeland jars (Fisher). Each holds five slides, so the number needed depends on the size of the experiment.
22. 4% Perchloric acid (diluted from stock 60% perchloric acid [Fisher]). **Caution:** store in a fume hood; can be explosive. Need about 60 mL per Copeland jar.

2.2. Slide Processing I: Dipping in Emulsion

1. Rectangular glass slide jars with glass slide holders (Fisher). Each holds 10 slides.
2. Distilled water.
3. Paper towels.
4. Sealed darkroom (*see* **Note 8**).
5. Kodak Radiography Emulsion NTB-2, approx 4.0 oz, stored at 4°C (*see* **Note 9**).
6. 48°C Water bath in the darkroom.
7. Lab tape.
8. 50-, 400-, and 1000-mL beakers.
9. Amersham dipping chamber (Piscataway, NJ).
10. Darkroom drying box (*see* **Fig. 3**).
11. Light-tight slide boxes containing desiccant at one end behind a glass slide.
12. Regular and heavy-duty aluminum foil.
13. Refrigerator.

2.3. Slide Processing II: Developing Emulsion

1. Four rectangular glass slide dishes (Fisher).
2. Three lab timers (VWR, Pittsburgh, PA).
3. Tap water and ice.
4. Medium-sized plastic developing tray (Gage Industrial, Lake Oswego, OR).
5. Thermometer.
6. Kodak D-19 Developer, stored at 4°C (Eastman Kodak, Rochester, NY).
7. Kodak fixer, stored at 4°C (Eastman Kodak).
8. Two glass staining dishes for slides (Copeland jars).
9. 0.5 g Giemsa powder (Fisher).
10. Glycerol.
11. 60°C Water bath.
12. Methanol.
13. Stirring plate.
14. Parafilm.
15. Whatman filter paper (3-mm CHR) and funnel.
16. 100-mL Brown glass bottle.

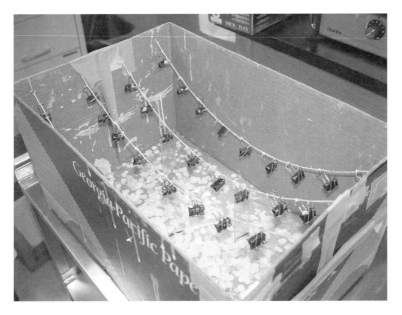

Fig. 3. An example of a drying box for slides just dipped in emulsion. It is best to have a box with a removable lid (in this example, a copier paper box). Four pieces of string are strung across the length of the box like a clothes line, with nine small bulldog clips evenly spaced on the knotted string, to hang the slides until they are dry and ready to be boxed.

17. Giemsa stock solution (*see* **Note 10**).
18. 0.1 *M* Citric acid.
19. 0.2 *M* Na_2HPO_4.
20. Staining solution: 0.015% (w/v) Giemsa, 0.6 *M* methanol, 7 m*M* citric acid, 0.02 *M* Na_2HPO_4, pH 5.75. For 100 mL: 2 mL Giemsa stock solution, 2.4 mL methanol, 6.8 mL 0.1 *M* citric acid, 9.2 mL 0.2 *M* Na_2HPO_4, and 80 mL distilled H_2O.
21. Rinse buffer: 7 m*M* citric acid, 0.02 *M* Na_2HPO_4. For 100 mL: 6.8 mL 0.1 *M* citric acid and 9.2 mL 0.2 *M* Na_2HPO_4. Bring up to 100 mL with distilled H_2O.
22. Upright microscope with oil immersion 100× objective (e.g., Zeiss Axioskop, Oberkochen, Germany).

2.4. Grain Counting and Normalization

1. Create a standardized counting sheet, with columns for grains over nuclei and background (grains over a nucleus-sized area of the acellular field). Several other pieces of data that we suggest should be recorded include: total number of cells in the microscope field (countable nuclei and S-phase cells), S-phase cells, and morphology of the cells. These parameters may be correlated with NER, or may define differential cell populations.
2. Grain counts can be processed with any suitable statistical software, such as StatView (SAS Institute, Cary, NC) or the statistical package included in the Excel spreadsheet program (Microsoft, Redmond, WA).

3. Methods

3.1. Cell Irradiation, Labeling, and Fixation

1. All cells should be placed into culture at least 2 d before the performance of the UDS assay. Ideally, cells on the final slides should be easy to find, but not identifiable as clumps or clones (i.e., the slides should be less than semiconfluent on the day of the assay). Therefore, seed appropriate numbers of each experimental and control cell population (*see* **Notes 2–4**) into both chambers of four two-chamber slides (total volume of 1 mL, free of dimethylsulfoxide, trypsin, and so on.

2. Place each chamber slide into a 10-cm² round cell culture dish with a piece of dampened sterilized filter paper (*see* **Note 11**).

3. Incubate at 37°C in a standard humidified tissue culture incubator with 5% CO_2 for 2 d.

4. Turn on UV bulbs on the UV delivery device (**Fig. 2**), and allow them to warm up for at least 1 h. Test the dose-delivery rate under experimental conditions with a short-wave (254-nm) UV meter, and adjust if necessary (time of exposure and/or distance from bulbs (*see* **Note 12**).

5. Thaw radioactive label, and allow to warm to room temperature.

6. Feed all cells (replace with fresh medium) 1 h before UV exposure. Label all slides in pencil.

7. Thoroughly mix the [³H]thymidine label by vigorous vortexing. For up to 20 slides, add 200 μL label to 20 mL medium with serum to create "hot incubation media" with a final concentration of 10 μCi/mL. Vortex until foam appears.

8. Remove regular medium from all chamber slides. Divide experimental and control chamber slides into groups of four, ensuring there is a positive control slide (and a negative control slide [un-irradiated control], if necessary) in each group.

9. Leave the chamber of each slide closest to the ground glass label covered with the plastic lid, and uncover the other chambers.

10. Start the turntable (set at "mid" speed) to equalize exposure. Expose slides in sets of four, as determined in **step 8**.

11. Immediately after irradiation, add 0.5 mL of "hot incubation medium" to each chamber of each chamber slide, for a total of 1 mL of media per slide. Ten to 12 slides should be handled at a time to prevent the cells from drying out, with a maximum of 40 slides per experiment.

12. Incubate slides for 2 h at 37°C in tissue culture incubator. (You may wish to designate a "radioactive" incubator and/or a "radioactive" shelf; *see* **Note 13**).

13. Add FCS to the "cold chase medium."

14. After 2 h, using the radioactive hood, remove the "hot incubation medium" from all chamber slides by pipeting, and replace with 0.5 mL of "cold chase media."

15. Incubate slides for 2 h at 37°C in a tissue culture incubator.

16. Prepare fresh 70% ethanol and fixative solutions (33% acetic acid in 100% ethanol).

17. In the radioactive hood, remove the "cold chase medium" by aspiration, and gently rinse each side of the chamber slides with 1 mL of 1X SSC.

18. Remove the 1X SSC immediately by aspiration, and replace it with 0.5 mL fixative solution in each chamber. Leave at room temperature for 15 min.

19. Remove fixative by aspiration and leave slides to dry partially for 5 min. Add 0.5 mL of 70% ethanol to each chamber, and leave at room temperature for 15 min.

20. Remove the ethanol by aspiration. Remove the chambers and rubber gaskets from the slides, using a sharp scalpel to loosen one corner of the rubber gasket. Once the corner is free, use a pair of hemostats to pull the remaining gasket away from the slide. Any remain-

ing gasket can be lightly scraped off with the scalpel. All traces of the gasket must be removed, or it will cause the emulsion to be too thick on the edges of the slide.

21. Place slides in radioactively labeled Copeland jars with 4% perchloric acid. Then place the jars in a refrigerator overnight.

3.2. Slide Processing I: Dipping in Emulsion

Caution: all steps in the dipping process must be done in complete darkness (with no safe lights) until the slides are dry, packaged, and wrapped three times in foil (*see* **Note 8**).

1. Remove slides from Copeland jars and rinse by letting them sit in distilled H_2O for 3–4 min. Then allow the slides to dry in the hood for 24 h in glass slide holders sitting on paper towels.

2. Melt emulsion, and heat to 48°C in a water bath in the darkroom. First, place the emulsion in a 1000-mL beaker with 400 mL of water, and then place the beaker into the water bath for 1.5 h. To keep the emulsion container from floating, fill a 50-mL beaker, and place it on top of the emulsion container. Swirl the emulsion container every 30 min, to ensure complete thawing.

3. Prepare a drying box in which to hang and dry the slides (*see* **Fig. 3**).

4. Before taking the slides into the darkroom, place a triangular piece of lab tape on the upper right corner of each slide on the ground glass. This is to allow the slides to be oriented by touch in the dark while dipping. At this time, select one slide of each type of control to be "tester" slides. These slides will be placed in a separate drying box and will be developed first to determine when the emulsion on the slides from the entire experiment have exposed sufficiently for scoring.

5. Place an Amersham slide-dipping container in a beaker half full of 48°C water. In the darkroom, with all the lights off including the red ("safe") light, carefully pour the emulsion into the dipping container. Use your ungloved little finger to ensure that the emulsion has filled the dipping container to the top. (The emulsion is nontoxic.)

6. Orienting the slides using the piece of tape from **step 4**, take each slide and slide it into the dipping container. (Lightly tap the slide on both sides of the container to ensure it is fully immersed in the dipping container.)

7. Allow each slide to drip for a few seconds after removing it from the dipping container, and then hang the slide in the box with the bulldog clips clamped onto the ground glass labeling portion of the slide in the mouth of the slip.

8. The "tester" slides should be hung exclusively on the first string and all subsequent slides hung on the other three pieces of string. The emulsion will have to be refilled every 15–20 slides.

9. After all slides have been dipped, the lid should be placed over the box. Allow the slides to dry in the box in complete darkness for 1 h.

10. Preparation of plastic slide boxes.

    a. Place a clean glass slide at one end of the box. Tape the edges of the slide to prevent its removal.
    b. In the space behind the slide, add desiccant to the end of the box.
    c. Place a piece of tape on the lid of the slide box to orient the front of the box in the dark.
    d. For each box, have three layers of aluminum foil ready to wrap the boxes in the dark after the slides have been placed in them (two regular layers and one heavy duty).

11. Place the tester slides only in the first slide box, close the lid, wrap it in foil, and mark it with a "T" (for testers) on the foil, with the date.

12. Remove the remaining slides from the drying box, and place them in the other slide boxes, wrapping them in foil and marking them "E" (for experimental) and dating them.
13. Place the emulsion back in its original box and wrap it with foil three times as well. The emulsion is very light-sensitive, so any measures that are taken to lessen the exposure to light will prolong the useful lifetime of the emulsion and maintain low background on the slides.
14. Place the slide boxes in a refrigerator until developing.

3.3. Slide Processing II: Developing Emulsion

1. Develop the tester slides 12 d after dipping (d 1 being the day after dipping).
2. Take all slide boxes out of the refrigerator, and allow to warm to room temperature for a minimum of 5 h.
3. In the darkroom, create a 15°C water bath using cold water and a small amount of ice in a medium-sized developing tray. Use a thermometer to verify the temperature.
4. Place four slide dishes into the 15°C water bath. In the first dish, place D19 developer (1:1 mixed with dH_2O), distilled H_2O in the second dish, fixer in the third dish, and distilled water in the fourth dish (each slide dish holds 250 mL of liquid). The red light may be on while these solutions come to temperature (approx 2 h).
5. Set three timers (one for 4 min and two for 5 min) before you enter the darkroom. It helps if the timers beep when the start button is pressed as well as when the time has expired.
6. In complete darkness, place the tester slides in a glass slide holder, and attach the wire holder. Lower the slide holder into the first dish (developer), and start the timer set for 4 min.
7. After 4 min, dip the slides into the second dish (water) for a count of 10 s, and then dip them into the third dish (fixer) for 5 min (using a pre-set timer).
8. After 5 min dip the slides into the fourth dish (water again), and start the second timer set for 5 min. The lights can then be turned back on, as long as there are no other open slide boxes or unexposed slides.
9. After 5 min dry the tester slides for at least 1 h on the bench at room temperature.
10. Giemsa-stain the slides for 7 min in Copeland jars (*see* **Note 14**).
11. Rinse the slides in rinse buffer for 3 min, and allow to air-dry in a dust-free environment for 2–3 h.
12. Score the tester slides according to **Subheading 3.4.** If the emulsion on the slides is determined to have been exposed long enough (*see* **Note 15**), develop the experimental slides in batches of 5–10 according to **Subheading 3.3., steps 1–9**. The experimental slides can dry overnight in a dust-free environment, to be stained the following day. If exposure is not sufficient, return the experimental slides to the refrigerator, and allow the emulsion to be exposed longer (*see* **Note 13**).

3.4. Grain Counting and Normalization

Once all the slides have been stained, the nuclei of the cells can be counted (**Fig. 4**). There should be at least two slides per type of cell. Two criteria must be met for both the controls and the experimental slides for a successful experiment:

1. There must be a reasonable number of grains per nucleus, particularly with regard to the background (25–50 for the irradiated chamber, and 1–5 in the unirradiated chamber).
2. There must be sufficient cells (or nuclei) on at least two slides (100 scorable nuclei is ideal, and less than 20 is insufficient).

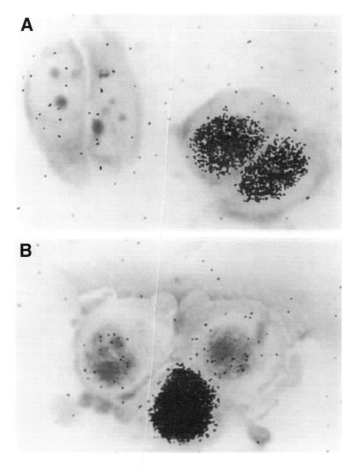

Fig. 4. Micrographs of Giemsa-stained MCF-7 cells after performance of the UDS assay. (**A**) Unirradiated cells. (**B**) Irradiated cells. In both panels, heavily labeled S-phase cells are evident as well as cells labeled only during repair synthesis. (Original magnification ×100.)

The counting procedure is as follows:

1. Orient the slide to be counted on the microscope stand so that the ground glass is to the left. (The unirradiated side of the slide will now always be to the left and the irradiated to the right.)
2. Scan both sides of the slide with a low-power objective before counting, to ensure there are at least 20 cells on both sides. If less than 20 cells are visible in each chamber, then it will be necessary to pool multiple slides of the same exposure time to obtain 20 unirradiated nuclei and 20 irradiated nuclei. If multiple slides do not exist, then this specimen cannot be evaluated for repair capacity. It is best to count a minimum of 100 cells on both sides of a slide. There should be some nuclei that are black with grains indicating cells that are in S phase (*see* **Fig. 4**). The number of these cells can be tallied in a separate column on the counting sheets but it is impossible to score them for silver grains.

3. If the slide is scorable, view it under oil immersion at a total magnification of 1000× (10× eyepiece × 100× objective) to resolve individual silver grains.

4. The Giemsa stain should provide three shades of purple at high magnification. The lightest purple is the cytoplasm of the cells. There should be few to no grains in this area (*see* **Note 16**). The nuclei are the second darkest purple. The silver grains in this area represent the [³H]thymidine incorporated into the cell's DNA. The number of grains in the nuclei is proportional to the amount of repair. These are the grains that are counted (*see* **Note 17**). For the positive control and the experimental slides, if the positive control is appropriate, the average number of grains per nuclei should be approx 50 on the irradiated side of the slide. The third, deeper purple, is often manifested in the nucleolus of the cell nucleus.

5. To determine the background grain count outside the nuclei, the counter should define an acellular area that is about the same size as the nuclei in that field; count the number of grains in that area. Background counts should be usually 5 grains or less. For evaluation of tester slides, *see* **Note 15**.

6. For each experiment, two slides should be counted for each type of cell, and two individuals should count each slide. Slides of the same cell type analyzed in the same experiment and developed on the same day should have a coefficient of variance of 10–15%. Counters on the same slide should have results that are within 10–15% as well.

7. After the unirradiated and irradiated sides of a slide are counted, statistical analysis may be completed. To arrive at the corrected value for the individual nuclei, take the counts per nucleus and subtract the background for that field for both the unirradiated and irradiated counts. To find the mean number of grains for each slide, take the corrected value for the unirradiated cells and divide by the total number of nuclei counted (not including S-phase cells). Do the same for the irradiated cells, then take the average number of grains per nucleus for the unirradiated nuclei, and subtract it from the average number of grains for the irradiated nuclei.

$$\frac{\text{Corrected irradiated grains per nucleus} - \text{Corrected unirradiated grains per nucleus}}{\text{Total number nuclei counted}}$$

$$= \text{Average number of grains per nucleus}$$

8. To compare the experimental slides with the control, take the average number of grains per nucleus for the experimental slide, and divide by the average number of grains per nucleus for the control. Multiply this number by 100 to arrive at the percent repair for the experimental slide compared with the control.

$$\frac{\text{Average number of grains per nucleus of experiment}}{\text{Average number of grains per nuclei of control} \times 100} = \% \text{ Repair compared with control}$$

9. To compare the experimental slides with a *population of controls*, take the percent repair compared with the concurrent control (run in the same experiment), and multiply this by the ratio of the concurrent control divided by the average repair for the population. Multiply this number by 100 to arrive at the percent repair for the experimental slide compared with the average of the control population.

$$\frac{\dfrac{\% \text{ Repair compared with}}{\text{concurrent control}} \times \dfrac{\text{Average number of grains per}}{\text{nucleus of concurrent control}}}{\text{Average number of grains per nucleus of average of control population} \times 100}$$

$$= \% \text{ Repair compared with average of control population.}$$

4. Notes

1. There is a perception that the host cell reactivation (HCR) assay is specific for the transcription coupled repair (TCR) component of NER, whereas the UDS assay is specific for global genomic repair (GGR). The specificity of the HCR assay (*see* Chap. 28) comes from the fact that repair is detected through repair of a reporter gene (although it is a foreign gene in an unnatural context). However, to be specific for TCR, the GGR machinery would also have to specifically avoid or exclude repairing damage in transcribed sequences, and there is no evidence that GGR has such specificity. Indeed, it has been estimated that approx 10% of the repair measured in the HCR assay occurs through the incidental activity of GGR on the reporter gene *(30–32)*. The specificity of the UDS assay, if it has any, comes simply from the fact that the vast majority of the genome is either noncoding, or nontranscribed in any particular cell type. Indeed, given the faster kinetics of TCR, the UDS assay probably quantitates a greater proportion of this type of repair than actual GGR; however, how much this contributes to the final result is unknown.

2. The UDS assay has traditionally been performed on monolayer cell cultures, such as skin fibroblasts, transformed fibroblastic cell lines, or hepatocytes. The stable attachment of such cells to glass slides (generally coated with some sort of substratum) allows the entire assay to be performed as described, on cells cultured on chamber slides. However, irradiation and labeling can be done prior to the attachment of the cells to a slide for quantification if such attachment is impossible. Indeed, with cells such as lymphocytes that have a weaker attachment to the slides themselves, we see a significant attrition in scorable cells through slide processing. Thus, we have coated the slides to enhance their attachment *(23,33)*. Similarly, we have attached single-layer sheets of cells to slides for processing, or even isolated labeled nuclei and attached them to the slide *(24)*. We have also found that 3D cellular structures can be analyzed, as long as only the outer layer of cells is scored, since they are the only ones that receive an unattenuated dose of UV and that are directly exposed to the emulsion *(23)*.

3. Since the UDS assay is affected by the strength of the radiolabel as well as the number of times the emulsion has been thawed, it cannot be considered an absolute assay of DNA repair, and raw grain counts in and of themselves are relatively meaningless (although they are often reported). *Instead, repair capacity should be reported relative to a standardized positive control, analyzed concurrently in each experiment.* Foreskin fibroblasts (FFs) have traditionally been used as the positive control for the UDS assay (*see* **Note 18** for a protocol for establishing FF cultures). Besides being relatively easy to acquire, FFs under 13 passages are described as having relatively high levels of repair *(18)*, suggesting that NER declines with age, which some studies have observed *(34)*, but not our own *(23)*. The positive control should ideally provide two different, but related, references: first, it should provide a baseline measure of the "normal" level of NER for the experimental samples to be compared against, and second, it should provide a guide as to when the experiment, specifically the exposure of the emulsion, can be successfully concluded (*see* **Notes 4** and **15**). FFs have long been considered to provide both references, both for analyses of cell lines and for fibroblast samples taken from patients for diagnosis. However, it is significant that diagnostic studies of PBLs have used normal PBLs as controls; we have recently shown that there is a 20-fold difference in the baseline NER capacity of these two cell types *(23)*. In addition, a single "normal" sample, often randomly acquired, usually serves as the control, whereas we have also shown that there is considerable interindividual variability in NER capacity in the "normal" population. Mixtures of FFs

from several babies have sometimes been used to attempt to account for possible interindividual differences. Instead, we suggest that a population of normal samples should first be analyzed, with the "concurrent" control included. The final grain counts can then be normalized not just against the concurrent normal sample but, through it, to the normal population, as described in **Subheading 3.4., step 9**.

If lymphocytes are being run in the experiment, an appropriate control appears to be the lymphoblastoid cell line TK6 (although transformed cells, in general, cannot be assumed to have "normal" repair). Lymphocytes need to be developed for a longer period because of their low repair, usually 15–18 d instead of 12. The accuracy of the final determination is based on the number of grains scored, not the number of cells. Thus, if the slides are developed too early (which would be the case if lymphocyte slides were developed on a timetable based on FF controls), they have very few grains, making it difficult to establish unambiguously a difference between the irradiated and unirradiated populations. In general, grain counts of 50–100 should be projected prior to emulsion development, and we regularly count 200–300 nuclei per slide.

4. Tester slides are extra positive control slides that must be designed into an experiment to determine the optimal exposure time for the emulsion. The freshness of the label and of the emulsion, as well as the changing conditions of the darkroom, can all be variables in terms of the length of time autoradiographic slides should be developed for maximal signal-to-noise ratio. Generally two extra FFs (or other control) slides are made for this purpose and are packaged separately for development at 12 d, to be grain counted before the slides from the rest of the experiment have been developed. If the rest of the experimental slides are developed on the same day as the tester slides, then the tester slides can be used as additional positive control slides in the experiment. If the tester slides are developed on a day other than the experimental slides, they may not be included (as positive standards of comparison) in the analysis of the experimental slides.

5. If the experiment is designed to document repair deficiency, "negative" controls, i.e., repair-deficient cells, may be included, in addition to the standardized positive controls. Indeed, a second set of slides may be prepared and developed using the negative controls slides as guides, although these will not in any way replace the unirradiated chamber controls. Three human diseases have been found to be associated with defects in the NER genes: XP, with seven complementation groups, Cockayne's syndrome, with five complementation groups, three of which overlap with those of XP, and trichothiodystrophy, with three complementation groups, two of which overlap with XP *(1)*. UDS has historically been used to diagnose XP in skin fibroblasts or in PBLs, since these patients are more or less deficient in NER depending on their complementation group. Cockayne's syndrome affects TCR. There is a considerable range of residual activity amongst patients in these various complementation groups (<10% in groups A, B, and G, up to 50% in groups D and E), with none exhibiting complete deficiency *(35)*. Complete NER deficiency may be a prenatal lethal condition; mutations in *ERCC1*, the first NER gene cloned, have never been identified in a patient, perhaps because they are inviable at the organismal level *(36)*. XP cell lines (immortalized both with and without the use of exogenous agents) can be purchased from the American Type Culture Collection (ATCC, Manassas, VA) or Coriell Cell Repositories (Camden, NJ) for negative control use.

6. Date the label when it arrives, and discard 1 mo from the arrival date, owing to chemical deterioration. Label should be stored at –20°C.

7. Cold thymidine media should be stored without the presence of serum, which can bind and effectively lower the bioavailable thymidine. For 100 mL of medium, add 24.2 mg of

thymidine. (This solution can be stored at 4°C for a period of 3 mo as long as it lacks serum.)

8. This portion of the assay is extremely light-sensitive. All light sources must be covered or removed, including lights on water baths, temperature control for the room, light leaks from doorways and light fixtures, and any other sources in the darkroom including fluorescent watches. Spend 20 min in the room with all the lights off to identify light sources, and cover them before the procedure is begun if you are uncertain of the integrity of your darkroom. The assay can also be affected by static electricity from gloves and clothing during the winter months.

9. Reuse of previously melted emulsion can cause higher background in sequential experiments, owing to factors like static electricity that expose it with each use. Use the same emulsion at most three times to avoid increasing spurious background grains.

10. Giemsa stock solution: 0.8% (w/v) Giemsa in 1:1 glycerol/methanol. Warm glycerol in a 60°C water bath, add 0.5 g Giemsa powder to 33 mL glycerol, and place it on a stir plate overnight without heat. The following morning, add 33 mL methanol and cover with Parafilm and Saran Wrap. The next day, filter the solution using Whatman filter paper, and store in a dark bottle at room temperature. The filtration step takes several hours.

11. The Petri dish also provides an extra layer of protection against air-borne contamination. The moistened filter paper creates an additional humidity chamber for the cells growing in chamber slides.

12. The recommended dosage of UVC light at 254 nm is 14 J/m^2 to produce the desired amount of DNA damage, although a dose-dependence curve should be performed at the start of any study of NER. For a desired dose of 14 J/m^2, with a mean fluence of 1.2 J/m^2/s from the UV bulbs, a 12-s exposure of the cells is generally used by our laboratory (dose in J/m^2 = fluence [read from the meter] × number of seconds). The readout from the Spectroline meter will be μW/cm^2 (e.g., 210 μW/cm^2 = 2.1 J m^{-2} sec^{-1})

13. This allows sufficient time for the cells to repair the 6-4 photoproducts that were created by the UVC light but not the pyrimidine dimers. (To effectively quantitate the repair of pyrimidine dimers would require an 8-h incubation) *(37,38)*.

14. Slides may be stained as many times as needed in order to view the nuclei clearly. Alternatively, methanol can be used to lighten the stain if it is too heavy. Some cells such as CHO cells only need to be stained for 2 min instead of 7 min.

15. For the tester slides, once the slides have dried, view under an oil immersion lens at a total magnification of 1000×, and count 25 nuclei on both the irradiated and unirradiated sides of the slide. This will allow a decision to be made as to whether or not the experimental slides should be developed that same day. If no grains are observed, then the radioactive label was not added to the incubation mixture, and the experiment is unusable. If an average of approx 50 grains/nucleus or more above background are observed in the irradiated chamber of the positive control, the experimental slides are ready to be developed. However, a set of controls and the experimental slides must be counted and developed at the same time under the same conditions in order to perform the normalization. S-phase cells should be visible on both sides of the slide (in approximately equal numbers). If the controls do not exhibit the required number of grains/nucleus, the remaining control and experimental slides should be developed 24–72 h later. If longer development seems necessary, it is likely that the signal-to-noise (background) ratio will be too high to determine NER capacity accurately. If background grains appear to be unevenly distributed, or distributed in a pattern, there is probably a light leak in the slide boxes used to store the dipped slides. Background counts of 8–10 or above are too high for accurate analysis.

16. If the cytoplasm is covered with grains and the nucleus is relatively uncovered, it is most likely a result of *Mycoplasma* contamination. These slides are not scorable, and the cell population will have to be reacquired or rendered free of contamination in order to be assayed.

17. If the tester slides have been used correctly and the experimental slides average about 50 grains/nucleus, nuclei with more than approx 90 grains should be considered to be in S phase.

18. FFs can be generated in large quantities from a single foreskin by finely mincing the tissue and stirring it in trypsin for 5 h at room temperature, followed by repeated trituration with a 25-mL pipet and subsequent plating in tissue culture dishes. The first few passages should be performed to remove cell clumps and create even monolayers of fibroblasts. Then these early-explant passages can be frozen in 10% dimethylsulfoxide for use in many UDS experiments. FF repair capacity is stable for about 18 passages, so we recommend the use of FFs only up to passage 13 to retain consistency *(19)*.

References

1. Thompson, L. H. (1998) Nucleotide excision repair: its relation to human disease, in *DNA Damage and Repair,* vol. 2: *DNA Repair in Higher Eukaryotes* (Nickoloff, J. A. and Hoekstra, M. F., eds.), Humana, Totowa, NJ, pp. 335–393.
2. Wood, R. D., Mitchell, M., Sgouros, J., and Lindahl, T. (2001) Human DNA repair genes. *Science* **291,** 1284–1289.
3. Reed, E. (1998) Platinum-DNA adduct, nucleotide excision repair and platinum based anti-cancer chemotherapy. *Cancer Treat. Rev.* **24,** 331–344.
4. Kaneko, M. and Cerutti, P. A. (1980) Excision of *N*-acetoxy-2-acetylaminofluorene-induced DNA adducts from chromatin fractions of human fibroblasts. *Cancer Res.* **40,** 4313–4319.
5. Andersson, B. S., Sadeghi, T., Siciliano, M. J., Legerski, R., and Murray, D. (1996) Nucleotide excision repair genes as determinants of cellular sensitivity to cyclophosphamide analogs. *Cancer Chemother. Pharmacol.* **38,** 406–416.
6. Gamesik, M. P., Dolan, M. E., Andersson, B. S., and Murray, D. (1999) Mechanisms of resistance to the toxicity of cyclophosphamide. *Curr. Pharmaceut. Des.* **5,** 587–605.
7. Mullenders, L. H. F. and Berneberg, M. (2001) Photoimmunology and nucleotide excision repair: impact of transcription coupled and global genome excision repair. *J. Photochem. Photobiol. B* **56,** 97–100.
8. Covertey, D., Kenney, M. K., Rupp, W. D., Lane, D. P., and Wood, R. D. (1991) Requirement of the replication protein SSB in human DNA excision repair. *Nature* **347,** 538–541.
9. Huang, J. C., Svoboda, D. L., Reardon, J. T., and Sancar, A. (1992) Human nucleotide excision nuclease removes thymine dimers from DNA by incising the 22nd phosphodiester bond 5' and the 6th phosphodiester bond 3' to the photodimer. *Proc. Natl. Acad. Sci. USA* **89,** 3664–3668.
10. Shivji, K. K., Kenney, M. P., and Wood, R. D. (1992) Proliferating cell nuclear antigen is required for DNA excision repair. *Cell* **69,** 367–374.
11. Grossman, L. and Thiagalingam, S. (1993) Nucleotide excision repair, a tracking mechanism in search of damage. *J. Biol. Chem.* **268,** 16871–16874.
12. Satoh, M. S., Jones, C. J., Wood, R. D., and Lindahl, T. (1993) DNA excision-repair defect of xeroderma pigmentosum prevents removal of a class of oxygen free radical-induced base lesions. *Proc. Natl. Acad. Sci. USA* **90,** 6335–6339.
13. Huang, J. C., Hsu, D. S., Kazantsev, A., and Sancar, A. (1994) Substrate specificity of human exinuclease: repair of abasic sites, methylated bases, mismatches, and bulky adducts. *Proc. Natl. Acad. Sci. USA* **91,** 12213–12217.

14. Bohr, V. A., Smith, C. A., Okumoto, D. S., and Hanawalt, P. C. (1985) DNA repair in an active gene: removal of pyrimidine dimers from the DHFR gene of CHO cells is much more efficient than in the genome overall. *Cell* **40**, 359–369.

15. Bootsma D. and Hoeijmakers J. H. J. (1994) The molecular basis of nucleotide excision repair syndromes. *Mutat. Res.* **307**, 15–23.

16. Cleaver, J. E. (1968) Defective repair replication of DNA in xeroderma pigmentosum. *Nature* **218**, 652–656.

17. Painter, R. B. and Cleaver, J. E. (1969) Repair replication, unscheduled DNA synthesis and the repair of mammalian DNA. *Radiat. Res.* **37**, 451–466.

18. Cleaver, J. E. and Thomas, G. H. (1981) Measurement of unscheduled synthesis by autoradiography, in *DNA Repair: A Laboratory Manual of Research Procedures,* vol. I (Friedberg, E. C. and Hanawalt, P. C., eds.), Marcel Dekker, New York, pp. 277–287.

19. Michalopoulos, G., Sattler, G. L., O'Connor, L., and Pitot, H. C. (1978) Unscheduled DNA synthesis induced by procarcinogens in suspensions and primary cultures of hepatocytes on collagen membranes. *Cancer Res.* **38**, 1866–1871.

20. Williams, G. M., Mori, H., and McQueen, C. A. (1989) Structure-activity relationships in the rat hepatocyte DNA-repair test for 300 chemicals. *Mutat. Res.* **221**, 263–286.

21. Killary, A. M. and Fournier, R. E. K. (1984) A genetic analysis of extinction: trans-dominant loci regulate expression of liver-specific traits in hepatoma hybrid cells. *Cell* **38**, 523–534.

22. Clarke, R., Leonessa, F., Brunner, W. N., and Thompson, E. W. (2000) In vitro models, in *Diseases of the Breast* (Harris, J. R., Lippman, M. E., Morrow, M., and Osborne, C. K., eds.), Lippincott Williams & Wilkins, Philadelphia, pp. 347–348.

23. Latimer, J. J., Nazir, T., Flowers, L. C., et al. (2003) Unique tissue-specific level of DNA nucleotide excision repair in primary human mammary epithelial cultures. *Exp. Cell Res.* **291**, 111–121.

24. Latimer, J. J., Hultner, M. L., Cleaver, J. E., and Pederson, R. A. (1996) Elevated DNA excision repair capacity in the extraembryonic mesoderm of the midgestation mouse embryo. *Exp. Cell Res.* **228**, 19–28.

25. Rasmussen, R. E. and Painter, R. B. (1964) Evidence for repair of UV damaged deoxyribonucleic acid in cultured mammalian cells. *Nature* **203**, 1360–1362.

26. Kam, E. Y. and Pitts, J. D. (1984) Computer-assisted grain counting for autoradiography. *Comput. Programs Biomed.* **19**, 81–83.

27. Schellart, N. A., Zweijpfenning, R. C., van Marle, J., and Huijsmans, D. P. Computerized pattern recognition used for grain counting in high resolution autoradiographs with low grain densities. *Comput. Methods Programs Biomed.* **23**, 103–109.

28. Mize, R. R., Thouron, C., Lucas, L., and Harlan, R. (1994) Semiautomatic image analysis for grain counting in in situ hybridization experiments. *Neuroimage* **1**, 163–172.

29. Steier, H. and Cleaver, J. E. (1969) Exposure chamber for quantitative ultraviolet photobiology. *Lab Prac.* **18**, 1295.

30. Carreau, M., Eveno, E., Quilliet, X., et al. (1995) Development of a new easy complementation assay for DNA repair deficient human syndromes using cloned repair genes. *Carcinogenesis* **16**, 1003–1009.

31. Qiao, Y., Spitz, M. R., Shen, H., et al. (2002) Modulation of repair of ultraviolet damage in the host-cell reactivation assay by polymorphic XPC and XPD/ERCC2 genotypes. *Carcinogenesis* **23**, 295–299.

32. Svetlova, M., Solovjeva, L., Pleskach, N., et al. (2002) Clustered sites of DNA repair synthesis during early nucleotide excision repair in ultraviolet light-irradiated quiescent human fibroblasts. *Exp. Cell Res.* **276**, 284–295.

33. Forlenza, M., Latimer, J., and Baum, A. (2000) The effects of stress on DNA repair capacity. *Psychol. Health* **15,** 881–891.

34. Moriwaki, S., Ray, S., Tarone, R. E., Kraemer, K. H., and Grossman, L. (1996) The effect of donor age on the processing of UV-damaged DNA by cultured human cells: reduced DNA repair capacity and increased DNA mutability. *Mutat. Res.* **364,** 117–123.

35. Kraemer, K. H., Levy, D. D., Parris, C. N., et al. (1994) Xeroderma pigmentosum and related disorders: examining the linkage between defective DNA repair and cancer. *J. Invest. Dermatol.* **103(suppl. 5),** 96S–101S.

36. Hsia, K. T., Millar, M. R., King, S., et al. (2003) DNA repair gene *Ercc1* is essential for normal spermatogenesis and oogenesis and for functional integrity of germ cell DNA in the mouse. *Development* **130,** 369–378.

37. Roza, L., Vermeulen, W., Bergen Henegouwen, J. B., et al. (1990) Effects of microinjected photoreactivating enzyme on thymine dimer removal and DNA repair synthesis in normal human and xeroderma pigmentosum fibroblasts. *Cancer Res.* **15,** 1905–1910.

38. Ye, N., Bianchi, M. S., Bianchi, N. O., and Holmquist, G. P. (1999) Adaptive enhancement and kinetics of nucleotide excision repair in humans. *Mutat. Res.* **435,** 43–61.

28

Analysis of DNA Repair Using Transfection-Based Host Cell Reactivation

Jennifer M. Johnson and Jean J. Latimer

Summary

Host cell reactivation (HCR) is a transfection-based assay in which intact cells repair damage localized to exogenous DNA. This chapter provides instructions for the application of this technique using UV irradiation as a source of damage to a luciferase reporter plasmid. Through measurement of the activity of a reporter enzyme, the amount of damaged plasmid that a cell can "reactivate" or repair and express can be quantitated. Different DNA repair pathways can be analyzed by this technique by damaging the reporter plasmid in different ways. Because it involves repair of a transcriptionally active gene, when applied to UV damage the HCR assay measures the capacity of the host cells to perform transcription-coupled repair (TCR), a subset of the overall nucleotide excision repair pathway that specifically targets transcribed gene sequences.

Key Words: DNA damage; host cell reactivation (HCR); transcription-coupled repair (TCR); global genomic repair (GGR); nucleotide excision repair (NER); transfection; luciferase; UV irradiation; thymine dimers; 6-4 photoproducts.

1. Introduction

The term *host cell reactivation* (HCR) was first used to describe the survival of ultraviolet (UV)-irradiated bacteriophages in host cells that had been pretreated with UV irradiation. Survival of phages was increased in pretreated host cells compared with untreated hosts. Researchers first hypothesized that the mechanism that accounted for this "reactivation" of the phage involved homologous recombination between the phage and the bacterial genome. This hypothesis was later replaced by the idea of enzymatic repair *(1)*. In an adaptation of the use of viral DNA to measure inherent cellular repair capabilities, transient expression plasmid DNA vectors were used by Protic-Sabljic and Kraemer on SV40 transformed human fibroblasts in 1985 *(2)* and by Athas et al. on human lymphocytes in 1991 *(3)*.

The plasmid reactivation assay indirectly monitors cellular repair of transcriptional activity by measuring activity associated with a transfected enzymatic marker gene. In brief, cells are transfected with the damaged plasmid, allowed time to express the reporter enzyme, harvested for protein, and then assayed for the enzymatic activity of

From: *Methods in Molecular Biology, vol. 291, Molecular Toxicology Protocols*
Edited by: P. Keohavong and S. G. Grant © Humana Press Inc., Totowa, NJ

the reporter. Two levels of controls are utilized for the HCR assay. The first involves the use of damaged and undamaged versions of the same expression vector to determine the ratio of expression of the damaged (and repaired) plasmid divided by the expression of the undamaged vector. In addition, a plasmid distinguishable from the experimental plasmids is also necessary to control for transfection efficiency. To make the results of individual experiments comparable to each other, we also recommend that the absolute numbers expressed by the ratio of damaged (and repaired) over undamaged plasmid be divided by similar results derived from a standard cell line run in every experiment. In the protocol described in this chapter, the experimental reporter used is firefly luciferase, and the control is bacterial β-galactosidase. Other reporter systems such as bacterial chloramphenicol acetyltransferase can and have also been used.

The host repair system interrogated in the HCR assay depends entirely on the type of transcription-inhibiting damage introduced into the plasmid (*see* **Note 1**). In practice, the vast majority of studies of this type have involved repair of UV-induced DNA damage via the nucleotide excision repair (NER) pathway.

As discussed in Chapter 27, NER is one of a number of types of DNA repair acting to maintain the integrity of the genome. It is a particularly complex pathway, however, which can remediate many types of DNA damage. Indeed, unlike other DNA repair pathways, it is not the specific damage itself that activates NER, but the resulting distortion in the DNA helix, making it applicable to a broad spectrum of genotoxic insults. Human cells perform NER at two distinct levels. First, the rapid and efficient removal of lesions that block ongoing transcription and thus need to be eliminated quickly, also known as *transcription-coupled repair* (TCR), and second, the slower, less efficient, repair of bulk DNA, including the nontranscribed strand of active genes, also referred to as *global genome repair* (GGR) *(4)*. The former process links NER to transcription, and the latter process links it to replication. TCR therefore represents a subset of the overall repair that occurs in NER.

The HCR assay specifically provides researchers with a method of investigating the ability of a cell to perform TCR *(5)*. It is presumed that some of the damaged reporter plasmid makes its way into the nucleus, where repair occurs, and then gene transcription and translation occur via normal cellular trafficking.

The plasmid vectors used in this experiment include pGL3, used as the experimental vector, and pCH110, used as the control plasmid (**Fig. 1**). pGL3 codes for a luciferase gene derived from the firefly. It allows for high levels of expression because of the presence of an SV40 promoter upstream of the luciferase gene and a downstream SV40 enhancer and polyadenylation signal. The sensitivity of this system is generally 100-fold greater than that based on the chloramphenicol acetyltransferase (*CAT*) gene *(2)*. pCH110 codes for the β-galactosidase enzyme derived from the *E. coli lacZ* gene under the control of the SV40 early promoter.

In our hands, the pGL3 vector is irradiated using 700 J/m^2 of UV light to induce DNA damage in the form of 6-4 photoproducts and pyrimidine dimers that block transcription and cannot produce an active luciferase enzyme until it is repaired. The pCH110 plasmid, with *lacZ* as an internal reporter gene to control for transfection efficiency, remains undamaged.

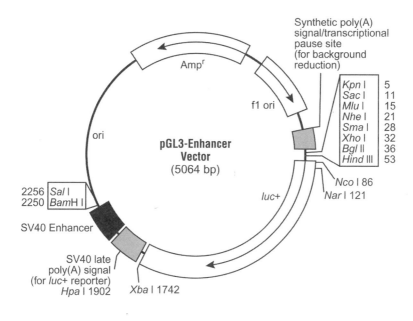

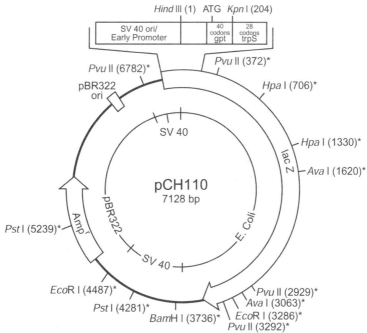

Published doses of UV irradiation utilized for HCR experiments in mammalian cells can range from 56 to 800 J/m^2. Protic-Sabljic and Kraemer *(2)* demonstrated that a dose as low as 56 J/m^2 was enough to inactivate a CAT reporter plasmid in repair-deficient xeroderma pigmentosum complementation group A (XPA) and XPD fibroblasts, whereas a dose of 680 J/m^2 was required to inactivate the same vector in normal human fibroblasts. Athas et al. *(3)* used incremental doses of 0, 200, 400, 600, and 800 J/m^2 in their field test of HCR on human lymphocytes. Their results showed a significant, 11-fold difference in repair capacities between normal peripheral blood lymphocytes and XPA and XPD lymphoblastoid cell lines at a UV dose of 200 J/m^2.

The ability of cells to repair UV-induced DNA damage is expressed as the percentage of the reactivated luciferase activity of damaged relative to the activity of undamaged (baseline expression) genes after a period of gene repair and expression.

$$\text{TCR capacity as an absolute number} = \frac{(\text{luciferase expression from damaged plasmid})}{(\text{luciferase expression from undamaged plasmid})}$$

A major advantage of this technique is that it minimizes the cytotoxic effects of damaging agents that might indirectly compromise the repair mechanisms of the cell *(6)*. Damage takes place in vitro and can be adapted to investigate specific damaging agents. Concerns arise from the fact that a nonmammalian reporter gene is being expressed in a mammalian cell, although most transfection-based assays utilize nonmammalian genes to minimize backgrounds.

2. Materials

2.1. Preparation of Host Cells

1. Experimental cells: 24 h before transfection the cells to be evaluated should be growing exponentially. They should be then harvested by trypsinization and replated so they are 90–95% confluent at the time of transfection. The number of cells required for this will vary significantly with cell type. Trypsinization must be performed at least 20 h prior to transfection to give the cells adequate time to anchor to the substratum. The cells should not be grown in the presence of antibiotics. Sufficient cells should be plated to fill one and one-half, 6-well culture dishes.
2. Positive control cells (*see* **Note 2**).
3. Negative control cells (*see* **Note 3**).
4. Cell culture incubator (e.g., ThermoForma Series II Water Jacketed CO_2 Incubator, Forma Scientific, Marietta, OH).
5. Appropriate growth media for each cell type, with the appropriate amount and type of serum.
6. 6-Well culture dishes (e.g., BD Falcon Tissue Culture Plates, Fisher Scientific, Pittsburgh, PA).
7. Photography equipment (MC100 Spot 35-mm camera, cat. no. 456014, Zeiss, attached to a Zeiss Axioskop, Oberkochen, Germany; optional).

2.2. UV Irradiation of Reporter Plasmid

1. Plasmid pGL3 (Promega cat. no. E1771, Madison, WI): approx 15 µg/cell line; however, batch irradiation is suggested. (Irradiated plasmids should be stored in 15–100-µg aliquots at –80°C.)

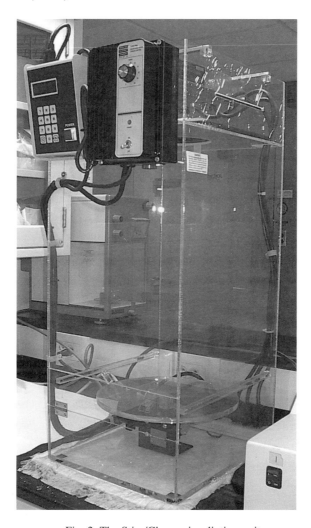

Fig. 2. The Stier/Cleaver irradiation unit.

2. 60-mm² Tissue culture dishes (Fisher).
3. Irradiation unit (**Fig. 2**; *see* **Note 4**).
4. TE: 0.25 *M* Tris-HCl, 5 m*M* EDTA (Sigma, St. Louis, MO), 500 mL, sterile filtered; store at 4°C.

2.3. Transient Transfection (Lipofection)

1. Appropriate growth media for each cell type, with and without serum.
2. LipofectAMINE (Gibco-BRL, Invitrogen cat. no. 11668-019, Carlsbad, CA).
3. Plasmid pGL3 (Promega): the amount required will vary with the ratio of reporter to control plasmid chosen, as well as the total amount of plasmid DNA chosen to be used per well (*see* **Note 5**). As a guideline, approx 30 µg of this reporter plasmid DNA per cell line

should be prepared if one is using a total of 5 µg per well and a ratio of 5:1 reporter/control plasmid.

4. Plasmid pCH110 (Amersham, cat. no. 27-4508-01, Piscataway, NJ). As a guideline, approx 5 µg of this plasmid DNA per cell line should be prepared if one is using a total of 5 µg per well and a ratio of 5:1 reporter/control plasmid.
5. UV-irradiated plasmid pGL3 (from **Subheading 3.2.**).

2.4. Protein Isolation

1. 1X Reporter lysis buffer (RLB). Prepare in bulk by dilution of 5X RLB (Promega; stored at –20°C) with 4 vol of dH$_2$O and mixing. Each well will require 500 µL. The 1X buffer should be equilibrated to room temperature prior to use.
2. Phosphate-buffered saline (PBS), Ca^{2+}/Mg^{2+}-free (CellGro, cat. no. 21-031-CV, Herndon, VA).
3. Rocking platform or orbital shaker (e.g., Red Rotor, Hoefer Scientific Instruments, San Francisco, CA)
4. Rubber policeman (one each for each well).
5. 1-mL Microcentrifuge tubes.
6. 1-mL Micropipetor and tips.
7. Refrigerated microcentrifuge (e.g., Sigma 2K 15, cat. no. 10810, Sigma Labzentrifugen, Germany).

2.5. Protein Quantification

1. BCA Protein Assay Kit (Pierce, cat. no. 23227, Rockford, IL): one kit will provide more than 50 assays.
2. Centrifuge tubes (1.5-mL Eppendorf tubes; Fisher).
3. TE: 0.25 M Tris-HCl, 5 mM EDTA, 500 mL, sterile filtered; store at 4°C.
4. Bovine serum albumin (BSA) stock (included in the BCA kit).
5. Micropipetors (200 and 20 µL) and appropriate tips.
6. Reagents A and B (included in the BCA kit).
7. 96-Well tissue culture plastic plates (Fisher): 18 wells are needed for the control + 36 wells for each cell line analyzed.
8. Rocking platform or orbital shaker.
9. Incubator: could be same as cell culture incubator, although it does not need to be humidified or in the presence of CO$_2$.
10. Microplate reader (e.g., Ceres 900 HDi, Bio-Tek Instruments, Winooski, VT).

2.6. Quantification of Luciferase Expression

1. Luciferase® Assay System (Promega, cat. no. E4030).
2. Luciferase assay reagent (LAR): resuspend the lyophilized luciferase assay substrate in 10 mL of luciferase assay buffer (both provided in the kit). The reagent should be green. The optimum temperature for luciferase activity is 20–25°C (approximately room temperature). Allow LAR to equilibrate fully to room temperature before using (*see* **Note 6**). Also ensure that samples to be measured are at room temperature.
3. 1X RLB.
4. Luminometer tubes (e.g., Sarstedt 5 mL, 75 × 12 mm, cat. no. 55526, Newton, NC).
5. Luminometer (e.g., Zylux Femtomaster FB15, Maryville, TN).

2.7. Quantification of β-Galactosidase Expression

1. Breaking buffer: 0.2 M Tris-HCl, 0.2 M NaCl, 0.01 M Mg acetate, 0.01 M 2-mercaptoethanol, 5% glycerol, pH 7.6 (all constituents from Sigma). Need approx 2.5 mL per cell line.
2. Z buffer: 0.06 M Na$_2$HPO$_4$, 0.04 M NaH$_2$PO$_4$, 0.01 M KCl, 0.001 M MgSO$_4$, 0.05 M 2-mercaptoethanol, pH 7.0 (all constituents from Sigma). Need approx 10 mL per cell line.
3. 4 mg/mL *o*-Nitrophenyl-β-D-galactosidase (ONPG) in dH$_2$O (Sigma).
4. 1 M Na$_2$CO$_3$ (Sigma).

3. Methods
3.1. Preparation of Host Cells

1. One day before transfection, trypsinize and count all cells to be transfected.
2. Replate cells in 6-well culture dishes so they will be 90–95% confluent on the day of transfection. (Best results are achieved when the cells are transfected at this high cell density). The number of cells required to achieve this will be different for each cell type or cell line. For each well, the appropriate number of cells should be resuspended in 2 mL of normal growth media containing serum and no antibiotics. For each experimental cell line, nine wells (1.5 dishes) will be required.

3.2. UV Irradiation of Reporter Plasmid (see Note 7)

1. For each cell line, 15 μg of reporter plasmid is necessary; however, batch irradiation can be performed (i.e., irradiation of reporter plasmid for the evaluation of a number of target cell populations can be performed at the same time).
2. Immediately before irradiation, dilute pGL3 DNA to 50 μg/mL in cold (4°C) distilled, sterile filtered water.
3. Pipet dilute plasmid solution into a 60-mm^2 tissue culture dish on ice. Four mL of diluted DNA solution is used per dish.
4. Irradiate with a dose of 700 J/m^2 of UVC light at 254 nm (*see* **Note 8**). The turntable should turn during the entire irradiation.
5. After exposure, cover the plate and keep on ice.
6. The damaged plasmid should be aliquoted and stored at –80°C. To ensure that additional damage is not done to the plasmid DNA, make sure aliquots are small enough so that each one is sufficient for a standardized experiment, with only a small volume remaining (i.e., aliquots of 15–100 μg). Aliquots should not be refrozen after use because refreezing will cause nicking of the plasmid.

3.3. Transient Transfection (Lipofection)

The following protocol is adapted from Invitrogen Life Technologies Lipofectamine 2000 CD Reagent instructions (*7*).

1. Every experiment and control is done in triplicate, i.e., in three wells. A minimum of nine wells (as prepared in **Subheading 3.1., step 2**) is therefore required for each host cell type to be assayed.
2. Several types of controls are used in these experiments. As an internal control of transfection efficiency, each well is transfected with undamaged pCH110 plasmid, which

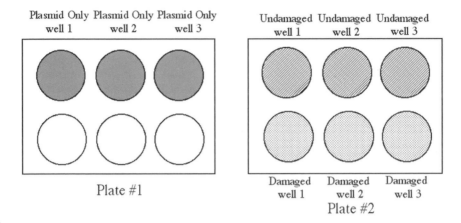

Fig. 3. Schematic for the setup of an HCR assay for one cell line.

expresses β-galactosidase. As another control for transfection, wells are mock transfected, not by withholding plasmid, as has been done traditionally, but by omitting the lipofectamine agent. The nine wells of each cell type are allocated as shown in **Fig. 3**.

3. On the day of transfection, feed each well of cells normal growth media complete with serum. It may be useful to capture an image of the cells prior to transfection as a reference for evaluating their condition later in the experiment. The plates should then be labeled as indicated in **Fig. 3**.

4. A total of 5.0 μg of DNA (which includes a 10:1 ratio of experimental [pGL3] to control plasmid [pCH110]) is required for every well, in 250 μL of medium without serum per well. (Charged proteins and lipids in serum may interfere with the formation of DNA–cationic lipid complexes; *see* **Note 5**.) These solutions can be prepared in bulk. For each experimental point, six wells will need a 10:1 ratio of undamaged pGL3 to pCH110, and three wells will need a 10:1 ratio of damaged pGL3 to (undamaged) pCH110.

5. Mix the Lipofectamine 2000 reagent (LF2000) gently before use. Do not vortex. Dilute 15 μL of LF2000 into 250 μL of medium (without serum) per well, and incubate for 3 min at room temperature. This dilution can also be prepared in bulk for multiple wells. For each experimental point, six wells will receive LF2000 and three wells will receive only medium. The LF2000 should sit no longer than 5 min after dilution in medium, as inactivation can occur.

6. Immediately mix the lipofectamine and plasmid solutions 1:1 in the following combinations:

   a. Plasmid-only row (no LF2000)
      3 wells: medium – LF2000 undamaged pGL3 + undamaged pCH110
   b. Undamaged row
      3 wells: medium + LF2000 undamaged pGL3 + undamaged pCH110
   c. Damaged row
      3 wells: medium + LF2000 damaged pGL3 +   undamaged pCH110

Incubate at room temperature for 20 min to allow DNA–LF2000 complexes to form. The solutions may begin to appear cloudy as the complexes form. These complexes are stable for at least 6 h at room temperature.

7. After the 20-min incubation, remove the media from each of the cell wells. Add 500 µL of the appropriate plasmid solution to each well, and mix gently by rocking the plate back and forth. Incubate the cells at 37°C in a CO_2 incubator for 1 h.

8. After the 1-h incubation, add 1.5 mL media with serum to each well. There will be no need to change the media again after this point.

9. At 24 h after transfection, observe and (if necessary) capture images of the cells. Transfected cells should appear damaged and unhealthy.

3.4. Protein Harvest and Quantification

The following protocol was adapted from Promega's Technical Manual No. 040, Dual Luciferase® Reporter Assay System, *(8)* and Pierce's BCA Protein Assay Reagent Kit manual (23227) *(9)*.

1. At 44 h after transfection, remove the growth media from each well of cultured cells and gently rinse each well with approx 500 µL of PBS to remove dead cells. To add the PBS, place the pipet tip on the side of the well, and allow the PBS to trickle down the side of the well and spread out across it. Completely remove this rinse solution by placing a pipet into the corner of each well and aspirating off the PBS.

2. Add 500 µL of prepared 1X RLB to each well. Place the plate on a rocking platform or orbital shaker with gentle rocking/shaking for 10 min (or longer if culture is overgrown) at room temperature.

3. After about 10 min, you should see a white clump forming in the middle of each well as the cells lyse. At this point, take a rubber policeman and scrape the cells from the bottom of the wells. Scrape in both the vertical and horizontal directions, paying special attention to the sides of the wells.

4. After scraping, return the plates to the orbital shaker for an additional 10 min. Check the plates under a microscope to verify that there are no whole cells remaining attached to the bottom of the wells.

5. Using a 1-mL micropipetor, transfer the lysate to the appropriate microcentrifuge tube. Disperse the white clump by pipeting up and down.

6. Clear the lysate by centrifuging for 30 s at the top speed of a refrigerated microcentrifuge.

7. Transfer cleared lysates to a fresh tube for further handling and storage. Proteins may be stored at this point at –80°C before continuing further.

3.5. Protein Quantification

1. Begin by preparing a standard consisting of a small set of serial dilutions of BSA. Label four centrifuge tubes with the following standardized concentrations: 1, 0.5, 0.25, and 0.125 µg/µL. Add 100 µL of TE to each tube. Add 100 µL of BSA stock to the "1-mg/mL" tube and mix. Transfer 100 µL of this solution to the "0.5-mg/mL" tube, and mix. Continue until serial dilutions are complete. Standards remain good for 1 week at 4°C.

2. Next, prepare "working reagent" by combining 50 parts reagent A with 1 part reagent B The working reagent will be green.

3. Pipet 10 µL of each BSA standard (including the 2 mg/mL stock and the blank, 10 µL of buffer) into appropriate 96-well microtiter plate wells, changing tips each time. Perform these standards in triplicate.

4. Pipette 10-µL samples of each lysate into fresh wells, in duplicate.

5. For 1:2 dilutions, pipet 5 µL of each lysate and 5 µL TE buffer into fresh wells, in duplicate.

6. Make a map showing where each standard and sample were placed.

7. Add 200 µL of working reagent to each well.
8. Cover the microtiter plate and shake at 200 rpm at room temperature for 30 s on an orbital shaker.
9. Incubate at 37°C for 30 min.
10. Using a plate reader, read the absorbance of each well at 562 nm. Average the absorbances of the three replicates of each standard, and create a standard curve for each plate using the controls by directly connecting the dots. (This curve should reflect the actual data, rather than relying on an idealized, computer-generated curve fit.) Average the absorbances of the two undiluted samples with the average of the two 1:2 dilutions multiplied by 2, and then determine the concentration of protein based on the absorbance vs concentration curve. Calculate the volume of each sample necessary to yield 26.0 ng of total protein.

3.6. Quantification of Luciferase Expression

The following protocol was adapted from Promega's Technical Manual No. 281, Luciferase® Assay System *(8)*.

1. If a manual luminometer is being used, proceed directly to **step 2**. If the luminometer being used has an automatic injector, place pump tubing into the reagent reservoir. Prime the injector with sufficient reagent before beginning. Settings for the automated luminometer should be as follows: measuring time: 10 s; delay: 3 s; injection delay: 1 s; injection volume: 100 µL.
2. To measure background (all measurements in relative light units [RLUs]), pipet 50-µL aliquots of 1X RLB into three luminometer tubes, and measure the luminescence. This background reading will automatically be subtracted from all subsequent readings.
3. To measure samples, pipet the amount of each calculated to give 26 ng of total protein into each of three luminometer tubes. Add sufficient 1X RLB to each tube to give a total volume of 50 µL.
4. For each sample, first pipet 100 µL of LAR into a luminometer tube. Then, add the amount of each sample calculated to give 26 ng of total protein, and mix by pipeting two or three times. Do not vortex. Vortexing will coat the sides of the sample tube with the luminescent mixture. After 10 s of reading, remove the tube and record the reading.

3.7. Quantification of β-Galactosidase Expression

The following protocol was adapted from **ref. *10***.

1. For each sample, pipet the amount calculated to give 26 ng of total protein (from **Subheading 3.5., step 10**) into a 15-mL conical tube, and add sufficient 1X RLB to provide a final volume of 50 µL.
2. Dilute this sample 1:100 in breaking buffer. (Sample volume is now 5 mL.)
3. Add 50 µL of this dilution to 1 mL Z buffer in a disposable cuvet, and equilibrate at 28°C.
4. Prepare a blank of breaking buffer in Z buffer as a control for spontaneous hydrolysis of ONPG.
5. To all samples and blank, add 0.2 mL ONPG solution, also equilibrated to 28°C.
6. Incubate samples for at least 10 min at 28°C, watching for a yellow color to develop.
7. As each sample becomes noticeably yellow, stop the reaction by adding 0.5 mL 1 *M* Na_2CO_3, and record the length of time required for the color change.

8. Read the OD_{420} against the negative control for spontaneous hydrolysis of ONPG control, and calculate the specific activity of each sample using the formula (*see* **Note 9**):

$$\frac{OD_{420} \times 380}{\text{min at } 28°C \times \text{mg protein in reaction}}$$

9. Subtract the average specific activity of the three mock-transfected wells from those of both the "damaged" and "undamaged" wells. This will control for the endogenous β-galactosidase activity present in some cell types.

3.8. Calculating Relative TCR Capacities

1. For each sample, divide the luciferase RLU by the β-galactosidase specific activity to correct for transfection efficiency.
2. Find the average of the mock-transfected wells, the wells transfected with undamaged plasmid, and the wells transfected with damaged plasmid for each sample.
3. Subtract the average of the mock-transfected wells from the average of the undamaged and the average of the damaged wells.
4. The ratio of damaged to undamaged wells is a measure of TCR.
5. If desired, divide again by positive control to express as % normal.
6. If normal control has been evaluated in the context of a population of normals, normalize again by the ratio of the experimental normal to the average of the normal population to express your experimental data relative to the normal population.

4. Notes

1. Next to UV, X-irradiation is the most common damaging agent used in the HCR assay *(11)*. Under most conditions, this treatment results in a mixture of DNA double-strand breaks and lesions caused by ionization of the medium, followed by its interaction with the DNA target. In this simple system, DSB repair probably involves mostly nonhomologous end joining, although more complicated HCR assays specific for homologous recombinational repair have also been developed *(12; see* also Chap. 31).

   UV damage creates primarily pyrimidine dimers and 6-4 photoproducts, both of which involve covalent binding of adjacent bases from the same DNA strand and result in an obvious constriction of the DNA helix. A number of other agents have been used to generate such intrastrand crosslinks (ICL) in the plasmid target of an HCR assay, including *cis*-platinum *(13)*, L-phenylalanine mustard (L-PAM) *(14)*, and mechlorethane *(15)*. Like 8-methoxypsoralen *(16)*, however, some of these agents also cause interstrand crosslinks, which in turn block replication at S phase or cause double-strand breaks during mitotic chromosome segregation.

   NER also repairs so-called bulky adducts, such as those induced by 2-amino-1-methyl-6-phenylimidazole[4,5]pyridine (PhIP) and *N*-acetyl-2-aminofluorene (AAF), and these have also been used to damage plasmids for HCR analysis of repair *(17)*. 4-Hydroxy-aminoquinoline-1-oxide, the proximate form of 4-nitroquinoline-1-oxide (4NQO) has also been used to study NER by HCR *(18)*, as has benzo[*a*]pyrene diol epoxide, a derivative of the tobacco smoke mutagen benzo[*a*]pyrene *(19)*. These compounds illustrate the fact that since the plasmid is exposed outside of a biological system, chemicals that require metabolic activation are not operative in this assay. If the carcinogenic derivatives of a chemical are known, however, as in the above examples, they can be studied instead of the parental species; there is also no reason why pretreatment of the parental chemical with microsomal S9 couldn't be used, although this would be expected to produce a mixed exposure. Plasmid treatment with monofunctional alkylating reagents such as 2-chloroethyl ethyl sulfide would also be expected to generate bulky adducts *(20)*. Finally, rather than simply expose the plasmid to a damaging agent, an altered base can also be specifically incorporated during its synthesis, such as the free-radical–induced bulky adduct 8,5'-(S)-cyclo-2'-deoxyadenosine *(21)*, or even a simple fluorescein label *(22)*.

Base excision repair (BER) has also been analyzed by HCR, using either nonspecific methylating agents such as *N*-methyl-*N*'-nitro-*N*-nitrosoguanidine (MNNG) *(23)* or very specific methylating agents known to produce substrates for specific BER glycosylases, such as 5-(3-methyl-1-triazeno)imidazole-4-carboxamide (MTIC) *(24)*. BER is also known to remediate some of the damage caused by exposure of DNA to oxidative agents, such as ozone and sources of singlet oxygen *(25,26)*. The steps in BER beyond the initial glycosylation can be analyzed by acid/heat treatment of the plasmid to produce apurinic sites *(27)*, or apurinic sites can be specifically introduced *(28)*.

A specific modification of the HCR assay has been developed to allow for analysis of DNA mismatch repair via generation of microsatellite instability following exposure of the reporter plasmid to etoposide or fotemustine *(29)*. This is not a very quantitative assay, however, and it seems strange that HCR plasmids have not simply been generated with single or multiple base mismatches by isolation of heteroduplexes. Further guidance in the creation of site-specifically modified templates can be found in Perlow et al. *(30)*.

2. Appropriate positive control cells would include: fibroblasts or lymphocytes derived from healthy adult patients, or skin fibroblast cultures derived from patients with xeroderma pigmentosum complementation group C (XPC). These cell types are all known to be competent in TCR. (The deficiency in XPC cells is specific to GGR.) It is important to consider the fact that NER has been shown to be tissue-specific *(31–33)* and that the choice of a positive control should reflect this tissue specificity, if possible. In addition, when a putative disease specimen is being tested, this sample should be placed into the context of the normal range. This can be accomplished by running several normal controls for comparison or by comparing with a previously established range of normal *(3)*. "Normal" human fibroblasts or lymphocytes can be obtained from the Coriell Cell Repositories (Camden, NJ; http://locus.umdnj.edu/ccr). It should be noted, however, that some of these cell lines have been immortalized using exogenous agents and that several of these agents have been shown to alter the original DNA repair capacity of the cells *(34,35)*. Several cell lines that have not been treated with exogenous agents are available.

3. The most appropriate negative controls for this experiment are fibroblasts or lymphocytes that have been derived from Cockayne syndrome (CS) patients, either type I or type II. Patients with deficiencies in XP complementation groups A, D, F, and G share their inability to perform TCR *(36)*. Explant cultures as well as immortalized cell lines of fibroblasts and lymphocytes derived from patients with these inborn diseases can be obtained from Coriell Cell Repositories (*see* **Note 2**).

4. A specialized machine has been created to deliver the damaging dosage of UVC light (or any UV-based light) accurately (**Fig. 2**) *(37)*. The machine consists of a turntable, an electronically timed shutter, and three Wistam bulbs (General Electric, Nela Park, OH) placed above the turntable behind the shutter. An issue that has arisen involves the length of time required to irradiate the plasmids: it is too long to use on the electrically timed

shutter, making it necessary to turn the light sources on and off manually. The company that produced this instrument (Design Specialties, Bethel Park, PA) is being consulted for an alternate timer that encompasses a longer time period.

5. The amount of DNA used in each well, the ratio of experimental to control plasmid, and the amount of Lipofectamine 2000 reagent may be different for every cell type. Cell lines may vary by several orders of magnitude in their ability to take up DNA. Experiments to optimize these amounts can be carried out per recommendations by Invitrogen *(7)*. Ratios of 10:1 to 50:1 experimental-to-control vector are recommended by Promega *(37)*, as they minimize potential *trans* effects between promoter elements.

6. The reconstituted LAR can be frozen at –80°C for 1 mo. The components are heat-labile, and frozen aliquots should be thawed in a water bath at room temperature. Mix thawed reagent prior to use by inverting several times or gently vortexing.

7. UV bulbs should be turned on 2 h prior to use and tested with a Spectroline short-wave (252 nm) UV meter (Spectroline DM-254XA Short Wave Ultraviolet Meter, Spectronics, Westbury, NY). After determining fluence, use the formula fluence × time = dose to determine the amount of time needed for irradiation. The readout from the Spectroline meter will be in $\mu W/cm^2$ (e.g., 210 $\mu W/cm^2$ = 2.1 J m^{-2} sec^{-1}).

8. For 700 J/m^2 with a mean fluence of 2.1 J/m^2s from the UV bulbs, a 333-s exposure of the plasmid is required. In order for such a long exposure time to be undertaken with the machine described above, the latch on the shutter must be unhooked and the lights themselves turned on and off for timing (*see* **Note 4**).

9. For example, if the assay was conducted for 10 min and the OD_{420} was 0.500, the specific activity would be:

$$\frac{0.500 \times 380}{10.0 \times 0.026} = 730 \text{ units/mg}$$

References

1. Rupert, C. and Harm, W. (1966) Reactivation after photobiological damage. *Adv. Radiat. Biol.* **2,** 1–81.

2. Protic-Sabljic, M. and Kraemer, K. H. (1985) One pyrimidine dimer inactivates expression of a transfected gene in xeroderma pigmentosum cells. *Proc. Natl. Acad. Sci. USA* **82,** 6622–6626.

3. Athas, W. F., Hedayati, M. A., Matanoski, G. M., Farmer, E. R., and Grossman, L. (1991) Development and field-test validation of an assay for DNA repair in circulating human lymphocytes. *Cancer Res.* **51,** 5786–5793.

4. Bohr, V. A., Smith, C. A., Okumoto, D. S., and Hanawalt, P. C. (1985) DNA repair in an active gene: removal of pyrimidine dimers from the DHFR gene of CHO cells is much more efficient than in the genome overall. *Cell* **40,** 359–369.

5. Matijasevic, Z., Precopio, M. L., Snyder, J. E., and Ludlum, D. B. (2001) Repair of sulfur mustard-induced DNA damage in mammalian cells measured by a host cell reactivation assay. *Carcinogenesis* **22,** 661–664.

6. Berwick, M. and Veneis, P. (2000) Markers of DNA repair and susceptibility to cancer in humans: an epidemiologic review. *J. Natl. Cancer Inst.* **92,** 847–897.

7. Invitrogen Life Technologies Lipofectamine 2000 CD Reagent, pp. 1–2; available at http://www.invitrogen.com.

8. Promega Luciferase Assay System Instructions, Technical Bulletin No. 281, pp. 1–13; available at http://www.promega.com.

9. BCA Protein Assay Reagent Kit 23227 Instructions, pp. 1–8; available at http://www.piercenet.com.

10. Miller, J. H. (1972) *Experiments in Molecular Genetics*, Cold Spring Harbor Laboratory, Cold Spring Harbor, NY, pp. 352–355.

11. Rainbow, A. (1975) Host-cell reactivation of irradiated human adenovirus. *Basic Life Sci.* **5B,** 753–754.

12. Slebos, R. J. and Taylor, J. A. (2001) A novel host cell reactivation assay to assess homologous recombination capacity in human cancer cell lines. *Biochem. Biophys. Res. Commun.* **281,** 212–219.

13. Hansson, J. and Wood, R. D. (1989) Repair synthesis by human cell extracts in DNA damaged by cis- and trans-diamminedichloroplatinum(II). *Nucleic Acids Res.* **17,** 8073–8091.

14. Yen, L., Woo, A., Christopoulopoulos, G., et al. (1995) Enhanced host cell reactivation capacity and expression of DNA repair genes in human breast cancer cells resistant to bi-functional alkylating agents. *Mutat. Res.* **337,** 179–189.

15. Dean, S. W., Sykes, H. R., and Lehmann, A. R. (1988) Inactivation by nitrogen mustard of plasmids introduced into normal and Fanconi's anaemia cells. *Mutat. Res.* **194,** 57–63.

16. Sun, Y. and Moses, R. E. (1991) Reactivation of psoralen-reacted plasmid in Fanconi anemia, xeroderma pigmentosum, and normal human fibroblast cells. *Somat. Cell Mol. Genet.* **17,** 229–238.

17. Stevnsner, T., Frandsen, H., and Autrup, H. (1995) Repair of DNA lesions induced by ultraviolet irradiation and aromatic amines in normal and repair-deficient human lymphoblastoid cell lines. *Carcinogenesis* **16,** 2855–2858.

18. Tanooka, H. and Tada, M. (1975) Reparable lethal DNA damage produced by enzyme-activated 4-hydroxyaminoquinoline 1-oxide. *Chem. Biol. Interact.* **10,** 11–18.

19. Cheng, L., Eicher, S. A., Guo, Z., Hong, W. K., Spitz, M. R., and Wei, Q. (1998) Reduced DNA repair capacity in head and neck cancer patients. *Cancer Epidemiol. Biomarkers Prev.* **7,** 465–468.

20. Matsijasevic, Z., Precopio, M. L., Snyder, J. E., and Ludlum, D. B. (2001) Repair of sulfur mustard-induced DNA damage in mammalian cells measured by a host cell reactivation assay. *Carcinogenesis* **22,** 661–664.

21. Kuraoka, I., Bender, C., Romieu, A., Cadet, J., Wood, R. D., and Lindahl, T. (2000) Removal of oxygen free-radical-induced 5',8-purine cyclodeoxynucleosides from DNA by the nucleotide excision repair pathway in human cells. *Proc. Natl. Acad. Sci. USA.* **97,** 3832–3837.

22. Iakoucheva, L. M., Walker, R. K., van Houten, B., and Ackerman, E. J. (2002) Equilibrium and stop-slow kinetic studies of fluorescently labeled DNA substrates with DNA repair proteins XPA and replication protein A. *Biochemistry* **41,** 131–143.

23. Day, R. S. III and Ziolkowski, C. H. (1979) Human brain tumour cell strains with deficient host-cell reactivation of N-methyl-N'-nitro-N-nitrosoguanidine-damaged adenovirus 5. *Nature* **279,** 797–799.

24. Maynard, K., Parsons, P. G., Cerny, T., and Margison, G. P. (1989) Relationships among cell survival, O^6-alkylguanine-DNA alkyltransferase activity, and reactivation of methylated adenovirus 5 and herpes simplex virus type 1 in human melanoma cell lines. *Cancer Res.* **49,** 4813–4817.

25. L'Herault, P. and Chung, Y. S. (1982) Host cell reactivation of ozone-treated T3 bacteriophage by different strains of *Escherichia coli*. *Experentia* **38,** 1491–1492.

26. Diem, C. and Runger, T. M. (1997) Processing of three different types of DNA damage in

cell lines of a cutaneous squamous cell carcinoma progression model. *Carcinogenesis* **18,** 657–662.

27. Protic-Sabljic, M. and Kraemer, K. H. (1986) Host cell reactivation by human cells of DNA expression vectors damaged by ultraviolet radiation or by acid/heat treatment. *Carcinogenesis* **7,** 1765–1770.

28. Matsumoto, Y. (1999) Base excision repair assay using *Xenopus laevis* oocyte extracts, in *Methods in Molecular Biology*, vol. 113, *DNA Repair Protocols: Eukaryotic Systems* (Henderson, D. S., ed.), Humana, Totowa, NJ, pp. 289–300.

29. Runger, T. M., Emmert, S., Schadendorf, D., Diem, C., Epe, B., and Hellfritsch, D. (2000) Alterations of DNA repair in melanoma cell lines resistant to cisplatin, fotemustine, or etoposide. *J. Invest. Dermatol.* **114,** 34–39.

30. Perlow, R. A., Schinecker, T. M., Kim, S. J., Geacintov, N. E., and Scicchitano, D. A. (2003) Construction and purification of site-specifically modified DNA templates for transcription assays. *Nucleic Acids. Res.* **31,** e40.

31. Latimer, J. J., Hultner, M. L., Cleaver, J. E., and Pedersen, R. A. (1996) Elevated DNA excision repair capacity in the extraembryonic mesoderm of the mid-gestation mouse embryo. *Exp. Cell Res.* **228,** 19–28.

32. Cheng, L., Guan, Y., Li, L., et al. (1999) Expression in normal human tissues of five nucleotide excision repair genes measured simultaneously by multiplex reverse transcription-polymerase chain reaction. *Cancer Epidemiol. Biomarkers Prev.* **8,** 801–807.

33. Latimer, J. J., Nazir, T., Flowers, L. C., et al. (2003) Unique tissue-specific level of DNA nucleotide excision repair in primary human mammary epithelial cultures. *Exp. Cell Res.* **291,** 111–121.

34. Ford, J. M., Baron, E. L., and Hanawalt, P. C. (1998) Human fibroblasts expressing the human papillomavirus E6 gene are deficient in global genomic nucleotide excision repair and sensitive to ultraviolet irradiation. *Cancer Res.* **58,** 599–603.

35. Bowman, K. K., Sicard, D. M., Ford, J. M., and Hanawalt, P. C. (2000) Reduced global genomic repair of ultraviolet light-induced cyclobutane pyrimidine dimers in simian virus 40-transformed human cells. *Mol. Carcinogen.* **29,** 17–24.

36. Fututa, T., Ueda, T., Aune, G., Sarasin, A., Kraemer, K. H., and Pommier, Y. (2002) Transcription-coupled nucleotide excision repair as a determinant of cisplatin sensitivity of human cells. *Cancer Res.* **65,** 4899–4902.

37. Steier, H. and Cleaver, J. E. (1969) Exposure chamber for quantitative ultraviolet photobiology. *Lab Prac.* **18,** 1295.

38. Promega Transfection Guide, pp. 1–56; available at http://www.promega.com.

29

An Immunoassay for Measuring Repair
of Ultraviolet Photoproducts

Shirley McCready

Summary

A method is described that makes use of a polyclonal antiserum to measure repair of the principal photoproducts induced in DNA by short-wave ultraviolet light (UVC)—pyrimidine-pyrimidone 6-4 photoproducts ([6-4]PPs) and cyclobutane pyrimidine dimers (CPDs). DNA extracted from irradiated cells is applied to a nitrocellulose dot blot and quantitated using an enzyme-conjugated secondary antibody and a color assay. Although the polyclonal antiserum contains antibodies to both [6-4]PPs and CPDs, repair of these can be measured separately by differential destruction or repair of one or other photoproduct. The method is useful for measuring repair in total genomic DNA and is sufficiently sensitive to measure repair of damage induced by doses of 10 J/m^2 of UVC and less. The method is very versatile and has been used to measure repair in human cells, yeasts, plants, archaea, bacteria, and filamentous fungi.

Key Words: UV damage; DNA repair; cyclobutane dimers; 6-4 photoproducts; immunoassay; dot blot.

1. Introduction

The dot blot method described here can be used to measure repair of the principal photoproducts induced in DNA by short-wave ultraviolet light (UVC)—pyrimidine-pyrimidone 6-4 photoproducts ([6-4]PPs), and cyclobutane pyrimidine dimers (CPDs). These photoproducts are also induced by midwave UV light (ultraviolet-B [UVB]), and the method given here can be used to measure UVB damage induced, for example, by Westinghouse FS-20 lamps. The method is used to measure the overall rate of repair in total genomic DNA. One of the advantages it has over other methods is its sensitivity—the assay is sufficiently sensitive to measure repair of damage induced by doses of 10 J/m^2 of UVC with ease and could be used for lower doses. It is also very versatile and has been successfully used to measure repair in human cells, in yeasts, and in a variety of other organisms (*1–3*; McCready, unpublished data). In addition, the DNA does not have to be especially intact for this assay, unlike polymerase chain reaction (PCR) methods and alkaline gel methods that rely on high and uniform integrity of the extracted DNA.

From: *Methods in Molecular Biology, vol. 291, Molecular Toxicology Protocols*
Edited by: P. Keohavong and S. G. Grant © Humana Press Inc., Totowa, NJ

To use the method, it is necessary to raise polyclonal antiserum to UV-irradiated DNA. The antiserum must then be characterized for its ability to recognize damage that can be photoreactivated by *E. coli* photolyase (CPDs) and damage that is not photoreactivated (predominantly [6-4]PPs and the Dewar isomer of [6-4]PPs *[4,5]*). Antisera containing activities against both CPDs and [6-4]PPs can be used to measure total lesions. Alternatively, it can be used to measure each type of photoproduct individually, by destroying one or the other lesion in the DNA before carrying out the assay. [6-4]PPs can be destroyed by treating DNA samples with hot alkali prior to the blotting. CPDs can be destroyed in the DNA after it has been transferred to the blot by treating the entire membrane with *E. coli* photolyase and visible light.

To perform the assay, cells are irradiated with UV, and samples are harvested immediately and after suitable incubation periods. DNA can be extracted from the cells by a variety of procedures—commercially available kits or the phenol or phenol-chloroform methods. It is of crucial importance to equalize the amounts of DNA in samples from the different time-points, and this is best done by running aliquots on an agarose gel and estimating relative amounts by densitometry. Concentrations must be adjusted and checked on gels for as many times as necessary until the DNA concentrations are uniform. Each DNA sample is then divided in two, and one-half is treated with hot alkali to destroy [6-4]PPs. Dilution series of the samples are then applied to duplicate dot blots. One blot is exposed to a crude preparation of photolyase and illuminated with visible light to destroy CPDs. The blots are then exposed to the polyclonal antiserum, then to a biotinylated secondary antibody, and then to alkaline phosphatase-conjugated avidin. Nitroblue tetrazolium is used as substrate, so that a blue color stains the DNA containing UV lesions. Over a certain range, the amount of blue color is proportional to the amount of damage. Blots contain their own built-in calibration curves, namely, the dilution series of the time-zero samples. The amount of damage remaining in postincubation samples is quantitated by densitometry and reference to the time-zero dilution series.

The method was originally developed for measuring repair rates in yeast, and the details that follow are as used for budding yeast. Exactly the same method can be used for measuring repair in human or other mammalian cells. The difference is only in the protocol for the repair experiment and DNA extraction.

2. Materials

All growth media and buffers are sterilized by autoclaving. If not otherwise attributed, all chemicals and reagents are available from Sigma-Aldrich (Dorset, UK).

2.1. Production of Polyclonal Antiserum

1. High-molecular-weight calf thymus DNA: make 10 mL by dissolving at 1 mg/mL in isotonic saline. Can store at –20°C for up to 1 yr.
2. Isotonic saline: 0.15 *M* NaCl (should be pH 7.0 without needing adjustment). Make up 100 mL stock and sterilize by autoclaving; stable at 4°C for up to 1 mo.
3. Microcentrifuge tubes.
4. TE-equilibrated phenol.
5. Microcentrifuge (e.g., Eppendorf model 5415D, Fisher, Loughborough, UK).
6. 100% Ethanol.

7. Midwave ultraviolet light (UVB) source (e.g., Westinghouse FS20 sunlamp, Philadelphia, PA).
8. 95°C Heating block or water bath.
9. 2X Isotonic saline: 0.30 M NaCl (should be pH 7.0 without needing adjustment). Make up 100 mL stock and sterilize by autoclaving; stable at 4°C for up to 1 mo.
10. Methylated bovine serum albumin (MBSA): 1 mL should be made fresh for each experiment by dissolving at 2 mg/mL in sterile water and adding an equal volume of 2X isotonic saline (final concentration 1 mg/mL in isotonic saline).
11. 1-mL Syringe.
12. 4.5-μm Syringe filter.
13. 2–5-mL Syringes and needles.
14. Complete Freund's adjuvant.
15. Incomplete Freund's adjuvant.
16. Poly(dA)·poly(dT).

2.2. Preparation of Crude Photolyase

1. Luria broth (LB) with 20 mg/mL tetracycline. Make 1 L of LB as required. Store at 4°C for up to 1 wk, adding 2 mL of tetracycline stock to each liter of LB immediately before inoculating with *E. coli*. The tetracycline stock consists of 100 μg of tetracycline dissolved in 10 mL 50% (v/v) ethanol. It should be stored at 4°C shielded from light.
2. 840 mM Isopropylthio-β-D-galactopyranoside (IPTG; 0.2 g/mL in water): make 20 mL and store in 1-mL aliquots at –20°C.
3. Lysis buffer: 50 mM Tris-HCl, pH 7.4, 1 mM EDTA, 100 mM NaCl, 10 mM β-mercaptoethanol. Stock of 100 mL should be autoclaved before adding β-mercaptoethanol; may be stored at 4°C for up to 1 mo.
4. 20-mL Glass universal (McCartney) bottles (Fisher).
5. Sonicator (e.g., Ultrasonic disintegrator, Fisher).
6. Centrifuge (e.g., Sorvall RC-5B with SS-34 rotor, Fisher).
7. Ultracentrifuge (e.g., Beckman Optima with a Ti50 rotor (Beckman Coulter, Fullerton, CA).
8. Corex centrifuge tubes (Fisher).
9. Storage buffer: 50 mM Tris-HCl, pH 7.4, 1 mM EDTA, 50% glycerol, 10 mM dithiothreitol (DTT). Stock of 100 mL should be autoclaved before adding DTT; may be stored at 4°C for up to 1 mo.
10. *E. coli* strain PMS 969 PHR1; kindly provided by Dr. Aziz Sancar *(6) (see* **Note 1***)*.

2.3. Repair Experiments and DNA Isolation

1. YEPD medium: 1% yeast extract, 1% peptone, 2% dextrose. Make 100 mL and store at 4°C for up to 1 mo after sterilizing.
2. 50-mL Tubes (e.g., BD Biosciences, Franklin Lakes, NJ).
3. 10-mL (or larger) pipets.
4. 100% Ethanol (ice cold).
5. Ice and appropriate container.
6. 10X YEPD: 10% yeast extract, 10% peptone, 20% dextrose. Make 100 mL and divide into 10-mL aliquots in glass universal (McCartney) bottles. May be stored for up to 3 mo at 4°C.
7. 28°C Temperature controlled water bath or orbital shaker.
8. Centrifuge (e.g., Sorvall RC-5B with SS-34 rotor, Fisher).
9. Set of micropipetors and appropriate tips.
10. Tris-EDTA (TE): 10 mM Tris-HCl, pH 8.0, 1 mM EDTA. Make 1 L and store for up to 1 mo at 4°C.

11. Microcentrifuge tubes.
12. Microcentrifuge.
13. 1 *M* Sorbitol: make 1 L and store at 4°C for up to 1 mo after autoclaving.
14. Zymolyase: zymolyase 20T (ICN Biochemicals, Basingstoke, UK) dissolved in sterile water at 10 mg/mL. Make 10 mL and store at –20°C as 0.5-mL aliquots in sterile microcentrifuge tubes.
15. Phase contrast microscope.
16. 10% Sodium dodecyl sulfate (SDS): 10% (w/v) SDS in water. Make 100 mL in a sterile glass bottle; heat at 65°C for 1 h to sterilize. Can be stored at room temperature for up to 1 yr.
17. Phenol-chloroform: 50 mL of TE-equilibrated phenol, 50 mL of chloroform, 2 mL of isoamyl alcohol.
18. 3 *M* Sodium acetate, adjusted to pH 5.2 with glacial acetic acid. Make 100 mL and store at room temperature for up to 6 mo after autoclaving.
19. RNaseA solution (DNase-free; Sigma no. 4642). Store at –20°C.
20. Agarose and agarose gel apparatus (e.g., Bio-Rad, Hemel Hempstead, UK)
21. 5 µg/mL Ethidium bromide: 100 mL are necessary to stain a gel, but may be reused. **Caution:** Ethidium bromide is a powerful carcinogen.
22. Gel scanner and image analysis system suitable for quantitative analysis of color intensity on dot blots (e.g., Bio-Rad Molecular Imager).

2.4. Preparation and Processing of Dot Blots

1. Microcentrifuge tubes.
2. Set of micropipetors and appropriate tips.
3. Control DNA containing CPDs: irradiate 10 mL herring sperm DNA (0.1 mg/mL) in 10 n*M* acetophenone in an open Petri dish with midwave ultraviolet light. Under these conditions, the only detectable photoproducts are CPDs *(7)*. Store at –20°C in 1-mL aliquots in microcentrifuge tubes.
4. 1 *N* NaOH. Always make 10 mL fresh.
5. 90°C Water bath.
6. Ice and appropriate container.
7. Neutralizing solution: 3 *M* potassium acetate in 5 *M* acetic acid. Make 20 mL and store at room temperature for up to 3 mo after autoclaving.
8. Siliconized microtiter plates (e.g., 96-well V-bottomed plates—siliconization is done using Sigmacote according to the manufacturer's instructions).
9. 1 *M* Ammonium acetate: make 1 L and store at room temperature for up to 1 mo.
10. Dot blot apparatus (e.g., Bio-Rad or Schleicher and Schuell, London, UK).
11. Nitrocellulose membrane (e.g., Schleicher and Schuell; *see* **Note 2**).
12. 5X SSC: 0.75 *M* sodium chloride, 0.075 *M* sodium citrate (should be pH 7.0 without needing adjustment). Make 1 L and store at room temperature for up to 1 mo.
13. 1% Gelatin: make 50 mL per blot fresh as required. Warm to dissolve in water (i.e., 50–60°C. Do not boil).
14. Photoreactivation solution: 100 µL of crude photoreactivating enzyme (from **Subheading 3.2.**) in 20 mL of 50 m*M* Tris-HCl, pH 7.6.
15. Two standard desk lamps with 60-W bulbs.
16. Plate glass pieces the approximate size and shape of the blots. The edges should be beveled to minimize risk of injury.
17. Phosphate-buffered saline (PBS): 20 m*M* sodium phosphate, 150 m*M* NaCl. Make 1 L and store at room temperature for up to 1 mo.

18. PBNT: PBS containing 0.5% normal goat serum, 0.5% bovine serum albumin (BSA), 0.05% Tween-20. Make 50 mL per blot, as required. Do not store.
19. Carrier DNA: a scaled-up (20-mL) crude DNA preparation from yeast, prepared as in **Subheading 3.4.** Can be stored at –20°C for up to 1 yr.
20. Anti-UV-DNA polyclonal antiserum (from **Subheading 3.1., step 6**).
21. PBX: PBS containing 0.1% Tween-20. Make 1 L at 2X and store at room temperature for up to 1 mo.
22. Biotinylated antirabbit antiserum and alkaline phosphatase-conjugated ExtrAvidin (ExtrAvidin Alkaline phosphatase staining kit, Sigma EXTRA-3A; *see* **Note 3**).
23. Tris-buffered saline (TBS): 50 mM Tris-HCl, pH 7.4, 150 mM NaCl. Make 1 L and store at room temperature for up to 1 mo.
24. Alkaline phosphatase buffer: 100 mM NaCl, 5 mM MgCl$_2$, 100 mM Tris-HCl (should be pH 9.5 without needing adjustment). Make 1 L and store at room temperature for up to 1 mo.
25. 15 mL Alkaline phosphatase substrate (premixed solution of nitro blue tetrazolium and 5-bromo-4-chloro-3-indolylphosphate available from Invitrogen, Paisley, UK; *see* **Note 3**).
26. PBS-EDTA: PBS containing 0.75% (w/v) EDTA. Make 20 mL and store at –20°C for up to 1 yr.
27. Any image analysis system suitable for quantitative analysis of color intensity on dot blots (e.g., Bio-Rad Molecular Imager).

3. Methods

3.1. Preparation and Characterization of the Polyclonal Antiserum

The antiserum is raised in rabbits, following the protocol described by Mitchell and Clarkson *(4)*.

1. Dissolve freshly phenol-extracted and ethanol-precipitated calf thymus DNA (use standard procedure *[8]* or adaptation of the protocol in **Subheading 3.4., step 4**) in isotonic saline at a concentration of 1 mg/mL.
2. Irradiate 2 mL of the DNA solution in an open Petri dish on ice, giving a total dose of 100 kJ/m^2.
3. Adjust the concentration of the DNA to 0.4 mg/mL with isotonic saline.
4. Immediately prior to inoculation, heat-denature the irradiated DNA at 95°C for 5 min in a heating block or water bath. Prepare 1 mL of immunogen by mixing 0.5 mL of the heat-denatured irradiated DNA with 0.5 mL of MBSA. Mix gently but thoroughly and filter-sterilize by passing through a 4.5-µm syringe filter.
5. For the first injection, emulsify 1 mL of immunogen with 1 mL of complete Freund's adjuvant. Give four subsequent injections every 2 wk using incomplete adjuvant. Two weeks after the last injection, administer a booster of 200 µg of poly(dA)·poly(dT) DNA irradiated with a dose of 250 kJ/m^2. Preimmune serum and test bleeds taken after each injection must be checked for activity.
6. Harvest the antiserum 2 wk after the booster. The exact details of this protocol must be approved and possibly modified according to local rules for animal handling.
7. Test bleeds: prepare test strips by applying a dilution series of denatured herring sperm DNA, which has been irradiated with UVC at 50 J/m^2 to dot blots in the same way as for the repair assay (*see* **Subheading 3.5.**). Process the test strips in exactly the same way as for the repair assay (*see* **Subheading 3.6.**). The activity of the antiserum against total lesions and nondimer photoproducts should be monitored (**Fig. 1**).

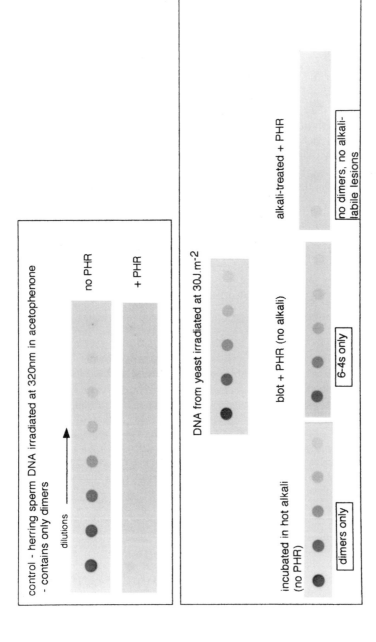

Fig. 1. Strip tests for polyclonal antiserum. The control DNA (top panel) contains only CPDs, which are completely removed by incubating the blot in photolyase (PHR) under visible light illumination (photoreactivation). Yeast DNA incubated in hot alkali (lower left) contains only CPDs, which are completely removed if the blot is treated with photolyase (lower right). Photolyase treatment alone removes CPDs (lower middle) and leaves alkali-labile sites, which are principally or entirely [6-4]PPs.

342

3.2. Preparation of Crude Photolyase

This method is based on the first part of the purification procedure for photolyase described by Sancar et al. *(6)*.

1. Grow *E. coli* (PHRl) in 1 L of LB containing tetracycline (25 mg/L) to an OD_{600} of approx 1.0–1.1. Add IPTG to 0.5 m*M*. Grow for a further 12 h.
2. Harvest the cells by centrifugation at 4000*g* and wash in lysis buffer.
3. Resuspend by pipeting in 20 mL of ice-cold lysis buffer. Divide the suspension into three aliquots in glass universal bottles, and sonicate (four 30-s pulses on ice). Keep the lysate cool.
4. Recombine the sonicated aliquots and spin at 31,000*g* at 4°C for 20 min.
5. Pour off the supernatent and spin at 120,000*g* at 4°C for 1 h.
6. Carefully pour the supernatant into a sterile 100-mL glass conical flask, and to 20 mL of supernatant, add 8.6 g of ammonium sulfate, slowly, over a 1-h period, keeping on ice and swirling to dissolve well.
7. Spin down the yellow precipitate, in a sterile Corex tube, at 8000*g* for 30 min at 4°C.
8. Dissolve the precipitate in 5 mL of ice-cold storage buffer. Add 100-mL aliquots to pre-cooled 0.5-mL microcentrifuge tubes and store at –70°C.
9. The photolyase preparation should be tested for photoreactivating activity on test strips (**Fig. 1**).

3.3. Repair Experiment

The method given here is for budding yeast, *Saccharomyces cerevisiae*. *See* **Note 4** for measuring repair in mammalian cells.

1. Irradiate mid-log–phase cells in sterile water at a cell density of $1–2 \times 10^7$/mL using a dose of 50 J/m^2. The cells should be irradiated as a 0.5-cm-deep suspension in an open plastic tray. Thirty milliliters of cell suspension will be necessary for each time-point (*see* **Notes 5** and **6**).
2. Immediately after irradiation, take a 30-mL sample and add 30 mL of ice-cold ethanol. This will serve as the time-zero sample.
3. Divide the remaining suspension into 30-mL aliquots. Add 3 mL of 10X YEPD to each, and incubate at 28°C with gentle shaking in a temperature-controlled water bath or orbital shaker. For each time-point, add one of the 30-mL cultures to 30 mL of ice-cold ethanol, and keep on ice for 5 min before harvesting by centrifugation at 27,000*g* for 10 min.
4. Resuspend the cells in 1 mL of TE by vortexing. Transfer to a microcentrifuge tube. Wash (resuspend as above, and then spin down in a microcentrifuge at 12,000*g* for 3 min) the cells in TE and then in 1 *M* sorbitol.

3.4. DNA Extraction

Various DNA extraction methods can be used. The method given here is for budding yeast, *S. cerevisiae*. A commercial kit for genomic DNA isolation can be used or, alternatively, DNA can be extracted by phenol/chloroform extraction as follows.

1. Resuspend the cells from **Subheading 3.3.**, **step 4** in 500 µL of 1 *M* sorbitol by vortexing, and add 25 µL of zymolyase to convert the cells to spheroplasts. After 10 min, begin checking the cells under the microscope—spheroplasts are round and dark under phase contrast, and they will swell and burst in water.

2. Spin down the spheroplasts in a microcentrifuge at 12,000*g* for 3 min.
3. Gently resuspend the spheroplasts by pipeting in 500 μL of TE and lyse by adding 50 μL of 10% SDS.
4. Add 500 μL of phenol/chloroform. Mix well by vortexing, and spin at 12,000*g* for 10 min in a microcentrifuge. Transfer the top (aqueous) layer to a 2-mL microcentrifuge tube and add 1 mL of room temperature ethanol. Precipitate the DNA at room temperature for 5 min.
5. Spin down the precipitate at 12,000*g* in a microcentrifuge at room temperature. Allow the precipitate to air-dry (can take anywhere from 30 min to several hours).
6. Dissolve the precipitate in 500 μL of water.
7. Add 50 μL of 3 *M* sodium acetate and 1 mL of room temperature ethanol.
8. Repeat **steps 5** and **6**. Add 2 μL of RNase A solution, and incubate for 30 min.
9. Repeat **step 7**, centrifuge at 12,000*g*, and dissolve the DNA in 450 μL of water.
10. Run 5-μL aliquots on 0.8% agarose gel(s), and stain by immersion in ethidium bromide solution. Scan the gel(s) and compare concentrations by densitometry using an appropriate image analysis system according to manufacturer's instructions. Adjust the concentrations, and run aliquots again. Repeat until all the samples have identical DNA concentrations (*see* **Note 7**).

3.5. Preparation of Dot Blots

The layout of the dot blots is shown in **Figs. 2** and **3**. Additional time-points are needed for mammalian cells (*see* **Note 4**).

1. Divide each 400 μL DNA sample into two 200-μL aliquots in microcentrifuge tubes on ice.
2. To one aliquot, add 22 μL of freshly made 1 *N* NaOH, incubate at 90°C for 30 min, and then cool on ice for 5 min.
3. Add 110 μL of neutralizing solution and 70 μL of water.
4. Treat the second 200-μL aliquot the same way, including the addition of NaOH, but omit the 90°C incubation.
5. Transfer 100-μL aliquots of all samples into siliconized microtiter plates, and set up a twofold dilution series in 1 *M* ammonium acetate in a 96-well microtiter plate, as indicated in **Fig. 2**.
6. Transfer samples onto nitrocellulose filters using a vacuum dot-blotting apparatus. Wash the filters by immersing and agitating briefly in 1 *M* ammonium acetate and then in 5X SSC, air-dry on filter paper (should take about 1 h after blotting off the excess on filter paper), and bake at 80°C for 2 h.

3.6. Developing the Dot Blots and Quantitating DNA Damage

This method is derived from that described by Wani et al. (*9*).

1. Incubate the blots overnight in 50 mL of a 1% gelatin solution at 37°C.
2. Incubate the blots destined for measurement of [6-4]PPs in 20 mL photoreactivation solution. Incubate the blots in individual plastic boxes for 5 min in the dark, followed by 1 h under two 60-W desk lamps, using a piece of plate glass to cut out wavelengths below 320 nm (*see* **Note 8**).
3. Rinse all blots in 50 mL PBS.
4. Incubate all blots at 37°C for 1 h in 20 mL of PBNT containing 1 mL of denatured crude unirradiated yeast carrier DNA (*see* **Notes 6** and **9**) and 1 μL/mL (i.e., 1:1000 dilution) anti-UV–DNA polyclonal antiserum.

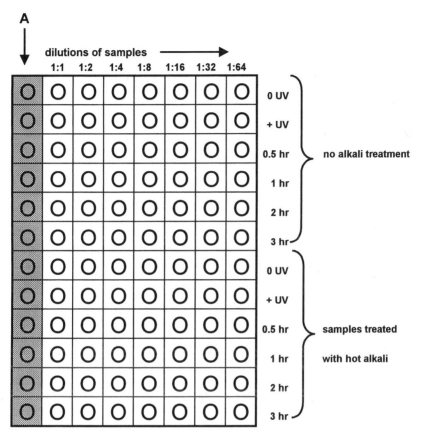

Fig. 2. Layout of dot blots for a typical repair experiment in yeast. Doubling dilutions in 1 *M* ammonium acetate are set up in microtiter plates, and samples are transferred to duplicate blotting membranes in the array illustrated.

5. Wash the blots four times in 100 mL PBX.
6. Incubate the blots for 1 h at 37°C in 20 mL PBNT containing 1:1000 biotinylated antirabbit antiserum.
7. Wash the blots three times in PBX followed by two washes in 100 mL TBS.
8. Incubate for 1 h at 37°C in 20 mL of TBS containing 1:1000 alkaline phosphatase-conjugated ExtrAvidin.
9. Wash the blots thoroughly in several changes of 100 mL TBS, and then incubate, in the dark, in 15 mL of substrate solution for 5–10 min. Watch the reaction and stop before the background begins to go blue, by adding 25 mL of PBS-EDTA. Rinse the blots in water (*see* **Note 10**). Examples of processed dot blots are shown in **Fig. 3**.
10. Air-dry the blots on filter paper and scan using a scanning densitometer with an image analysis facility (**Fig. 4**). Measure the intensity of the blue color in the dots and set up a calibration curve for each set of samples using the serial dilutions of the time-zero sample as standards. Calculate the lesions remaining in the samples from each of the time-points as a percentage of the lesions in the time-zero sample (**Fig. 5**; *see* **Note 11**).

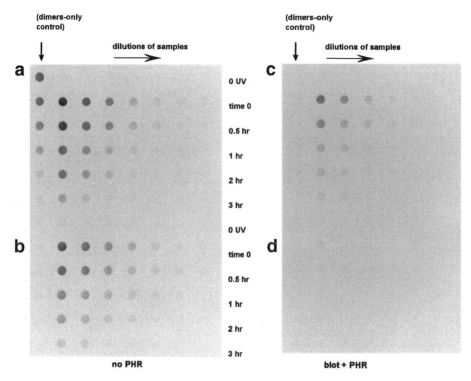

Fig. 3. Dot blots from a yeast repair experiment. Cells were irradiated with 50 J/m², and samples were taken immediately and at the postirradiation times indicated. Samples were applied in the array illustrated in **Fig. 2**. The blot on the right was incubated in photolyase (PHR) under visible light illumination to photoreactivate cyclobutane pyrimidine dimers (CPDs).

4. Notes

1. Available from the *E. coli* Stock Center, Yale University, New Haven, CT (http://cgsc.biology.yale.edu/cgsc.html).
2. Several types of membrane have been tried for this method. Nitrocellulose gives the lowest background and cleanest results. Nylon gives very high background and is not suitable.
3. Several different enzyme-linked assays and different substrates were used when developing this assay. The one described here gave a low background and good sensitivity.
4. For mammalian cells, postirradiation incubation times must be longer than for yeast. For example, human cells repair only 50% of CPDs during a 24-h incubation after UV, although [6-4]PPs are repaired within a few hours *(10)*.
5. The appropriate number and timing of sampling is organism- and dose-dependent and must be found by trial and error, or by reference to the relevant literature *(1)*.

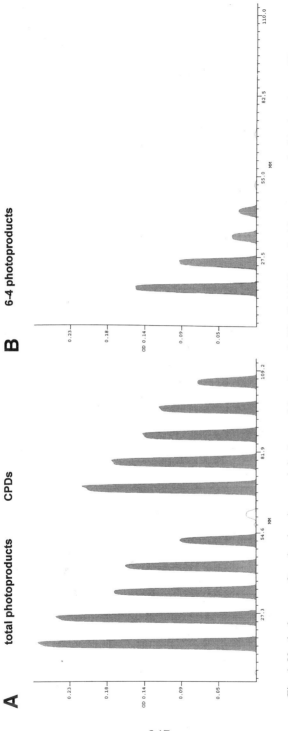

Fig. 4. Vertical scans of tracks showing repair in the two blots shown in **Fig. 3**. (**A**) From the blot not treated with photolyase. (**B**) From the photolyase-treated blot. CPD, cyclobutane pyrimidine dimmer.

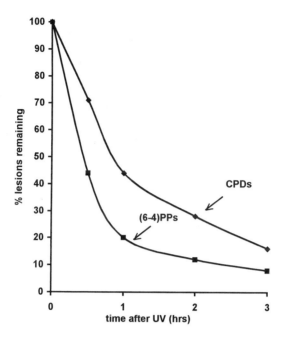

Fig. 5. Repair curve for cyclobutane pyrimidine dimers (CPDs) and 6-4 photoproducts ([6-4]PPs) calculated from scans of the blot in **Fig. 3**.

6. Unirradiated yeast carrier DNA is needed in the hybridization to be performed in **Subheading 3.6., step 4** and can be made alongside these irradiated samples. However, it is simpler to make it in bulk and store it frozen.

7. It is crucial to equalize the DNA in the samples from the various time-points. This cannot be done accurately with a spectrophotometer and is difficult to do accurately even with a fluorimeter. The gel method described is the only one we have found to be adequate.

8. These lamps provide photons of photoreactivating light at suitable wavelengths so the photolyase will repair the previously induced CPD. (The blue wavelengths required by the photolyase happen to be emitted by ordinary 60-W light bulbs.) Uncolored standard plate glass approx 0.3 cm thick can be used to protect the blot from further exposure to short wave UV.

9. Empirically, addition of yeast DNA seems to block nonspecific binding better than using herring sperm DNA alone, perhaps because the antiserum contains antibodies to proteins present in miniscule amounts in the original DNA samples used as antigen.

10. When incubating with the substrate, it is essential to keep the solution in the dark, to agitate the solution, to keep the blot well covered, and to stop the reaction before the background begins to go blue.

11. Although the method is only semiquantitative, it gives highly reproducible results provided care is taken to choose dilutions in which the intensity of the blue color is not near saturation, i.e., choose the linear part of the calibration curve.

References

1. McCready, S. J. and Cox, B. S. (1993) The repair of 6-4 photoproducts in *Saccharomyces cerevisiae. Mutat. Res.* **293,** 233–240.
2. McCready, S. J., Carr, A. M., and Lehmann, A. R. (1993) The repair of cyclobutane pyrimidine dimers and 6-4 photoproducts in *Schizosaccharomyces pombe. Mol. Microbiol.* **10,** 885–890.
3. McCready, S. J. (1996) Induction and repair of UV photoproducts in the salt-tolerant archaebacteria, *Halobacterium cutirubrum, Halobacterium halobium* and *Haloferax volcanii. Mutat. Res.* **364,** 25–32.
4. Mitchell, D. L. and Clarkson, J. M. (1981) The development of a radioimmuno-assay for the detection of photoproducts in mammalian cell DNA. *Biochem. Biophys. Acta* **655,** 54–60.
5. Mitchell, D. L. and Nairn, R. S. (1989) The biology of the (6-4) photoproduct. *Photochem. Photobiol.* **49,** 805–820.
6. Sancar, A., Smith, F. W., and Sancar, G. B. (1984) Purification of *Escherichia coli* DNA photolyase. *J. Biol. Chem.* **259,** 6028–6032.
7. Lamola, A. A. (1969) Specific formation of thymine dimers in DNA. *Photochem. Photobiol.* **9,** 291–294.
8. Moore, D. (1988) Purification and concentration of DNA from aqueous solutions, in *Current Protocols in Molecular Biology,* vol. 1 (Ausubel, F. M., Brent, R., Kingston, R. E., et al., eds.), Wiley Interscience, New York, pp. 2.1.1.
9. Wani, A. A., d' Ambrosio, S. M., and Nasir, A. K. (1987) Quantitation of pyrimidine dimers by immunoslot blot following sublethal UV-irradiation of human cells. *Photochem. Photobiol.* **46,** 477–482.
10. Cleaver, J. E., Cortes, F., Lutze, L., Morgan, W. F., Player, A. N., and Mitchell, D. L. (1987) Unique DNA repair properties of a xeroderma pigmentosum revertant. *Mol. Cell. Biol.* **7,** 3353–3357.

30

Analysis of DNA Double-Strand Break Repair by Nonhomologous End Joining in Cell-Free Extracts From Mammalian Cells

Petra Pfeiffer, Elke Feldmann, Andrea Odersky, Steffi Kuhfittig-Kulle, and Wolfgang Goedecke

Summary

Double-strand breaks (DSBs) in genomic DNA are induced by ionizing radiation or radiomimetic drugs, but they also occur spontaneously during the cell cycle at quite significant frequencies. In vertebrate cells, nonhomologous DNA end joining (NHEJ) is considered the major pathway of DSB repair. NHEJ is able to rejoin two broken DNA termini directly end-to-end irrespective of sequence and structure. Genetic studies in various radiosensitive and DSB repair-deficient hamster cell lines have yielded insights into the factors involved in NHEJ. Studies in cell-free systems derived from *Xenopus* eggs and mammalian cells have allowed the dissection of the underlying mechanisms. In the present chapter, we describe a protocol for the preparation of whole cell extracts from mammalian cells and a plasmid-based in vitro assay that permits the easy analysis of the efficiency and fidelity of DSB repair via NHEJ in different cell types.

Key Words: DSB repair; NHEJ (nonhomologous DNA end joining); ligation; illegitimate recombination; cell-free extracts; in vitro assays.

1. Introduction

Double-strand breaks (DSBs) in genomic DNA may arise spontaneously (mainly during DNA replication *[1,2]*) or after exposure to DNA-damaging agents, such as ionizing radiation (IR) or radiomimetic drugs. The estimation that mammalian cells suffer at least 10 DSBs per cell cycle spontaneously *(1)* implies that efficient DSB repair is critical for survival. Failure to do so can result in deleterious genome rearrangements, cell cycle arrest, or cell death.

Repair of DSBs is achieved by at least three different mechanisms, of which the first two are dependent on regions of extensive sequence homology, whereas the third is not *(2–5)*: (1) homologous recombination repair (HRR), a highly accurate process that usually restores the precise DNA sequence at the break; (2) single-strand annealing (SSA), a process that leads to the formation of deletions; and (3) nonhomologous

From: *Methods in Molecular Biology, vol. 291, Molecular Toxicology Protocols*
Edited by: P. Keohavong and S. G. Grant © Humana Press Inc., Totowa, NJ

DNA end joining (NHEJ), which joins two broken ends directly end-to-end. The latter mechanism is considered the major pathway of DSB repair in mammalian cells, and the present chapter focuses exclusively on the analysis of this type of DSB repair.

1.1. General Remarks on NHEJ

The fact that NHEJ is able to join virtually any two DSB ends, irrespective of their structure or sequence, has several important implications for the mutagenic potential of this pathway: (1) the original sequence is only restored if the two complementary ends are precisely religated; therefore, ligation of cohesive or blunt ends is the simplest form of NHEJ; (2) if two noncomplementary ends are rejoined, they first have to be converted to a ligatable form by enzymatic modifications that may cause base pair substitutions, insertions, and/or deletions; and (3) if, furthermore, the two ends originate from different chromosomes or distantly located regions of the same chromosome, genomic rearrangements such as translocations or interstitial deletions may occur *(6)*. Despite this mutagenic or "error-prone" element in the process, the consequences of DSB repair via NHEJ are probably tolerable in diploid somatic cells of multicellular organisms because (1) as long as the breaks are rare, originally related ends will be rejoined; (2) the chance that small-scale alterations at break points affect a critical region in an expressed gene is low owing to the high ratio of noncoding to coding DNA in the genome (~100:1); and (3) occasionally arising irreversibly damaged cells may be eliminated by apoptosis.

The analysis of radiosensitive rodent cell lines defective in DSB repair led to the identification of five gene products involved in NHEJ: the Ku70/80 heterodimer, which binds to DNA ends; the catalytic subunit of the DNA-dependent protein kinase (DNA-PK$_{CS}$); DNA ligase IV; and its associated cofactor, the XRCC4 protein *(7,8)*. This "Ku-dependent" NHEJ pathway is characterized by high efficiency and high accuracy of junction formation. In the absence of any of the five proteins, a second, less efficient and less well-characterized NHEJ pathway is still functional, which is inaccurate in that it creates deletions exhibiting small patches of sequence homology (microhomologies) at their breakpoints *(9,10)*.

Many studies of NHEJ have made use of restriction enzymes (REs) to introduce defined DSBs in the genomic DNA of cultured mammalian cells *(11,12)*, or in plasmids offered as DSB substrates in transfection assays *(13–16)*, or in cell-free extracts *(17,18)*. The fact that REs induce no other lesions but DSBs, which are exactly defined with respect to their structure (depending on the enzyme used: 5'- or 3'-overhangs or blunt ends; always 3'-hydroxyl and 5'-phosphate) and position within a given DNA sequence has greatly facilitated the study of the efficiency and fidelity of NHEJ in the above systems by comparing the original DSB termini and the resulting repair site (junction).

This chapter does not discuss any in vivo methods of measuring NHEJ, but describes only the methods used to analyze NHEJ in vitro in whole cell extracts from mammalian cells. It is worth mentioning that a number of different cell-free systems have been developed for this purpose that differ in their methods of extract preparation, the types of products formed, and the efficiency and fidelity of NHEJ *(17,19–30)*. Although these are not discussed here, the interested reader is referred to an excellent review that has recently summarized the specific features of all of these different cell-free systems *(31)*.

The first cell-free extract described was prepared from *Xenopus laevis* eggs *(18)* and is characterized by an extremely high efficiency and reproducible fidelity of the NHEJ reaction that has not yet been reached by other cell-free systems. Based on the method used for preparation of the *Xenopus* extract, we have developed a protocol that allows the preparation of whole cell extracts from human and rodent cells that form, at only slightly reduced efficiency and fidelity, all types of products seen in the *Xenopus* system *(9,17)*.

1.2. The NHEJ In Vitro Assay

1.2.1. Substrates

The most commonly used in vitro assay for NHEJ employs plasmid DNA linearized with REs to mimic DNA molecules with a defined DSB. Plasmid substrates generated by cleavage with a single RE have complementary ends that allow measurement of the efficiency and fidelity of ligation of cohesive 5'- or 3'-ends, or blunt ends (**Fig. 1A**). Substrates generated by cleavage with two different REs have noncomplementary DNA ends (5'/5'; 3'/3'; blunt end/5'; blunt end/3'; 5'/3') that allow measurement of the efficiency and fidelity of genuine nonhomologous DNA end joining (**Fig. 1B** and **C**). This type of NHEJ is more complex, and requires more factors, than "simple" cohesive or blunt end ligation because the ends must be converted first into a ligatable form by fill-in DNA synthesis and/or exonucleolytic removal of unpaired bases.

1.2.2. NHEJ Products: Efficiency and Fidelity

The extract-mediated NHEJ reaction converts all types of RE-cleaved plasmid substrates into monomeric open circular (oc) intermediates, covalently closed circles (ccc), and various linear multimers, which can be separated by agarose gel electrophoresis (**Fig. 2**). In the case of substrates containing noncomplementary ends, it is important to note that only the circular monomers represent truly nonhomologously joined products, in which two different ends are joined to each other (always head to tail [H:T]), whereas linear multimers can arise by both ligation of complementary ends (head-to-head [H:H] and tail-to-tail products [T:T]) and joining of noncomplementary ends (H:T products). The different products formed can best be detected by Southern blot analysis or *in situ* gel hybridization, which are much more sensitive than direct staining with ethidium bromide and allow easy determination of the efficiency of the NHEJ reaction on different substrate types by measurement of the relative band intensities of the corresponding products in a phosphoimager.

The fidelity of the NHEJ reaction can be accomplished by sequence analysis of the junctions created in the extract. NHEJ fidelity is of particular interest for the comparison of the different NHEJ pathways in wild-type cells and in cells deficient in certain factors involved in the NHEJ machinery. In this context, it is important to define the term "accurate NHEJ." Although it is obvious that "accurate ligation" of complementary cohesive or blunt restriction ends restores the original restriction site used to create the DSB (**Fig. 1A**), the definition of "accurate NHEJ" is not self-evident, because

terminus configurations	ends	mechanism	proteins
(A) 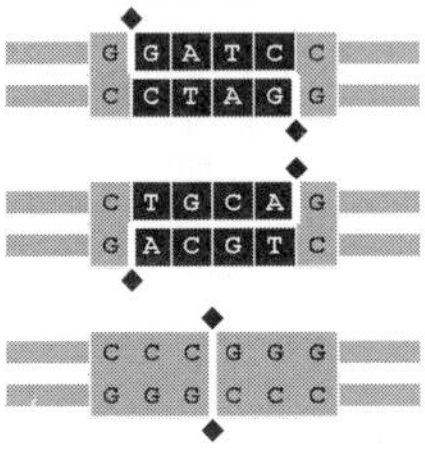	5'-coh. / 3'-coh. / blunt	<u>accurate ligation</u>	Ku70/80 DNA-PK_{CS} XRCC4 DNA ligaseIV
(B) 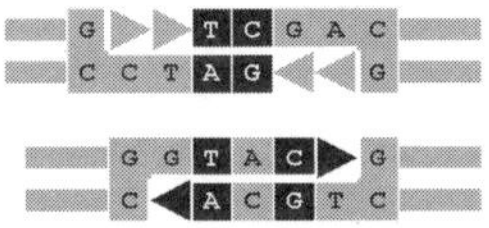	5'/5' / 3'/3'	<u>accurate NHEJ:</u> overlap of anti-parallel ends	Ku70/80 DNA-PK_{CS} XRCC4 DNA ligase IV DNA polymerase 5'-3' and/or 3'-5' exonuclease
(C) 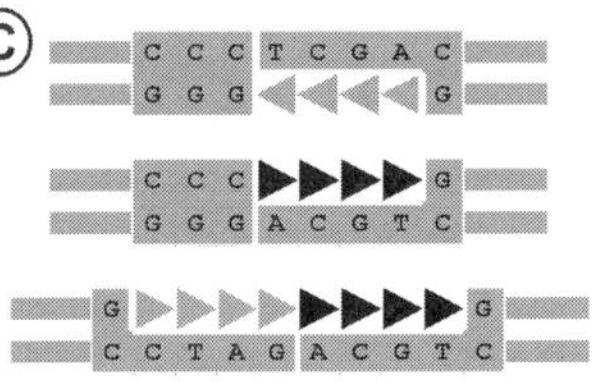	bl/5' / bl/3' / 5'/3'	<u>accurate NHEJ:</u> fill-in of abutting ends	Ku70/80 DNA-PK_{CS} XRCC4 DNA ligase IV DNA polymerase
(D) 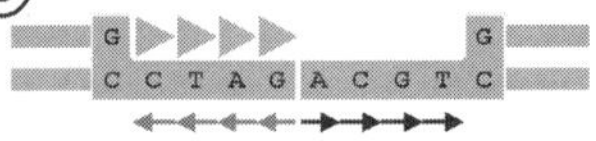	any	<u>inaccurate NHEJ:</u> blunting of 5' or 3' ends in any configuration	DNA ligase DNA polymerase 5'-3' and/or 3'-5' exonuclease
(E) 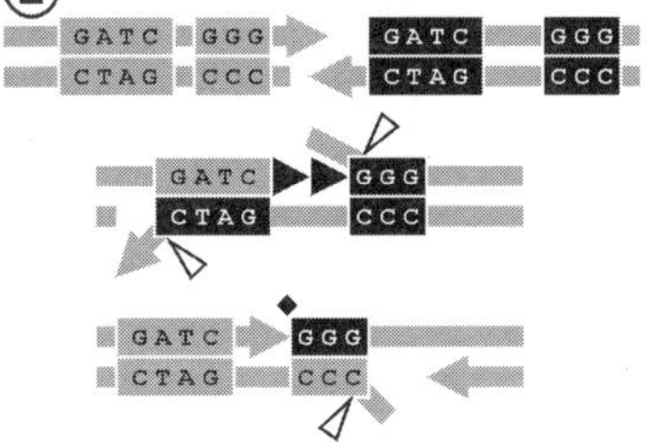	any	<u>inaccurate NHEJ:</u> μhom-SSA / μhom priming / μhom ligation	DNA ligase DNA polymerase 5'-3' and/or 3'-5' exonuclease DNA helicase flap endo-nuclease

Fig. 1. Types of different nonhomologous DNA end joining (NHEJ) pathways as observed in the cell-free system described here and their predicted protein requirements (for details, see **Subheading 1.2., item 2**). The thick gray lines represent the plasmid duplex adjacent to the DSB termini, which were induced by different REs (see different structures [blunt vs 5'- or 3'-overhang and sequences]). White letters on black background indicate complementary base pairs in (**A**) accurate ligation (black diamonds) of complementary cohesive (coh) or blunt ends;

joining of noncomplementary restriction ends necessarily causes a change in the original sequence. Still, general rules have been established for the Ku-dependent NHEJ of noncomplementary ends, because extracts from *Xenopus* eggs *(18)* and mammalian cells *(9,17)* generate highly reproducible spectra of junctions using two main joining modes (*overlap* and *fill-in* mode). The mode used is determined by the structure of the ends being joined: whereas the overlap mode typically joins DNA ends containing 5'- or 3'-antiparallel single-stranded overhangs (5'/5'; 3'/3'; **Fig. 1B** *[32]*), the fill-in mode joins abutting DNA ends [5'/blunt end; 3'/blunt end; 5'/3'; **Fig. 1C** *[33]*).

In the first case, the ends form incompletely matched overlaps by pairing of single fortuitously complementary bases, and the overlap structure determines the patterns of subsequent repair reactions. In the second case, the sequences of participating 5'- or 3'-overhangs are preserved fully by fill-in DNA synthesis, in a process in which the ends are transiently held together (presumably by the Ku70/80 heterodimer *[9]*) so that the 3'-hydroxyl group of the 5'-overhang or blunt end can serve as a primer to direct repair synthesis of the 3'-overhang. In addition to this accurate Ku-dependent NHEJ, less accurate NHEJ can occur, e.g., by blunting of 5'- or 3'-overhangs and subsequent blunt end ligation (**Fig. 1D**). While 5'-overhangs can be blunted by either fill-in or 5'-3'-exonucleolytic degradation, 3'-overhangs can be blunted only by 3'-5'-exonucleolytic degradation. The dependence of this joining mode on the Ku heterodimer and other cofactors is not yet clear. Another inaccurate NHEJ pathway, most likely independent of Ku and cofactors, generates small deletions by using fortuitous complementary bases in the duplex region adjacent to the DSB for microhomology-mediated SSA (**Fig. 1F** *[9,10]*).

Fig. 1 (*continued from page 4*) (**B**) accurate NHEJ of antiparallel ends by the overlap mode *(32)*; (**C**) accurate NHEJ of abutting ends by the fill-in mode (gray arrowheads indicate fill-in of 5'-overhang and black arrowheads fill-in of 3'-overhangs) *(33)*; (**D**) inaccurate NHEJ by blunting of 5' or 3'-overhangs by fill-in of 5'-overhangs or exonucleolytic degradation of 5'- (small gray arrows) or 3'-overhangs (small black arrows); (**E**) inaccurate NHEJ by microhomology-mediated (μhom) SSA *(10)*, which can occur at any terminus configuration. Fortuitous microhomology patches present in the duplex adjacent to the DSB are exposed on long single strands by helicase unwinding and/or exonucleolytic degradation of the ends and used for annealing. In the microhomology-priming model, the gray GATC patch of the trimmed left-hand duplex is located directly at a 3'-end, which can serve, upon annealing, as a primer for DNA fill-in synthesis (black arrowheads). In the microhomology-ligation model, the black GGG patch of the trimmed right-hand duplex comes into direct adjunction with the recessed strand of the left-hand duplex facilitating nick ligation (black diamond). In the following step, unpaired flap ends (oblique lines) can be removed by exonucleolytic digestion or a flap endonuclease (open oblique arrowheads). The NHEJ modes shown in (A–C) are dependent on the Ku70/80 heterodimer, the catalytic subunit of protein kinase (DNA-PK$_{CS}$); ligase IV, XRCC4, and additional, as not yet identified, enzymatic activities. Whether the NHEJ mode shown in (D) is also dependent on the Ku system is not known yet; the NHEJ pathway shown in (E) is apparently not dependent on the Ku system *(9,10,24)*.

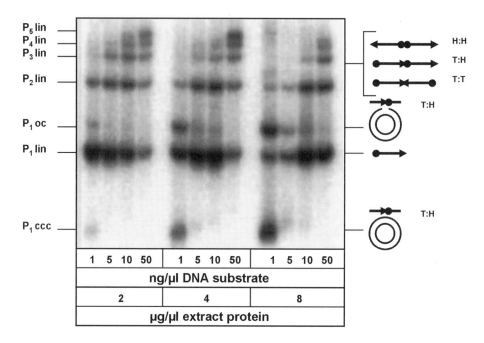

Fig. 2. Agarose gel separation of a typical NHEJ reaction (with different concentrations of substrate DNA and extract protein tested). Incubation of linear plasmid substrate (P_1 lin) yields open circle (P_1 oc) and covalently closed circular monomers (P_1 ccc), linear dimers (P_2 lin), and several higher linear multimers (P_{3-5} lin). The corresponding orientations of H:T, H:H, and T:T junctions is shown on the right side). The balance between circular monomers and linear multimers is dependent on the DNA/protein ratio used in the assay; the optimal balance is achieved with a low ratio of DNA/protein (e.g., 1 ng/µL DNA and 4–8 µg/µL extract protein as the final concentration in a standard 10-µL NHEJ assay. Note that equal amounts of DNA were loaded in each lane).

Isolation of single NHEJ events for sequence analysis of the junctions can be achieved by two different strategies: (1) transfection of total products in *E. coli*, resulting in preferential cloning of the junctions in circular products (with decreasing efficiency for ccc > oc >> linear); and (2) polymerase chain reaction (PCR) amplification of gel-purified linear multimers and subsequent sub-cloning in *E. coli* to produce single clones suitable for sequencing.

The advantage of the cell-free system described here is that both NHEJ pathways (the "Ku-dependent" and "Ku-independent") are fully active, so that both mechanisms can be studied in parallel. Interestingly, the two mechanisms can be distinguished by the products they form: the Ku-dependent pathway forms circular and multimeric products, and the Ku-independent pathway forms mainly linear multimers, so that extracts made from cells deficient in the Ku-dependent pathway can be easily identified by the absence of ccc products (**Fig. 3** *[9,10,24]*). Although linear multimers can, in principle, arise by ligation of corresponding complementary ends, it is worth mentioning

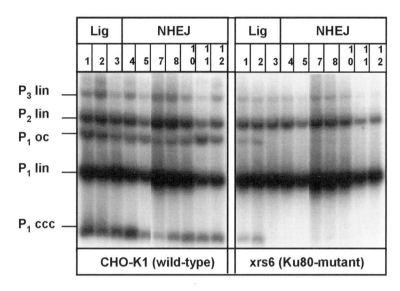

Fig. 3. Comparison of the NHEJ efficiencies of two Chinese hamster ovary (CHO) cell lines with different plasmid substrates. The xrs6 mutant cell line (right panel) is defective in Ku80 *(35)* and was derived from wild-type CHO-K1 (left panel). Numerals (1–5, 7, 8, 10–12) on top of each panel refer to the numbers of the different substrate types given in **Fig. 5**; band designations are as in **Fig. 2**. Note that xrs6 is able to form oc and ccc products only from substrates with cohesive 5'- (1) or 3'-ends (2), but not from blunt ends (3) or any of the noncomplementary substrates (4, 5, 7, 8, 10–12). The absence of circular products is a hallmark of extracts prepared from cells defective in the Ku-dependent NHEJ pathway *(9,10,24)*. The multimers observed in xrs6 are not formed by simple ligation of complementary ends but mainly by microhomology-mediated SSA, as shown in **Fig. 1**.

that the multimers in Ku-deficient cells are not formed by ligation, but by inaccurate NHEJ, which leads to the formation of small deletions exhibiting microhomologies at their breakpoints (**Fig. 1E**). This issue is particularly interesting with respect to extracts from mutant cell lines deficient in one of these pathways, because this allows performance of biochemical complementation or inhibition of certain components involved in one or the other pathway.

2. Materials

2.1. Cells and Cell Collection

1. At least 5×10^8 cells are required for each extract preparation. (This will yield about 0.5–1 mL of whole cell extract, which is sufficient for 50–100 NHEJ assays.)
2. 50- and 15-mL Screw-cap plastic tubes (e.g., Sarstedt, Nümbrecht, Germany).
3. Phosphate-buffered saline (PBS; ice-cold): 4 mM Na$_2$HPO$_4$, 2 mM KH$_2$PO$_4$, pH 7.4, 136 mM NaCl, 3 mM KCl (all chemicals from Sigma, Taufkirchen, Germany).

4. 10-mL Pipets.
5. Refrigerated centrifuge (e.g., Heraeus Biofuge; Kendro Laboratory Products, Hanau, Germany).

2.2. Extract Preparation

1. Source of ice and container for ice.
2. Set of 10 self-made calibrated 15-mL reference tubes (containing from 0.5 to 5.0 mL water in increments of 0.5 mL, water levels indicated with a permanent marker) to measure the packed cell volume (PCV).
3. Solution I (hypotonic; ice-cold; 50 mL is sufficient for two to three extract preparations; use 50-mL plastic screw-cap tube; Sarstedt): 10 mM Tris-HCl, pH 8.0, 1 mM EDTA, 5 mM dithiothreitol (DTT) (all chemicals from Sigma).
4. Set of micropipetors and appropriate tips (Eppendorf, Wesselinng-Berzdorf, Germany).
5. Protease inhibitors:

   a. 100 mM (200X) Phenyl-methyl-sulfonyl-fluoride (PMSF; Serva, Heidelberg, Germany): 170 mg in 10 mL isopropanol (keeps for up to 6 mo at room temperature).
   b. 1 mM (1000X) Leupeptin (Serva): 0.5 mg in 1 mL double-distilled (dd) H$_2$O (keeps for up to 6 mo at –20°C).
   c. 1 mM (1000X) Pepstatin A (Serva): 5 mg in 7.14 mL methanol (keeps for up to 2 wk at –20°C; isopropanol, methanol from Sigma).

6. Phase-contrast microscope (e.g., Olympus type CH2, Olympus-Deutschland, Hamburg, Germany).
7. Optional: 5-mL glass homogenizer (with a tightly fitting glass pestle; e.g., Merck Eurolab, Lohmar, Germany; *see* **Note 1**.)
8. Cold room (4–6°C).
9. 20-, 30-, and 50-mL glass beakers.
10. Magnetic stirrer and stirring bar.
11. 10-mL Pipets.
12. Solution II (ice-cold; 50 mL is sufficient for two to three extract preparations; use 50-mL plastic screw-cap tube): 50% glycerol (take 100% stock and pour the equivalent volume in the tube—do not pipet); 25% sucrose (pour the equivalent volume of a 70% stock on the glycerol); 50 mM Tris-HCl, pH 8.0; 10 mM MgCl$_2$; 2 mM DTT (all from Sigma).
13. Saturated ammonium sulfate solution (ice-cold): 10.3 g ammonium sulfate in 20 mL ddH$_2$O; adjust to pH 7.0 with just a few drops of 2 N NaOH (check with pH paper-sticks with pH optimum at 7.0 [Merck Eurolab]; chemicals from Sigma).
14. 10–12-mL polyallomer centrifuge tubes (e.g., Beckman Coulter, Krefeld, Germany).
15. Ultracentrifuge (e.g., Beckman L8-80, Beckman Coulter) with swing-out rotor for 10–12-mL polyallomer tubes (e.g., SW41, Beckman Coulter).
16. Very fine mortared solid ammonium sulfate (Sigma).
17. 1 mL 1 N NaOH, freshly diluted from a higher concentration stock (Sigma).
18. 30-mL Centrifuge tubes with cap (Beckman Coulter).
19. Refrigerated centrifuge (e.g., Avanti J25, Beckman Coulter) with rotor for 30-mL plastic tubes (e.g., JA-18, Beckman Coulter).
20. Dialysis tubing (3/4 inch; Invitrogen, Karlsruhe, Germany; store at 4°C) and four tightly fitting clamps for each sample to be dialyzed.
21. 300 mL of 100 mM β-sodium-glycerol-phosphate (Sigma), pH 7.0 stock solution; make fresh, sterilize by filtering through 0.22 μm 250-mL bottle-top filter (Millipore, Eschborn, Germany), and store at 4°C.

22. Storage buffer (2 L is sufficient for three extract preparations): 20% glycerol, 30 m*M* Tris-HCl, pH 8.0, 90 m*M* KCl, 10 m*M* β-sodium-glycerol-phosphate, pH 7.0, 2 m*M* EGTA, pH 8.5, 1 m*M* EDTA, pH 8.0, 1 m*M* DTT, 2 m*M* MgCl$_2$ (Sigma).
23. 2-mL Cryotubes with screw caps (e.g., Greiner Bio-One, Frickenhausen, Germany); different color caps can be used for identifying extracts from different cell lines.
24. Liquid nitrogen.
25. Kit for determination of protein concentration according to Bradford (e.g., Bio-Rad, München, Germany). Dilute Bradford solution 1:5 in ddH$_2$O and filter through paper filter (e.g., 185 mm diameter, Whatman-Biometra, Gottingen, Germany).
26. 1:20 Dilution in ddH$_2$O of a 10 mg/mL bovine serum albumin (BSA) stock solution (New England Biolabs, Frankfurt, Germany) for calibration curve to measure a range of 1–10 μg protein.
27. Spectrophotometer (e.g., Eppendorf Bio Photometer, Eppendorf, Hamburg, Germany).
28. Disposable 2-mL plastic cuvets (220–16 nm, Eppendorf).

2.3. Substrate Preparation

1. Plasmid with polylinker (e.g., pSP65 or pUC18; Promega, Mannheim, Germany) for the generation of substrates with complementary ends.
2. Plasmid harboring an approx 1-kb fragment of any DNA in the middle of the polylinker for the generation of substrates with noncomplementary ends (**Fig. 4**).
3. Restriction enzymes of choice (e.g., Roche Diagnostics, Mannheim, Germany).
4. Set of micropipetors and appropriate tips (e.g., Eppendorf).
5. 1.5- and 0.5- (or 0.2)-mL Microcentrifuge tubes.
6. Variable temperature heating block(s) or water bath(s) for incubation of restriction digests (usually at or near 37°C). Same or dedicated incubator set at 65°C for DNA denaturation prior to electrophoresis.
7. Source of ice and container for ice.
8. 1X TA electrophoresis buffer (dilute from a 50X stock; make up 1 L containing 0.5 μg/mL ethidium bromide): 40 m*M* Tris-base, 12 m*M* sodium acetate, adjusted to pH 7.4 with acetic acid.
9. Preparative 1% agarose gel (~12 cm in length, with large narrow slots) in 1X TA buffer containing 0.5 μg/mL ethidium bromide (*see* **Note 2**).
10. Gel electrophoresis apparatus (*see* **Note 3**) and power supply (e.g., Consort 3-300W/6-600V/10-1000mA, Merck Eurolab).
11. 10X Loading buffer: 2.5 m*M* Tris-HCl, pH 8.0, 50 m*M* EDTA, pH 8.0, 90% glycerol, 0.01% bromophenol blue (BPB), 0.01% xylene cyanol (XC).
12. UV transilluminator (e.g., Merck Eurolab), goggles, gloves, and scalpel.
13. Gel extraction kit (e.g., Qiagen, Hilden, Germany).
14. TE buffer: 10 m*M* Tris-HCl, pH 7.5, 0.1 m*M* EDTA.

2.4. In Vitro NHEJ Assay

1. Frozen aliquot(s) of cell-free extract. (At least 5 μg protein/μL; 8 μL are required per 10 μL standard NHEJ assay; check size of aliquot needed and use economically.)
2. Frozen aliquots of linear plasmid substrate of choice, at a concentration of 10 ng/μL in TE (from **Subheading 3.2.**, **step 8**; 1 μL required per assay.)
3. Source of ice and container for ice.
4. Cold room (4–6°C).
5. M buffer (reaction buffer; 50 mL, ice-cold): 50 m*M* MOPSO-NaOH, pH 7.5, 40 m*M* KCl, 10 m*M* MgCl$_2$, 5 m*M* β-mercaptoethanol (Sigma). Dilute freshly from stock solutions

pSP65

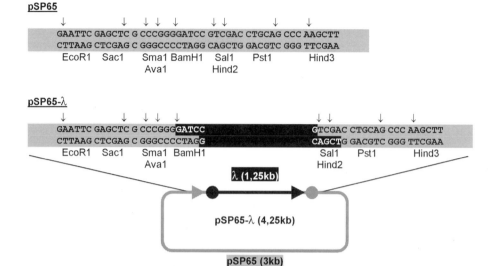

Fig. 4. Schematic presentation of the plasmids used in our laboratory for the preparation of linear substrates. Top: polylinker of pSP65 (highlighted in gray); bottom: polylinker of pSP65-λ (4.25 kb), which harbors a 1.25-kb fragment of λ-DNA (highlighted in black) cloned into the *Bam*H1 and *Sal*1 sites *(32)*. Small vertical arrows mark the cleavage sites of the restriction enzymes indicated. Complete excision of the λ-insert yields a 3-kb plasmid band and a 1.25-kb λ-band (check in the analytical gel that no residual linear 4.25-kb band and no ccc band is left) and indicates a generation of a clean linear plasmid substrate containing two noncomplementary restriction ends. Insertion of additional linkers into pSP65-λ (not shown) has enlarged the spectrum of RE sites in our substrate system (*see* **Fig. 5**).

directly prior to use (500 m*M* MOPSO-NaOH, pH 7.5 [light-sensitive!] stock should be stored in aliquots at –20°C; keeps for approx 6 mo; each aliquot should be used only once). Add protease inhibitors (i.e., to 1X PMSF/leupeptin/pepstain) directly before dialysis.

6. Protease inhibitors (*see* **Subheading 2.2., item 5**).
7. 10-cm Petri dishes.
8. Microdialysis filters (0.025-μm pore diameter; Millipore, Eschborn, Germany, cat. no. VSPWPO2500).
9. Set of micropipetors and appropriate tips.
10. Microcentrifuge tubes.
11. 65°C Heating block or water bath (necessary for both initial substrate DNA denaturation and later termination of the NHEJ reaction; therefore, should not be adjusted and used for NHEJ reaction itself).
12. 10X LNB (make up 1 mL and store in 10–100-μL aliquots at –20°C; keeps for at least 1 yr): 10 m*M* Tris-HCl, pH 8.0, 1.2 m*M* MgCl$_2$, 10 m*M* KCl, 1 m*M* β-mercaptoethanol, supplemented with 10 m*M* ATP, pH 7.0, 2 m*M* dNTPs (0.5 m*M* each), 0.5 mg/mL BSA.
13. Variable temperature heating block(s) or water bath(s) for incubation of substrate DNA with protein extracts at optimal temperature (*see* **Note 2**).

14. 2X TE-Stop/SDS: 40 mM Tris-HCl, pH 7.5, 2 mM EDTA, 2% sodium dodecyl sulfate (SDS) (10 μL required for each standard 10-μL NHEJ assay).
15. Table top microcentrifuge (e.g., Eppendorf 5415R).

2.5. Analytical Agarose Gel Electrophoresis (see Notes 3 and 4)

1. Set of micropipetors and appropriate tips.
2. Mini-stop: 2.5 mM Tris-HCl, pH 8.0, 50 mM EDTA, pH 8.0, 77% glycerol, 0.01% BPB, 0.01% XC.
3. Proteinase K (Sigma): 20 mg/mL in ddH$_2$O; store in small aliquots (~50 μL) at –20°C. (Each aliquot should be used only once.)
4. Pro-stop: 1 mg/mL proteinase K in loading buffer. Prepare as follows: for 400 μL, add 250 μL Mini-stop and 112.5 μL ddH$_2$O to 37.5 μL proteinase K.
5. Microcentrifuge tubes.
6. Table top microcentrifuge (e.g., Eppendorf 5415R).
7. 37°C and 65°C heating blocks or water baths.
8. Source of ice and container for ice.
9. 1% Agarose (e.g., Biozym, Oldendorf, Germany) gel in 1X TA buffer containing 1 μg/mL ethidium bromide. The gel should be very thin (4–5 mm), be at least 10 cm long, and contain small slots (preferably ~1 × 2.5 mm).
10. Gel electrophoresis apparatus and power supply (*see* **Subheading 2.3., item 10**).
11. Supercoiled and linear plasmid DNA (1 ng/μL) as marker.
12. Zipper-lock plastic bags for storing gels.

2.6. In Situ Gel Hybridization (Instead of Southern Blotting)

1. Gel-soak solutions:

   a. GS0: 1.5 M NaCl, 0.25 N HCl, pH 0–1.0.
   b. GS1: 1.5 M NaCl, 0.5 N NaOH, pH 13.0–14.0.
   c. GS2: 1.5 M NaCl, 1 M Tris-HCl, pH 7.5.

2. Gel dryer (e.g., model 583, Bio-Rad, München, Germany).
3. Whatman 3MM filter paper (Whatman-Biometra, Göttingen, Germany).
4. Plastic wrap (e,g., Saran wrap).
5. 50–100 ng Linear plasmid DNA (the same as used for substrate preparation in **Subheading 2.3., item 2**) in 25 μL ddH$_2$O.
6. Set of micropipetors and appropriate tips.
7. Boiling water bath.
8. [^{32}P]α-dCTP (5000 Ci/mmol; Amersham-Pharmacia, Freiburg, Germany).
9. Random priming kit (Amersham-Pharmacia).
10. Nick™ columns (Amersham-Pharmacia).
11. Sheered denatured salmon sperm DNA (0.2 mL; 10 mg/mL).
12. 20X SSC: 3 M NaCl, 300 mM sodium citrate.
13. Hybridization solution (50 mL): 6X SSC, 1% SDS, 50 mM Tris-HCl, pH 7.5, 4 mM EDTA.
14. Hybridization box: heat-resistant plastic box with tightly closing lid whose area is slightly larger than the gel to be hybridized.
15. 65°C Water bath with shaking facility or hybridization oven (e.g., Julabo, Seebach, Germany).
16. 10% SDS (Sigma).
17. Washing solution (WS; need 300 mL): 6X SSC, 0.5% SDS.
18. Room temperature shaker (e.g., Duomax 1030, Heidolph Instruments, Schwabach, Germany).

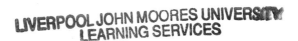

19. Portable Geiger counter for monitoring ^{32}P (e.g., Impo RM3, Novodirect, Kehl, Germany).
20. Phosphoimaging facility (e.g., Cyclone, Packard Bioscience, Dreieich, Germany) or X-ray film (e.g., Kodak, through B.W. Plus Roentgen, Kamp-Lintford, Germany).

2.7. Transformation in E. coli and Preparation of Cloned Junctions

1. Set of micropipetors and appropriate tips.
2. Microcentrifuge tubes.
3. Source of ice and container for ice.
4. 1X TE-Stop/PK (100 µL per NHEJ assay): 20 mM Tris-HCl, pH 7.6, 1 mM EDTA, containing 1 µg/µL proteinase K.
5. Table top microcentrifuge.
6. 37°C and 65°C Heating blocks or water baths.
7. TE-equilibrated phenol, pH 7.5–8.0 (e.g., Roth, Karlsruhe, Germany).
8. Vortex mixer.
9. Chloroform (Sigma).
10. Phenol/chloroform (1:1).
11. 20 mg/mL Glycogen (Roche Diagnostics, Mannheim, Germany)
12. 100% and 70% Ethanol (Sigma).
13. –20°C Freezer for DNA precipitation incubation.
14. Electrocompetent *E. coli* cells (e.g., strain DH5α). Buy (Invitrogen) or make yourself *(34)*.
15. LB medium (10 g NaCl, 10 g Bacto-tryptone, 5 g yeast per L of water) and agar (15 g Bacto-agar per L of LB; medium) plates containing the appropriate antibiotics (usually ampicillin [Roth], prepare 1000X stock [100 mg/mL] in ddH$_2$O, and store in 1-mL aliquots at –20°C).
16. Electroporator (e.g., Eppendorf) and corresponding cuvets.
17. 37°C Incubator for agar plates (e.g., Heraeus B15, Kendro Laboratory Products).
18. 37°C Shaker for incubation of overnight bacterial cultures (e.g., Certomat, Melsungen, Germany).
19. Plasmid miniextraction kit (e.g., Qiagen).

2.8. Sequence Analysis

1. Sequencing primer that binds approx 50–100 bp upstream of the polylinker region of the plasmid used as substrate. May be ordered from an oligo synthesizing service, e.g., Invitrogen. For pSP65, we use: 5'-CTACAATTAATACATAA CCTTA.
2. For sequencing, the cheapest and least time-consuming alternative is a sequencing service (e.g., Seqlab, Göttingen, Germany).

3. Methods

3.1. Extract Preparation (see Notes 1 and 2)

1. All steps must be performed on ice. **Caution:** Gloves should be worn at all times, owing to the toxicity of the protease inhibitors.
2. Collect thawed cells (5–10 × 10^8) in PBS in a 50-mL screw-top plastic tube. Wash twice with ice-cold PBS.

   a. For the first wash, resuspend the cells by gentle pipeting in a total volume of 50 mL of PBS and collect by centrifugation for 5 min at 4°C at 180g.
   b. For the second wash, resuspend the cells in 15 mL PBS, transfer into a 15-mL plastic tube, and centrifuge again under the same conditions.

3. Estimate the PCV of the cell pellet by comparison with calibrated set of reference tubes.
4. Resuspend the cell pellet in 4 PCV of solution I and add protease inhibitors immediately (i.e., to a PCV of 1 mL, add 4 mL of solution I; to the total volume of 5 mL, add 25 µL of PMSF and 12.5 µL each of leupeptin and pepstatin). Do not vortex, but gently pipet cells and shake the tube "overhead."
5. Incubation:

    a. Incubate the cell suspension on ice for about 20 min (time varies with the cell type).
    b. Depending on the cell type, cells should start to swell and break after approx 5 min, and the cell suspension should be periodically checked under a phase contrast microscope after approx 10 min.
    c. The incubation is complete when 80–90% of the nuclei have been released from the cytoplasm and are still intact. At this stage (after ~20–30 min), add another 0.5X PMSF (12.5 µL if original volume was 5 mL).
    d. All subsequent steps should be performed in the cold room (4–6°C).

6. Pour cell lysate into a precooled 30–50-mL glass beaker, and stir slowly on a magnet stirrer.
7. Add 4 PCV of solution II slowly by dripping from a 10-mL pipet. If the phases do not mix properly, pour the lysate into a fresh, precooled beaker.
8. Very slowly add 0.8 PCV of the saturated ammonium sulfate solution with a 1-mL micropipetor. Stir slowly for 30 min or longer (check stirring repeatedly, because the lysate is very viscous).
9. Transfer suspension into a precooled polyallomer centrifuge tube, one extract preparation per 12-mL tube. Centrifuge at 212,000g for 3 h at 2°C.
10. Transfer the high-speed supernatant to a 15-mL plastic tube with a 1-mL micropipetor. The remaining viscous material (~2 mL) at the bottom of the centrifuge tube should be discarded.
11. Estimate the volume of the high-speed supernatant by comparison with a set of calibrated reference tubes, and transfer it to a precooled 20-mL glass beaker.
12. Place beaker on a magnet stirrer, and slowly add solid fine mortared ammonium sulfate (0.33 g/mL supernatant) under constant gentle stirring.
13. Neutralize the solution by addition of 10 µL of freshly diluted 1 N NaOH per mg of added solid ammonium sulfate.
14. Stir slowly for 30 min.
15. Transfer solution into a precooled 30-mL centrifuge tube without transferring unresolved ammonium sulfate crystals.
16. Centrifuge at 27,000g for 30 min at 2°C.
17. Wearing gloves, and using sterilized scissors, cut an approx 10-cm piece of dialysis tubing for each extract preparation, and stir for 30 min in ice-cold sterile ddH$_2$O to remove residual ethanol.
18. Remove the supernatant and resuspend the low-speed pellet quickly in 1/20 vol (based on the high-speed supernatant) of storage buffer freshly supplemented with protease inhibitors (i.e., to 1X PMSF/leupeptin/pepstain). To avoid extreme foaming, do not vortex, but wash the pellet repeatedly with the buffer by allowing it to run down the tube wall onto the pellet with a 1-mL micropipetor.
19. Transfer the protein solution into the watered dialysis tubing (still wearing gloves) and securely tighten two clamps, one at each end of the tube.
20. Dialyze overnight in 1 L of storage buffer, with one change of buffer after 1 h. Add protease inhibitors (1X PMSF/leupeptin/pepstatin) only directly prior to dialysis.
21. Transfer the dialyzed extract with a 1-mL micropipetor into a 1.5-mL microcentrifuge tube.

22. Clear the turbid extract by centrifugation at 16,000*g* (full speed for the Heraeus Biofuge) for 5 min at 4°C.

23. Distribute the cleared extract (50- and 100-μL aliquots; *see* **Note 5**) into precooled cryotubes. Keep 10 μL separate for determination of protein concentration.

24. Shock-freeze aliquots by immersion in liquid nitrogen (**Caution:** use gloves, goggles, and forceps to prevent injury) and store at –80°C, or preferably in liquid nitrogen, in which aliquots remain active for at least 9 mo.

25. Measure the protein concentration of the extract: add 950 μL of diluted, filtered Bradford solution to 50 μL each of 1:50 and 1:100 dilutions of the extract sample, leave for 5 min at room temperature, transfer into disposable plastic cuvets, measure the OD at 595 nm, and compare with a calibration curve made with BSA on the same day. The protein concentration should range between 4 and 12 μg/μL.

3.2. Substrate Preparation (see Notes 6 and 7)

1. Digest 10 μg of plasmid DNA with one or two different REs according to the manufacturer's specifications.

2. Mix completely digested DNA sample with an appropriate volume of 10X loading buffer, incubate at 65°C for 5 min, chill on ice, and load directly on a preparative 1% agarose gel.

3. Run electrophoresis at 5 V/cm (or at 1 V/cm overnight), until the BPB dye has reached the bottom edge of the gel.

4. Cut out the linear 3-kb plasmid band under UV light using a scalpel.

5. Extract DNA from agarose with a gel extraction kit according to the manufacturer's instructions.

6. Measure DNA concentration in a spectrophotometer at 260 nm.

7. Dilute linear substrate DNA in TE to 10 ng/μL.

8. Distribute in small aliquots (e.g., 20 μL) and store at –20°C.

3.3. In Vitro NHEJ Assay (see Note 8)

1. Thaw the amount of extract needed on ice (7–8 μL extract per NHEJ assay).

2. Pour approx 20 mL of freshly prepared ice-cold M buffer containing 1X protease inhibitors (PMSF/leupeptin/pepstatin) in a Petri dish placed on ice in the cold room.

3. Place microdialysis filter on the surface of the buffer (glossy side up).

4. Pipet extract onto the filter (maximum of 150 μL per filter; maximum of three filters per Petri dish), and let stand for 30 min.

5. Place an appropriate number of microcentrifuge tubes (one for each NHEJ reaction) in a rack on ice.

6. Incubate the substrate DNA at 65°C for 5 min, and chill on ice to avoid sticking of complementary ends.

7. Pipet 1 μL of substrate DNA (10 ng/μL) and 1 μL of 10X LNB into each assay tube.

8. Remove extract from the filter using a 100-μL micropipetor.

9. Add 8 μL of extract, and mix by pipeting.

10. Incubate at the optimal temperature for the optimal time (*see* **Note 2**).

11. Terminate NHEJ reactions by addition of 10 μL 2X TE-Stop/SDS and immediate incubation at 65°C for 5 min.

12. Centrifuge briefly (e.g., for 20 s in a microcentrifuge at full speed) to spin down condensation droplets, and freeze at –20°C.

3.4. Measurement of NHEJ Efficiency by Analytical Agarose Gel Electrophoresis (see *Notes 9 and 10*)

1. Pipet 4 µL of Pro-stop in each of an equivalent number of microcentrifuge tubes on ice.
2. Microcentrifuge thawed NHEJ samples for 5 min to pellet protein and SDS.
3. Pipet 4 µL of the supernatant (equivalent to 2 ng of substrate input) into the prepared tubes.
4. Incubate samples for 30 min at 37°C and then at 15 min at 65°C. Microcentrifuge briefly and chill in ice.
5. Load each sample (2 ng of DNA in 8 µL) and appropriate markers (1 ng of DNA per lane) on a thin analytical 1% agarose gel.
6. Run electrophoresis at 10 V/cm until the BPB dye has reached the bottom edge (~2 h for 10 cm) to achieve optimal band separation.
7. Pass the gel through the three GS solutions: GS0: 5 min; GS1: 30 min; GS2: 10 min.
8. Place the soaked gel on a piece of filter paper and cover with plastic wrap.
9. Dry gel on a gel dryer for 30 min at 80°C.
10. Store dried gel in a plastic bag at room temperature.

3.5. In Situ *Gel Hybridization* (see *Notes 10 and 11*)

1. Label 50–100 ng of linear denatured plasmid DNA (25 µL) with [^{32}P]α-dCTP by random priming using a kit according to the manufacturer's instructions.
2. Purify radioactively labeled plasmid probe over a "nick" column according to the manufacturer's instructions (resulting probe volume 400 µL).
3. Add 200 µL of denatured salmon sperm DNA to radioactively labeled probe.
4. Pipet the probe plus salmon sperm DNA into a plastic screw-cap tube containing 50 mL hybridization solution, and mix.
5. Boil for 10 min.
6. Remove filter paper from the dried gel by rinsing in tap water.
7. Place the gel in a hybridization box containing the boiled hybridization mix.
8. Incubate at 65°C for at least 6 h or overnight.
9. Wash the hybridized gel twice in 100 mL of WS with shaking for 20 min at room temperature.
10. *Optional*: wash the gel once in 100 mL of WS with shaking for 10 min at 65°C.
11. Place the gel on filter paper and cover with plastic wrap.
12. Expose the gel to a phosphoimager screen or X-ray film.

3.6. Transformation of E. coli (see *Note 12*)

1. Pipet 100 µL TE-Stop containing 1 µg/µL proteinase K into each of an equivalent number of microcentrifuge tubes on ice.
2. Microcentrifuge thawed NHEJ samples (from **Subheading 3.3.**) for 5 min at full speed.
3. Pipet 4 µL of the supernatant (equivalent to 4 ng of substrate DNA) into the prepared tubes.
4. Incubate samples for 30 min at 37°C and then 15 min at 65°C. Microcentrifuge briefly to consolidate sample.
5. Extract once with 100 µL of phenol: add 100 µL of phenol, vortex, microcentrifuge for 5 min at full speed to separate the organic phase (bottom) from the aqueous phase (top), remove the bottom phase with a 250-µL micropipet, and discard into organic waste.
6. Extract once as in **step 5** with 100 µL of 1:1 phenol/chloroform. (Discard the bottom organic phase.)

7. Extract once with 100 μL of chloroform and transfer the top (aqueous) phase to a new microcentrifuge tube.
8. Add 1 μL of glycogen solution, and mix by vortexing.
9. Add 250 μL of 100% ethanol and mix "overhead."
10. Incubate for at least 30 min at –20°C.
11. Microcentrifuge at full speed for 30 min.
12. Discard the supernatant and wash the pellet by pipeting 100 μL of 70% ethanol onto it and then removing the ethanol. Do not vortex or otherwise disturb the pellet.
13. Resuspend the dried pellet in 5 μL ddH₂O by repeated pipeting.
14. Add 5 μL purified DNA sample to 50 μL of electrocompetent cells, and perform electroporation according to the manufacturer's instructions.
15. Spread an equivalent volume (up to 500 μL; *see* **Note 12**) of transformed cells on an agar plate containing ampicillin or another suitable selective compound.
16. Incubate overnight at 37°C.
17. Check plate for colonies.

3.7. Preparation of Cloned Junctions

1. Grow 5 mL overnight cultures from randomly picked single colonies in LB medium containing the appropriate antibiotics.
2. Prepare plasmid DNA using a miniextraction kit according to the manufacturer's instructions.

3.8. Restriction Analysis (see Note 13)

1. Check miniprep DNA for the presence of accurate junctions by cleavage with the appropriate RE and subsequent separation of products in analytical agarose gels (**Fig. 5**).

3.9. Sequence Analysis (see Note 13)

1. Clones that are resistant to RE cleavage can be subjected to sequencing (commercially or do-it-yourself) for further analysis.

4. Notes

1. Not more than three extract preparations should be made on any one day. In most cases, a glass homogenizer is not required (only needed for very robust cells), because swelling in the hypotonic solution I breaks the cells and releases the nuclei in a much more gentle manner than homogenizing. The incubation time in solution I varies with the cell type used.
2. When preparing extracts from a new cell line for the first time, it is necessary to determine the optimal conditions by performing kinetics at different incubation temperatures and times (25°C and 37°C; 0, 5, 15, 60, and 360 min) and different ratios of DNA/protein. (We routinely prepare 10-μL samples containing 1 ng/μL of DNA and 4–6 μg/μL of extract protein in each NHEJ assay; optimization usually consists of testing a series of samples made by keeping the amount of DNA constant at 1 ng/μL and testing final extract protein concentrations of 2, 4, 6, 8, and 10 μg/μL.) The latter is especially important to achieve a balanced formation of circular monomers and linear multimers (*see* **Fig. 2**).
3. We use self-built agarose gel chambers (buffer volume of ~1 L) that accommodate our gels (*see* **Note 4**); something comparable is not commercially available. A system is needed that allows for the casting of thin gels with many slots: a minielectrophoresis system (10 × 11.5-cm gels) containing 20 slots available from Roth is probably the best fit.

substrate	terminus configuration	main junctions			RE-cut
1. BamH1 / BamH1 5'-coh. end Lig	CGGG GATCCTCT GCCCCTAG CAGA	a) b)	CGGGGATC | GATCCTCT CGGGGATC | CTCT	0/0: fill-in 0/-4: ovlp; acc LIG	a) no b) Bam (0/-4)
2. Pst1 / Pst1 3'-coh. end Lig	GACCTGCA GCCC CTGG ACGTCCCC	a) b)	GACCTGCA | GCCC GACC | GCCC	0/-4: ovlp; acc LIG -4/-4: bl/bl	a) Pst (0/-4) b) no
3. Sma1 / Sma1 blunt end Lig	TCGCCC GGGGAT AGCGGG CCCCTA	a)	TCGCCC | GGGGAT	0/0: bl/bl: acc. LIG	a) Sma (0/0)
4. BamH1 / Asp718 5'/5' NHEJ	CGGG GTACCGGA GCCCCTAG GCCT	a) b)	CGGGGATC | GTACCGGA CGGGG(AT)C | CGGA	0/0: fill-in 0/-4: ovlp; acc NHEJ	a) no b) Bam and / or Asp (ovlp)[1]
5. BamH1 / Sal1 5'/5' NHEJ	CGGG TCGACCTG GCCCCTAG CGAC	a) b)	GGGGGATC | TCGACCTG CGGGGATC | GACCTG	0/0: fill-in 0/-2: ovlp; acc NHEJ	a) no b) no
6. BstX1 / BstX1 3'/3' NHEJ	CCACTAAG GTGG GGTG AAACCACC	a) b)	CCACT(AA)C | GTGG CCAC | GTGG	0/-4: ovlp; acc NHEJ -4/-4: bl/bl	a) BstX1 (ovlp)[2] b) no
7. Kpn1 / Pst1 3'/3' NHEJ	GGGGTAC GCCC GGGC ACGTCGGG	a) b) c) d)	CCCGGT(A)C | AGCCC CCCGG(T)A | GCCC CCCG | GCCC CCCG	0/-3: ovlp; acc NHEJ -1/-4: ovlp; acc NHEJ -4/-4: bl/bl -4/-8: μhom SSA	a) no[3] b) no[4] c) no d) no
8. Sma1 / Sal1 bl/5' NHEJ	TCGCCC TCGACCTG AGCGGG GGAC	a) b)	TCGCCC | TCGACCTG TCG | ACCTG	0/0: fill-in; acc NHEJ -3/-6: μhom SSA	a) no b) no
9. Ava1 / Hind2 5'/bl NHEJ	TCGC GACCTG AGCGGGCC GTCGAC	a)	TCGCCCGG | GACCTG	0/0: fill-in; acc NHEJ	a) Ava (0/0)
10. Sma1 / Pst1 bl/3' NHEJ	TCGCCC GCCC AGCGGG ACGTCGGG	a) b) c)	TCGCCC | TGCAGCCC TCGCCC | GCCC TCGCCC	0/0: fill-in; acc NHEJ 0/-4: bl/bl 0/-8: μhom SSA	a) Pst (0/0; -1/0; -2/0) b) no c) no
11. Bam1 / Pst1 5'/3' NHEJ	CGGG GCCC GCCCCTAG ACGTCGGG	a)	CGGGGATC | TGCAGCCC	0/0: fill-in; acc NHEJ	a) Pst (0/0)
12. Sac1 / Sal1 3'/5' NHEJ	TTCGAGCT TCGACCTG AAGC GGAC	a) b) c)	TTCGAGCT | TCGACCTG TTCG | TCGACCTG TTCGA | CCTG	0/0: fill-in; acc NHEJ -4/0: bl/fill -3/-4: μhom SSA	a) no b) Sal (-4/0) c) no
13. EcoR1 / Kpn1 5'/3' NHEJ	ACGG CGGA TGCCTTAA CATGGCCT	a) b) c)	ACGGAATT | GTACCGGA ACGGAATT | CGGA ACGG | GTACCGGA	0/0: fill-in; acc NHEJ 0/-4: bl/fill -4/0: bl/fill	a) no b) Eco (0/-4) c) Kpn (-4/0; -5/0)
14. Sac1 / Hind3 3'/5' NHEJ	TTCGAGCT AGCTTGGC AAGC ACCG	a) b)	TTCGAGCT | AGCTTGGC TTCGAGCT | TGGC	0/0: fill-in; acc NHEJ -4/0: bl/fill or μhom SSA	a) no b) no
15. Ava1 / Kpn1 5'/3' NHEJ	TCGC CGGA AGCGGGCC CATGGCCT	a) b)	TCGCCCGG | GTACCGGA TCGCCCGG | A	0/0: fill-in; acc NHEJ 0/-7: μhom SSA	a) Kpn (-1/0; 0/0) b) no

[1] the T:T and A:A mismatches segregate in T:A and A:T (Asp[S]) and A:T and T:A (Bam[S]);
[2] the two A:A mismatches segregate in A:T and A:T (BstX[S]) and T:A and T:A (BstX[S]);
[3] the A:C mismatch segregates in A:T and G:C;
[4] the T:G mismatch segregates in A:T and G:C

Fig. 5. List of substrates with complementary (1–3), noncomplementary antiparallel (4–7), and abutting (8–15) ends used in our laboratory. Substrates 1–3 can be prepared from pSP65, substrates 5, 8–12, and 14 can be prepared from pSP65-λ (*see* **Fig. 4**), and substrates 4, 6, 7, 13, and 15 are derived from modified pSP65-λ containing additional linkers for *Kpn* (=*Asp718*) or *BstX*1 (not shown). Corresponding structures and sequences of ends are shown in column 2, "terminus configuration," with the RE sequence highlighted in light gray and complementary base pairs marked in white letters on black background; microhomology patches in the adjacent duplex are shown in dark gray. The main types of junctions resulting from accurate (acc) ligation or NHEJ (fill-in or overlap [ovlp] mode; *see* **Fig. 1**) and microhomology-mediated (μhom) single-strand annealing are shown as top strand sequences with vertical lines indicating the junction breakpoint. Negative numerals indicate the number of bases lost from the left and right termini, respectively. Underlined sequences mark restored RE sites that can be used for RE analysis (also see right column). Note that segregation in *E. coli* of the mismatches in the junctions of substrates 4, 6, and 7 leads to two different sequences (*see* footnotes 1–4) and, in the case of substrate 4, to sensitivity to cleavage with *Bam* or *Asp* or both (*36*).

4. We routinely use 12 × 12-cm gels (4–5-mm thick) containing 30 slots (each 1 × 2.5 mm). A Teflon comb with 30 slots is placed with the help of two small clamps at a distance of approx 1 mm from the surface and 1 cm from the top edge of a clean, polished, sharp-edged glass plate on which 45 mL of almost boiling agarose are poured (two fillings of a 25-mL pipet).

5. The size and number of aliquots frozen after overnight dialysis of freshly prepared extract batches depends on the number of NHEJ assays planned for a single experiment (50-μL aliquots are sufficient for six to seven NHEJ assays if the extract is used in undiluted form) and the available space in the liquid nitrogen tank (or –80°C freezer): principally, many small aliquots are better than few large aliquots in terms of economizing extract. (Each extract aliquot that has been thawed should not be frozen again, so that excess thawed extract has to be discarded.) However, many small aliquots will take more space in the freezer.

6. For generation of substrates with complementary ends, a plasmid (~3 kb) containing a polylinker is required (e.g., pSP65; **Fig. 4**). Quantitative digestion with a single RE should yield only linear 3-kb DNA (no residual oc and ccc). For generation of substrates containing noncomplementary ends, it is advantageous to use a plasmid haboring a fragment (~1 kb) of any DNA in the polylinker (**Fig. 4**). Excision of the insert with a combination of two REs cleaving 5' and 3' of the fragment allows control of quantitative digestion, which should yield linear equal amounts of 3-kb plasmid DNA and the 1-kb insert, with no residual 4 kb oc or ccc. In this way, it is verified that the resulting 3-kb plasmid substrate indeed carries two different ends.

7. It is important that the plasmid used for substrate preparation is digested to completion, because residual oc and ccc DNA may yield false-positive results in the NHEJ assay. Therefore, completeness of digestion should be verified with an analytical agarose gel before loading the DNA on the preparative gel. Use sufficiently large slots and do not overload the preparative gel to avoid smearing of bands. Before loading, it is advantageous to heat the sample for 5 min to 65°C to avoid sticking of cohesive ends (which yield linear dimers). Run the gel slowly over a long distance (~10 cm) to achieve good separation of the linear substrate band from the closely migrating contaminating residual oc DNA (and the released diagnostic fragment).

8. When using extracts from different cell lines (e.g., wild-type and mutant) in the NHEJ assay, all extracts should be adjusted to the same protein concentration (usually that of the extract with the lowest protein concentration) by addition of an appropriate volume of storage buffer. Then dialyze the extract volume needed to perform the planned number of NHEJ assays against M buffer by carefully spotting the extract on the glossy side of a microdialysis filter. Note that the extract volume will increase upon dialysis. When removing the extract from the dialysis filter, take care not to submerge the filter in the buffer. After dialysis against M buffer, the extract should be placed on ice and used immediately in the assays. Therefore, depending on the number of NHEJ reactions to be performed, it may be better to start preparing the tubes before thawing the extract. If a given DNA substrate is used in several assays, an appropriate volume of a 1:2 mixture of the DNA substrate with 10X LNB (1 μL of DNA at 10 ng/μL plus 2 μL of 10X LNB per NHEJ assay) can be prepared, which is distributed in the tubes (2 μL per tube) to which the extract (8 μL) is added.

9. The gels and *in situ* hybridization described here help keep the NHEJ sample volumes small, so they are used very economically and a large number of NHEJ assays can be performed with one batch of extract. The standard reaction volume for an NHEJ assay is 10 μL (equivalent to 10 ng of substrate input), which is sufficient for analytical gel electrophoresis (measurement of NHEJ efficiency; 2 ng of substrate input per slot required; two gels can be run) and transformation in *E. coli* for subsequent analysis of cloned junc-

tions by restriction digestion and sequencing (measurement of NHEJ fidelity; 2–4 ng of substrate input per transformation required; one or two transformations can be performed). First determine efficiency, and then fidelity.

10. For gel electrophoresis, samples do not need to be particularly clean. (Proteinase K digest is sufficient; phenol extraction is not required.) The ethidium bromide in the gel is required to achieve optimal separation of oc and ccc DNA. (The extract produces relaxed ccc, which is converted to a positive supercoiled form by the ethidium bromide.) Before soaking the gel in the GS solutions, check their pH with pH paper: if GS0 is not sufficiently acid and GS1 not sufficiently alkaline, the ccc band will not denature and thus not hybridize properly. (To control this, a ccc plasmid marker should be loaded on each gel.) It might also be helpful to mark the number of gels soaked in a particular batch of GS solution on the corresponding bottle. (One liter of any GS solution can be used for 10–15 gels, and then new solutions should be prepared.)

11. Two gels can be hybridized simultaneously in the same hybridization mix. If stored at 4°C, the mix can be used repeatedly for up to five gels within 2 wk. Note that the mix must be adjusted to 50 mL with ddH$_2$O and incubated in a boiling water bath for 10 min prior to each round of hybridization. Check gels for excess radioactivity after each washing step of with a portable monitor. (The edges of the gel should be "cold," whereas the lanes containing the DNA bands should be "hot.") The last washing step at 65°C is only necessary if the gel is still "hot" at the edges outside of the lanes. Instead of gel *in situ* hybridization, a Southern blot can also be performed. Note, however, that blotting is more time-consuming. The advantages of gel *in situ* hybridization (or Southern blotting) over the use of ethidium bromide staining are the high sensitivity of both techniques and the fact that less DNA substrate (and thus less extract) per assay is required.

12. For transformation of *E. coli*, clean DNA is needed, so that proteinase K digestion followed by phenol extraction and ethanol precipitation is recommended. Only ccc (and oc) products but not linear multimer products (and linear substrate input) will generate bacterial colonies (transformation efficiency: ccc > oc >> linear). Owing to the low yield of ccc in extracts from NHEJ mutant cell lines, electroporation is recommended as the transformation method. When using only extracts from NHEJ wild-type cells, other, less efficient, transformation protocols may be used. The number of bacteria to be spread on each agar plate depends on the efficiency of the NHEJ reaction: for extracts from NHEJ wild-type cells (high NHEJ efficiency—high transformation efficiency), less bacteria need to be spread than for extracts from NHEJ mutant cells (low NHEJ efficiency—low transformation efficiency: ~10–50 times lower). Each colony obtained represents a single cloned junction.

13. Most of the substrates listed in **Fig. 5** allow an easy check of large, statistically significant numbers of cloned junctions for accurate NHEJ by restriction analysis, which is much cheaper than sequencing. Only the junctions not cleaved by RE then have to be subjected to sequence analysis. The cheapest and least time-consuming solution is to send the samples to a sequencing service. Short run sequences, which show approx 300 bp (often cheaper than long run sequences) are more than sufficient, because NHEJ generates only small sequence alterations within the polylinker region.

References

1. Haber, J. E. (1999) DNA recombination: the replication connection. *Trends Biochem. Sci.* **24,** 271–275.
2. Pfeiffer, P., Goedecke, W., and Obe, G. (2000) Mechanisms of DNA double-strand break repair and their potential to induce chromosomal aberrations. *Mutagenesis* **15,** 289–302.

3. Haber, J. E. (1999) DNA repair. Gatekeepers of recombination. *Nature* **398**, 665–667.
4. Haber, J. E. (2000) Partners and pathways repairing a double-strand break. *Trends Genet.* **16**, 259–264.
5. Haber, J. E. (2000) Recombination: a frank view of exchanges and vice versa. *Curr. Opin. Cell Biol.* **12**, 286–292.
6. Pfeiffer, P. (1998) The mutagenic potential of DNA double-strand break repair. *Toxicol. Lett.* **96–97**, 119–129.
7. Critchlow, S. E. and Jackson, S. P. (1998) DNA end-joining: from yeast to man. *Trends Biochem. Sci.* **23**, 394–398.
8. Featherstone, C. and Jackson, S. P. (1999) DNA double-strand break repair. *Curr. Biol.* **9**, R759–R761.
9. Feldmann, E., Schmiemann, V., Goedecke, W., Reichenberger, S., and Pfeiffer, P. (2000) DNA double-strand break repair in cell-free extracts from Ku80-deficient cells: implications for Ku serving as an alignment factor in non-homologous DNA end joining. *Nucleic Acids Res.* **28**, 2585–2596.
10. Göttlich, B., Reichenberger, S., Feldmann, E., and Pfeiffer, P. (1998) Rejoining of DNA double-strand breaks in vitro by single-strand annealing. *Eur. J. Biochem.* **258**, 387–395.
11. Bryant, P. E. (1984) Enzymatic restriction of mammalian cell DNA using *Pvu* II and *Bam* H1: evidence for the double-strand break origin of chromosomal aberrations. *Int. J. Radiat. Biol.* **46**, 57–65.
12. Natarajan, A. T. and Obe, G. (1984) Molecular mechanisms involved in the production of chromosomal aberrations. III. Restriction endonucleases. *Chromosoma* **90**, 120–127.
13. Kabotyanski, E. B., Gomelsky, L., Han, J. O., Stamato, T. D., and Roth, D. B. (1998) Double-strand break repair in Ku86- and XRCC4-deficient cells. *Nucleic Acids Res.* **26**, 5333–5342.
14. King, J. S., Valcarcel, E. R., Rufer, J. T., Phillips, J. W., and Morgan, W. F. (1993) Noncomplementary DNA double-strand-break rejoining in bacterial and human cells. *Nucleic Acids Res.* **21**, 1055–1059.
15. Roth, D. B., Porter, T. N., and Wilson, J. H. (1985) Mechanisms of nonhomologous recombination in mammalian cells. *Mol. Cell. Biol.* **5**, 2599–2607.
16. Roth, D. B. and Wilson, J. H. (1986) Nonhomologous recombination in mammalian cells: role for short sequence homologies in the joining reaction. *Mol. Cell. Biol.* **6**, 4295–4304.
17. Daza, P., Reichenberger, S., Göttlich, B., Hagmann, M., Feldmann, E., and Pfeiffer, P. (1996) Mechanisms of nonhomologous DNA end-joining in frogs, mice and men. *Biol. Chem.* **377**, 775–786.
18. Pfeiffer, P. and Vielmetter, W. (1988) Joining of nonhomologous DNA double strand breaks in vitro. *Nucleic Acids Res.* **16**, 907–924.
19. Baumann, P. and West, S. C. (1998) DNA end-joining catalyzed by human cell-free extracts. *Proc. Natl. Acad. Sci. USA* **95**, 14066–14070.
20. Boe, S. O., Sodroski, J., Helland, D. E., and Farnet, C. M. (1995) DNA end-joining in extracts from human cells. *Biochem. Biophys. Res. Commun.* **215**, 987–993.
21. Cheong, N., Okayasu, R., Shah, S., Ganguly, T., Mammen, P., and Iliakis, G. (1996) In vitro rejoining of double-strand breaks in cellular DNA by factors present in extracts of HeLa cells. *Int. J. Radiat. Biol.* **69**, 665–677.
22. Cheong, N., Perrault, A. R., Wang, H., et al. (1999) DNA-PK-independent rejoining of DNA double-strand breaks in human cell extracts in vitro. *Int. J. Radiat. Biol.* **75**, 67–81.
23. Derbyshire, M. K., Epstein, L. H., Young, C. S., Munz, P. L., and Fishel, R. (1994) Nonhomologous recombination in human cells. *Mol. Cell. Biol.* **14**, 156–169.

24. Labhart, P. (1999) Ku-dependent nonhomologous DNA end joining in *Xenopus* egg extracts. *Mol. Cell. Biol.* **19,** 2585–2593.
25. Lakshmipathy, U. and Campbell, C. (1999) Double strand break rejoining by mammalian mitochondrial extracts. *Nucleic Acids Res.* **27,** 1198–1204.
26. Mason, R. M., Thacker, J., and Fairman, M. P. (1996) The joining of non-complementary DNA double-strand breaks by mammalian extracts. *Nucleic Acids Res.* **24,** 4946–4953.
27. Nicolas, A. L. and Young, C. S. (1994) Characterization of DNA end joining in a mammalian cell nuclear extract: junction formation is accompanied by nucleotide loss, which is limited and uniform but not site specific. *Mol. Cell. Biol.* **14,** 170–180.
28. Nicolas, A. L., Munz, P. L., and Young, C. S. (1995) A modified single-strand annealing model best explains the joining of DNA double-strand breaks mammalian cells and cell extracts. *Nucleic Acids Res.* **23,** 1036–1043.
29. North, P., Ganesh, A., and Thacker, J. (1990) The rejoining of double-strand breaks in DNA by human cell extracts. *Nucleic Acids Res.* **18,** 6205–6210.
30. Sathees, C. R. and Raman, M. J. (1999) Mouse testicular extracts process DNA double-strand breaks efficiently by DNA end-to-end joining. *Mutat. Res.* **433,** 1–13.
31. Labhart, P. (1999) Nonhomologous DNA end joining in cell-free systems. *Eur. J. Biochem.* **265,** 849–861.
32. Pfeiffer, P., Thode, S., Hancke, J., and Vielmetter, W. (1994) Mechanisms of overlap formation in nonhomologous DNA end joining. *Mol. Cell. Biol.* **14,** 888–895.
33. Thode, S., Schäfer, A., Pfeiffer, P., and Vielmetter, W. (1990) A novel pathway of DNA end-to-end joining. *Cell* **60,** 921–928.
34. Sharma, R. C., and Schimke R. T. (1996) Preparation of electrocompetent *E. coli* using salt-free growth medium. *BioTechniques* **20,** 42-44.
35. Zdzienicka, M. Z. (1999) Mammalian X-ray-sensitive mutants which are defective in non-homologous (illegitimate) DNA double-strand break repair. *Biochimie* **81,** 107–116.
36. Pfeiffer, P., Thode, S., Hancke, J., Keohavong, P., and Thilly, W. G. (1994) Resolution and conservation of mismatches in DNA end joining. *Mutagenesis* **9,** 527–535.

Measuring Recombination Proficiency in Mouse Embryonic Stem Cells

Andrew J. Pierce and Maria Jasin

Summary

A method is presented to measure homologous recombination in mouse embryonic stem cells by both gene targeting and short-tract gene conversion of a double-strand break. A fluorescence-based reporter is first gene targeted to the *Hprt* locus in a quantifiable way. A homing endonuclease expression vector is then introduced to generate a double-strand break, the repair of which is also quantifiable.

Key Words: Recombination; double-strand break; *Hprt*; mouse embryonic stem cell; GFP (green fluorescent protein); flow cytometry; gene targeting; gene conversion; I-*Sce*I; homing endonuclease.

1. Introduction

Homologous recombination (HR) is an important process in mitotically dividing mammalian cells *(1)*. Although poorly defined mechanistically, two processes involving HR are gene conversion and gene targeting. In these related processes, a particular chromosomal locus (the "recipient") is altered such that it becomes modified to that of a different locus (the "donor"). In both cases, there is a necessity that the recipient and donor sequences possess significant lengths of sequence homology, which is thought to "guide" transfer of information from the donor locus into the recipient locus through some as yet undetermined base-pairing mechanism. In gene conversion, the donor is located in the genome, whereas in gene targeting the donor is exogenously supplied.

Gene conversion is an important DNA repair mechanism for maintaining genomic integrity in mammalian cells, and, reflecting its role in DNA repair, it is strongly stimulated by a double-strand break in the recipient locus *(2)*. Gene targeting is a valuable molecular biology tool for the generation of mutant cell lines and potentially for gene therapy, since in a gene targeting reaction the exogenously supplied DNA is used to alter a specific chromosomal sequence in a defined way (for review, *see* **ref. 3**).

This chapter describes the use of the plasmid phprtDRGFP *(4)* (**Fig. 1**) in a system for assaying double-strand break (DSB)-mediated gene conversion in a mouse *Hprt*

From: *Methods in Molecular Biology, vol. 291, Molecular Toxicology Protocols*
Edited by: P. Keohavong and S. G. Grant © Humana Press Inc., Totowa, NJ

hprtDRGFP

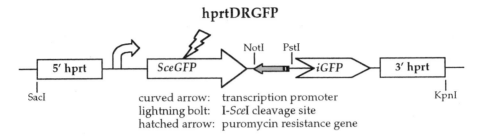

curved arrow: transcription promoter
lightning bolt: I-*Sce*I cleavage site
hatched arrow: puromycin resistance gene

Fig. 1. Schematic of the conversion of the mouse *Hprt* gene. Curved arrow, transcription promoter; lightening bolt, I-*Sce*I cleavage site; gray arrow, puromycin resistance gene. See text for details.

gene targeting context. In this system, the DR-GFP reporter is first gene targeted to the mouse *Hprt* locus in a quantifiable way, and then cells successfully targeted with the reporter are transfected with a separate plasmid (pCbASce) *(5)*, which encodes the I-*Sce*I homing endonuclease that will generate the gene conversion-triggering double-strand break. The efficiency of this gene conversion is also quantifiable.

When cells are supplied with an exogenous gene targeting construct, the construct can integrate either into random loci (nontargeted) or into the homologous locus (targeted). Gene targeting efficiency is usually expressed as the percentage of targeted to total integrations (nontargeted plus targeted). In an organism like yeast, this approaches 100%. In mammalian cells, the gene targeting efficiency seems to be strongly influenced by genomic context, but is usually on the order of a few percent. When the hprtDRGFP fragment is introduced into mouse embryonic stem cells, the *Hprt* targeting arms can direct integration of the construct to the *Hprt* locus *(6)*. When this occurs, exon 2 of the *Hprt* gene is replaced by the DR-GFP reporter. This deletion of *Hprt* exon 2 inactivates the gene, rendering cells resistant to the nucleotide analog 6-thioguanine (6-TG). Incorporation of the DR-GFP reporter carries with it a gene conferring resistance to puromycin. Hence, the efficiency of gene targeting can be determined by the fraction of transfected cells that are resistant to puromycin and 6-TG (targeted integration at *Hprt*) vs cells that are resistant to puromycin in the absence of 6-TG selection (nontargeted integration anywhere in the genome).

After identification of cells that have successfully integrated the DR-GFP reporter at the *Hprt* locus, DSB-induced gene conversion can be quantitated by assaying green fluorescent protein (GFP) after transfection of these cells with an expression vector for the I-*Sce*I endonuclease (pCbASce) *(7)*. The upstream GFP repeat (*SceGFP*) is nonfunctional owing to insertion of a recognition sequence for I-*Sce*I; hence, I-*Sce*I expression will generate a DSB in this repeat. The break can then be repaired by several mechanisms including nonhomologous end joining, single-strand annealing, and gene conversion. Gene conversion can be further mechanistically subdivided into short or long tract, with or without crossing over. Short-tract gene conversion without crossing over represents the majority of these events *(8)* and results in repair of the DSB using the downstream internal fragment GFP repeat *(iGFP)* as a template. The result is that *SceGFP* becomes a constitutively expressed functional *GFP+* gene, and cells acquire green fluorescence. The fraction of I-*Sce*I-transfected cells that repair the break by short-tract gene conversion without crossing over then becomes easily quantifiable by flow cytometry. In wild-type mouse embryonic stem cells, this fraction is on the order of several percent.

Thus, using the hprtDRGFP/pCbASce system, it is possible to quantify both gene targeting and recombinagenic repair of DSBs in cells of differing genotypes, especially of DNA repair genes. This approach also works effectively using wild-type cell lines transfected to express dominant-negative constructs of DNA repair genes and presumably also can be adapted for the use of small inhibitory double-stranded RNA molecules (siRNA) *(9)*.

2. Materials

2.1. Embryonic Stem Cell Culture

1. A well-characterized line of mouse embryonic stem (ES) cells (e.g., J1, E14, available from Dr. Jasin, m-jasin@ski.mskcc.org).
2. Tissue culture incubator.
3. Laminar flow tissue culture hood.
4. 10-cm Tissue culture plates.
5. 70% Ethanol.
6. Ca^{2+}/Mg^{2+}-free phosphate-buffered saline (PBS): 200 mg/L KCl, 200 mg/L KH_2PO_4, 8 g/L NaCl, 2.16 g/L $Na_2HPO_4 \cdot 7H_2O$. Filter-sterilize and store at room temperature indefinitely (also available commercially from Gibco, Gaithersburg, MD).
7. ES cell medium: mix 500 mL high-glucose Dulbecco's modified Eagle's medium (DMEM), 75 mL ES cell qualified fetal bovine serum (FBS; *see* **Note 1**), 6 mL 100X penicillin/streptomycin (10,000 U/mL each stock), 6 mL 100X nonessential amino acids (10 m*M* each stock), 6 mL 100X L-glutamine (200 m*M* stock), 6 mL dilute 2-mercaptoethanol (dilution is 21.6 mL of stock 2-mercaptoethanol in 30 mL of PBS), and 60 mL leukemia inhibitory factor (LIF; stock 10^7 U/mL; available as ESGRO from Chemicon, Temecula, CA). Store at 4°C for up to several weeks. Store all stock solutions at 4°C for routine use, or freeze at –20°C for long-term storage.
8. Trypsin/EDTA solution: 0.2% trypsin, 1 m*M* EDTA in PBS. Store at 4°C for routine use. For long-term storage freeze at –20°C.
9. Clinical centrifuge (e.g., Marathon model 8K, Fisher, Pittsburgh, PA).
10. 4 mg/mL Puromycin (Sigma, St. Louis, MO) in PBS.
11. 10 mg/mL 6-TG (Sigma) in 1 *N* NaOH.
12. Dimethyl sulfoxide (DMSO).
13. Cryovials.
14. 100% Methanol.
15. Giemsa stain.

2.2. Preparation and Analysis of Targeting Plasmid

1. Plasmid phprtDRGFP (available from Dr. Jasin).
2. Restriction enzymes: *Sac*I, *Kpn*I, *Eco*RV (e.g., New England Biolabs, Beverly, MA).
3. Agarose (molecular biology grade, e.g., Invitrogen, Carlsbad, CA) and agarose gel apparatus, including power supply (e.g., Owl Scientific, Portsmouth, NH).

4. Gel loading buffer: mix 600 mL 50% glycerol, 100% ethanol, 50 mL 1% bromophenol blue in ethanol, 50 mL 1% xylene cyanol in ethanol, 60 mL Tris-HCl buffer, pH 8.0, 60 mL 500 mM EDTA, pH 8.0, and 180 mL water. Store at room temperature.
5. DNA size markers (e.g., λ DNA digested with *Bst*EII; Invitrogen).
6. 8 M LiCl.
7. 100% and 75% Ethanol.
8. Tabletop microfuge (e.g., Eppendorf 5415 D, Fisher).
9. 1/10X TE: 1 mM Tris-HCl, 0.1 mM EDTA, pH 8.0. Filter-sterilize and store at room temperature.

2.3. Transfecting ES Cells With the Targeting Plasmid

1. Electroporator (e.g., GenePulser II, Bio-Rad, Hercules, CA).
2. Electroporation cuvets (0.8 mL with a gap width of 0.4 cm; Fisher).
3. 96-, 24-, and 6-Well tissue culture plates

2.4. Preparing Genomic DNA From Transfectants

1. SALT-X genomic DNA extraction solution: 400 mM NaCl, 10 mM Tris-HCl, 2 mM EDTA, pH 8.0, 2% sodium dodecyl sulfate (SDS), 0.4 mg/mL proteinase K. Freeze 10-mL aliquots at –20°C.
2. Hybridization oven.
3. Saturated NaCl solution.
4. Isopropanol.
5. 75% Ethanol (room temperature).
6. Spectrophotometer.

2.5. Southern Hybridization

1. Restriction enzymes: *Hin*dIII, *Pst*I, *Sac*I, *Not*I (New England Biolabs).
2. Gel purification kit (e.g., GFX PCR DNA and Gel Band Purification Kit, Amersham Biosciences, Piscataway, NJ).
3. Blotting membrane (e.g., GeneScreen Plus charged nylon membrane [NEN, Boston, MA] works well when following the alkaline transfer instructions provided by the manufacturer).
4. Radiolabeling kit (e.g., Prime-It II Random Primer Labeling Kit, Stratagene, La Jolla, CA).
5. ProbeQuant G-50 Micro Column (size exclusion; Amersham).
6. Southern blot hybridization solution: mix equal amounts of 1 M Na$_2$HPO$_4$ and 2 mM EDTA, pH 8.0, 2% bovine serum albumin (BSA), 10% SDS. Stock solutions can be stored at room temperature indefinitely. The SDS in the mixed stock solutions will tend to precipitate at room temperature. It will go back into solution when heated to 65°C.
7. 20X SSC (3 M NaCl, 0.3 M Na citrate, pH 7.0): mix: 175.3 g NaCl, 88.2 g Na citrate, and 800 mL H$_2$O.
8. Adjust to pH 7.0 with HCl, if necessary, and adjust volume to 1 L. Store indefinitely at room temperature.

2.6. Measuring Homologous Recombination at a Double-Strand Break

1. Plasmid pCbASce (available from Dr. Jasin).
2. High-capacitance electroporator (e.g., Gene Pulser II with Capacitance Extender Plus; Bio-Rad).
3. Flow cytometer (e.g., FACScan [488-nm argon laser], BD Biosciences, San Jose, CA).

3. Methods

Mouse ES cells grow very well in culture. Log-phase growth has a doubling time on the order of 18 h. It is necessary to culture ES cells in the presence of LIF to prevent their spontaneous differentiation and loss of pluripotency. ES cells preferentially grow in clumps piled on top of each other. A healthy, nondifferentiated culture of ES cells will show discrete large "patches" of cells with individual cells not distinguishable within the patch. Additionally, the patches should show sharp, bright borders under a phase contrast microscope on low power, indicative of their 3D piled-up nature. Nonhealthy and/or differentiated ES cells will show flat monolayers of individually distinguishable cells that appear dull under phase contrast.

Caution: All manipulations must be carried out in a laminar flow tissue culture hood.

3.1. Preparing a Tissue Culture Plate for ES Cells

1. Completely coat the bottom of a tissue culture plate with a 0.1% gelatin solution, e.g., use 3 mL for a 10-cm-diameter plate. Make sure the bottom of the plate is completely covered by tilting the plate back and forth a few times. Let the gelatin sit on the plate for a minute or two. Store sterile gelatin solution at room temperature.
2. Completely aspirate off the gelatin solution but do not allow the plate to dry out. Leaving too much gelatin on the plate will "drown" the ES cells.
3. Add an appropriate volume of ES cell media to the plate; 8–10 mL for a 10-cm plate works well (*see* **Note 2**).

3.2. Thawing Frozen ES Cells

1. Remove the vial of cells from frozen storage, and wipe down the vial with a 70% ethanol solution.
2. Open and then reclose the vial briefly to allow air pressure to equilibrate. (Skip this step if using a sealed glass vial.)
3. Wearing gloves, hold the vial of cells in your hand until it is partially thawed.
4. Mix the partially thawed cells by inverting the vial a few times.
5. Pour the partially thawed cells into the ES cell medium on a prepared tissue culture plate.
6. Thaw the cells completely by swirling in the medium in the plate.
7. Place immediately in a 37°C humidified tissue culture incubator with 5% CO_2.

3.3. Subculturing ES Cells

1. Remove the plate of ES cells from the incubator to a laminar flow tissue culture hood.
2. Aspirate the medium from the plate.
3. Add an appropriate volume of trypsin/EDTA solution to the cells, and tilt the plate back and forth several times to ensure even treatment; 2 mL for a 10-cm plate works well.
4. When most of the cells detach from the plate with gentle rocking (usually a minute or two), add at least 2 vol of tissue culture medium to the trypsinized cells, and pipet up and down several times to disperse the cell clumps and generate a single cell suspension. Do not allow cells to sit in the trypsin/EDTA solution longer than necessary as they will lyse. Cells will be stable after dilution into medium, as the serum in the medium stops the action of the trypsin. After addition of the medium, the cell density of the cellular suspension can be measured with a hemocytometer if desired.
5. Add an appropriate volume of the dispersed ES cells to the medium on a prepared tissue culture plate, and replace in the incubator. Split ratios of 10:1 work well, and 20:1 splits are possible, if necessary. Splits of greater than 20:1 are not recommended.

3.4. Freezing ES Cells

1. Trypsinize cells from a 50% confluent 10-cm plate as described above in **Subheading 3.3., step 3**.
2. Centrifuge the single-cell suspension of ES cells in medium for 5 min at 500g in a clinical centrifuge.
3. Aspirate the trypsin/EDTA/medium from the cell pellet.
4. Resuspend the cell pellet completely in 1 mL of 90% ES medium/10% sterile dimethyl-sulfoxide (DMSO).
5. Add to a labeled freezer vial.
6. Freeze slowly by either using a freezing container at –80°C or by placing the cell-containing vial directly in the *vapor* phase of a liquid nitrogen freezer. Do *not* place cells directly in the liquid phase of a liquid nitrogen freezer for the actual freezing process.
7. Short-term storage (several days) at –80°C is acceptable. For long-term storage (more than 1 wk), store in a liquid nitrogen-cooled freezer. Either liquid or vapor phase storage works fine. Cells stored in liquid nitrogen remain viable for several years.

3.5. Determining ES Cell Drug Sensitivity

It is necessary to determine for each ES line what level of drug selection will kill nonresistant cells. For hprtDRGFP, the selective drugs are puromycin and 6-TG. In general, we find that a final concentration of 10 µg/mL 6-TG works for all cell lines but that the concentration of puromycin must be determined empirically.

1. Prepare ten 10-cm tissue culture plates with 9 mL ES cell medium on each plate.
2. Trypsinize a 50% confluent 10-cm plate of ES cells, add medium, and centrifuge for 5 min at 500g in a clinical centrifuge.
3. Aspirate the medium from the pellet, resuspend the pellet in 10 mL medium, and add 1 mL of the cell suspension to each of the prepared 10-cm plates for a total volume of medium and cells of 10 mL per plate.
4. Add puromycin to each plate to give final concentrations of 0, 0.1, 0.18, 0.32, 0.56, 1.0, 1.8, 3.2, 5.6, and 10.0 µg/mL puromycin.
5. Incubate cells at 37°C in a humidified incubator with 5% CO_2 for 5 d.
6. Note minimal concentration of puromycin that was necessary to kill *all* the cells, i.e., no viable attached cells on the plate. For most ES cell lines, this is typically in the range of 1–2 µg/mL puromycin.

3.6. Staining Colonies on a Tissue Culture Plate

1. Aspirate medium from the plate.
2. Treat with 100% methanol for 30 s.
3. Rinse briefly with water.
4. Stain with dilute Giemsa solution (typically a 10:1–20:1 dilution of stain in water—consult instructions from the supplier) until colonies are stained dark blue
5. Rinse away the stain completely with water, and let the plate air-dry.

3.7. Preparation of the Targeting Plasmid

The vast majority of mouse ES lines in current use are derived from male mice. The goal is to target the hemizygous (X chromosome-linked) *Hprt* locus in male ES cells with the hprtDRGFP targeting construct to (1) determine the targeting efficiency at this locus, and (2) derive stable integrants that contain the DR-GFP reporter at a defined locus in order to perform the gene conversion assay.

1. Linearize the plasmid phprtDRGFP at the ends of the targeting arms (**Fig. 1**): Digest 70 μg of plasmid for each cell line to be transfected in a total restriction digest volume of 400 μL with 100 U of *Sac*I and 100 U of *Kpn*I overnight at 37°C.
2. Verify that the plasmid has been correctly linearized: Digest 1 μL of the *Sac*I/*Kpn*I-digested DNA with *Eco*RV (4 U) in a total digestion volume of 15 μL at 37°C for 1 h. As a control, add 1 μL of the *Sac*I/*Kpn*I-digested DNA to 14 μL of water.
3. Add 3 μL of gel loading buffer to the *Eco*RV digest and the control. Load and run on a 0.8% agarose gel with suitable DNA site markers.
4. If the *Sac*I/*Kpn*I digest was complete, the control lane should have two bands of 9611 and 2856 bp. The *Eco*RV-digested DNA should give three bands of 4982, 4629, and 2856 bp.
5. If the *Sac*I digest was incomplete, the *Eco*RV digest will show a higher band at 7485 bp and under-representation of the 4629-bp band. If the *Kpn*I digest was incomplete, the *Eco*RV digest will show a higher band at 7838 bp and under-representation of the 4982-bp band. In either case, the control DNA will show a higher band at 12,467 bp. In the event of an incomplete digest, add another 20 U of the appropriate enzyme, and digest again overnight. Then repeat *Eco*RV treatment and gel analysis.
6. Ethanol-precipitate the complete *Sac*I/*Kpn*I digest by adding 40 μL of 8 *M* LiCl and 800 μL 100% ethanol. Vortex briefly, incubate at room temperature for 3 min, and then microfuge at 12,000g for 3 min.
7. A white DNA pellet should be clearly visible. Decant the supernatant and add 500 μL 75% ethanol. Invert the tube several times to mix, and then centrifuge briefly to get the pellet back to the bottom of the tube.
8. Pipet off the 75% ethanol, allow the pellet to air-dry (do *not* "SpeedVac" the pellet), and dissolve the pellet completely in 70 μL 1/10X TE overnight at room temperature.

3.8. Transfecting ES Cells With the Targeting Plasmid

1. Two days before electroporation, seed 2×10^6 ES cells onto a 10-cm tissue culture plate. Incubate at 37°C in a humidified incubator with 5% CO_2.
2. Warm bottles of ES cell medium trypsin/EDTA solution to 37°C.
3. Aspirate the medium from the cells to be transfected, and add prewarmed medium. Incubate cells for 4 h at 37°C after this change to fresh medium.
4. Prepare 10 10-cm tissue culture plates with 9 mL medium each.
5. Place 70 μL of linearized targeting plasmid in a 1.0 × 0.4-cm electroporation cuvette.
6. Add 10 mL prewarmed medium to a sterile 15-mL tube.
7. Aspirate the medium from the ES cells, and add 2 mL warmed trypsin/EDTA.
8. When cells start to detach, add 4 mL warmed ES medium. Resuspend the cells well, and then centrifuge for 5 min at 500g in a clinical centrifuge.
9. Resuspend the cell pellet in 650 μL room temperature PBS by pipeting up and down. Add the cell suspension in PBS to the electroporation cuvet with the added plasmid DNA, and mix by pipeting up and down (*see* **Note 3**).
10. Electroporate the plasmid into the cells with an electroporator set to 0.8 kV, 3 μF (*see* **Note 4**). Immediately add 1300 μL (2X 650 μL) of medium from the 15-mL tube to the electroporation cuvet. Pipet up and down to mix, and add the entire contents back to the 15-mL tube.

11. Add 1 mL of the electroporated cell suspension to each of the 10 prepared 10-cm plates for a final volume of medium and cells of 10 mL, and incubate overnight at 37°C in a humidified incubator with 5% CO_2.

12. Add an appropriate amount of puromycin (*see* **Subheading 3.5.**) to each of the transfected plates, and replace in the incubator for an additional 3 d.

13. There should be significant cell killing after 3 d of puromycin selection. Replace the medium on all plates with fresh puromycin-containing medium, and continue to incubate until colonies are barely visible to the naked eye (another 3 d typically).

14. After colonies start to become visible (approx 6 d post transfection), add 6-TG stock solution to a final concentration of 10 µg/mL to 9 of the 10 transfected plates, leaving 1 plate with puromycin without 6-TG.

15. After colonies on the plate with puromycin alone are easily visible to the naked eye (an additional 2 or 3 d typically for a total of 8–10 days post transfection), stain the plate and count the colonies. This count represents the total of both random and targeted integration. At this time, also change medium on the remaining nine plates to fresh medium with puromycin and 6-TG.

16. When the puromycin/6-TG resistant (doubly resistant) colonies are 2–3 mm in diameter, they are ready to pick. First count how many of the doubly resistant colonies there were on the nine doubly selected plates in total. The gene targeting efficiency is the ratio of the number of these targeted colonies to the total number of stable integrants (from the plate with puromycin alone) normalized to the total number of cells transfected under each drug selection condition. For wild-type cells, this value is on the order of a few percent.

17. Replace the medium on the nine targeted (doubly-selected) plates with PBS. With a sterile pipet tip, remove 18 of the doubly resistant colonies to individual wells in a 96-well plate, each well containing 20 µL trypsin/EDTA solution.

18. Incubate at 37°C for 5 min, then add 180 µL fresh medium, and disperse the colonies by pipeting up and down. Transfer the cell suspensions to individual wells of a gelatin-pretreated 96-well plate. Place in the incubator for several days until cells are well established in the wells.

19. Expand these individual colonies progressively through growth on 24-well plates, 6-well plates, and finally, individual 10-cm plates.

20. After expansion, freeze stocks of the clones, and prepare genomic DNA for verification of targeting by Southern blot.

3.9. Preparing Genomic DNA From Transfectants

There are many procedures for preparing genomic DNA from tissue culture cells, but this one is included because it is particularly simple and inexpensive *(10)*. Adequate DNA is isolated from mouse ES cells from either a semiconfluent well of a 6-well plate, or from about one-fourth of a 10-cm plate.

1. Trypsinize and suspend cells in medium as in **Subheading 3.3., step 3**.
2. Pellet an appropriate volume of cells, and remove supernatant.
3. Add 400 µL SALT-X solution. Resuspend by agitation, and incubate at 55–65°C in hybridization oven until the solution clears completely, typically from overnight to several days (*see* **Note 5**).
4. Remove digested cells to a 1.5-mL microcentrifuge tube. Add 300 µL NaCl-saturated water, and shake the tube vigorously. Do not vortex. A white precipitate should form immediately.

5. Centrifuge for 3 min to pellet proteins. If the pellet is not solid, shake vigorously again and repeat this step.

6. Remove all the supernatant to a new 1.5-mL microcentrifuge tube and recentrifuge. This step is optional but recommended.

7. Remove 600 μL of the supernatant to a new microcentrifuge tube. Avoid any pellet and/ or cloudiness.

8. Add 420 μL room temperature isopropanol, and mix by repeated gentle inversion. Precipitated DNA should be evident. Let sit for 3 min at room temperature.

9. Pellet genomic DNA in a microfuge at 12,000g for 3 min. Rinse the pellet with room temperature 75% ethanol, carefully aspirate the ethanol, let air-dry, and resuspend in 100 μL 1/10X TE overnight at room temperature.

10. Ensure that the genomic DNA is well dissolved, measure the DNA concentration by taking an OD_{260} reading in a spectrophotometer, and adjust the concentration of genomic DNA to 1 μg/mL with water and gentle agitation. The DNA will be stable at room temperature for several weeks or can be frozen for long-term storage.

3.10. Verifying Targeted Integration of HprtDRGFP by Southern Blot

Individual clones are screened by Southern blot to verify that the reporter has integrated in an intact manner into the *Hprt* locus. A radiolabeled probe consisting of the *GFP* coding sequence is used, and genomic DNA is digested with enzymes that cut between the *GFP* repeats in hprtDRGFP (e.g., *Pst*I, *see* **Fig. 1**) and in the genome outside the construct. If the reporter integrated correctly, two bands (and only two bands) of well-defined length should be observed. For a *Pst*I digest, the bands should be 8177 and 3755 bp, corresponding to targeted integration on the 5' and 3' sides respectively. For a *Sac*I/*Not*I digest, the bands should be 7488 and 5126 bp, corresponding to correct integration on the 3' and 5' sides respectively. Colonies resistant to both puromycin and 6-TG typically show greater than 95% correct targeted integration in wild-type cells.

1. Isolate *GFP* coding sequence for use as a probe. Plasmid phprtDRGFP, when digested with *Hind*III, will yield three fragments of 9363, 2298, and 806 bp. Gel-purify the 806-bp fragment using a suitable kit according to manufacturer's instructions.

2. Digest 8 μg of genomic DNA from each isolated 6-TG-resistant clone with *Pst*I or with a combination of *Sac*I and *Not*I. Run the digestion products on a 0.8% agarose gel with suitable size markers. Take a picture of the gel to locate the size markers.

3. Blot the gel onto a suitable membrane.

4. Radiolabel 15 ng of the *GFP* coding sequence probe with $\alpha[^{32}P]dCTP$ or $\alpha[^{32}P]dATP$. Ten picograms of whatever size marker you used in **step 2** above can be included in the reaction to radiolabel the marker bands.

6. Purify the radiolabed probe from the unincorporated radionucleotides and primers using a ProbeQuant G-50 Micro Column.

7. Hybridize the probe with the membrane in hybridization solution overnight at 65°C.

8. Rinse the membrane using successive 30-min rinses with 2X SSC/0.1% SDS (twice), 1X SSC/0.1% SDS (twice), and finally 0.5X SSC/0.1% SDS (once), all at 65°C. Dry the membrane and expose to film for several days.

3.11. Measuring Homologous Recombination at a Double-Strand Break

Transfection of hprtDRGFP-targeted cells with the pCbASce expression vector for the I-*Sce*I homing endonuclease will generate a DSB in the *SceGFP* gene (*see* **Fig. 1**). Homologous recombination via short-tract gene conversion without crossing over involving the downstream *iGFP* repeat will generate a functional *GFP+* gene, giving rise to cells that constitutively express GFP. The quantity of cells expressing functional GFP can be easily measured by flow cytometry. A flow cytometry core facility can perform this analysis if you do not have direct access to a flow cytometer. The practical limit of detection with this procedure is on the order of 0.01% fluorescent cells. Wild-type cells generally show homologous repair of a few percent.

1. Two days before electroporation, seed 2×10^6 hprtDRGFP-targeted ES cells onto a 10-cm tissue culture plate. Incubate at 37°C in a humidified incubator with 5% CO_2.
2. Warm a bottle each of ES cell medium, trypsin/EDTA solution, and PBS to 37°C.
3. Aspirate the medium from the cells to be transfected, and add back prewarmed medium. Incubate cells for 4 h at 37°C after this change to fresh medium.
4. Add 50 μg pCbASce in a volume less than 80 μL to a 1.0 × 0.4-cm electroporation cuvet.
5. Prepare two 10-cm tissue culture plates with 10 mL medium each.
6. Aspirate the medium from the cells, and add 2 mL warmed trypsin/EDTA solution. When cells have substantially detached from the plate, add 4 mL warmed medium, and resuspend cells thoroughly.
7. Add 0.5 mL of the cell suspension to one of the prepared 10-cm plates. This will serve as the untransfected control. Place this plate back in the incubator.
8. Centrifuge the remaining cell suspension at 500*g* for 5 min in a clinical centrifuge.
9. Aspirate the medium from the pellet. Add 650 μL of warmed PBS to the pellet, and resuspend by pipeting up and down. Add the cells suspended in the PBS to the electroporation cuvet with the pCbASce DNA and thoroughly mix by pipeting up and down.
10. Immediately electroporate in a high-capacitance electroporator at 1000 μF, 0.25 kV (*see* **Note 6**).
11. Immediately add 2 × 650 μL of medium from the prepared 10-cm plate to the electroporation cuvet. Pipet vigorously up and down to resuspend the electroporated cells. Pour back onto the 10-cm plate, swirl, and immediately place in the 37°C humidified incubator with 5% CO_2.
12. The following day, rinse the electroporated plate with warmed PBS, removing as much cellular debris as possible, and add back fresh medium.
13. Split the unelectroporated control plate if necessary, while the cells on the electroporated plate grow to a semiconfluent state (usually 2–3 d).
14. Trypsinize cells from the untransfected and transfected plates into a cellular suspension. Replate 1/10 vol of cells suspended in medium from each plate onto a freshly prepared 10-cm plate.
15. Analyze 1/10 vol of the cells suspended in medium by flow cytometry for the presence of green fluorescence. This is the preliminary analysis. We use a Becton Dickinson FACScan (488-nm argon laser) with settings as in **Table 1**.

Table 1
Argon Laser Settings

Parameter	Voltage	Amplification	Scale
FSC (forward scatter)	10^{-1}	4.8X	linear
SSC (side scatter)	380 V	1.0X	linear
FL1 (green fluorescence)	460 V	1.0X	log
FL2 (orange fluorescence)	525 V	1.0X	log

We set the threshold to FSC 52 and use 25% FL2–FL1 compensation. Your settings will depend on your particular instrument.

16. Set up a gate on SSC vs FSC to select for cells with a well-defined size and shape, taking care to eliminate debris and clumps. We typically collect fluorescent information from 10,000 cells within the gated SSC vs FSC population.

17. From this gated population, plot FL1 (green fluorescence) vs FL2 (orange fluorescence). The nonfluorescent cells will fall on the FL1/FL2 diagonal. Cells that underwent homologous recombination to restore a functional *GFP* gene will form an obvious discrete population shifted "greenward" on the FL1 axis, away from the FL1/FL2 diagonal. Set a gate to quantitate these cells (**Fig. 2**).

18. When the split cells have grown to a semiconfluent state, trypsinize, resuspend in medium, and reanalyze by flow cytometry (**steps 15–17**) to get the final values for green fluorescence.

4. Notes

1. This serum has been specifically tested for the ability to support undifferentiated ES cell growth (e.g., Gibco).

2. The recommended depth of the medium is 3 mm. Less medium tends to have nutrients consumed and pH altered too rapidly whereas greater depths lead to poor gas exchange.

3. The PBS is actually slightly hypotonic to the cells. Extended suspension in PBS will render the cells more fragile and lead to greater cell killing and lower transfection efficiencies.

4. These electroporation conditions are very mild. There should be almost no cell killing. These conditions are suitable for electroporation of linearized plasmid DNA only—circular or supercoiled plasmid will not transfect under these conditions.

5. The digestion process can be enhanced by periodically agitating the mixture. If the digestion process was incomplete, the proteins will not pellet cleanly in subsequent steps, and genomic DNA will be difficult to recover.

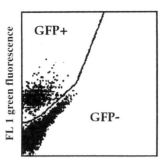

FL 2 orange fluorescence

Fig. 2. Flow cytometry of a transfected recombinant clone showing reconstitution of a functional *GFP* gene. GFP, green fluorescent protein. *See* text for details.

6. These conditions, suitable for efficient electroporation of circular and supercoiled plasmid, are quite harsh and should kill approx 50% of the cells. If excessive cell killing is noted, reduce the electroporation voltage, typically in 20-V increments. If little cell killing is noted, the electroporation voltage can be increased to give greater transfection efficiency.

References

1. Liang, F., Han, M., Romanienko, P. J., and Jasin, M. (1998) Homology-directed repair is a major double-strand break repair pathway in mammalian cells. *Proc. Natl. Acad. Sci. USA* **95**, 5172–5177.
2. Rouet, P., Smih, F., and Jasin, M. (1994) Introduction of double-strand breaks into the genome of mouse cells by expression of a rare-cutting endonuclease. *Mol. Cell. Biol.* **14**, 8096–8106.
3. Ledermann, B. (2000) Embryonic stem cells and gene targeting. *Exp. Physiol.* **85**, 603–613.
4. Pierce, A. J., Hu, P., Han, M., Ellis, N., and Jasin, M. (2001) Ku DNA end-binding protein modulates homologous repair of double-strand breaks in mammalian cells. *Genes Dev.* **15**, 3237–3242.
5. Richardson, C., Moynahan, M. E., and Jasin, M. (1998) Double-strand break repair by interchromosomal recombination: suppression of chromosomal translocations. *Genes Dev.* **12**, 3831–3842.
6. Donoho, G., Jasin, M., and Berg, P. (1998) Analysis of gene targeting and intrachromosomal homologous recombination stimulated by genomic double-strand breaks in mouse embryonic stem cells. *Mol. Cell. Biol.* **18**, 4070–4078.
7. Pierce, A. J., Johnson, R. D., Thompson, L. H., and Jasin, M. (1999) XRCC3 promotes homology-directed repair of DNA damage in mammalian cells. *Genes Dev.* **13**, 2633–2638.
8. Johnson, R. D. and Jasin, M. (2000) Sister chromatid gene conversion is a prominent double-strand break repair pathway in mammalian cells. *EMBO J.* **19**, 3398–3407.
9. Elbashir, S. M., Harborth, J., Lendeckel, W., Yalcin, A., Weber, K., and Tuschl, T. (2001) Duplexes of 21-nucleotide RNAs mediate RNA interference in cultured mammalian cells. *Nature* **411**, 494–498.
10. Aljanabi, S. M. and Martinez, I. (1997) Universal and rapid salt-extraction of high quality genomic DNA for PCR- based techniques. *Nucleic Acids Res.* **25**, 4692–4693.

VI

ARRAY TECHNOLOGIES

32

Strategies for Measurement of Biotransformation Enzyme Gene Expression

Marjorie Romkes and Shama C. Buch

Summary

The analysis of gene expression is an integral part of any research characterizing gene function. A wide variety of techniques have been developed for this purpose, each with their own advantages and limitations. This chapter seeks to provide an overview of some of the most recent as well as conventional methods to quantitate gene expression. These approaches include Northern blot analysis, ribonuclease protection assay (RPA), reverse transcription polymerase chain reaction, expressed sequence tag (EST) sequencing, differential display, cDNA arrays, and the serial analysis of gene expression (SAGE). Current applications of the information derived from gene expression studies require assays to be adaptable for the quantitative analysis of a large number of samples and end points within a short period coupled with cost effectiveness. A comparison of some of these features of each analytical approach as well as their advantages and disadvantages has also been provided.

Key Words: mRNA expression; RT-PCR; TaqMan; serial analysis of gene expression; cDNA microarrays; Northern blot; ribonuclease protection assay (RPA); expressed sequence tag sequencing; differential display; pharmacogenomics; biotransformation enzymes.

1. Introduction

Gene expression analyses have long been used to provide insights into gene function. Many environmental pollutants, toxicants, and heavy metals affect cellular function by causing drastic changes in gene expression patterns. For both toxicological screening and chemical-specific mechanism of action studies, a wide range of approaches is available to evaluate changes in gene expression at the molecular level that may occur because of a toxic response. These approaches are not unique to the analysis of endpoints of interest in molecular toxicology, as for example, the expression of biotransformation enzymes, but are extremely valuable tools for all genomic studies. The recent rapid technological advances in this field were prompted by the ability to identify genes at the nucleic acid level, rather than proceeding from a known protein to its chromosomal counterpart. Expression studies have previously relied on

From: *Methods in Molecular Biology, vol. 291, Molecular Toxicology Protocols*
Edited by: P. Keohavong and S. G. Grant © Humana Press Inc., Totowa, NJ

techniques such as Northern blot analyses or the ribonuclease protection assay, each of which measures the expression of only a small set of genes at a given time. More recent technologies, including serial analysis of gene expression (SAGE), quantitative reverse transcription polymerase chain reaction (RT-PCR), cDNA microarrays, and high-resolution 2D gel electrophoresis, allow for the expression levels of tens to thousands of genes to be screened at once. As summarized in **Table 1** and **Fig. 1**, depending on both the number of samples and number of genetic endpoints to be analyzed and taking into account both cost and throughput capability, one analytical approach for RNA expression analysis may be more appropriate for a particular application or research study.

Prior to any expression analyses, it is essential to verify the integrity of the RNA and to obtain accurate measurement of RNA concentration levels. The feasibility of obtaining meaningful quantitative gene expression data is dependent on the utilization of a validated approach with multiple quality control measures in place. These include the inclusion of either endogenous or exogenous standards or positive controls to assess reproducibility of all steps of the assay; verification of the absence of genomic DNA contamination by DNase treatment and/or in the case of PCR-based methods, the use of primers that span intron/exon junctions for amplification of cDNA only; quantitation analysis of samples collected during the exponential phase of PCR amplification; and negative controls to verify absence of contamination and specificity of the probe used for detection of target mRNAs. Several techniques used for the quantitation of gene expression are reviewed in the following sections.

2. Northern Blot Analysis

Northern blotting was developed as the RNA counterpart of Southern blotting *(1)*. This technique mainly involves separation of RNA species on the basis of size by denaturing gel electrophoresis followed by transfer of the RNA onto a membrane by capillary, vacuum, or pressure blotting. The RNA is then permanently bound to the membrane either by heating at 80°C or by UV crosslinking. These membranes are then probed with partial or complete cDNA oligonucleotides that are labeled by radionucleotides or chemiluminescent moieties. Nonspecific hybridization is removed by washing, and then the blots are audioradiographed. The resulting visible band(s) indicates the size of the RNA, and the intensity corresponds to the relative amounts of the RNA. The band intensities are quantitated by densitometry using the appropriate image analysis software. Northern blotting is perhaps one of the few techniques that permits mRNA size determination and therefore is useful for the detection of alternatively spliced transcripts or mutations that result in modified mRNA sizes. One of the primary drawbacks of Northern blotting, however, is that the technique yields semiquantitative results. The other limitations involve the requirement of very high quality intact RNA concentrations, variability in transfer efficiencies, and high background levels on the audioradiograms *(2)*. Typically, the expression of various housekeeping genes with similar copy numbers are used as external controls for sample loading variability and blot-to-blot comparisons. However, the expression of these housekeeping genes may vary with different stages in the cell cycle or among different

Table 1
Summary of Techniques for RNA Expression Analysis

Technique	Minimum total RNA required	Throughput			Advantages	Disadvantages
		No. of samples	No. of endpoints			
Northern blot	1–10 µg	Low	Low		Can be used to estimate size differences in RNA transcripts	Poor sensitivity Semiquantitative
RT-PCR						
Gel-based	50–100 ng	Low	Low		Extremely specific and sensitive	Semiquantitative
FRET-based	5–100 ng	Medium	Medium		Extremely specific and sensitive, quantitative	
EST	1.0–5.0 µg	Low	High		Redundant sequencing of highly expressed sequences is minimized	Full-length cloning may be required for novel genes
Differential display	10–100 ng	Low	High		Every gene in the cell can be potentially identified	Full-length cloning may be required for novel genes
Microarrays	1.0 µg or more	Medium	High		High throughput	Data interpretation requires specialized software
SAGE	1.0–5.0 µg	Low	High		High specificity	Sequencing errors

Abbreviations: EST, expressed sequence tag; FRET, fluorescence resonance energy transfer; RT-PCR, reverse transcription polymerase chain reaction; SAGE, serial analysis of gene expression.

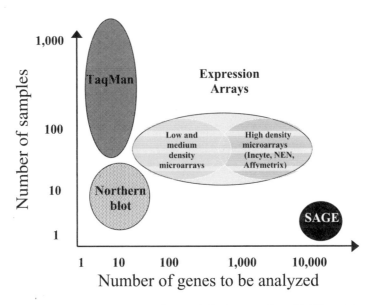

Fig. 1. Comparison of mRNA expression analytical approaches. SAGE, serial analysis of gene expression.

cell, tissue, or disease types. Variations of the Northern blot such as dot, slot, and fast blots have been developed in an attempt to increase quantitation and simplify the assay *(3)*. However, before any of these alternate procedures can be used, it is imperative to demonstrate, via the Northern blot, that the probe used in the application is specific to the target RNA, as there is no scope for size fractionation with these methods.

3. Ribonuclease Protection Assay (RPA)

The ribonuclease protection assay (RPA) is a variation of the Northern blot approach, except that it is performed in a solution containing a labeled antisense target RNA probe and the target mRNA without prior gel fractionation or blotting *(4)*. The unhybridized probe and the sample RNA are degraded enzymatically following incubation for several hours. The remaining hybrids are electrophoresed on a denaturing polyacrylamide gel and visualized by autoradiography. Alternatively the RNase-resistant hybrids are precipitated and bound to filters for direct quantitation by scintillation counting *(5)*. RPA is considered to be 10-fold more sensitive than Northern blot analysis.

Several issues need to be taken into account when one is designing RPA probes. If the RPA products are to be analyzed using gel electrophoresis, the RPA probe should contain some terminal sequences that will not hybridize with the target mRNA, so that undigested probe can be distinguished from probe-RNA hybrids on the basis of size. As is the case with Northern analysis, quantitation requires the concurrent hybridization of an invariant control mRNA. Probes may be multiplexed together in a single hybridization reaction if the sizes of the products do not overlap. This holds true if the products are analyzed by electrophoresis. However, if RPA products are going to be analyzed by the scintillation counter method, then the use of two different radio-nucleotides solves this problem. The two main advantages to RPA are sensitivity and the ability to determine absolute RNA levels. The disadvantages are difficulties encountered in designing adequately sensitive internal controls, and the high quantity/ quality of RNA required for the assay.

4. Expressed Sequence Tag (EST) Sequencing

The concept of expressed sequence tag (EST) sequencing was first described in 1991 *(6)*. The underlying goal was to create cDNA libraries, pick random clones, and then carry out a single sequencing reaction with a large number of clones. Each reaction generates approx 300 bp of sequences that represent a unique sequence tag for a particular transcript. EST sequencing can be carried out using both normalized (in which each transcript is represented in more or less equal numbers) and nonnormalized cDNA libraries *(7)*. The advantage of using normalized libraries is that redundant sequencing of highly expressed genes is minimized *(8)*. The advantage of nonnormalized libraries is that the abundance of the transcript in the original cell is accurately reflected in the frequency of clones in the library *(9)*. Hence these libraries can be used to identify highly expressed but unknown genes as well as to compare the expression of highly expressed genes in different cells or tissues.

There are currently over 1.5 million human ESTs in the publicly available database of ESTs (dbEST) provided by the National Center for Biotechnology Information (NCBI, Baltimore, MD; release 082799). These ESTs are derived from approx 1200 human cDNA libraries. In addition to public databases, several companies have generated larger collections of ESTs. These include Human Genome Sciences (Rockville, MD), Incyte Pharmaceuticals (Palo Alto, CA), and Celera Genomics Group (South San Francisco, CA).

5. Subtractive Cloning by Representational Difference Analysis (RDA)

Subtractive cloning methods have been in use for many years and offer an inexpensive and flexible alternative to EST sequencing and cDNA array hybridization. The PCR-based method commonly used is known as representational difference analysis (RDA) *(10,11)*. In this analysis, double stranded-cDNA is created from the two cell or tissue populations of interest (for example, tumor and normal tissue), linkers are ligated to the end of the cDNA fragments, and then the cDNA pools are amplified by PCR. The cDNA pool from which unique clones are desired is designated as the "tester," and the cDNA pool that is used to subtract shared sequences is designated as the "driver." Following PCR amplification, the linkers are removed from both cDNA pools, and unique linkers are ligated to the tester sample. The tester is then hybridized to an excess of driver DNA, and sequences that are unique to the tester cDNA pool are amplified by PCR. The primary limitation of this method is that subtle quantitative differences are missed because the cDNAs identified are usually those that differ significantly in expression level between the cell populations. In addition, because each experiment is a pairwise comparison, and the subtractions are based on a series of sensitive biochemical reactions, it then becomes difficult to compare a series of RNA samples directly.

6. Reverse Transcription-Polymerase Chain Reaction (RT-PCR)

RT-PCR is an in vitro method for amplifying defined target sequences of RNA *(12)*. It is an extremely sensitive method and can be used to compare levels of mRNA in different sample populations and to characterize patterns of mRNA expression. RT-PCR analyses have been modified to increase its sensitivity and accuracy; some of the modifications include semi-nested *(13)*, nested *(14)*, and even three-step nested *(15)* RT-PCR techniques. There are also a number of detection methods that can be used, yielding either semiquantitative or quantitative results. All of the components of an RT-PCR reaction and subsequent product detection are interdependent and require careful optimization to ensure specificity, sensitivity and reproducibility of the assay. Typically, all measurements are standardized to a calibrator sample so that data collected at different time points can be compared directly.

The first step in RT-PCR is the reverse transcription (RT) of the RNA template into cDNA, followed by its exponential amplification in a PCR reaction. Separation of the RT and the PCR steps is advantageous for long-term storage of the cDNA or analysis of multiple targets. The RT step can be primed using specific primers, random hexamers, or oligo-dT primers. Specific primers can sometimes cause marked variation in estimates of mRNA copy numbers; while random hexamers can overestimate mRNA copy numbers by about 19-fold. Numerous RT enzyme preparations are commercially available and vary in terms of efficiency and in range of primers that can be used for first-strand synthesis. In all RT-PCR applications, it is critical to include a no-RT template control to avoid the quantitation of false positives.

Like other methods for RNA quantitation, RT-PCR can be used for relative or absolute quantitation. Absolute quantitation, using competitive RT-PCR, measures the absolute amount or number of copies of a specific target mRNA sequence in a sample *(16)*. In competitive RT-PCR, increasing amounts of DNA highly homologous to the target, but distinguishable by either size or restriction sites, are added to the PCR, and both target and competitive template are quantified. It is assumed that the amplification efficiency of both templates is identical; however, this may not be the case. Most gene expression analysis studies utilize a relative expression calculation similar to those used in standard assays such as the Northern blot. Expression of the gene of interest is reported relative to expression of an endogenous control gene, which is assumed to have equal expression in all tissues in the study. In this way, expression levels can be compared from tissue to tissue. The endogenous internal control in relative RT-PCR may be analyzed in a multiplexed reaction or in two separate reactions. Common internal controls include 18S rRNA, β-actin, β-glucuronidase, and GAPDH mRNAs *(17)*.

Critical to either absolute or relative RT-PCR is quantitation of the product during the exponential phase of PCR. This represents a challenge because internal control RNAs are typically constitutively expressed housekeeping genes of high abundance, and their amplification reaches the plateau phase with very few PCR cycles. It is therefore difficult to identify comparable exponential phase conditions in which the PCR product from a rare target mRNA is detectable. Detection methods with low sensitivity, like ethidium bromide staining of agarose gels, are therefore not recommended. Detecting a rare message while staying in exponential phase with an abundant message can be achieved in several ways: (1) by improving the sensitivity of product detection; (2) by decreasing the amount of input template in the RT or PCR reactions; and/or (3) by decreasing the number of PCR cycles.

Modifications involving the application of fluorescence probes and instrumentation have led to the development of kinetic RT-PCR methodologies that facilitate the quantitation of nucleic acids with improved sensitivity and throughput and overcome many of the problems described above. There are currently at least three manufacturers of fluorescence resonance energy transfer detection (FRET)-based instrumentation systems.

The ABI PRISM 7700 (Perkin Elmer Applied Biosystems, Foster City, CA) contains a built-in thermal cycler with 96 wells and a fluorescence reader that can read wavelengths between 500 and 660 nm. The fluorescent light source in this case is a laser, and the emission is directed to a spectrograph with a charge-coupled device (CCD). The most recent commercially available model, ABI PRISM 7000, uses a tungsten–halogen lamp, and the fluorescence emission is directed through four optical filters to a CCD camera. The rest of the features are similar to the 7700. On the other hand, the ABI PRISM 7900HT has a 384-well capacity and allows the use of multiple fluorophores in a single reaction owing to the feature of continuous wavelength detection *(18)*.

The LightCycler (Roche Molecular Biochemicals, Mannheim, Germany) uses small-volume glass capillary tubes that are heated and cooled by an airstream. A blue light-emitting diode is the light source, and the fluorescence is read by three photodetection diodes with different filters. It can analyze up to 32 samples per run *(19)*.

Bio-Rad has recently launched an optical module that fits into their conventional thermal cycler. This device can scan up to 96 samples simultaneously and at present can monitor four different fluorescent reporters.

To date, there are four different competing techniques available to detect the amplified product with the same sensitivity. The simplest method employs fluorescent dyes that bind specifically to double-stranded DNA. The other three utilize the hybridization of fluorescently labeled probes to specific amplicons. These four methods are molecular beacons, DNA binding dyes, hybridization probes, and hydrolysis probes.

6.1. Molecular Beacons

Molecular beacons are probes that have a loop structure complementary to the target nucleic acid molecule and a stem structure that is formed by the annealing of complementary sequences on the ends of the probe sequence *(20)*. A fluorescent marker is attached to one arm, and a quencher is attached to another. In solution, the free molecular beacons have a hairpin structure, with the stem keeping the arms in close proximity, thereby resulting in the efficient quenching of the probe. On encountering a complementary target, they undergo a conformational change that results in the formation of a probe-target hybrid. This hybrid forces the stem apart, leading to the separation of the fluorophore and the quencher and consequently the restoration of fluorescence, while the free molecular beacons remain nonfluorescent. The main drawback of molecular beacons is their ability to form alternate conformations that fail to place the fluorophore next to the quencher, resulting in large background signals.

6.2. DNA-Binding Dyes

DNA-binding dyes such as SYBR green, which exhibit no fluorescence alone in solution, can be incorporated into double-stranded DNA during the PCR elongation step *(21)*. Detection of the fluorescence of the DNA-binding dyes therefore increases during the elongation step and decreases during denaturation. The specificity of target detection largely depends on the specificity of the PCR primers, and a separate probe is not added. An important failing of this method is that the number of dye molecules that are incorporated into the PCR product may vary with each PCR cycle and from sample to sample, and therefore the analysis is semiquantitative at best.

6.3. Hybridization Probes

The LightCycler™ uses hybridization probes. One probe has at its 3' end a fluorescein donor, whose emission spectrum overlaps the excitation spectrum of an acceptor fluorophore, which is attached to the 5' end of the second probe *(19)*. This acceptor labeled probe is blocked at its 3' end to prevent its extension during PCR. Fluorescent light is produced from FRET following excitation of the donor. The two dyes are apart when in solution; however, following hybridization of the probes to the target sequence, they are brought into close proximity, and FRET occurs. Therefore, the increasing intensity of wavelength of the second dye is directly proportional to the amount of DNA synthesized. Furthermore, a melting curve analysis can also be performed for multiplex analysis, as the probes are not hydrolyzed.

6.4. Hydrolysis Probes

Hydrolysis probes are usually used in TaqMan™ assays; they use the 5' nuclease activity of the DNA polymerase to hydrolyze a hybridization probe after it has bound to its target *(22)*. The PCR step, which follows the RT step, increases the specificity of the reaction by the use of three oligonucleotides complementary to the DNA. Two primers amplify a specific amplicon, followed by the use of a probe that hybridizes to the product during annealing/extension. The probe has a fluorescent dye at the 5' end and a quencher at the 3' end. If no complementary amplicon is generated, the probe remains intact. Conversely, if the probe binds to the complementary sequence as it is being amplified, it is eventually cleaved, thus separating the reporter and quencher dyes, causing emission of fluorescence. Because of the high Tms of the probe, the TaqMan system PCR annealing and extension steps can be combined and most reactions are carried out at 60–62°C. This also ensures maximum 5'-3' exonuclease activity of the *Taq* polymerase. The increase in the length of the annealing/extension step, coupled with increased Mg^{2+} or Mn^{2+} for longer amplicons, makes this system less efficient and flexible than others. Real-time RT-PCR assays are conclusively more reliable than conventional ones and can easily be adapted to a high-throughput setup.

7. Differential Display

Another widely used PCR-based method that is extremely popular is differential display or RNA fingerprinting *(23,24)*. Differential display involves RT primed with either an oligo-dT or an arbitrary primer, in conjunction with the RT primer to amplify cDNA fragments that are then separated on a polyacrylamide gel. The presence or absence of bands on the gel visualizes differences in gene expression. Differential display has also been adapted for use in fluorescent DNA sequencing machines. It is efficient for analyzing as little as 5–10 ng of total RNA. A limitation of this method is the generation of false positives either during PCR or in the cloning of differentially expressed PCR products. Large amounts of RNA are required to discriminate true positives from false positives. A modification of the technique based on the analysis of 3'-end restriction fragments claims to result in fewer false-positive signals *(25)*. In this method, double-stranded cDNA is prepared and digested with a restriction enzyme with a four-base recognition site. Linkers are then ligated to the restriction fragments, and the entire pool of transcripts is amplified by PCR. Gel electrophoresis of the 3'-end fragments reveals the differences in gene expression. The distinct advantage this modification offers is that every gene in the cell can be identified by the use of a series of restriction enzymes; furthermore, because the migration of the bands in the gel is determined by the restriction site at the 3'-end, known genes can simply be identified by measuring the size of the restriction fragment.

8. cDNA Microarrays

In a cDNA array, many gene-specific polynucleotides derived from the 3'-end of RNA transcripts are individually arrayed on a single matrix *(26)*. This matrix is then simultaneously probed with fluorescently tagged cDNA representations of total RNA pools from test and reference samples, allowing one to determine the relative amount of transcript present in the pool by the type of fluorescent signal generated. An internal control is provided for each measurement. The adaptable nature of the fabrication of the array and hybridization methods allow the technique to be widely applied—the limitations being cost, the availability of clones for the solid phase, and the quality of the RNA extracted from cell lines or tissues. The targets for the arrays are labeled representations of cellular mRNA pools. A labeled product from the 3'-end of the gene is produced by RT with an oligo-dT primer. The purity of the RNA is critical, particularly when using fluorescence, as cellular proteins, lipids, and carbohydrates can mediate significant nonspecific binding of fluorescently labeled cDNAs to slide surfaces. For adequate fluorescence, the total RNA required per target, per array, is 50–200 ng. For mRNA present as a single transcript per cell, application of target derived from 100 ng of total RNA over an 800-mm^2 hybridization area containing 200-μm-diameter probes will result in approx 300 transcripts being sufficiently close to the target to have a chance to hybridize. Therefore, if the fluorescently tagged transcripts are 600 bp, have an average of 2 fluor tags per 100 bp, and hybridize to their probe, approx 12 fluors will be present in a 100-μm^2 scanned pixel. Such low levels of signal are at the lower limit of fluorescence detection and can easily be rendered undetectable by assay noise. A variety of means by which to improve signal from limited RNA have been proposed. For example, efficient mixing of the hybridization fluid should bring more molecules into contact with their cognate probe, increasing the number of productive events. Posthybridization amplification methods have also been reported in which detectable molecules are precipitated at the target by the action of enzymes "sandwiched" to the cDNA target *(27)*.

A critical challenge of the high-throughput technologies available to measure gene expression is the accurate and adequate analysis of the vast amounts of data generated. At present the most widely used computational approach for analyzing microarray data is cluster analysis. This analysis groups genes based on similar expression profiles and compares them with other clustered genes, providing clues to the function or regulation of the genes. The three broad categories of cluster analysis include a tree-based approach that uses a measure of the distance between genes such as a correlation coefficient to group genes into hierarchical trees *(28,29)*. The second category minimizes variation within clusters so that between-cluster variation is maximized *(30)*. The third category groups genes into two basic blocks, one in which the correlation is maximized and one in which the correlation is minimized *(31)*. All these categories basically utilize the intensity differences between the mean intensity for each of the groups. However, relative mean comparisons ignore the premise that differences in expression level of less than 100% may exert meaningful biological effects. Various statistical models have been designed to approach the problem of gene expression data analysis, and several problems still remain associated with each of the strategies *(32)*. Although technological advances have simplified the ability to study thousands of genes at once, the interpretation of this data and its subsequent analysis continue to pose a challenge.

9. Serial Analysis of Gene Expression (SAGE)

Serial analysis of gene expression (SAGE) utilizes isolated sequence tags from individual mRNAs that are concatenated serially into long DNA molecules that are then sequenced *(33)*. Initially double-stranded cDNA is synthesized from mRNA using a biotinylated oligo-dT primer. The cDNA pool is then cleaved by a restriction enzyme, also known as an anchoring enzyme, and is then separated on a polyacrylamide gel. The total number of tags identified by this method to date number close to 5 million. SAGE requires relatively higher concentrations of RNA compared with RT-PCR or microarray analyses, and it is relatively technically difficult to create tag libraries. There are two major concerns when using SAGE. One concern is identifying sequencing errors, and the second is making valid tag to gene assignments. Several modifications have been developed to increase the utility of SAGE in terms of both methodology and data interpretation *(34)*.

References

1. Sambrook, J., Fritsch, E. F., and Maniatis, T. (1989) *Molecular Cloning: A Laboratory Manual*, 2nd ed. Cold Spring Harbor Laboratory, Cold Spring Harbor, NY.
2. Reue, K. (1988) mRNA quantitation techniques: considerations for experimental design and application. *J. Nutr.* **128,** 2038–2044.
3. Costanzi, C. and Gillespie, D. (1987) Fast blots: immobilization of DNA and RNA from cells. *Methods Enzymol.* **152,** 582–587.
4. Azrolan, N. and Breslow, J. L. (1990) A solution hybridization/RNase protection assay with riboprobes to determine absolute levels of apo B, apo A-I and apo E mRNA in human hepatoma call lines. *J. Lipid Res.* **31,** 1141–1146.
5. Melton, D. A., Kreig, P. A., Rebagliati, M. R., Maniatis, T., Zinn, K., and Green, M. R. (1984) Efficient in vitro synthesis of biologically active RNA and DNA hybridization

probes from plasmids containing a bacteriophage SP6 promoter. *Nucleic Acids Res.* **12,** 7035–7056.

6. Adams, M. D., Kelley, J. M., Gocayne, J. D., et al. (1991) Complementary DNA sequencing: expressed sequence tags and the human genome project. *Science* **252,** 1651–1656.

7. Patanjali, S. R., Parimoo, S., and Weissman, S. M. (1991) Construction of a uniform-abundance (normalized) cDNA library. *Proc. Natl. Acad. Sci. USA* **88,** 1943–1947.

8. Bonaldo, M. F., Lennon, G., and Soares, M. B. (1996) Normalization and subtraction: two approaches to facilitate gene discovery. *Genome Res.* **6,** 791–806.

9. Ji, H., Liu, Y. E., Jia, T., et al. (1997) Identification of a breast cancer-specific gene, BCSG1, by direct differential cDNA sequencing. *Cancer Res.* **57,** 759–764.

10. Hubank, M. and Schatz, D. G. (1994) Identifying differences in mRNA expression by representational difference analysis of cDNA. *Nucleic Acids Res.* **22,** 5640–5648.

11. Diatchenko, L., Lau, Y. F.-C., Campbell, A. P., et al. (1996) Suppression subtractive hybridization: a method for generating differentially regulated or tissue-specific cDNA probes and libraries. *Proc. Natl. Acad. Sci. USA* **93,** 6025–6030.

12. Rappolee, D. A., Mark, D., Banda, M. J., and Werb, Z. (1988) Wound macrophages express TGF-α and other growth factors *in vivo*: analysis by mRNA phenotyping. *Science* **241,** 708–712.

13. Wasserman, L., Dreilinger, A., Easter, D., and Wallace, A. (1999) A seminested RT-PCR assay for HER2/neu: initial validation of a new method for the detection of disseminated breast cancer cells. *Mol. Diagn.* **4,** 21–28.

14. Israeli, R. S., Miller, W. H. Jr., Su, S. L., et al. (1994) Sensitive nested reverse transcription polymerase chain reaction detection of circulating prostatic tumor cells: comparison of prostate-specific membrane antigen and prostate-specific antigen-based assays. *Cancer Res.* **54,** 6306–6310.

15. Funaki, N. O., Tanaka, J., Itami, A., et al. (1997) Detection of colorectal carcinoma cells in circulating peripheral blood by reverse transcription polymerase chain reaction targeting cytokeratin-20 mRNA. *Life Sci.* **60,** 643–652.

16. Wang, A. M., Doyle, M. V., and Mark, D. F. (1989) Quantitation of mRNA by the polymerase chain reaction. *Proc. Natl. Acad. Sci. USA* **86,** 9717–9721.

17. Suzuki, T., Higgins, P. J., and Crawford, D. R. (2000) Control selection for RNA quantitation. *BioTechniques* **29,** 332–337.

18. www. appliedbiosystems.com

19. Wittwer, C. T., Ririe, K. M., Andrew, R.V., David, D. A., Gundry, R. A., and Balis, U. J. (1997) The LightCycler: a microvolume multisample fluoimeter with rapid temperature control. *BioTechniques* **22,** 176–181.

20. Tyagi, S. and Kramer, F. R. (1996) Molecular beacons: probes that fluoresce upon hybridization. *Nat. Biotechnol.* **14,** 303–308.

21. Morrison T. B., Weiss, J. J., and Wittwer, C. T. (1998) Quantifiaction of low-copy transcripts by continuos SYBR Green I monitoring during amplification. *BioTechniques* **29,** 954–962.

22. Livak, K. J., Flood, S. J., Marmaro, J., Giusti, W., and Deetz, K. (1995) Oligonucleotides with fluorescent dyes at opposite ends provide a quenched probe system useful for detecting PCR product and nucleic acid hybridization. *PCR Methods Appl.* **4,** 357–362.

23. Liang, P. and Pardee, A. B. (1992) Differential display of eukaryotic messenger RNA by means of the polymerase chain reaction. *Science* **257,** 967–970.

24. Welsh, J., Chada, K., Dalal, S. S., Cheng, R., and McClelland, M. (1992) Arbitrarily primed PCR fingerprinting of RNA. *Nucleic Acids Res.* **20,** 4965–4970.

25. Kato, K. (1995) Description of the entire mRNA population by a 3' end cDNA fragment generated by class IIS restriction enzymes. *Nucleic Acids Res.* **18,** 3685–3690.
26. Duggan, D. J., Bittner, M., Chen, Y., Meltzer, P., and Jeffrey, T. (1999) Expression profiling using cDNA microarrays. *Nat. Genet.* **Suppl. 21,** 10–14.
27. Marshall, A. and Hodgson, J. (1998) DNA chips: an array of possibilities. *Nat. Biotechnol.* **16,** 27–31.
28. Tamayo, P., Slonim, D., Mesirov, J., et al. (1999) Interpreting patterns of gene expression with self-organizing maps: methods and application to hematopoietic differentiation. *Proc. Natl. Acad. Sci. USA* **96,** 2907–2912.
29. Eisen, M. B., Spellman, P. T., Brown, P. O., and Botstein, D. (1998) Cluster analysis and display of genome-wide expression patterns. *Proc. Natl. Acad. Sci. USA* **95,** 14863–14868.
30. Tavazoie, S., Hughes, J. D., Campbell, M. J., Cho, R. J., and Church, G. M. (1999) Systematic determination of genetic network architecture. *Nat. Genet.* **22,** 281–285.
31. Ben-Dor, A., Shamir, R., and Yakhini, Z. (1999) Clustering gene expression patterns. *J. Comput. Biol.* **6,** 281–297.
32. Thomas, J. G., Olson, J. M., Tappscott, S. J., and Zhao, L. P. (2001) An efficient and robust statistical modeling approach to discover differentially expressed genes using genomic expression profiles. *Genome Res.* **11,** 1227–1236.
33. Velculescu, V. E., Zhang, L., Vogelstein, B., and Kinzler, K. W. (1995) Serial analysis of gene expression. *Science* **270,** 484–488.
34. Carulli, J. P., Artinger, M., Swain, P. M., et al. (1998) High throughput analysis of differential gene expression. *J. Cell. Biochem.* **Suppl. 30/31,** 286–296.

33

Genotyping Technologies

Application to Biotransformation Enzyme Genetic Polymorphism Screening

Marjorie Romkes and Shama C. Buch

Summary

Pharmacogenomics encompasses several major areas: the study of polymorphic variations in drug response and disease susceptibility, identification of the effects of drugs/xenobiotics at the genomic level, and genotype/phenotype associations. The most common type of human genetic variations is single-nucleotide polymorphisms (SNPs). Several novel approaches to detection of SNPs are currently available. The range of new methods includes modifications of several conventional techniques, such as PCR, mass spectrometry (ms), and sequencing, as well as more innovative technologies such as fluorescence resonance energy transfer (FRET) and microarrays. The application of each of these techniques is largely dependent on the number of SNPs to be screened and sample size. The current chapter presents an overview of the general concepts of a variety of genotyping technologies, with an emphasis on the recently developed methodologies, including a comparison of the advantages, applicability, cost efficiency, and limitations of these methods.

Key Words: Genotyping; SNP detection; pharmacogenomics; biotransformation enzymes; genetic polymorphisms; PCR; microarray.

1. Introduction

The human genome is made up of approx three billion nucleotides that code for all the macromolecules necessary for human life. The most common types of human genetic variations are single-nucleotide polymorphisms (SNPs), which are defined as DNA sequence variations that occur when a single nucleotide (A, T, C, or G) in the genome sequence is changed *(1)*. It is estimated that only one in every thousand bases is different, or that the DNA code is approx 99.9% identical between human subjects. SNPs occur in both coding and noncoding regions and may or may not result in altered

From: *Methods in Molecular Biology, vol. 291, Molecular Toxicology Protocols*
Edited by: P. Keohavong and S. G. Grant © Humana Press Inc., Totowa, NJ

gene expression or gene products. Even SNPs that do not themselves change protein expression and cause disease may be in close physical proximity on the chromosome, or "linked" to deleterious mutations. Because of this linkage, SNPs may be shared among groups of people with harmful but unknown mutations and serve as markers for them. Such markers can help uncover the actual functional mutations and accelerate efforts to find therapeutic drugs.

One of the initial applications of the recent advances in the human genome sequencing project is the emerging field of pharmacogenomics. Pharmacogenomics encompasses several major areas: the study of polymorphic variations to drug response and disease susceptibility, identification of the effects of drugs/xenobiotics at the genomic level, and genotype/phenotype associations. The promise of pharmacogenomics is that studies using genome-based technology will lead to the identification of novel SNPs and the characterization of their impact on human health. The development and application of screening technologies is therefore of high priority.

The last decade or so has witnessed a veritable explosion in the design and development of molecular genetic technologies that can be used in pharmacogenomic and molecular toxicological studies to understand the biological basis of complex traits and diseases and their relationship to environmental exposures. It is well-recognized that characterization of DNA sequence variation will enable the identification of novel genetic risk factors for disease, novel targets for drug therapies, and avoidance of adverse drug reactions. The SNP consortium (a group of pharmaceutical and bioinformational companies, five academic centers, and a charitable trust) is currently producing an ordered high-density SNP map of the human genome *(2)*. Furthermore, mapped SNPs are being placed regularly into public domain websites *(see*, for example, http://snp.cshl.org).

For the last 25 yr, the most commonly used approach to identify genes that influence traits has been meiotic or linkage mapping. All linkage analysis methods involve the assessment of the transmission and cosegregation of alleles at regions on the genome known as marker loci, with disease alleles assumed to be carried by family members exhibiting the disease of interest *(3)*. Unfortunately, linkage analysis has not proved powerful enough to detect genes influencing many common multifactorial diseases, primarily because the study of genes with a small to moderate effect on a trait or a disease requires the collection of hundreds if not thousands of families for reliable results.

There are a variety of reasons why SNPs have emerged as an alternative form of sequence variation for gene identification and mapping studies. Primary among them is the high frequency with which SNPs are found in the genome, lending utility for the discovery of disease-related genes. SNPs are found throughout the genome, in exons, introns, intergenic regions, promoters, enhancers, and so on. Therefore, they are likely to be associated with a functional or physiologically relevant allele. Because SNPs occur in such great abundance over the genome, groups of neighboring SNPs may have alleles that show distinctive patterns of linkage disequilibrium and may create a haplotypic diversity that can be exploited in both genetic linkage and direct association epidemiologic studies. Another advantage to studying SNPs is that since they typically have only two variant alleles, SNPs will have allele frequencies that will drift as a function of the dynamics of different populations, creating allele frequency differences that can be exploited in population-based studies. Lastly and most importantly, owing to their simple structure, the development of technologies that enable rapid, efficient, and cost-effective genotyping of thousands of individuals for hundreds of SNPs has become possible.

A number of novel, high-throughput genotyping technologies have recently been developed, including various microarray formats, matrix assisted laser desorption/ionization time of flight (MALDI-TOF) mass spectrometry (MS), and TaqMan® allele discrimination approaches. However, these current state-of-the-art approaches do not yet meet all of the requirements for maximum utilization of genotyping information. A major issue with each of these approaches is the cost per SNP detection. Currently, most procedures involve polymerase chain reaction (PCR) amplification of a target sequence, a somewhat costly and time-consuming method that limits possibilities for automation. As the scale of genotyping analyses increases, the cost per genotype will need to decrease from the current level of approx $1–3 to pennies or tenths of pennies. A second key requirement for any genotyping technology is flexibility. As new SNPs are identified, there will be a need for rapid inclusion of the novel SNP within the screening procedure. For several currently commercially available, preconfigured microarrays, this is a major problem. Although it is now possible to reconfigure an existing microarray or develop a new custom array more rapidly, these technologies are still associated with high costs for synthesis and further assay validation requirements. Additional requirements for an optimal genotyping approach include sensitivity (requiring less than 1 ng genomic DNA/genotype), scalability and automation compatibility, and efficient turnaround times. For most of these newer technologies, DNA template amount is not a problem, although the amount of input DNA for microarray analysis is relatively higher.

An overview of many of the genotyping approaches currently available, ranging from those developed in the late 1980s to those in development today, is given below.

2. PCR-Based Techniques

2.1. SSCP-PCR

Single-strand conformational polymorphism (SSCP) analysis is one of the most widely used methods for mutation detection. DNA regions with potential polymorphisms are amplified by PCR, the products are denatured, and the single strands thus formed are electrophoresed on a polyacrylamide gel *(4,5)*. A fragment with a single base modification migrates differently than wild-type DNA. Alternative conformation-based mutation screening methods include conformation-sensitive gel electrophoresis, chemical or enzymatic mismatch cleavage detection *(6)*, denaturing gradient gel electrophoresis (DGGE) *(7)*, and denaturing high-performance liquid chromatography (HPLC) *(8)*. The underlying principle of these methods is that the melting characteristics of double-stranded DNA are defined by its sequence, and hence a single-base mismatch can produce conformational changes in the double helix that cause the differential migration of homoduplexes and heteroduplexes containing base mismatches during gel electrophoresis. This method is highly sensitive for identifying mutations in areas of highly GC-rich sequences (*see* Chap. 23).

2.2. PCR Mismatch Cleavage Detection

Mismatch cleavage detection takes advantage of the fact that mismatched bases are sensitive to cleavage by enzymes and chemicals *(6)*. After PCR amplification, wild-type and variant alleles are subjected to denaturation/renaturation to create heteroduplex molecules. The products are electrophoresed side by side to detect the presence of mismatch cleaved molecules following incubation with resolvases.

2.3. Denaturing Gradient Gel Electrophoresis (DGGE)

In denaturing gradient gel electrophoresis, the PCR products are resolved on a denaturing gradient gel containing formamide and urea under temperature control *(7)*. SNPs are revealed by their migrational differences from wild-type homoduplexes. The major advantage of this method is its accuracy; however, its disadvantages are low throughput and difficulty of optimization (*see* Chap. 20).

2.4. Denaturing HPLC

In this method, polymorphisms are detected by analyzing the mobility of DNA heteroduplexes using chromatography under denaturing conditions *(8)*. The variant sample is first hybridized with wild-type DNA to form a mixture of homo- and heteroduplexes. The heteroduplexes can be separated from the homoduplexes by column chromatography at a temperature that partially denatures the mismatched DNA.

2.5. Restriction Fragment Length Polymorphism (RFLP)-PCR Analysis

For restriction fragment length polymorphism (RFLP)-PCR analysis, a specific target region of genomic DNA is amplified by PCR. The product is then digested with appropriate restriction enzyme(s) and visualized after being gel-electrophoresed *(9)*. If the SNP produces a gain or loss of restriction site, the restriction pattern is altered, and homozygous wild-type, mutant, or heterozygote carriers are easily identified. A major limitation of this method is the requirement that the polymorphisms result in an altered restriction enzyme site.

2.6. Oligonucleotide Ligation Assay (OLA) Genotyping

The oligonucleotide ligation assay (OLA) approach is based on the premise that hybridization with specific oligonucleotide probes effectively discriminates between wild-type and variant sequences *(10)*. Three probes are used in this assay, two allele-specific probes and a common fluorescent probe. The 5'-end of the common probe is immediately adjacent to the 3'-end of the allele-specific probe. The PCR product is incubated with the three probes in the presence of thermally stable DNA ligase. Ligation of the fluorescently labeled probe to the allele-specific probe occurs only when there is a perfect match between the probe and the template. The wild-type and the variant genotypes are differentiated following electrophoresis of the ligated products. The major disadvantage of this method is that highly GC-rich regions make the allele-specific ligation step difficult to optimize.

2.7. Branch Migration Inhibition (BMI)

The branch migration inhibition (BMI) technique is based on the fact that spontaneous strand exchange is inhibited by sequence differences between two DNA molecules *(11)*. Genomic DNA is amplified using four primers. The two forward primers are 5'-labeled with either biotin or digoxigenin. The two reverse primers have similar priming sequences but different tail sequences, which consist of 20 nucleotides that are not complementary to the genomic target but are incorporated into the PCR products. The PCR products are then subjected to heat denaturation and reannealing of single strands to form, eventually, a doubly labeled, four-stranded cruciform DNA structure. When there is no mutation, the two arms of this structure are identical, and strand exchange via branch migration leads to its complete dissociation into two duplex molecules, producing no signal. In the presence of a sequence difference, as in mutation or polymorphism, branch migration in the presence of Mg^{2+} is inhibited, and the cruciform structure does not get resolved. Thus, the stable association of biotin and digoxigenin is detected by standard enzyme-linked immunosorbent assay (ELISA) techniques. One of the primary limitations of BMI is that it cannot distinguish between homozygotes for two alternative alleles. It only detects heterozygotes and therefore requires an additional step, in which a reference amplicon is added to each amplified sample corresponding to one of the two possible homozygotes. The denaturation and branch migration steps are then repeated *(11)*.

3. Pyrosequencing

Pyrosequencing is a DNA sequencing technique based on the detection of released pyrophosphate (PPi) during DNA synthesis *(12)*. In a cascade of enzymatic reactions, visible light is generated that is proportional to the number of incorporated nucleotides. The cascade starts with a nucleic acid polymerization reaction in which inorganic PPi is released as a result of polymerase-mediated incorporation of nucleotides. The released PPi is subsequently converted to ATP by ATP sulfurylase, which provides the energy to luciferase to oxidize luciferin and produce light. Since the added nucleotide is known, the sequence of the template can be determined. Pyrosequencing uses the Klenow fragment of *E. coli* DNA *Pol*I. The ATP sulfurylase used in pyrosequencing is a recombinant version from the yeast *Streptomyces cerevisiae*, and the luciferase is from the American firefly *Photinus pyralis*. One picomole of DNA yields 6×10^{11} ATP molecules, which generates more than 6×10^9 photons at a wavelength of 560 nm. A charge-coupled device (CCD) camera easily detects this light. Two different pyrosequencing strategies are currently available: solid and liquid phase *(13)*. Solid-phase pyrosequencing utilizes immobilized DNA, and the excess substrate is washed off after each nucleotide addition. In liquid-phase pyrosequencing, a pyrase, a nucleotide-degrading enzyme is introduced, thereby enabling the removal of the solid phase support and intermediate washing. For SNP analysis using pyrosequencing, the 3'-end of the primer is designed to hybridize one or a few bases before the polymorphic position. Each allele combination provides a distinct pattern on the program readout. These programs can be analyzed manually or by pattern recognition software *(14)*.

3.1. Array Pyrosequencing

Pyrosequencing can be applied to both ordered and random arrays; for example, the PSQ™ 96 System (Pyrosequencing AB, Westborough, MA) employs a DNA array, a nucleotide delivery module, and a CCD camera. A sprayer is used to deliver all four different nucleotides. Current imaging technologies require a minimum of more than 5000 template molecules. Several optimizations are still under way to allow the use of this technology for reliable high-throughput DNA sequencing, but the range of applications is growing as more institutions acquire the technology.

Specialized software has been designed to automate the classification of genotypes for samples screened by pyrosequencing in a microtiter plate using a SNP genotyping algorithm. Based on pattern recognition, this algorithm both scores the genotype and provides a value for the quality of each SNP that is scored *(14)*. The assignment of this value is based on a number of different parameters, including differences in expected and obtained sequences around the SNP, signal-to-noise ratio, and variance in peak height and peak width.

4. Dynamic Allele-Specific Hybridization (DASH)

Dynamic allele-specific hybridization (DASH) is essentially an enhanced form of allele-specific hybridization that uses a convenient microtiter plate format, a simple duplex-DNA intercalation for signal production, and a dynamic low–high temperature sweep to capture all phases of probe–target–DNA melting *(15)*. For the purpose of DASH assay design, one needs to anticipate target-DNA secondary structure problems, and a maximum negative threshold of –4.0 kcal/mol should be expected. Furthermore, probe target ratios of C+G percentages should be more than 1.0. Two probes are designed for each SNP, representing both allelic sequences complementary to the biotinylated strand of the PCR product. The plates containing the bound product, the probes, and a DNA intercalating dye are subjected to a range of different temperatures, to follow the decrease in fluorescence as the temperature increases. The assay is repeated by using alternative allele-specific probes, and genotypes are scored from the fluorescence curves obtained. Devices that support the DASH procedure have been used to analyze 89 intragenic SNPs *(15)*.

5. Allele Discrimination Using Fluorescence Resonance Energy Transfer Detection (FRET)

Fluorescence resonance energy transfer (FRET) occurs when two fluorescent dyes are in close proximity to one another and the emission spectrum of one dye molecule overlaps the excitation spectrum of the other fluorophore. Commonly used FRET-based technologies include the TaqMan™ assay (Applied Biosystems, Foster City, CA) and Molecular Beacons™ (Integrated DNA Technologies, Skokie, IL).

5.1. TaqMan® Genotyping

The basis for FRET allele discrimination and quantitation is to measure PCR product accumulation continuously using a dual-labeled fluorogenic oligonucleotide probe, called a TaqMan® probe *(16)*. This probe is composed of a short (~20–30-base) oligodeoxynucleotide labeled with two different fluorescent dyes. On the 5'-terminus is a reporter dye, and on the 3'-terminus is a quenching dye. This oligonucleotide probe sequence is homologous to an internal target sequence present in the PCR amplicon. When the probe is intact, energy transfer occurs between the two fluorophors, and emission from the reporter is quenched by the quencher. During the extension phase of PCR, the probe is cleaved by the 5'-nuclease activity of DNA polymerase, thereby releasing the reporter from the oligonucleotide quencher and producing an increase in reporter emission intensity. The Applied Biosystems Sequence Detection systems use fiberoptic systems that connect to each well in a 96-well PCR tray format. The laser light or tungsten–halogen lamp excitation source excites each well, and a CCD camera measures the fluorescence spectrum and intensity from each well to generate real-time data during PCR amplification. The system software examines the fluorescence intensity of reporter and quencher dyes and calculates the increase in normalized reporter emission intensity over the course of the amplification. The results are then plotted vs time, represented by cycle number, to produce a continuous measure of PCR amplification *(16)*. Several other companies also market real-time PCR detection systems including Stratagene (La Jolla, CA) and Bio-Rad (Hercules, CA).

Lee et al. *(17)* first demonstrated that the 5'-nuclease assay could be used for allelic discrimination. In the assay, two TaqMan probes as described above are included in the reaction, one specific for each allele. The probes are distinguished through the use of different fluorescent reporter dyes (usually 6-carboxy-fluorescein [FAM] and 6-carboxy-4,7,2',7'-tetrachlorofluorescein [TET]). A mismatch between probe and target greatly reduces the probe hybridization efficiency and specific cleavage. Following PCR, an increase in the level of a FAM fluorescent signal without an increase in the TET-specific signal indicates that only the FAM-specific sequence (allele) was present and that the sample is homozygous (and vice versa). An increase in both reporter signals indicates heterozygosity. The software makes three separate calculations to arrive at the result for allele discrimination. First, using multicomponent analysis, the software determines the contribution of each component dye to the observed fluorescence spectrum. Following this, these dye component results are normalized based on control reactions (which have no template), known allele 1 template, or known allele 2 template, which are run on the same plate. An allele 1 score (on a scale of 0–1) and an allele 2 score are calculated for each sample. Finally, the allele 1 and 2 scores are normalized for the extent of the reaction, based on the results of the no-template control *(18)*. A number of factors contribute to allelic discrimination based on a single mismatch. First is the thermodynamic contribution owing to the disruptive effect of a mismatch on hybridization. A mismatched probe will have a lower melting temperature than a perfectly matched probe. Second, the assay is performed under competitive conditions; therefore the mismatch is prevented from binding because stable binding of an exact match probe blocks hybridization of the mismatch. Third, the 5'-end of the probe must start to be displaced before cleavage occurs. Once a probe starts to be displaced, complete dissociation occurs faster with a mismatch than with an exact match.

5.2. Molecular Beacons

Molecular beacons are oligonucleotide probes that have two complementary DNA sequences flanking the target DNA sequence and a donor/acceptor dye pair at opposite ends of each probe *(19)*. The probe adopts a hairpin loop conformation with the reporter and the quencher dyes close together when it is not hybridized to the target, and therefore, no donor fluorescence is generated. When hybridized to the right target sequence, the two dyes are separated and the fluorescence increases. Thermal instability of the mismatched hybrids increases the specificity of molecular beacons. For SNP genotyping, two molecular beacons with exact sequence matches to the wild-type and variant alleles are used in the same PCR. The use of two differentially labeled molecular beacons in the same PCR reaction allows the simultaneous detection of three possible allelic combinations.

6. Multiplex Automated Primer Extension Analysis (MAPA)

Multiplex automated primer extension analysis (MAPA) is a semiautomated fluorescent method that can accurately and easily genotype multiple SNPs simultaneously *(20)*. This technique is a modification of a commercially available protocol (SNaPshot, Applied Biosystems) that uses the extension of a primer designed to end one nucleotide 5' of a given SNP with fluorescent ddNTPs, followed by automatic sequencing on an ABI PRISM 377 Sequencer. The MAPA modification includes the incorporation of several primers corresponding to several SNPs in the same reaction and loading the primer extension products on a single gel lane. There is a limit to the number of SNPs one can multiplex with this method, dictated by the range of primer lengths (16–50 nucleotides) and the minimum spacing in the primer length that allows for separation. Therefore, the maximum number of SNPs this method can multiplex is approx 10–12 SNPs per sample. Another drawback is that primer orientation appears to affect the accuracy of genotyping heterozygotes, perhaps because of the formation of strand-specific secondary structures *(20)*.

7. Capillary Electrophoresis

In 1981, Jorgenson and Lukacs *(21)* were the first to demonstrate electrophoretic separation of samples inside narrow-bore capillaries filled with electrophoretic media. Capillary electrophoresis (CE) was found to separate small molecules with a very high resolution. In recent years this technique has been modified for the detection of point mutations and SNPs. The most widely employed of several modifications is a technique known as constant denaturant capillary electrophoresis (CDCE), coupled with high-fidelity PCR. This application has lent itself extremely well to high-throughput analysis of samples. CDCE combines the principles of CE and denaturing gradient gel electrophoresis (DGGE) in linear polyacrylamide matrices. The denaturing conditions in CDCE are achieved by heating a section of capillary in a temperature-controlled water jacket. CDCE offers high resolution and amenability to automation, and, coupled with high-fidelity PCR, it is possible to measure point mutations at frequencies as low as 10^{-6} in human genomic DNA *(22)*. The CDCE instrument has been further improved by the addition of a two-wavelength detector. This allows the use of two sets of samples labeled with two different fluorescent dyes, thus permitting comparison of two separate channels. Separation of PCR products is generally conducted in capillaries with an internal diameter of 75 µm at a constant current of 9 µA. Future integration of multiple capillary arrays and automation systems should increase the speed and the scale of this technique.

8. MALDI-TOF Mass Spectrometry

Karas and Hillenkamp *(23)* first introduced MALDI-TOF MS in 1988 as a revolutionary method for ionizing and mass-analyzing large biomolecules. They discovered that irradiation of crystals formed by suitable small organic molecules (called the matrix) with a short laser pulse at a wavelength close to a resonant absorption band of the matrix molecules caused an energy transfer and desorption process, producing gas phase matrix ions. They also found that when a low-concentration of a nonabsorbing analyte, such as a protein or a nucleic acid molecule, was added to the matrix in solution and embedded in the solid matrix crystals, the nonabsorbing, intact analyte molecules were also desorbed into the gas phase and ionized upon irradiation, allowing their mass analysis.

Originally, MALDI-TOF MS was proposed as an alternative high-throughput technology for DNA sequencing to replace the conventional method. Enzymatic DNA sequencing coupled with MALDI-TOF MS analysis has been shown to be effective at discovering previously unknown SNPs *(24)*. However, there is a loss of signal intensity and mass resolution with increasing DNA size, owing to the size-dependent tendency of the phosphodiester backbone of DNA to fragment during the MALDI process. Consequently a robust MALDI-based approach to SNP discovery, which requires sequencing of PCR products up to 300 bp in length, has not been demonstrated. This limitation has also hampered attempts to analyze PCR amplicons containing SNPs directly. Additionally, during the MALDI process, double-stranded PCR products can dissociate into single strands of slightly different masses, which as a result are poorly resolved. Minisequencing has become the most widely used MALDI-TOF MS-based method for SNP analysis. It involves annealing of a primer to a template PCR amplicon downstream of a SNP. A mix of deoxynucleotide triphosphates and dideoxynucleotide triphosphates are added to a PCR template and primer, along with a DNA polymerase. The polymerase extends the 3'-end of the primer by specifically incorporating nucleotides that are complementary to the sequence of the PCR product. Extension terminates at the first position in the template where a nucleotide complementary to one of the ddNTPs in the mix occurs. MALDI-TOF MS-based methods have been developed in which extended primers are solid phase-purified and detected by MS; the identity of the polymorphic nucleotide is determined by measuring the mass of the extended primer *(25)*.

The greatest promise of MALDI-TOF MS for SNP analysis lies in its ability to genotype many SNPs rapidly, accurately, and simultaneously. Recently, another approach to MALDI-TOF MS has been developed that does not require a PCR amplification step. This direct approach (Invader assay, Third Wave Technologies, Madison, WI) involves the sequence-specific hybridization of two oligonucleotides to form an overlapping structure at the polymorphic position *(26)*. Enzymatic cleavage and amplification of an allele-specific, short oligonucleotide signal molecule, which is derived from this overlap structure, follow this. The signal molecules produced in this reaction contain a biotin group, enabling solid-phase sample preparation by capturing these molecules on streptavidin-coated magnetic beads. They are then washed to remove contaminants, and the clean signal molecules are eluted for MALDI-TOF MS analysis.

9. Microarrays

The DNA microarray chip has revolutionized the application of high-throughput genotyping in the last few years. A DNA microarray is a small chip, generally about a square centimeter, most commonly made of glass, plastic, or silicon. SNP analysis with the DNA microarray chip is a hybridization-based genotyping technique that allows the simultaneous analysis of many polymorphisms. High-density microarrays are created by attaching hundreds of thousands of oligonucleotides to a solid surface in an ordered array. The DNA of interest is PCR-amplified to incorporate fluorescently labeled nucleotides and then hybridized to the chip *(27)*. Each oligonucleotide in the array acts as an allele-specific probe. Well-matched sequences hybridize more efficiently than mismatched sequences and therefore give stronger fluorescent signals. The signals are quantitated by high-resolution fluorescent scanning and analyzed by sophisticated software programs. Many biotechnology companies have developed and are marketing DNA microarrays. The unique features for several different microarray approaches currently available are described in the following sections.

9.1. Affymetrix GeneChip® Technology

Affymetrix (Santa Clara, CA) uses light-directed synthesis for the construction of high-density DNA probe arrays using two methods: photolithography and solid-phase DNA synthesis *(28)*. Synthetic linkers modified by photochemically removable groups are attached to a glass substrate, and light is directed through a photolithographic mask to specific surface areas to produce photodeprotection. This is followed by the chemical coupling of hydroxyl-protected deoxynucleosides at the illuminated sites. Next, light is directed to different regions of the substrate by a new mask, and the chemical cycle is repeated. Thus, for a given reference sequence, a DNA probe array can be designed that consists of a highly dense collection of complementary probes. The amount of nucleic acid information encoded on the array in the form of different probes is limited only by the physical size of the array and the achievable lithographic resolution. Because the arrays are constructed on a rigid material (glass), they can be inverted and mounted in a temperature-controlled hybridization chamber. A fluorescent-tagged nucleic acid sample injected into the chamber hybridizes to complementary oligonucleotides on the array. Laser excitation enters through the back of the glass support, focused at the interface of the array and the target solution, and the fluorescence emission is collected by a lens and passes to a sensitive detector through a series of optical filters. A quantitative 2D fluorescence image of hybridization intensity is obtained by simply scanning the laser beam or translating the array *(28)*.

Different flow-through systems have been developed to allow a continuous measurement of real-time hybridization to an array, by adding cell lysis and amplification to a miniaturized fluidics system. This approach extends the two dimensions of the lateral microarray resolution by the time-resolved analysis of the binding process as a third dimension *(28)*. Real-time hybridization also allows the calculation of binding kinetics for every spot under different temperatures and changed hybridization conditions.

9.2. Nanogen Biochip Cartridges

Nanogen (San Diego, CA) has developed a microchip cartridge, called the Nanochip™, to facilitate rapid identification and precise analyses of biological molecules using a process based on the electrical properties of biological molecules *(29)*. This technology, termed *electronic addressing*, places DNA fragments at selective sites on a silicon microchip and involves active hybridization as opposed to the passive hybridization process described above. After the DNA is addressed, a test site or multiple test sites are electronically activated with a positive charge. The negatively charged probes move to the positively charged test sites, where they are concentrated and bound by a chemical process to that site. The microchip is then washed, another set of DNA probes is added on, and different sites are activated. Therefore, an array of specifically bound DNA probes can be assembled or addressed in a user-defined order. The highly advantageous feature of the Nanochip compared with other array approaches is its flexibility in experimental design. Because you can hybridize only the sites you want by specifying particular sites for electronic concentration and hybridization, you can run multiple experiments on the same chip. The current configuration of the Nanochip contains 100 sites on a single cartridge.

9.3. Single-Base Extension-Tag Array on Glass Slides

Also called minisequencing or template-directed incorporation, single-base extension-tag array on glass slides (SBE-TAGS) involves extension of a primer located adjacent to the position of the SNP, using DNA polymerase in the presence of fluorescently labeled ddNTP *(30)*. The SBE-TAGS method marks each primer with distinct 5'-end sequence tags that allows separation of a multiplexed SBE reaction by hybridization to a microarray. Depositing unmodified nucleotides on a glass slide with routine spotting equipment can easily generate these arrays. Arrays are scanned using external argon lasers, and a matrix is applied to correct for the crosstalk between multiple overlapping fluorophores. This method has been used to genotype over 100 SNPs accurately *(30)*.

10. Microsphere-Based Technology

Microsphere-based techniques have been described in the literature for a number of applications but have been further developed by Luminex (Austin, TX). The Luminex technology couples existing flow cytometric technology with color-coded microspheres, each of which carries an individual assay. The approach is rapid and extremely flexible. The first use of flow cytometry for analysis of microsphere-based immunoassays was published in 1977 *(31)* and was reviewed by McHugh in 1994 *(32)*. The flow cytometer is able to discriminate different particles based on size or color, providing the potential for multiplex analysis. The Luminex system is based on the principle that panels are created by combining up to 100 different microsphere-based assays into a single sample test. Multiplexed assays can be run on sample volumes as small as 5 µL. Each assay is individually constructed around a single microsphere set with its own identifying fluorescent color. Each set of microspheres is manufactured with unique relative proportions of red and orange fluorescent dyes. The system consists of 100 distinct sets of fluorescent microspheres and a standard benchtop flow cytometer interfaced with a personal computer containing a digital signal-processing board. Individual sets of microspheres can be modified with reactive components such as oligonucleotides, antigens, or antibodies and then mixed to form a multiplexed assay set. A further advantage is that the system is extremely flexible and permits easy incorporation of new endpoint measures. This contrasts with DNA microarray chip technology, which is not only more expensive but has less flexibility in making new probes available as new polymorphic alleles are identified. So instead of requiring the reconfiguration and synthesis of a new chip when a new allele is to be added to the screening panel, the Luminex system simply requires the addition of an additional oligonucleotide-hybridized microsphere *(33)*.

The Luminex technology is very amenable to studies of SNP genotyping owing to its flexible format. One can visualize an assay in which a bank of prelabeled probes is held in reserve and an investigator or clinician can pick and choose the SNPs for which to screen. One drawback of the technology, however, is that it requires a considerable amount of time for assay optimization and validation, particularly in the multiplex format. For this reason, many investigators have decided to wait for the availability of commercial kits for use on the instrument.

Another method using the microsphere-based Luminex assays has also been developed for successful multiplexing of SNPs. The conventional Luminex assay using single base chain extension (SBCE) has been modified into an allele-specific primer extension reaction (ASPE) *(33)*. This method utilizes a pair of allele-specific primers that differ from each other at the 3'-end and encode different "ZipCode" sequences at the 5'-end, in the same reaction. The DNA polymerase extends only one primer if the template DNA sequence is homozygous, whereas both primers are extended in heterozygotes. The ASPE reaction eliminates the necessity of post-PCR cleanup and the addition of unlabeled nucleotides.

11. Example Application: Genotyping Analysis of the *CYP2D6* Gene

As mentioned above, the application of SNP genotyping analyses to pharmacogenetic endpoints is of growing clinical importance. The genetic polymorphisms associated with specific human CYP and phase II enzymes typically occur with variable frequency in different populations or ethnic groups and may result in poor metabolizers (PMs) or extensive metabolizers (EMs) for specific substrates. CYP2D6 metabolizes up to 20% of commonly prescribed medications, including antidepressant/psychotics, antiarrhythmics, and β-blockers, as well as many environmental agents *(34)*. There is a wide intersubject variability in the pharmacokinetics of all CYP2D6-metabolized substrates, which exhibit variations in clearance over a 20–200-fold range depending on the agent under study. To date, over 74 allelic variants in the human *CYP2D6* gene have been identified, many of which are associated with either decreased or enhanced metabolic activity *(35)*. The *CYP2D6* gene represents a challenge for genotyping: the numerous known polymorphisms are not caused only by single-nucleotide substitutions or deletions but also by gene deletions, duplications, and the presence of pseudogenes.

For *CYP2D6*, the 74 known variants are associated with 60 different polymorphic regions. The number of SNPs within a particular variant allele range from a single SNP (for example, *CYP2D6*1B*) to eight SNPs (for example, *CYP2D6*4G*). Four unique SNPs in exons 3, 4, 8, and 9 are observed among the *6 variant allele subfamily. Although the T1707Del SNP would identify a *6 variant, genotyping analysis would require the screening of all four of these SNPs to distinguish among the *6 A, B, C, and D variant alleles. Screening for only 4 of the 60 currently known possible SNPs results in redundant variant allele classifying information, i.e., screening for 56 SNPs is required for the accurate and complete elucidation of the *CY2D6* genotype.

A number of novel, high-throughput genotyping approaches have recently been developed, yet these do not yet meet all the requirements for maximum utilization of genotyping information. For example, PCR-based techniques such as PCR-RFLP, PCR SSCP, OLA, and others are time-consuming and labor-intensive and do not provide large amounts of information quickly, i.e., it is not possible to multiplex using any of these techniques. Furthermore, gene duplications and gene deletions such as those present in *CYP2D6* cannot be identified.

Sequencing-based techniques such as minisequencing and pyrosequencing are extremely accurate but, again, are laborious and not cost-effective. Furthermore, when multiple SNPs are necessary to define a variant allele and they lie in different regions of the gene, as they do in *CYP2D6*, numerous fragments would have to be sequenced in order to genotype an individual. FRET-based techniques do not provide a solution for multiplexing either, as the time and cost of optimizing assays far outweighs the ability to genotype for all the various SNPs. However, TaqMan-based assays are extremely useful in genotyping for the common variants of *CYP2D6* using commercially available kits. Microsphere-based methods using both SBCE and ASPE techniques coupled with flow cytometry and microtiter-based assays are promising in their applications for multiplexing. Multiple PCR products can be screened simultaneously using specific probes, thus allowing detection of SNPs that are far apart. *CYP2D6* genotyping, for example, therefore poses a great challenge, especially since none of the latest techniques allows for the detection of gene duplications and deletions in a speedy and cost-effective manner.

12. Summary

A major challenge for large-scale pharmacogenetic studies is to compare thousands of polymorphisms among numerous individuals. Therefore, its success depends on user-friendly and cost-effective technology that can be applied on a large scale. Furthermore, the availability and screening of large populations will be required to validate and discover new SNPs. In addition, data management and interpretation continue to pose a challenge, as we are faced with new technology that provides us with vast amounts of information. We provide a comparison of the different SNP detection techniques along with their advantages and disadvantages in **Table 1**.

Table 1
Advantages and Disadvantages of Different SNP Detection Techniques

Factor	Gel-based technologies	FRET	MS-based methods	Microarray technology	Microsphere technology
High throughput	Not applicable	96 samples in 3 h, requires a PCR step	Cannot be used for more than one sample at a time	100 samples/h	96 samples in 2–3 h
Cost effectiveness	$1–10/SNP/sample	$1–3/SNP/sample	$.50–5/SNP/sample	$.50–5/SNP/sample	$.50–2/SNP/sample
Ability to multiplex	Cannot be used for multiplexing	Difficult to multiplex	A robust multiplexed PCR product is required	Can be used quite easily for multiplexing coupled with high-throughput analyses	Has excellent applications for multiplexing.
Advantages	Ease of optimization if the sample size is small	Eliminates tedious steps of restrictions digestion, gel visualization and so on. Offers accurate detection of single SNPs	Specific and accurate without the use of specifically labeled probes and primers	Can screen 100s–1000s of SNPs for a single sample within one array	Extremely accurate and easy to perform whether screening for many SNPs on one sample or one SNP on many samples.
Disadvantages	RFLPs not present for all SNPs For PCR-based techniques the quality of amplification depends on the presence of secondary structures	Optimization is time-consuming and therefore cannot be used to study multiple markers in a small number of samples	Requires pure samples free of ions and other impurities	Depending on format, flexibility in adding novel SNPs may be difficult.	Optimizations is tedious and time-consuming, requires very specific probe design as the success of the assay depends on the sequence content surrounding the polymorphic sites.

Abbreviations: FRET, fluorescence resonance energy transfer; PCR, polymerase chain reaction; RFLP, restriction fragment length polymorphism; SNP, single-nucleotide polymorphism.

References

1. Cooper, D. N., Smith, B. A., Cooke, H. J., Niemann, S., and Schmidtke, J. (1985) An estimate of unique DNA heterozygosity in the human genome. *Hum. Genet.* **69,** 201–205.
2. Marshall, E. (1999) Drug firms to create public database of genetic mutations. *Science* **284,** 406–467.
3. Lander, E. S. and Schork, N. J. (1994) Genetic dissection of complex traits. *Science* **265,** 2037–2048.
4. Orita, M., Suzuki, Y., Sekiya, T., and Hayashi, K. (1989) Rapid and sensitive detection of point mutations and DNA polymorphisms using the polymerase chain reaction. *Genomics* **5,** 874–879.
5. Makino, R., Yazyu, H., Kishimoto, Y., Sekiya, T., and Hayashi, K. (1992) F-SSCP: fluorescence-based polymerase chain reaction-single-strand conformation polymorphism (PCR-SSCP) analysis. *PCR Methods Appl.* **2,** 10–13.
6. Youil, R., Kemper, B. W., and Cotton, R. G. (1995) Screening for mutations with enzyme mismatch cleavage with T4 endonuclease. *Proc. Natl. Acad. Sci. USA* **92,** 87–91.
7. Myers, R. M., Maniatis, T., and Lerman, L. S. (1987) Detection and localization of single base changes by denaturing gradient gel electrophoresis. *Methods Enzymol.* **155,** 501–527.
8. O'Donovan, M. C., Oefner, P. J., Roberts, S. C., et al. (1998) Blind analysis of denaturing high-performance liquid chromatography as a tool for mutation detection. *Genomics* **52,** 44–49.
9. Shi, M. M., Bleavins, M. R., and de la Iglesia, F. A. (1999) Technologies for detecting genetic polymorphisms in pharmacogenomics. *Mol. Diagn.* **4,** 343–351.
10. Baron, H., Fung, S., Aydin, A., Bahring, S., Luft, F. C., and Schuster, H. (1996) Oligonucleotide ligation assay (OLA) for the diagnosis of familial hypercholesterolemia. *Nat. Biotech.* **14,** 1279–1282.
11. Panyutin, I. G. and Hsieh, P. (1993) Formation of a single base mismatch impedes spontaneous DNA branch migration. *J. Mol. Biol.* **230,** 413–424.
12. Ronaghi, M., Karamohamed, S., Petersson, B., Uhlen, M., and Nyren, P. (1996) Real-time DNA sequencing using detection of pyrophosphate release. *Anal. Biochem.* **242,** 84–89.
13. Ronaghi, M., Uhlen, M., and Nyren, P. (1998) A sequencing method based on real-time pyrophosphate. *Science* **281,** 363–365.
14. Ronaghi, M. (2001) Pyrosequencing sheds light on DNA sequencing. *Genome Res.* **11,** 3–11.
15. Stoneking, M., Hedgecock, D., Higuchi, R. G., Vigilant, L., and Ehrlich, H. A. (1991) Population variation of human mtDNA control region sequences detected by enzymatic amplification and sequence-specific oligonucleotide probes. *Am. J. Hum. Genet.* **48,** 370–382.
16. Livak, K. J., Marmaro, J., Giusti, W., and Deetz, K. (1995) Oligonucleotides with fluorescent dyes at opposite ends provide a quenched probe system useful for detecting PCR product and nucleic acid hybridization. *PCR Methods Appl.* **4,** 357–362.
17. Lee, L. G., Connell, C. R., and Bloch, W. (1993) Allelic discrimination by nick-translation PCR with fluorogenic probes. *Nucleic Acids Res.* **21,** 3761–3766.
18. Lie, Y. S. and Petropoulos, C. J. (1998) Advances in quantitative PCR technology: 5' nuclease assays. *Curr. Opin. Biotech.* **9,** 43–48.
19. Tyagi, S., Bratu, D. P., and Kramer, F. R. (1998) Multicolor molecular beacons for allele discrimination. *Nat. Biotechnol.* **16,** 49–53.
20. Makridakis, N. M. and Reichardt, J. K. V. (2001) Multiplex automated primer extension analysis: simultaneous genotyping of several polymorphisms. *BioTechniques* **31,** 1374–1380.
21. Jorgenson, J. W. and Lukacs, K. D. (1981) Zone electrophoresis in open tubular glass capillaries. *Anal. Chem.* **53,** 1298–1302.

22. Jin, L. J., Ferrance, J., and Landers, J. P. (2001) Miniaturized electrophoresis: an evolving role in laboratory medicine. *BioTechniques* **31**, 1332–1353.

23. Karas, M. and Hillenkamp, F. (1988) Laser desorption ionization of proteins with molecular masses exceeding 10000 daltons. *Anal. Chem.* **60**, 2299–2303.

24. Kirpekar, F., Nordhoff, E., Larsen, L. K., Kristainsen, K., Roepstorff, P., and Hillenkamp, F. (1998) DNA sequence analysis by MALDI mass spectrometry. *Nucleic Acids Res.* **26**, 2554–2559.

25. Griffin, T. J. and Smith, L. M. (2000) Single nucleotide polymorphism analysis by MALDI-TOF mass spectrometry. *Trends Biotechnol.* **18**, 77–84.

26. Griffin, T. J., Hall, J. G., Prudent, J. R., and Smith, L. M. (1999) Direct genetic analysis by matrix-assisted laser desorption/ionization mass spectrometry. *Proc. Natl. Acad. Sci. USA* **96**, 6301–6306.

27. Lipshutz, R. J., Fodor, S. P. A., Gingeras, T. R., and Lockhart, D. J. (1999) High density synthetic oligonucleotide arrays. *Nat. Genet.* **21**, 20–24.

28. Blohm, D. H. and Guiseppi-Elie, A. (2001) New developments in microarray technology. *Curr. Opin. Biotechnol.* **12**, 41–47.

29. Huang, Y., Ewalt, K. L., Tirado, M., et al. (2001) Electric manipulation of bioparticles and macromolecules on microfabricated electrodes. *Anal. Chem.* **73**, 1549–1559.

30. Hirschhorn, J. N., Sklar, P., Linblad-Toh, K., et al. (2000) SBE-TAGS: an array-based method for efficient single-nucleotide polymorphism genotyping. *Proc. Natl. Acad. Sci. USA* **97**, 12164–12169.

31. Fulton, R. J., McDade, R. L., Smith, P. L., Kienker, L. J., and Kettman, J. R. J. (1997) Advanced multiplexed analysis with the FlowMetrix system. *Clin. Chem.* **43**, 1749–1756.

32. McHugh, T. M. (1994) Flow microsphere immunoassay for the quantitative and simultaneous detection of multiple soluble analytes. *Methods Cell Biol.* **42**, 575–595.

33. Chen, J., Iannone, M. A., Li, M., et al. (2000) A microsphere-based assay for multiplexed single nucleotide polymorphism analysis using single base extension. *Genome Res.* **10**, 549–557.

34. Nebert, D. W., Adesnik, M., Coon, M. J., et al. (1991) The P450 superfamily: update on new sequences, gene mapping and recommended nomenclature. *DNA* **11**, 1–12.

35. http://www.imm.ki.se/CYPalleles/cyp2d6.html.

34

TaqMan® Fluorogenic Detection System to Analyze Gene Transcription in Autopsy Material

Kaori Shintani-Ishida, Bao-Li Zhu, and Hitoshi Maeda

Summary

Real-time RT-PCR using a TaqMan® fluorogenic detection system is a simple and sensitive assay for quantitative analysis of gene transcription. This method is of potential usefulness in quantifying mRNA of a target gene in autopsy material that has undergone only a small amount of postmortem degradation. The TaqMan fluorogenic detection system can monitor PCR in real time using a dual-labeled fluorogenic hybridization probe (TaqMan probe) and a polymerase with 5'-3' exonuclease activity. The procedures of the quantitative RT-PCR are as follows: RNA is extracted from autopsy material and used to synthesize cDNA by an RT reaction, and the target of interest is amplified and detected by the real-time PCR. The absolute amount of target mRNA in the sample is then determined relative to a standard curve. This chapter describes the methodology of the TaqMan fluorogenic detection system in handling autopsy material in the gene transcription assay.

Key Words: Real-time PCR; TaqMan fluorogenic detection system; RT-PCR; quantification; mRNA; autopsy material; TaqMan probe.

1. Introduction
1.1. Real-Time Quantitative RT-PCR

Northern blot hybridization *(1)*, ribonuclease protection *(2,3)*, primer extension *(4)*, and reverse transcription-polymerase chain reaction (RT-PCR) *(5)* assays are in general used for the analysis of gene expression. The RT-PCR assay may be the simplest and most sensitive method to analyze gene transcription in autopsy material. Quantitative RT-PCR is a combination of an optimized system for the RT reaction and PCR amplification followed by the detection, discrimination, and quantification of the PCR products. There are two standard quantification strategies: competitive and kinetic PCR *(6,7)*. In competitive PCR *(6)*, adequate numbers of preliminary experiments are necessary to control the PCR efficiency and the initial target amount, because the standard cDNA is coamplified with the target. Furthermore, the endpoint detection of the PCR products limits the detection range owing to the "plateau effect" of the PCR. On the other hand, kinetic PCR *(7)*, taking data points from a series of PCR cycles,

From: *Methods in Molecular Biology, vol. 291, Molecular Toxicology Protocols*
Edited by: P. Keohavong and S. G. Grant © Humana Press Inc., Totowa, NJ

makes these preliminary experiments simple and the detection range wide. The TaqMan® fluorogenic detection system automatically performs kinetic PCR by monitoring the PCR in real time *(8)*. Using this system, which has a high sample throughput and is protected from contamination owing to elimination of post-PCR sample handling, the quantitative assay of mRNA has become more practical. This method also appears to have potential value in the gene expression analysis of autopsy material *(9,10)*.

1.2. Methodology of the TaqMan Fluorogenic Detection System

The TaqMan fluorogenic detection system is based on the use of fluorescence resonance energy transfer (FRET) of the dual-labeled fluorogenic hybridization probe *(11)* and 5'-3' exonuclease activity of the *Taq* polymerase that cleaves the probe during the extension phase of PCR *(12)*. The TaqMan probe consists of an oligonucleotide with a 5'-reporter dye and a 3'-quencher dye. The reporter fluorescence dye (fluorescein) linked to the 5'-end of the oligonucleotide is quenched by the quencher fluorescence dye (rhodamine) located at the 3'-end. During PCR, if the target of interest is present, the probe specifically anneals between the forward and reverse primer sites. The 5'-3' exonucleolytic activity of the *Taq* polymerase cleaves the probe only if the probe hybridizes to the target. The nuclease degradation of the hybridization probe releases the quenching by the 3'-quencher dye, resulting in an increase in fluorescent emission of the 5'-reporter dye.

The ABI PRISM® sequence detector allows continuous measurement of the fluorescent spectra of all 96 wells of the thermal cycler during the PCR amplification. Therefore, the PCR reactions are monitored in real time. A computer algorithm compares the amount of the 5'-reporter dye emission (R) with the 3'-quencher dye emission (Q) during the PCR amplification, generating a ΔRn value (R/Q). The ΔRn value reflects the amount of hybridization probe that is degraded. The algorithm fits an exponential function to the ΔRn values of every PCR extension cycle, generating an amplification plot (**Fig. 1A**). The algorithm calculates the cycle (C_T) at which each PCR amplification reaches a significant threshold, which is proportional to the amount of target present in the sample (**Fig. 1B**). Therefore, the C_T value is a measurement of the concentration of the target cDNA found in each sample. The TaqMan fluorogenic detection system is performed using an ABI PRISM® 7000, 7700, or 7900HT sequence detector (Applied Biosystems, Foster City, CA); similar real-time kinetic quantitative PCR is available from other companies, including the LightCycler™ (Roche Diagnostics, Mannheim, Germany), iCycler iQ™ (Bio-Rad, Hercules, CA), and Smart Cycler® (TaKaRa, Kyoto, Japan) systems.

1.3. Determination of the Target Amount

The amount of target nucleic acid is determined from a standard curve and normalized to an endogenous reference, which is usually a housekeeping gene, e.g., glyceraldehyde-3-phosphate dehydrogenase *(13)*, β-actin *(14)*, or 18S ribosomal RNA *(15)*. It is possible to perform both absolute and relative quantifications. In a study of drug effects on gene expression, the relative quantification, which expresses the target amount as an *n*-fold difference from the appropriate control (e.g., untreated sample)

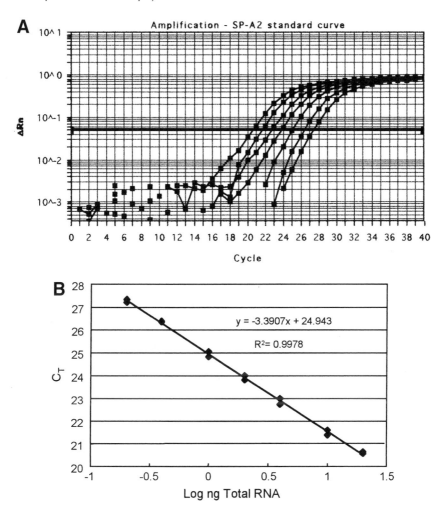

Fig. 1. Construction of a relative standard curve. (**A**) Amplification plot for the target gene, pulmonary surfactant-associated protein A2. Various concentrations (0.2, 0.4, 1.0, 2.0, 4.0, 10, and 20 ng) of total RNA isolated from human cadaveric lung were performed using real-time RT-PCR. The threshold ΔRn value was determined to be 0.05 in the exponential phase of the amplification plot. (**B**) Relative standard curve plotting log total RNA amount vs C_T value calculated from the amplification plot.

may be the more suitable method. For the relative quantification of RNA, any stock RNA or DNA (PCR product) can be used to prepare standards, because the unit from the standard curve and the efficiency of the RT step drop out when the sample quantity is divided by the control quantity.

2. Materials

2.1. Tissue Collection

1. RNA*later*™ (Ambion, Austin, TX).

2.2. Isolation of Total RNA

1. ISOGEN (Nippon Gene, Toyama, Japan).
2. Chloroform.
3. Isopropanol.
4. 70% Ethanol.
5. High-salt preparation solution: 1.2 M NaCl, 0.8 M sodium citrate in RNase-free water.
6. RNase-free water.
7. Mixer Mill MM 300 (Qiagen, Hilden, Germany).
8. 3-mm Tungsten carbide bead (Qiagen).

2.3. Reverse Transcription

1. TaqMan Reverse Transcription Reagents (Applied Biosystems).
2. Custom RT primer.
3. RNase-free water.

2.4. Real-Time PCR

1. TaqMan PCR Core Reagents Kit with AmpliTaq Gold (Applied Biosystems).
2. Custom primers.
3. Custom TaqMan probe.
4. RNase-free water.
5. MicroAmp Optical Tube (Applied Biosystems).
6. MicroAmp Optical Cap (Applied Biosystems).
7. MicroAmp 96-well Tray/Retainer Set (Applied Biosystems).

3. Methods

3.1. Tissue Collection

1. Cut a tissue specimen to a maximum thickness in any one dimension of 0.5 cm (e.g., 0.5 × 1 × 1 cm).
2. Immerse the fresh tissue in 5 vol of RNA*later* (*see* **Note 1**).
3. Store at 4°C until RNA isolation.

3.2. Isolation of Total RNA (see Note 2)

1. Remove tissue from the storage solution with sterile forceps.
2. Submerge 50 mg of the tissue in 1 mL ISOGEN in a 2-mL polypropylene microtube with a 3-mm tungsten carbide bead.
3. Disrupt the tissue by shaking at 1800 oscillations/min for 1 min using the Mixer Mill MM 300 (*see* **Note 3**).
4. Leave sample for 5 min at room temperature.
5. Add 0.2 mL of chloroform to the sample, mix by vortexing for 15 s, and leave for 2–3 min at room temperature.
6. Centrifuge at 12,000g for 15 min at 4°C.
7. Transfer the upper aqueous phase (carefully avoiding the interphase, which contains DNA and proteins) to a fresh 1.5-mL polypropylene microtube, add half volumes (~300 µL) of isopropanol and high-salt preparation solution, and leave for 5 min at room temperature.

8. Centrifuge at 12,000g for 10 min at 4°C. The RNA pellet should be visible at the bottom of the tube.
9. Decant the supernatant, and wash the pellet by adding 1 mL of 70% ethanol followed by centrifugation at 7500g for 5 min at 4°C.
10. Remove the supernatant, and allow the pellet to dry with the tube open at room temperature.
11. Resuspend the pellet in 100 μL of RNase-free water.
12. Calculate RNA purity and the concentration of the sample by measuring UV absorbance.

3.3. Primer and Probe Design for Real-Time PCR

1. Design primer pair and probe according to the guidelines described by Applied Biosystems, using Primer Express software. The most important points to remember are as follows:

   a. The maximum amplicon size should not exceed 400 bp.
   b. No G on the 5'-end of a probe.
   c. The estimated T_m for the probe should be 5–10°C higher than the estimated T_m for the primers.

2. Design any primer and probe to span an exon–intron junction to avoid the amplification of contaminating genomic DNA (*see* **Note 4**).

3.4. Reverse Transcription (see Note 5)

1. Make a 10-fold dilution of each RNA sample with RNase-free water (*see* **Note 6**).
2. Prepare the RT mix for the number of samples to be analyzed: 1X TaqMan RT buffer, 5.5 mM magnesium chloride, 500 μM of each dNTP, 2.5 μM or 200 nM RT-primer (*see* **Note 7**), 0.4 U/μL RNase inhibitor, and 1.25 U/μL MultiScribe Reverse Transcriptase (Applied Biosystems), for 9 μL final volume per sample.
3. Add 1 μL of RNA (up to 200 ng of total RNA) to each RT mix, and spin in a microfuge to remove air bubbles and to collect the liquid at the bottom of the tube.
4. Incubate at 25°C for 10 min, 48°C for 30 min, and 95°C for 5 min (*see* **Note 8**).

3.5. Real-Time PCR

1. Thaw all reagents except the enzyme and the RNase inhibitor, mix by vortexing, spin down the tube contents, and keep on ice. Keep the enzyme and the RNase inhibitor in a freezer until immediately prior to use. Protect the TaqMan Probe from excessive exposure to light.
2. Prepare the PCR mix for the number of samples to be analyzed: 1X TaqMan buffer A, 5.5 mM MgCl$_2$ (*see* **Note 9**), 200 μM dATP, 200 μM dCTP, 200 μM dGTP, 400 μM dUTP (*see* **Note 10**), 100 nM TaqMan probe, 200 nM forward primer (*see* **Note 9**), 200 nM reverse primer (*see* **Note 11**), 0.01 U/μL AmpErase Uracil N-glycosylase (UNG; *see* **Note 10**), and 0.025 U/μL AmpliTaq Gold DNA Polymerase, for a final volume of 40 μL per sample.
3. Place MicroAmp Optical Tubes in a MicroAmp 96-well tray, and transfer 40 μL of the PCR mix to the tubes.
4. Add 10 μL of cDNA to the PCR mix in the corresponding tubes (*see* **Note 11**) and mix by pipeting up and down.
5. Using fresh MicroAmp Optical Caps, cap the tubes, briefly spin down to remove bubbles, and collect the liquid at the bottom of the tube.
6. Transfer the plate to thermal cycler block of the sequence detector, and perform real-time quantitative PCR: 2 min at 50°C (incubation of UNG); 10 min at 95°C (activation of AmpliTaq Gold DNA Polymerase); and 40 cycles at 95°C for 15 s and 65°C for 1 min.

3.6. Determination of the Target Amount

1. The amounts of the target and endogenous reference are determined from the appropriate standard curves.
2. The target amount is then divided by the endogenous reference amount to obtain a normalized target value.   .
3. The normalized target value is then divided by the normalized control value to generate the relative expression level (*see* **Note 12**).

4. Notes

1. RNA*later* is a tissue storage reagent, which rapidly permeates tissue to stabilize and protect cellular RNA. RNA*later* is particularly useful for gene analysis in autopsy material, releasing the user from the obligation to process tissue specimens immediately or to freeze samples in liquid nitrogen for later processing. RNA*later* preserves RNA in tissues for 1 mo or more at 4°C. Tissues in RNA*later* can also be stored at –20°C or –80°C long-term.
2. Total RNA may be prepared by any of the established methods provided that the resulting preparation are essentially devoid of proteins.
3. The Mixer Mill MM 300 provides rapid and efficient disruption of up to 192 biological samples in a few minutes. Disruption is achieved through the beating and grinding effects of beads on the sample material as they are shaken together in the grinding vessel. The grinding vessels and beads used are disposable. The Mixer Mill is a high sample throughput and biosafety system for disruption of autopsy material.
4. To check for the amplification of contaminating genomic DNA, the negative control (without RT reaction) should be examined concomitantly during PCR.
5. Reverse transcription can be performed as a separate reaction from the PCR (two-step RT-PCR) or can be coupled to the PCR in the same tube (one-step RT-PCR). Two-step RT-PCR has the advantage of producing a stock of cDNA that can be used for multiple PCR assays.
6. The optimal concentration of the template is essential for an efficient RT reaction. However, particularly in small and degraded RNA from autopsy material, it may be difficult to calculate the amount of the template for RT-PCR by UV absorbance. Therefore, a 10-fold diluted sample should be determined concomitantly.
7. A random hexamer, oligo $d(T)_{16}$, or sequence-specific reverse primer can be used. If a random hexamer or an oligo $d(T)_{16}$ primer is used, the final concentration is 2.5 μM. The final concentration of a sequence-specific reverse primer is 200 nM.
8. If a sequence-specific reverse primer is used, the first incubation at 25°C for 10 min is not necessary.
9. A few variables may have to be optimized to achieve an accurate result on a TaqMan fluorogenic detection system. The optimum concentrations of the primers and of magnesium chloride should be specifically determined by empirical testing for optimizing PCR and hybridization of the TaqMan probe.
10. UNG is a nuclease, which acts on single- and double-stranded dU-containing DNA. It has no activity on RNA or dT-containing DNA. Therefore, UNG treatment can prevent the reamplification of carryover PCR products that have been previously synthesized using dUTP instead of dTTP.
11. Do not label the tubes and the caps.
12. If the PCR efficiencies of target and endogenous reference are approximately equal, the comparative C_T method is available. The comparative C_T method is similar to the relative

standard curve method, except it uses arithmetic formulae, not a standard curve. Refer to the user bulletin from Applied Biosystems *(16)* for the arithmetic formulae.

References

1. Alwine, J. C., Kemp, D. J., and Stark, G. R. (1977) Method for detection of specific RNAs in agarose gels by transfer to diazobenzyloxymethyl-paper and hybridization with DNA probes. *Proc. Natl. Acad. Sci. USA* **74**, 5350–5354.
2. Hod, Y. (1992) A simplified ribonuclease protection assay. *BioTechniques* **13**, 852–854.
3. Saccomanno, C. F., Bordonaro, M., Chen, J. S., and Nordstrom, J. L. (1992) A faster ribonuclease protection assay. *BioTechniques* **13**, 846–850.
4. Boorstein, W. R. and Craig, E. A. (1989) Primer extension analysis of RNA. *Methods Enzymol.* **180**, 347–369.
5. Freeman, W. M., Walker, S. J., and Vrana, K. E. (1999) Quantitative RT-PCR: pitfalls and potential. *BioTechniques* **26**, 112–122.
6. Becker-Andre, M. and Hahlbrock, K. (1989) Absolute mRNA quantification using the polymerase chain reaction (PCR). A novel approach by a PCR aided transcript titration assay (PATTY). *Nucleic Acids Res.* **17**, 9437–9446.
7. Wiesner, R. J. (1992) Direct quantification of picomolar concentrations of mRNAs by mathematical analysis of a reverse transcription/exponential polymerase chain reaction assay. *Nucleic Acids Res.* **20**, 5863–5864.
8. Gibson, U. E., Heid, C. A., and Williams, P. M. (1996) A novel method for real time quantitative RT-PCR. *Genome Res.* **6**, 995–1001.
9. Ishida, K., Zhu, B. L., and Maeda, H. (2000) Novel approach to quantitative reverse transcription PCR assay of mRNA component in autopsy material using the TaqMan fluorogenic detection system: dynamics of pulmonary surfactant apoprotein A. *Forensic Sci. Int.* **113**, 127–131.
10. Ishida, K., Zhu, B. L., and Maeda, H. (2002) A quantitative RT-PCR assay of surfactant-associated protein A1 and A2 mRNA transcripts as a diagnostic tool for acute asphyxial death. *Legal Med.* **4**, 7–12.
11. Kuimelis, R. G., Livak, K. J., Mullah, B., and Andrus, A. (1997) Structural analogues of TaqMan probes for real-time quantitative PCR. *Nucleic Acids Symp. Serv.* **37**, 255–256.
12. Longley, M. J., Bennett, S. E., and Mosbaugh, D. W. (1990) Characterization of the 5' to 3' exonuclease associated with *Thermus aquaticus* DNA polymerase. *Nucleic Acids Res.* **18**, 7317–7322.
13. Ercolani, L., Florence, B., Denaro, M., and Alexander, M. (1988) Isolation and complete sequence of a functional human glyceraldehyde-3-phosphate dehydrogenase gene. *J. Biol. Chem.* **263**, 15335–15341.
14. Nakajima-Iijima, S., Hamada, H., Reddy, P., and Kakunaga, T. (1985) Molecular structure of the human cytoplasmic β-actin gene: interspecies homology of sequences in the introns. *Proc. Natl. Acad. Sci. USA* **82**, 6133–6137.
15. Torczynski, R. M., Fuke, M., and Bollon, A. P. (1985) Cloning and sequencing of a human 18s ribosomal RNA gene. *DNA* **4**, 283–291.
16. Relative quantification of gene expression (1997) *ABI PRISM 7700 Sequence Detection System User Bulletin #2*, Perkin Elmer, Foster City, CA, pp. 11–13.

35

Development of Quantitative Reverse Transcriptase PCR Assays for Measuring Gene Expression

Tony E. Godfrey and Lori A. Kelly

Summary

Real-time, quantitative reverse transcriptase (RT)-PCR is a very useful and powerful technology for analysis of gene expression. At a first pass, real-time PCR appears to be a simple extension of regular PCR, and it should therefore be easy for an experienced PCR user to convert to quantitative assays. In practice, however, our experience would indicate that this is not usually the case, and most novice real-time PCR users run into problems even though they are very capable at regular PCR. One problem is that, unlike Northern blots, which are technically difficult but typically either work or do not, real-time PCR assays, even poorly designed ones, usually give data. Unfortunately, these data, or their interpretation, may be erroneous, since there are many potential pitfalls that need to be avoided when designing and using real-time PCR for measurement of gene expression. The purpose of this chapter is not to try to discuss the complexities of real-time PCR in detail (which would require a whole book), but, instead, to provide a simple outline for the development of real-time PCR assays. If followed, these guidelines should allow the reader to develop real-time PCR assays that avoid the most common pitfalls and that are capable of producing reliable and accurate gene expression data.

Key Words: Real-time PCR; relative gene expression; assay development.

1. Introduction

The seminal papers describing quantification of gene expression using real-time polymerase chain reaction (PCR) were published in 1996 *(1,2)*, but a literature search for articles using real-time PCR, TaqMan® or 5'-nuclease PCR in the years from 1996 to 1998 reveals that this technology was initially slow to make its way into routine use. From 1999 to 2001, however, the number of studies using this technology increased exponentially, and by July of 2002, more than 700 such articles had already been published that year alone. There are several reasons for this dramatic increase. First, real-time PCR has become widely accepted by journals and reviewers as an acceptable way of quantifying gene expression using reverse-transcription PCR (RT-PCR). Initially, all real-time PCR data had to be verified by other, more standard techniques,

From: *Methods in Molecular Biology, vol. 291, Molecular Toxicology Protocols*
Edited by: P. Keohavong and S. G. Grant © Humana Press Inc., Totowa, NJ

such as Northern blots, but more and more, real-time PCR is itself being used as a confirmatory technique, particularly for validation of cDNA microarray expression data. Second, the original real-time PCR instrumentation (the ABI 7700 or TaqMan [Applied Biosystems, Foster City, CA]) sold for upwards of $80,000 in 1996. The last 3 yr, however, have seen the introduction of many new real-time PCR instruments, some costing less than $30,000. This reduction in cost has made real-time PCR affordable for most researchers; whereas real-time instruments used to be the toys of industry, or confined to core facilities in academic institutions, it now seems that almost every major lab or department has real-time PCR capability. Third, and perhaps most importantly, researchers themselves have reached a certain degree of comfort with this maturing technology and are consequently using real-time PCR as their method of choice for gene expression analysis.

Unfortunately, to date, very few publications have provided detailed methods and potential pitfalls of real-time PCR for measurement of gene expression *(3,4)*. In part, this is because of the many complexities of real-time PCR experiments, and the even greater variety of experimental questions and designs to which this technique can be applied. In addition, even so-called experts in the field often disagree over procedural details, such as the use of standard curves or relative expression calculations, the need for precisely matching PCR efficiencies of all genes, the ability to obtain absolute quantification, and the validity of multiplexing in quantitative PCR. Although these are important issues for some, most researchers can obtain accurate and reliable information from real-time PCR experiments by following a few simple guidelines. For the purposes of this chapter, therefore, we have chosen to describe what we consider to be the basics of real-time RT-PCR assay development. The chapter is broken into sections that cover (1) design of PCR primers and probe, (2) cDNA synthesis, (3) initial testing of PCR primers, (4) optimization of the PCR conditions, (5) PCR sensitivity and efficiency testing, and (6) testing for quantitative RT. Finally, the last section briefly discusses some important considerations for experimental design and data analysis.

2. Materials

2.1. PCR Primer and Probe Design

1. Software design program such as Primer Express™ from Applied Biosystems or free software available on the web such as PrimerQuest™ (IDT, Coralville IA, http://www.idtdna.com/).
2. cDNA sequence of the genes that you wish to analyze. If possible, this should include information on location of exon junctions and any alternate splice forms for which you need to account. In addition, it is often very informative to run a BLAST search of the entire cDNA sequence. This may identify splice variants, sequence motifs, and areas of homology with similar genes that should be avoided in order to obtain an amplicon specific to the desired target.

2.2. cDNA Synthesis

1. PCR machine (e.g., Applied Biosystems 9600, 9700, or 2700, MJ Research PTC series [Waltham, MA], Bio-Rad I-Cycler [Hercules, CA], or any other thermal cycler).
2. 10X PCR buffer supplied with *Taq* enzyme, either Gibco-BRL Platinum *Taq* buffer (Gaithersburg, MD), or Applied Biosystems PCR buffer II.

3. MgCl$_2$ solution (supplied with *Taq* enzyme).
4. PCR tubes and caps.
5. Total RNA from a source known to express your target gene (positive control RNA). RNA should be at 50 ng/µL.
6. SuperScript II RNase H⁻ Reverse Transcriptase (Invitrogen, Carlsbad, CA), or other murine moloney leukemia virus (MMLV)-based reverse transcriptase (MMLV Reverse Transcriptase [Epicentre, Madison, WI] or MuLV Reverse Transcriptase [Applied Biosystems]).
7. 100 m*M* dNTP set: dATP, dCTP, dGTP, and dTTP (Gibco-BRL). Mix equal volumes to make a mixture of 25 m*M* each.
8. 40 U/µL RNase Inhibitor (Promega, Madison, WI).
9. Random hexamers (Roche, Indianapolis, IN).

2.3. Primer Testing

1. Tris-EDTA (TE) buffer, pH 8.0 (from 100X TE stock; Sigma, St. Louis, MO; *see* **Note 1**).
2. Non-diethylpyrocarbonate (DEPC) treated nuclease-free water (Ambion, Austin, TX).
3. 0.5-, 1.5-, and 2.0-mL RNase-free microcentrifuge tubes (Ambion).
4. DNA-free solution (Ambion).
5. PCR primers (*see* **Notes 2** and **3**).
6. Thermostable DNA polymerase (such as Amplitaq Gold from Applied Biosystems or Platinum *Taq* from Gibco-BRL).
7. Genomic DNA (Promega).
8. Positive control cDNA from **Subheading 3.2., step 1**.
9. No-RT control template from **Subheading 3.2., step 2**.
10. Polyacrylamide gel electrophoresis apparatus and power supply (e.g., Mini Protean 3 Cell, Bio-Rad; Xcell SureLock Mini-Cell, Invitrogen).
11. Ethidium bromide (0.5 µg/mL) or other DNA label, such as SYBR green.
12. 100-bp DNA ladder (Gibco-BRL).
13. Gel visualization equipment (UV lightbox and camera system such as Gel Doc 2000, Bio-Rad).
14. 5X Tris-borate-EDTA (TBE) buffer: 0.445 *M* Tris-borate, pH 8.3, 0.01 *M* EDTA (Sigma).
15. 6X Gel loading solution (Sigma).

2.4. Primer/Probe Optimization and PCR Efficiency Testing

1. PCR primers (5 µ*M* each).
2. Dual-labeled probe (10 µ*M*).
3. Real-time PCR instrument (e.g., Applied Biosystems 7700, 7900, or 7000, Opticon [MJ Research], SmartCycler [Cepheid, Sunnyvale, CA], MX4000 [Stratagene, La Jolla, CA], or others).
4. PCR tubes/plates and caps suitable for your real-time instrument.
5. GeneAmp 10X PCR buffer A and MgCl$_2$ solution (supplied in the TaqMan 200 or 1000 Rxn Gold Packs from Applied Biosystems).
6. Amplitaq Gold (supplied in the TaqMan 200 or 1000 Rxn Gold Packs from Applied Biosystems).
7. Nuclease-free water (Ambion).
8. Positive control cDNA, from RNA described in **Subheading 2.2., item 5**, as processed in **Subheading 3.2.**
9. 25 m*M* Mix of nucleotides prepared as described in **Subheading 2.2., item 7**.

2.5. Quantitative Reverse Transcription

1. Reverse transcription reagents as described in **Subheading 2.2.**
2. PCR reagents and instrumentation as described in **Subheading 2.4.**
3. 13 µg Positive control RNA at 500 ng/µL.

3. Methods

3.1. PCR Primer and Probe Design

For the purposes of this chapter, we will describe the original and most commonly used real-time PCR chemistry, the use of 5'-nuclease hydrolysis probes (TaqMan probes). These probes are short oligonucleotides (typically 20–35 bases) designed to be complementary to a target sequence between the PCR primers, on one strand of the generated PCR product. To prevent the probe from acting as a primer in the PCR, the 3'-end of the oligonucleotide is blocked with a 3'-phosphate group instead of a 3'-hydroxyl group. Then 5'-nuclease probes are labeled on the 5'-end with a fluorescent reporter dye and on the 3'-end with a quencher molecule that can be either fluorescent or nonfluorescent. Although the labels do not necessarily have to be on the 5'- and 3'-nucleotides (*5*), this is the most common and effective probe design. When the probe is in solution and single stranded, it is able to adopt conformations whereby the 5' and 3' dyes are very close together. When the probe is in these conformations, any light absorbed by the reporter dye is transferred by fluorescence resonance energy transfer (FRET) to the quencher dye. If the quencher is a fluorescent molecule, then the transferred energy is released as light of a longer wavelength (determined by the specific dye), whereas nonfluorescent quenchers dissipate the energy as heat. In either scenario, the shorter wavelength fluorescence that would typically be emitted by the reporter dye is quenched when the probe is intact and single-stranded.

At the beginning of a PCR reaction, there is very little specific probe target present, and therefore almost all the probe molecules are single-stranded and quenched. As the PCR proceeds, target sequences are amplified and accumulate exponentially. During the annealing/extension phase of each cycle, probe molecules bind to the homologous strand of the target sequences and form short stretches of double-stranded (ds)DNA. *Taq* polymerase extends the PCR primers until it reaches the dsDNA fragment, where the probe is bound, and then the 5'-nuclease activity of the enzyme cleaves the probe. This is done first by displacing a few bases from the 5'-end of the probe/target duplex to form a bifurcation or "fork-like" structure that is recognized by the 5'-nuclease component of *Taq* polymerase. The polymerase then cuts the probe at the bifurcation site, releasing a short oligonucleotide with the 5' reporter dye attached. This process repeats until the remaining probe is too short to remain hybridized and dissociates from the target sequence, allowing polymerization to be completed. Because the released reporter dye is no longer physically attached to the quencher dye, it is unable to transfer its energy to the quencher. Thus, when excited by light of an appropriate wavelength, it now emits fluorescence that can be detected and distinguished from quencher dye fluorescence based on its different emission wavelength. In this way, reporter dye fluorescence increases at each cycle in a cumulative fashion and is therefore propor-

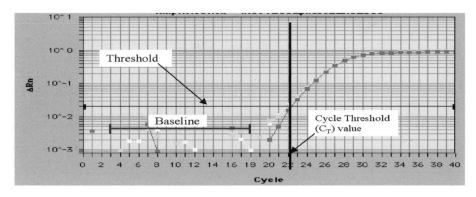

Fig. 1. Typical amplification plot from a real-time PCR amplification.

tional to the amount of PCR product generated. It is this increase in reporter dye fluorescence that is used to generate the PCR amplification plots that have become so familiar (**Fig. 1**).

1. For measurement of relative expression, it is necessary to compare expression of the target gene(s) (gene[s] of interest) with the expression of an endogenous control gene. The purpose of the endogenous control gene is to (1) control for the quantity and quality (integrity and to some degree purity) of the RNA in the reaction, and (2) control for the RT step of the RT-PCR. This is analogous to the use of actin or GAPDH as a control for loading and transfer in a Northern blot experiment. Before proceeding further, a suitable endogenous control gene should be chosen for your experiments (*see* **Note 4**), and primers and probes for this gene should be designed in parallel with primers and probes for your target gene(s).
2. Using an appropriate primer design program, design the PCR primers and probes using the following guidelines (*see* **Fig. 2** and **Note 5**):
   a. Primer length should be 16–24 bp with 35–55% GC and a melting temperature (T_m) of 57–62°C.
   b. Avoid runs of four or more consecutive identical bases, e.g., four Gs.
   c. The five 3'-bases of the primers should consist of no more than two or three G or C residues.
   d. Probe length should be 22–32 bp with 35–55% GC and a T_m of 67–72°C.
   e. Avoid runs of four or more consecutive identical bases, e.g., four Gs, and avoid a 5' G residue, since this will quench the reporter dye.
   f. Keep the PCR amplicon length below 150 bp and, if possible, below 100 bp.
3. Run a BLAST search for each primer sequence and the probe sequence individually, and also run a BLAST search for the whole PCR amplicon. This will identify any short-sequence homologies that may have been missed when searching with the whole cDNA sequence (*see* **Note 6**).
4. Order PCR primers but not probe (*see* **Note 7**).

3.2. cDNA Synthesis

It is important to realize that for RT-PCR assays to be quantitative, both the RT and the PCR steps need to be quantitative, that is, if the reaction is begun with more

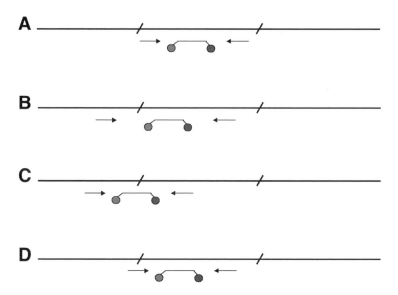

Fig. 2. Options for PCR primer and probe design in a target sequence comprised of three exons. (Exon junctions in the cDNA are indicated by the diagonal lines.) Option (**A**) shows a design in which the primers and probe are all in the same exon (intraexonic). This design will amplify both cDNA and genomic DNA equally well and should be avoided if possible. Option (**B**) shows a design in which the PCR primers are in different exons (intron-spanning design). This option will work well if the intron is large (preferably >2 kb) since amplification efficiency of the large genomic DNA product will be much lower than that of the short, cDNA product. If the intron is small, this design should be avoided since it will amplify, and generate, fluorescent signal, from both genomic DNA and cDNA. In option (**C**), the primers are also in different exons, but this time the probe also spans the exon junction. Regardless of intron size, this design should not generate fluorescent signal from genomic DNA. However, if the intron is small, genomic DNA PCR product will accumulate and may affect assay sensitivity. Although this design is intuitively the best, we try to avoid it unless the intron is large enough to eliminate amplification of genomic DNA effectively. In option (**D**), the reverse primer and probe are in the same exon, and the forward primer spans the exon junction. When properly designed, this option eliminates amplification of genomic DNA regardless of intron size.

RNA, there should be more cDNA produced and a lower (earlier) cycle threshold (C_T) value from the quantitative PCR. This will be addressed in more detail in **Subheading 3.6.**, but the RT reaction described below has been used by us on a variety of RNA sources (including RNA isolated from formalin-fixed, paraffin-embedded tissue blocks), and on more than 50 genes. This reaction should yield quantitative RT with up to 2 μg of total RNA and may be quantitative with even higher amounts (up to 10 μg in our hands).

1. Using the positive control RNA, set up (on ice) an RT reaction and a no-RT control as follows. Reactions should be set up in PCR tubes to fit your specific PCR instrument. For RT, set up a 100-μL reaction consisting of:

cDNA gDNA NTC   cDNA gDNA NTC   cDNA gDNA NTC

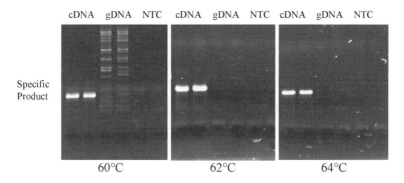

Specific
Product

60°C   62°C   64°C

Fig. 3. Acrylamide gel testing of primers. This example of gel-based primer testing illustrates how increasing the annealing temperature of the PCR reaction can eliminate nonspecific amplification from genomic DNA. Although the nonspecific products seen at 60°C may not generate signal and probe-based real-time PCR assay, they will certainly affect PCR efficiency and assay sensitivity. In this example, 62 or 64°C would be a better choice. NTC, no-template control.

10 µL 10X PCR buffer	1X final
30 µL of 25 m*M* MgCl$_2$ (Applied Biosystems)	
or	
15 µL of 50 m*M* MgCl$_2$ (Gibco-BRL)	7.5 m*M* final
4 µL dNTPs (25 m*M* each)	1 m*M* final
12.5 µL hexamers (100 µ*M*)	12.5 µ*M* final
1.25 µL SuperScript II (200 U/µL)	2.5 U/µL
1 µL RNase Inhibitor (40 U/µL)	0.4 U/µL

Add water to 90 µL. Add 10 µL of RNA (50 ng/µL).

2. For the no-RT reaction, use water in place of SuperScript II.
3. In the thermal cycler, incubate all reactions at 25°C for 10 min, 48°C for 30 min, 95°C for 5 min, and hold at room temperature.
4. Store cDNA at 4°C, or –20°C if long-term storage is required with infrequent access.

3.3. Primer Testing

Because primers are inexpensive, we prefer to test them using regular PCR and gel electrophoresis prior to ordering the more expensive probe. The purpose of this testing is to check that the primers amplify the expected size product from the cDNA, that they do not produce any visible secondary products, and that they do not amplify genomic DNA (see example in **Fig. 3**).

1. Clean work area and pipets with DNA-free solution.
2. Reconstitute all PCR primers to a stock concentration of 500 µ*M* in 1X TE. Store at –20°C.
3. Make a working dilution of the primers at 10 µ*M* in 1X TE. Store at 4°C.
4. Run duplicate PCR reactions on the positive control cDNA and on the no-RT control reaction product from **Subheading 3.2.**, **steps 1** and **2**, respectively. Also run duplicate reactions with 25 ng of genomic DNA and duplicate reactions with water (no-template controls [NTCs]) as template. The reagents and volumes (in µL) for setting up these reactions are given in **Table 1**:

Table 1
Reagents and Volume for Primer Testing

Reagents[a]	Positive control	No-RT control	Genomic DNA control	No-template control
Taq	0.5	0.5	0.5	0.5
10X PCR buffer	5	5	5	5
MgCl$_2$ (25 mM)[b]	7	7	7	7
dNTPs (2.5 mM)	4	4	4	4
Template				
RT cDNA	5	—	—	—
no-RT cDNA	—	5	—	—
H$_2$O	—	—	—	5
Genomic DNA (5 ng/µL)	—	—	5	—
Forward primer	5	5	5	5
Reverse primer	5	5	5	5
Water	to 50 µL	to 50 µL	to 50 µL	to 50 µL

[a]For reagents, *see* **Notes 8** and **9**.

[b]For MgCl$_2$, use half the volume if using the 50 mM MgCl$_2$ supplied with Platinum *Taq* (Gibco-BRL).

5. Incubate at 95°C for 12 min (if using *Taq* Gold; 2 min if using Platinum *Taq*) followed by 40 cycles of 95°C for 15 s and 60°C for 1 min (*see* **Note 10**).
6. Mix 5 µL of each PCR product with 1 µL of 6X loading dye and run on a 5% polyacrylamide gel along with a 100-bp ladder (*see* **Note 11**).
7. Stain with ethidium bromide (5 µL/100 µL TBE buffer) for 10–30 min.
8. Visualize under UV, verifying the size of the product for the gene of interest and the absence of amplification in genomic DNA, no-RT control, and NTC (*see* **Note 12**).
9. If the results are acceptable (*see* **Note 13**), order the dual-labeled probe(s) (*see* **Notes 14** and **15**), and reconstitute to 500 µM as previously described (*see* **Notes 2** and **3**). Store at –20°C.

3.4. Primer/Probe Optimization

The goal of these experiments is to find the primer and probe concentrations that give the most robust and reliable PCR amplification. They will also show that the probe is working as expected. For these experiments you should use the standard annealing temperature and magnesium chloride concentration described in **Subheading 3.2.**, **step 1**, unless these conditions had to be modified as described in **Note 13**.

The original probe and primer optimization recommendations from Applied Biosystems (some 5–6 yr ago) were to test a variety of different forward and reverse primer concentrations in combination with two probe concentrations. This resulted in a full 96-well PCR plate of reactions and was reasonably complex to set up. Current recommendations from Applied Biosystems are to use just 900 nM of each primer and 250 nM of probe and not to bother with optimization. Although these conditions do indeed work well in most cases, the high primer concentrations can result in some nonspecificity of the PCR and may limit sensitivity. Using higher oligo concentrations is also more expensive, and we find that very few primer/probe sets need these high concentrations to function with maximum efficiency and sensitivity. Therefore, we have chosen to compromise by performing a limited primer/probe optimization step as described below. For simplicity, the procedure outlined below is described specifically for use in the Applied Biosystems instruments and uses ABI buffers and reagents. Other buffers and enzymes can be used if desired.

1. Prepare 2X PCR master mix as described in **Note 8**.
2. Reconstitute probe to 500 μ*M* as described for the PCR primers in **Subheading 3.3., step 2** (*see* **Notes 2** and **3**).
3. Make a working concentration of probe at 10 μ*M* as described for the PCR primers in **Subheading 3.3., step 3**.
4. Set up duplicate PCR reactions with each of the following primer/probe combinations: 300, 500, and 900 n*M* for each pair of forward and reverse (F/R) primers with a 100-n*M* probe and 300, 500, and 900 n*M* for each pair of F/R primers with a 200-n*M* probe. The reaction setup for this experiment (in μL) when using Applied Biosystems reagents is given in the table following:

Primer/Probe Optimization Set-Up

	For 100-n*M* Probe			For 200-n*M* Probe		
n*M* F/R primers	300	500	900	300	500	900
Reagents (μL)						
2X PCR buffer A mix	25	25	25	25	25	25
Forward primer	3	5	9	3	5	9
Reverse primer	3	5	9	3	5	9
Probe	0.5	0.5	0.5	1	1	1
Water	13.5	9.5	1.5	13.5	9.5	1.5
Positive cDNA	5	5	5	5	5	5

5. Run 40 cycles of PCR with the following parameters: 95°C for 12 min, followed by 40 cycles of 95°C for 15 s and 60°C for 1 min.
6. Set the threshold at the lowest point above background (*see* **Figs. 4** and **5**) and within the linear portion of the amplification plot.
7. There are only two important things to look for in the data generated from this experiment: (1) the C_T value obtained from each primer/probe combination (lower is better), and (2) the absolute level of fluorescence reached at plateau for each combination (higher is better). Importantly, there should not be dramatic differences in either endpoint, particularly the C_T values. If C_T values differ significantly (more than one cycle) owing to primer or probe concentrations, *see* **Note 16**.

3.5. PCR Efficiency Testing

It is important to test the efficiency of your new PCR assay, primarily because a higher efficiency will generally result in a higher sensitivity and more robust assay.

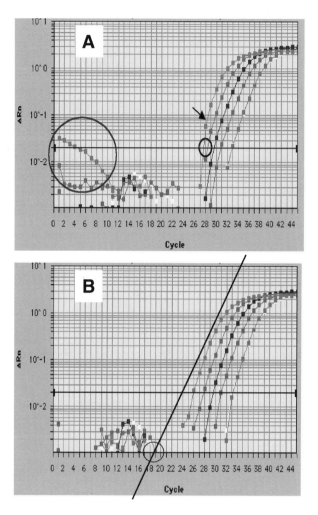

Fig. 4. Setting the baseline. The baseline area is used to calculate background fluorescence, which is then subtracted from all datapoints. In the example above, the baseline in (**A**) is set from 3 to 27. By cycle 27, however, real signal is being detected in the PCR reaction indicated by the arrow. This results in an artificially late C_T value for this reaction (circle). When the baseline settings are incorrectly set to include real signal, one frequently sees fluorescence above threshold in the early cycles (large oval), and this can be used as an indicator of incorrect baseline settings. In (**B**), the baseline is set from 3 to 22 cycles, and the problems in (**A**) are corrected. Extrapolation of the linear portion n the amplification plot (solid line) can be used as a guide to correct setting of the baseline cycles (described in **Note 24**).

Furthermore, a low PCR efficiency will not only limit the assay sensitivity but may also indicate other problems, such as nonspecificity. In general, we like our assays to have greater than 90% PCR efficiency, and most are closer to 95%.

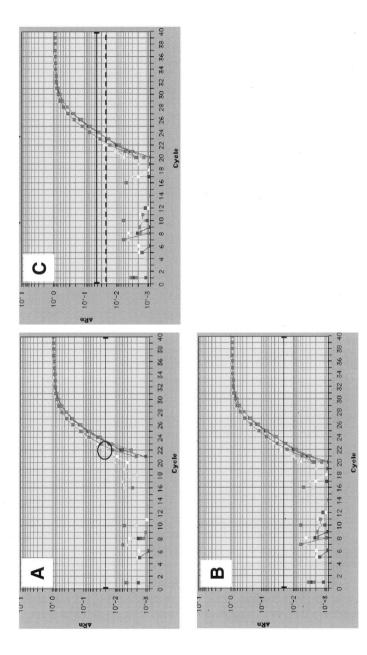

Fig. 5. Optimal setting of the baseline and threshold. This series of figures shows triplicate amplification plots from two samples. In (A), the baseline is set from 3 to 15 cycles (default on the ABI 7700), but there is some variability in the C_T values for the triplicate from the first sample (embedded oval). (B) Shows how setting the baseline area more appropriately (from 3 to 18 cycles in this case) can sometimes tighten up the C_T values. Finally, in (C), the threshold has been raised slightly to avoid the noise area that is still present in the first triplicate. These are now the optimal baseline and threshold settings for these two samples.

1. Make 3X serial dilutions of your positive control cDNA by mixing 15 µL of cDNA with 30 µL of nuclease-free buffer. Make at least four, and preferably five such serial dilutions, so that you have five or six dilution points (including the original cDNA; *see* **Note 17**).
2. Using the optimal primer/probe concentrations determined in **Subheading 3.4.**, set up triplicate 50-µL PCR reactions using 5 µL of each cDNA dilution as template (*see* **Note 18**).
3. In the real-time PCR machine, incubate at 95°C for 12 min, followed by 40 cycles of 95°C for 15 s and 60°C (or optimal temperature determined from **Subheading 3.3.**, **step 9**) for 1 min.
4. Set threshold and background parameters as previously described in **Subheading 3.4.**, **step 6**.
5. Using Microsoft Excel or a similar program, plot C_T value (*y*-axis) vs log cDNA concentration (*x*-axis). For 3X serial dilutions, this is easily done by arbitrarily assigning the most dilute cDNA sample a concentration value of 1, whereupon the first higher dilution will be 3, the second will be 9, and so on up to the highest concentration (which will be 243 in a 6-point curve). Plotting log cDNA concentration vs C_T should generate points on a line with a downward slope from left to right. Use the fit trendline option in Excel to fit a straight line through the datapoints and to calculate a slope and correlation coefficient (r^2; *see* **Note 19**). The PCR efficiency can be calculated from the slope using the following equation:

$$\text{Efficiency} = 10^{(1/-S)} - 1$$

where S = the slope of the standard curve. For example, for a slope of –3.4:

$$\text{Efficiency} = 10^{[(1/-(-3.4)]} - 1$$
$$= 10^{(1/3.4)} - 1$$
$$= 10\,(0.294) - 1$$
$$= 1.968 - 1$$
$$= 0.968 \text{ or } 97\%$$

3.6. Quantitative Reverse Transcription

A fundamental principle for the quantification of gene expression with RT-PCR is that once quantification is lost in a stage, it cannot be regained in subsequent stages of the experiment. Quantitative reverse transcription (QRT) refers to the principle that an increase in the starting RNA template concentration should result in a proportional increase in the amount of cDNA generated (and a lower C_T value on the subsequent PCR; *see* **Note 20**).

The RT protocol described in **Subheading 3.2.** has been tested extensively on many genes and many RNA sources. We find it to be more reliable and more quantitative than the RT protocols provided with the Superscript or MMLV RT enzymes. The purpose of the experiment outlined below is mainly to gain experience with the protocol and to get used to setting up multiple RT reactions at one time. It will also show you the quantitative RNA input range for your specific assay. All new researchers in our laboratory perform this experiment as a training exercise. Thus, this step is somewhat optional, and the experienced molecular biologist may feel comfortable proceeding directly to **Subheading 3.7.** The protocol below uses random hexamers to prime the RT reaction, because we feel that this method is suitable for a wide range of experimental scenarios and provides the most flexibility in terms of the genes that can be analyzed and requirements for RNA integrity. Oligo dT or gene-specific primers can be substituted in the protocol if desired (*see* **Note 21**).

1. Make five 2X serial dilutions (12 µL RNA + 12 µL water) of the stock RNA (500 ng/µL) in RNase-free water. This will result in dilutions in which a 10 µL vol contains 5, 2.5, 1.25, 0.61, 0.31, and 0.15 µg of RNA.
2. Perform RT reactions on each RNA dilution for the gene of interest and the endogenous control gene (*see* **Subheading 3.2.** for reaction setup, and **Note 22** for choice of RT primers).
3. In a 96-well plate, set up duplicate 50-µL PCR reactions for the genes of interest and the endogenous control, consisting of 1X TM buffer (*see* **Note 8**), the optimal concentration of forward and reverse primers and probe, and the primary PCR products (cDNAs) from **Subheading 3.6., step 2** (or water for NTCs).
4. Incubate at 95°C for 12 min, followed by 40 cycles of 95°C for 15 s and 60°C for 1 min in the TaqMan instrument (*see* **Note 23** for interpretation of results).

3.7. Some Comments on Experimental Design

If you follow the guidelines described so far in this chapter, chances are that you will have a real-time PCR assay capable of providing reliable, quantitative information on a set of samples. The next step, however, is to design the QRT-PCR experiments appropriately so that the data obtained are accurate and meaningful. At this point, you will need to decide whether you wish to perform your relative quantification using standard curves or comparative C_T calculations (target gene C_T – endogenous control gene C_T). Both approaches are described in detail in a User Bulletin available from Applied Biosystems (*6*) and will not be discussed here, other than to say that we almost exclusively use the comparative C_T approach. In either case, quantification of the target genes is calculated *relative* to the endogenous control, and, in our opinion, *absolute* quantification of mRNA copy number is unattainable with RT-PCR. Regardless of the approach you choose, the following section discusses some important considerations regarding experimental design for real-time PCR assays.

1. *Always try to run samples in batches.* For experiments in which a large number of samples are to be analyzed for gene expression, it is best to plan ahead and batch samples together. We typically batch 15–20 samples together for RT and then perform the PCR step one gene at a time on each RT batch. We try to avoid running multiple genes in the same PCR run whenever possible. Not only does batching result in more efficient use of the real-time PCR instrument, it also simplifies setup, data handling, and tracking of controls.
2. *Run appropriate controls along with each batch of samples.* Each RT-PCR run should contain duplicate or triplicate reactions for NTC and positive PCR controls. In most cases, we also run no-RT controls, even if we know that the assay design is cDNA-specific. The positive control should be a cDNA from an RNA sample known to express the target gene(s). The purpose of this control is to show that the PCR step was set up properly and functioned as expected. This is particularly useful when the samples show low or negative expression of the target gene. The NTC is used to detect PCR reagent contamination. The no-RT control may seem superfluous when the assay is designed to be cDNA-specific, but this control also detects RT reagent contamination if it is present.

3. *Use calibrator samples to allow comparison of data (not necessary when using standard curves).* Very few experiments can be completed in one RT-PCR run (one 96-well plate). Consequently it is typically necessary to compare data obtained on different days using different RT and PCR master mixes. A good way to do this is always to include a common (calibrator) RNA sample within each RT batch. Quantitative PCR for the endogenous control and target genes is then performed on this RNA sample along with the other RNA samples in the batch. Theoretically, the ΔC_T (C_T target gene – C_T endogenous control gene) for the calibrator sample should remain constant from run to run, but small variations can be corrected by using a Δ–Δ CT calculation, as described in a user bulletin from Applied Biosytems *(6)* and by us previously *(7)*. Alternatively, in large experiments, the variability in the calibrator ΔC_T can be tracked and used to determine reproducibility of the assay and to estimate error bars on samples that are analyzed only once instead of using replicates.

4. *Master-mix reagents whenever possible.* Data variability and pipeting errors can be greatly reduced by making master mixes of all common reagents whenever possible. In most cases, it should be possible to include all reagents in the master mix except the template. Try to avoid pipeting volumes less than 5 µL.

5. *Always run duplicate, or preferably triplicate, PCR reactions for each RT reaction.*

6. *Run replicate RT reactions, preferably on different amounts of RNA, for each sample.* Repeating the PCR on a cDNA sample only measures the variability inherent to PCR setup and instrumentation. In our experience, the most inconsistent part of real-time RT-PCR assays is the RT step. For this reason, we recommend that at least two, and preferably three, RT reactions be set up for each sample RNA. Furthermore, we prefer to put different amounts of RNA into each reaction (typically two- or three-fold different), thus generating a small dilution series for each sample. The ΔC_T between target and endogenous control gene should be consistent regardless of RNA input; if it is not, then the assay is not quantitative, and the data are unreliable. The most common reason for inconsistent ΔC_T values is poor RNA purity (presumably owing to RT inhibition caused by salt, protein, or phenol carryover from the RNA purification). In this case, inhibition increases along with increasing RNA in the RT reaction. Often, the inhibition affects target gene(s) and the endogenous control gene equally, and the ΔC_T remains constant. In this case, the only indicator of inhibition is that the endogenous control gene C_T values do not get lower with higher RNA input. Despite the constant ΔC_T in this instance, data from such samples should be viewed cautiously, and preferably one should clean up the RNA and repeat the RT-PCR.

7. *Be consistent with every step of the assay.* Always try to perform each part of the RT-PCR assay the same way every time, i.e., use the same RNA isolation procedure, quantify the RNA the same way (preferably by measuring OD_{260} on a spectrophotometer), track the $OD_{260/280}$ ratio, put the same amount(s) of RNA into each reaction, don't change reagent vendors without running controls to ensure that the data do not change, and set threshold values at the same point each time (this may vary gene by gene, but try to be consistent for any single gene). This level of consistency makes it much easier to identify when something goes wrong with an assay (which it will at some point!). For example, we typically use 400- and 200-ng RNA inputs for one large, ongoing study. Using our endogenous control gene, we expect to see C_T values from 23–35 cycles. If samples suddenly start to give different C_T values, then one can immediately identify that there is a problem and search for the solution (bad reagents, new primer/probe batch, and so on).

8. *Calculate error bars correctly.* Two common mistakes are made when calculating error

bars on real-time RT-PCR data. First, it is not correct to calculate error bars based on the replicate PCR reactions, since this only measures variability of the PCR setup and instrumentation (a typical PCR triplicate should have a standard deviation of less than 0.25 cycles). Instead, error bars should be calculated from the mean of duplicate or triplicate PCR reactions from replicate (preferably three or more) RT reactions on the same RNA. In many cases, one should actually take this a step further and analyze separate RNA samples from replicate, independent experiments. Second, error bars generated from PCR data should not be symmetric. PCR is exponential, and the data produced (C_Ts) have to be transformed in order to calculate relative expression. Calculation of error bars based on the transformed data is intuitively correct but generates symmetric error bars. Although this is not a major flaw, it does not truly represent the error in measurement inherent to the assay. A more appropriate way to calculate error bars is to calculate the mean and standard deviation using the C_T-based data and then transform the data. This concept is illustrated in the example shown in **Fig. 6.**

4. Notes

1. To avoid contamination of the stock primers and probes, it is important to use clean, fresh TE buffer for reconstitution. We purchase 100X TE (Sigma) and non-DEPC–treated, RNAse-free water (Ambion) and make up 100-mL batches of 1X TE in a separate laboratory using dedicated pipets. This is then aliquoted into 1.5-mL microcentrifuge tubes and frozen. A new aliquot is used to reconstitute each batch of primers and probes and to make the initial working dilution.

2. Most oligomer synthesis companies provide the absolute nanomol amount of each oligonucleotide in the tube. An easy way to obtain a 500 µM stock concentration is to add a volume (in µL) of 1X TE buffer, pH 8.0, that is two times the nmol amount of the respective primer/probe, e.g., for 25.2 nmol of primer, add 50.4 µL of TE.

3. High concentration (500 µM) stock primers should be stored at –20°C and only thawed occasionally to make a new working dilution. Working concentration primers (10 µM) should be stored at 4°C to avoid repeated freezing and thawing, which will damage them. Working primers are stable at 4°C in TE buffer for at least 1–2 mo.

4. Choosing an appropriate endogenous control is very important but can be difficult. The goal is to pick a gene whose expression is not expected to change from sample to sample in a given experiment. The following examples illustrate some of the factors to consider in some common experimental scenarios. Every system and experiment is unique, however, and these scenarios are simply intended to get readers thinking along the appropriate lines for choosing an endogenous control in their own experiments.

    a. When comparing expression in tissue culture cell lines of the same tissue origin, one should choose a gene whose expression is not cell cycle-dependent because cultures will express such a gene at different levels as they proceed through exponential growth and into confluence. Alternatively, always harvest cells at the same confluence level. This is also an issue when comparing tumor tissue with normal tissue, since tumors typically contain a higher percentage of actively cycling cells than normal tissue. GAPDH expression is particularly dependent on cell cycle and should be avoided in these scenarios.

    b. When comparing gene expression in cell lines or tissues of different tissue types, pick a gene that is expressed at similar levels in all tissue types. This is a very difficult scenario, but some commonly used genes include 18s rRNA, β-glucuronidase, β$_2$-microglobulin, cyclophilin A, and phosphoglycerate kinase 1.

Calculations based on transformed data →

	Relative Exp.	Mean Rel. Exp.	S.D.	Upper S.D. boundary	Lower S.D. boundary
Delta CT1	**-4.7**				
Delta CT2	**-4.9**				
Delta CT3	**-4.1**				
	25.992	24.333	6.515	30.847	17.818
	29.857				
	17.148				
Mean Delta CT	-4.567				
Relative Expression ($2^{-mean\,delta\,CT}$)					
S.D. of delta CT's	0.416				
Mean + S.D Delta CT	-4.150				
Mean - S.D Delta CT	-4.983				
Upper S.D. boundary	31.63				
Lower S.D. boundary	17.76				

Calculations based on delta C_T's, then transformed →

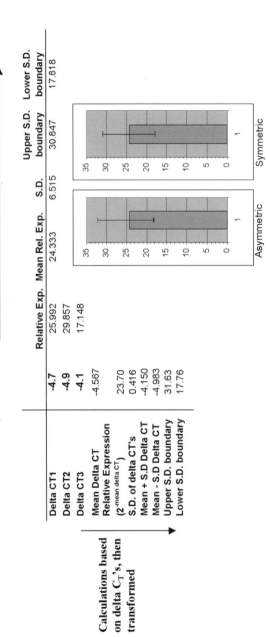

Fig. 6. Illustration of error bar calculation after data transformation (left to right) or before data transformation (top to bottom). When ΔC_T data are transformed into relative expression first, and mean and standard deviations (S.D.) are calculated from the transformed data, error bars are symmetric around the mean. This is incorrect. Mean and standard deviation should be calculated from ΔC_T values. The ΔC_T standard deviation is then added to or subtracted from the mean ΔC_T to generate the upper and lower ΔC_T standard deviation boundaries. These ΔC_T values are then transformed to generate error bars that are asymmetric about the mean.

Table 2
Suppliers of Custom Primer/Probe Oligonucleotides and Fluorescent Labels

Supplier	Web site	Phone Number
IDT	http://www.idtdna.com/	(800) 328-2661
Invitrogen	http://www.invitrogen.com/content.cfm?pageid=9714	(800) 955-6288
ABI	http://home.appliedbiosystems.com/index.cfm	(800) 327-3002
Synthegen (Houston, TX)	http://www.synthegen.com/catalog/index.lasso	(800) 949-8903
BioSource (Camarillo, CA)	http://www.keydna.com/	(800) 242-0607
Sigma-Genosys (The Woodlands, TX)	http://www.sigma-genosys.com/oligo.asp	(800) 234-5362

   c. When analyzing the response of a cell line (or animal) to an intervention or treatment (drug exposure, radiation, injury, and so on), the endogenous control gene expression must not be affected by the intervention or treatment. Again, this can be difficult, since the effects of many experimental treatments or interventions are not known. In many cases it may be therefore prudent to consider using more than one control gene until you have enough data to make an informed decision regarding which is most stable in your system (i.e., when using the same RNA input, which control gene gives the most stable C_T values under all experimental conditions). Alternatively, one could consider using total RNA input (measured by UV spectrophotometry or fluorimetry) as the reference point for measuring gene expression. In this case, expression of the target gene would be reported relative to total RNA input. This approach can be very attractive, but it has its own set of problems *(3)*.

5. When trying to design extremely sensitive RT-PCR assays, it is beneficial in the long run to try to avoid amplification of genomic DNA. This precludes the need for DNase treatment of RNA and ensures that no-RT control reactions are consistently negative. However, simply designing an amplicon to span an exon junction is not always enough. Placing the probe across the exon junction will eliminate the fluorescent signal, but this is not ideal because genomic DNA amplification is still occurring in the tube and can interfere with cDNA-specific amplification, particularly if the target gene has very low expression. If the intron is relatively short (<1000 bp), then genomic PCR product may still be efficiently amplified, and, if the probe is intraexonic, fluorescent signal will still be generated. Instead, we try to place one of the primers across the exon junction with less than six or seven of the 3' bases in one exon (**Fig. 2**). Often, this requires modification of the primer sequences preferred by the software program. In this case, most programs allow the user to define one or more of the primer sequences and then search for the opposite primer and probe. It is also a good idea to check the intronic sequence immediately adjacent to the exon to make sure there is not significant homology with the 3'-end of the PCR primer. In this way, the PCR primer cannot hybridize efficiently with genomic DNA, and amplification of genomic DNA is eliminated.

6. Most oligomer design programs will provide alternative primer and probe designs. If the BLAST search identifies significant homology of either primer or probe with an undesired sequence, it may be worthwhile investigating alternative designs.

7. PCR primers for QPCR do not need any special purification. Primers can be ordered from many sources including in-house oligomer synthesis facilities (*see* **Table 2** for a partial list of oligomer synthesis companies).

8. We recommend using the 2X master mix option for setting up PCR reactions. Prepare 5 mL of 2X TaqMan buffer (TM buffer) as follows using Applied Biosystems' 10X buffer A kit: 1 mL 10X buffer A, 2.43 mL nuclease-free water, 120 µL 25 mM dNTPs, 1.4 mL 25 mM MgCl$_2$, and 50 µL AmpliTaq Gold. Final concentrations: 2X buffer A, 7 mM MgCl$_2$, 600 µM dNTPs, 2.5 U AmpliTaq Gold. The 2X master mix can be made up in batches and stored at 4°C for up to 1 mo if necessary.

9. Bad dNTPs are probably the most common cause of failed or poor PCR reactions. We mix the four dNTPs together to make a 25-mM stock and freeze this in 125-µL aliquots, which are then used to make up 5-mL batches of 2X buffer. Alternatively, store the working aliquot at 4°C to avoid repeated cycles of freezing and thawing.

10. We strongly recommend using the same, or a very similar, PCR instrument for the primer testing as will be used for the actual quantitative runs. The PCR conditions listed above are a good starting point for all 96-well block PCR instruments. Instruments such as the Roche light cycler, Cepheid Smartcycler, and Corbett Research Rotor-Gene (Corbett Research, Mortlake, NSW, Australia) will require modification of the cycling parameters, in particular the hold times, and users of these instruments should contact their technical assistance representatives for guidelines.

11. When using PCR amplicons smaller than 100 bp, we find that 5% polyacrylamide gels are much more informative than higher percentage agarose. If a polyacrylamide gel apparatus is not available, some newer, high-resolution agarose products, e.g., Amplisize (Bio-Rad), work reasonably well.

12. The 6X dye will separate into two dye fronts: the slower running dye is xylene cyanole (XC), and the faster running dye is bromophenol blue (BPB). Run the gel at approximately 10–20 V/cm to a point at which the BPB dye is almost at the bottom of the gel. On a 5% polyacrylamide TBE gel (29:1, acrylamide/*bis*-acrylamide), the BPB dye corresponds to an approx 50-bp DNA product.

13. For the interpretation of gel-based PCR primer testing, *see* also **Table 3** and **Fig. 3**.

14. Dual-labeled probes can be ordered from a variety of sources (*see* **Table 3** for a partial listing). The choice of fluorescent label and quencher is determined by the instrument optics and personal preference. For most situations and instruments, a simple 6-carboxyfluorescein (FAM)/6-carboxytetramethyl rhodamine (TAMRA) or FAM/BHQ (Biosearch Technologies, Novata, CA) probe works very well. Check with technical support for your instrument to determine the best fluorophore combination for your needs.

15. Some oligomer synthesis companies offer two synthesis methods for dual-labeled probes, 5' NHS ester or 5' dye amidite. The 5' dye amidite probes are considerably cheaper than the N-hydroxysuccinimide (NHS) ester probes and in our hands work just as well.

16. If you see more than a one-cycle difference in C_T value under different primer concentrations, then your assay is going to be somewhat dependent on precise and reproducible setup. In this case, testing different MgCl$_2$ concentrations and annealing temperatures may help reduce the variability. The goal should be to find a primer concentration window (100–200 nM range) in which the C_T values do not change significantly. Similarly, if you see large C_T differences with probe concentration, this may indicate that your probe is not binding efficiently, and rather than increasing probe concentration it is worth trying higher MgCl$_2$ concentrations and/or lower anneal/extend temperatures. Increasing primer and probe concentrations often results in a higher absolute fluorescence at plateau. This may indicate a more robust assay, particularly at very low target concentrations, but we rarely choose the higher probe concentration for this reason alone, because of the increased cost for very little benefit.

17. To get a reasonably accurate estimate of PCR efficiency, it is necessary to have at least five, and preferably, six dilution points on the standard curve. The number of serial dilutions you can do, however, will depend on the expression level of your target gene in the positive control cDNA. Each 3X dilution will result in a C_T increase of approx 1.6 cycles, and points beyond a C_T of 35 cycles are often too variable to be reliable. Therefore, if your positive control cDNA gives a C_T of 30 cycles, you will have to do serial 2X dilutions. Conversely, if the C_T of your positive control cDNA is 20, you could do serial 4X or 5X dilutions. In general, a wider concentration range on the standard curve will give a more accurate estimate of PCR efficiency.

18. Because this experiment does not require that you vary the primer and probe concentrations, we suggest making a master mix of all reagents except the cDNA template. Calculate the number of reactions you need to run, and make enough master mix for that number plus 10% extra.

19. The correlation coefficient (r^2) indicates both the reproducibility of the triplicate reactions and the fit of the data to a straight line. The r^2 value is very important because it gives you an idea of the precision of your PCR efficiency estimate. Even with an r^2 more than 0.995, the error in the estimate of the slope may result in a ±5% error in estimation of the PCR efficiency. With r^2 values less than 0.99, the error is probably ±10% or more.

20. A loss in quantification for the RT can be seen as a constant C_T value, irrespective of the amount of RNA input. If all genes are affected equally, then the relative difference between any two remains unchanged, and the relative quantification method remains valid. If, however, the genes are not affected equally, for example, if the target gene RT plateaus before the endogenous control gene, then an abnormally low expression value will be obtained using the relative quantification approach. Probably the most common reason for a nonquantitative RT is an impure RNA preparation, presumably containing inhibitors of reverse transcription, such as phenol or certain proteins. Although $OD_{260/280}$ readings are only a crude measure of RNA purity, it is safe to say that ratios of less than 1.7 are likely to cause problems in the RT step, and one should consider a secondary purification, preferably one that does not use organic solvents. Ratios of 1.85 or higher generally provide good, quantitative RT, whereas ratios between 1.7 and 1.85 are a somewhat gray zone. Other, less common, reasons for nonquantitative RT include insufficient RT enzyme, primers, nucleotides, $MgCl_2$, or time, improper RT buffer, incorrect thermal protocol, and too much RNA input.

21. If using oligo-dT priming, use a final oligo-dT concentration of 200 nM. If using gene-specific priming, use a final primer concentration of 20–60 nM.

22. RTs extend a double-stranded oligonucleotide from a 5'-3' direction. As such, the synthesis of a cDNA strand from a single-stranded mRNA requires a primer (with DNA better than RNA). Traditionally, three primer systems have been used for this purpose:

    a. The first is hexamer oligonucleotides with random sequences. These primers bind to the RNA randomly and RT all RNA proportionately. The advantages of using this method are several. First, this method RTs ribosomal RNA as well as mRNA, allowing for use of 18S rRNA as the endogenous invariant gene control. Second, it does not require prior planning for the targets of choice for PCR amplification. Lastly, this approach is insensitive to sequence polymorphisms and mutations and can be somewhat beneficial when there is RNA degradation. The main disadvantage to this system is that one is limited to 1–2 µg of total RNA input before the reaction saturates and becomes nonquantitative.

Table 3
Interpreting Gel-Based Primer Testing

Observation	Possible problems	What to try
A. No band of expected size in positive control cDNA	Primers did not work	Check primer sequences were ordered correctly
	PCR reaction not set up correctly	Check reaction setup and calculations; repeat experiment
	Positive control RNA is not expressing target	Choose new positive control
	RT reaction failed	Check positive control gene PCR; if it also failed, repeat RT reactions
B. Product seen in NTC	Contamination of reagents	Repeat experiment using all new reagents; clean pipets and work area thoroughly
C. Specific product of same size as cDNA product seen in genomic DNA PCR reaction (but NTC is clean)	Primer design is not cDNA-specific	Redesign primers according to **Subheading 3.1.** or accept that you have to DNase-treat the samples and always run no-RT controls.
D. Products other than expected size seen in genomic DNA reaction	Nonspecific side reactions occurring	This may not be a major issue if the genomic DNA product bands are weak and the cDNA product is strong; try increasing the anneal/extend temperature to 62 or 64°C; alternatively, proceed to quantitative assays and see whether the genomic background PCR affects PCR efficiency and overall sensitivity (*see* **Subheading 3.5.**)
	Amplification across the intron	If the genomic DNA PCR product size matches the expected size for amplification across the intron, the options are as for **C** above
E. Multiple bands seen in cDNA reactions	Primers not specific	Recheck BLAST search results; try increasing annealing temperature to 62 or 64°C. Try reducing $MgCl_2$ concentration in 0.5 mM increments. Try sequencing the unexpected products to identify what is being amplified. Redesign primers if necessary
	Alternate splicing events	Sequencing the unexpected products may help identify this problem; consider redesigning PCR primers and probes in a different region of the mRNA

(continued on next page)

Table 3
Interpreting Gel-Based Primer Testing *(continued)*

Observation	Possible problems	What to try
F. Products seen in no-RT controls	Contamination of reagents	If this is the case, the no-template controls will also be contaminated; therefore follow instructions for **B** above.
	Genomic DNA contamination of RNA	This should only occur if the genomic DNA reaction is also giving unexpected PCR products (see **D** above for solutions)

b. The second primer system for cDNA synthesis is the use of oligo dT (15–20 base poly-T primer). This binds to the poly A sequence of mRNA and reverse transcribes mRNA from its 3' poly A tail in the 5' direction. The potential advantage of this system is that it can support a larger input of RNA, because it RTs only mRNA, which accounts for 2–5% of the total RNA. Similar to the hexamer method, this approach also allows one to examine any mRNA transcript, as well as evaluate the expression of new genes as they become important at future dates. However, the greatest disadvantage of this approach is that the results can vary based on the quality of the RNA. As more of the RNA is degraded, there are fewer full-length transcripts. Therefore, the evaluation of gene expression using sequences at the 5'-end of the message can be unreliable and even artifactual, especially when the possibility exists that the different samples may have slightly different RNA integrity (as is the case with most clinical samples). The other consideration when using relative quantification is the effect of the target and endogenous control gene sequences distance from the poly A tail. When one of the sequences is closer to the poly A tail, it will be affected to a lesser degree by variations in the RNA quality. Thus, it would be prudent to design all amplicons on the 3'-end of the mRNA template, as well as to verify the quality of the RNA (with gels) prior to the RT. Lastly, the evaluation of amplicons in the 5' end of the longer mRNAs could benefit by choosing an enzyme such as MMLV or its derivatives that generate longer cDNA transcripts.

c. The third and last method utilizes sequence-specific RT primers. Here, RT can be performed using gene-specific primers that are reverse-complemented to a region 3' of the region of interest for PCR. Also, because mRNA is single stranded, only one primer is needed. Owing to the relatively small number of mRNA molecules undergoing RT by this approach, RNA input in excess of 10 μg (dependent on the level of gene expression) can often be used in a single RT reaction using optimized protocols. Additionally, multiplex RT with several gene-specific primers can also be used without a loss in quantification. In using gene-specific primers for RT, the assay designer needs to be mindful of several issues. First, it is beneficial to place the RT primer as close to the PCR amplicon as possible to diminish the effect on RNA degradation in the sample. However, this also implies that regions 3' of the RT primer will not be reversed transcribed and thus cannot be used in the future. Second, it is important to design the assay for performance at higher temperatures that allow for the specific binding of the RT primer. Because RT is performed at 37–55°C, it is important to match the T_m of the RT primer to that of planned RT temperature. The practice of using the reverse PCR primer in the RT should be discouraged, because the high T_m of the PCR primer (~60°C) will result in nonspecific priming during the relatively low-temperature RT. Also, the use of an RT primer that lies external to the PCR amplicon helps overcome any effect the background nonspecific reverse trancription may have on the RT-PCR sensitivity. Third, the benefit of gene-specific RT in its ability to quantitatively RT high amounts of RNA will be lost if 18S rRNA is still used as the invariant endogenous control gene. A gene with lower expression, such as β-glucuronidase, $β_2$-microglobulin, cyclophilin A, or phosphoglycerate kinase 1 will better allow for a high RNA input RT. Fourth, the effect of RNA secondary structure is likely to influence the RT when using this primer method relative to the previously mentioned two methods. Thus validation of the efficiency of the RT-PCR using an RNA dilution standard curve must not be overlooked. Lastly, this method should not be used if there is a possibility that other, as yet undetermined, genes may need to be evaluated in the future from this aliquot.

23. For expression analysis by RT-PCR, the RT must be quantitative, i.e,, more RNA input should result in a proportional increase in cDNA product. The increase in C_T with more RNA input is exponential, i.e., a 2X dilution should give a ΔC_T of one cycle; a 4X dilution should give a ΔC_T of two cycles; an 8X dilution should give a ΔC_T of three cycles, and so on. In practice, one rarely sees data that perfectly fit these theoretical numbers. A difference of 0.8–1.2 cycles is probably acceptable for a two-fold difference in RNA input as long as the ΔC_T between target and control genes remains reasonably stable over the dilution series. If the RT is not quantitative, the concentrations of RT reaction components can be modified to optimize the dynamic range of the reaction. In our experience, the biggest single effect on RT linearity is achieved by increasing the nucleotide concentration. RT efficiency can be improved further by doubling the concentration of enzyme, hexamers, and $MgCl_2$. The RT linearity may have upper and lower limits; this is acceptable as long as experimental assays remain within the linear dynamic range.

24. Most real-time PCR instruments require the user to set a baseline area that is then used to calculate background fluorescence levels. The exact nomenclature and options for setting this baseline vary between manufacturers, but the underlying principles are the same. First, always view the amplification plots using a logarithmic *y*-axis scale. It may look "noisier," but it is easy to miss information when using a linear scale. Second, it is generally a good idea to exclude the first three to five cycles from the background calculation, as there can be some fluctuation in fluorescence levels. Third, and perhaps most importantly, be sure that the cycle range set for the baseline does not include any signal above background (i.e., signal generated as a result of amplification detection). In general, a good way to avoid this problem is to find the reaction with the earliest C_T value and extrapolate the linear portion of the amplification curve down to the *x*-axis. The baseline should not extend past the point that the extrapolated line crosses the *x*-axis. **Figures 4** and **5** show some examples of incorrectly and correctly set baselines using the ABI7700 software.

References

1. Heid, C. A., Stevens, J., Livak, K. J., and Williams, P. M. (1996) Real time quantitative PCR. *Genome Res.* **6,** 986–994.

2. Gibson, U. E., Heid, C. A., and Williams, P. M. (1996) A novel method for real time quantitative RT-PCR. *Genome Res.* **6,** 995–1001.

3. Bustin, S. A. (2000) Absolute quantification of mRNA using real-time reverse transcription polymerase chain reaction assays. *J. Mol. Endocrinol.* **25,** 169–193.

4. Ginzinger, D. G. (2002) Gene quantification using real-time quantitative PCR: an emerging technology hits the mainstream. *Exp. Hematol.* **30,** 503–512.

5. Livak, K. J., Flood, S. J., Marmaro, J., Giusti, W., and Deetz, K. (1995) Oligonucleotides with fluorescent dyes at opposite ends provide a quenched probe system useful for detecting PCR product and nucleic acid hybridization. *PCR Methods Appl.* **4,** 357–362.

6. PE Applied Biosystems (1997) *User Bulletin #2. Relative quantitation of gene expression.* Applied Biosystems, Foster City, CA.

7. Tassone, F., Hagerman, R. J., Taylor, A. K., Gane, L. W., Godfrey, T. E., and Hagerman, P. J. (2000) Elevated levels of FMR1 mRNA in carrier males: a new mechanism of involvement in the fragile-X syndrome. *Am. J. Hum. Genet.* **66,** 6–15.

VII

APOPTOSIS

36

Quantification of Selective Phosphatidylserine Oxidation During Apoptosis

James P. Fabisiak, Yulia Y. Tyurina, Vladimir A. Tyurin, and Valerian E. Kagan

Summary

Membrane phospholipids are gaining increasing attention as important mediators in a variety of signal transduction processes. Oxidation and changes in membrane topography of lipids are probably important elements in the regulation of phospholipid-dependent signaling. Phosphatidylserine (PS), in particular, is implicated in the regulation of macrophage-dependent clearance of apoptotic cell "corpses" in a pathway probably mediated by selective oxidation and translocation of PS in the plasma membrane. Here we describe our highly sensitive and specific assay to measure differential lipid peroxidation in individual phospholipid classes in live cells using metabolic integration of the fluorescent oxidation-sensitive fatty acid analog cis-parinaric acid (cis-PnA) and resolution of specific phospholipids by high-performance liquid chromatography (HPLC). These experimental approaches can provide insight into the roles and mechanisms of PS oxidation in the identification and clearance of apoptotic cells.

Key Words: Lipid peroxidation; phospholipids; phosphatidylserine; cis-parinaric acid (cis-PnA); high-performance liquid chromatography (HPLC); apoptosis; oxidative stress; aminophospholipids; fluorescence.

1. Introduction

Oxidative stress has been implicated as a functional component of the final common pathway of apoptosis execution, but the precise molecular events responsible for redox signaling and their functional consequences remain elusive. Membrane phospholipids are gaining increasing importance in our understanding of cell signaling phenomenon; by virtue of their content of polyunsaturated fatty acids, they are extremely sensitive to modification by low levels of oxidative stress. Thus, oxidation of various membrane phospholipids could play a role in the initiation or regulation of programmed cell death.

To characterize phospholipid oxidation during apoptosis more fully, we utilized cis-parinaric acid (cis-PnA), a naturally derived highly fluorescent fatty acid to label phospholipids metabolically in live cells. The presence of an extensive conjugated

From: *Methods in Molecular Biology, vol. 291, Molecular Toxicology Protocols*
Edited by: P. Keohavong and S. G. Grant © Humana Press Inc., Totowa, NJ

double-bond system in *cis*-PnA renders it highly sensitive to oxidation, with concomitant loss of its intrinsic fluorescence. Thus, comparison of the fluorescent content of various cellular derived phospholipid classes following their resolution by high-performance liquid chromatography (HPLC) can be used to assess site-selective phospholipid oxidation in the presence of various apoptotic stimuli *(1)*. Using 32D cells, we first described the selective oxidation of phosphatidylserine (PS) during paraquat-induced apoptosis *(2)*. Selective oxidation occurred early in the course of apoptosis, preceded PS externalization, and was blocked by overexpression of the antiapoptotic protein BCL-2. Further studies revealed that apoptosis-related PS oxidation was insensitive to vitamin E analogs, suggesting that PS oxidation proceeds via a unique mechanism different from randomly directed chain reactions among membrane lipids *(3)*. More recently, we confirmed that specific PS oxidation occurred in a multitude of cell types following a variety of stimuli, including those not directly associated with the ability to cause oxidative stress, such as Fas/FasL ligation *(4)* and staurosporine *(5)*. Thus, PS oxidation appears to be a nearly universal feature of apoptosis. Although its exact function remains elusive, we hypothesize that it may, in part, regulate PS translocation and/or its recognition by phagocytic macrophage. The utilization of directed oxidation of select phospholipids may represent a previously unappreciated feature of lipid-based signal transduction systems.

We describe here our highly sensitive method to measure oxidation in specific phospholipid classes based on the metabolic incorporation of *cis*-PnA. Its utility arises from the fact that it can report exceedingly low levels of oxidation in live cells, even in the presence of efficient phospholipid repair. We believe that this technique will greatly aid in studying the mechanistic connection between lipid peroxidation and translocation events during apoptosis.

2. Materials

2.1. Preparation of cis-PnA/hSA Complex

1. *cis*-PnA: 9Z, 11E, 13E, 15Z-octadecatetraenoic acid (Molecular Probes, Eugene, OR; *see* **Note 1**).
2. Dimethyl sulfoxide (DMSO; ACS grade or higher; Sigma, St. Louis, MO).
3. Fatty acid-free human serum albumin (hSA; Sigma).
4. Phosphate-buffered saline (PBS; Invitrogen, Gaithersburg , MD).
5. 0.45-μm Filter (e.g., Nalgene™, Nalge Nunc, Rochester, NY).

2.2. Metabolic Labeling of Cells With cis-PnA

1. Cells of interest (*see* **Note 2**).
2. Incubation media (tissue culture media formulation usually used for maintenance of the cell line of interest), without phenol red and fetal bovine serum (e.g., Sigma, Invitrogen, and others).
3. Trypan blue, 0.4% solution (Sigma).
4. Hemocytometer.
5. Tabletop centrifuge (e.g., CRU-5000 Centrit GE, Damon/IEC Division, Needham Heights, MA).
6. 37°C, 5% CO_2 Tissue culture incubator (e.g., Heraeus HERACell CO_2 Incubator, Kendro Lab Products, Newton, CT).

7. 0.5 mg/mL hSA in medium.
8. 15- and 50-mL Polypropylene centrifuge tubes (BD Falcon through Fisher Scientific, Pittsburgh, PA).

2.3. Lipid Extraction

1. PBS.
2. Tabletop centrifuge.
3. Methanol (HPLC grade; Sigma).
4. Butylated hydroxytoluene (ACS grade or higher; Sigma).
5. Chloroform (HPLC grade; Sigma).
6. Evaporation apparatus (e.g., Evap-O-Rac, Cole-Parmer, Chicago, IL).
7. 0.1 *M* NaCl (Sigma).
8. Vortex (e.g., Daigger Vortex Genie 2, Scientific Industries, Bohemia, NY).
9. 4:3:0.16 (v/v/v) Isopropanol/hexane/water (all HPLC grade; Sigma).
10. 13 × 100-mm Pyrex glass test tubes with screw-cap (Fisher).

2.4. HPLC Resolution of Phospholipid Classes

1. Shimadzu LC-600 high-performance liquid chromatograph equipped with in-line fluorescence detector (model RF-551) and UV-VIS detector (model SPD-10AV; Shimadzu, Columbia, MD). Apparatus is interfaced to a PC computer capable of acquiring the UV and fluorescence data in digital form and running Shimadzu EZChrom™ software.
2. 5 μm Supelcosil LC-Si column (Supelco, Bellefonte, PA).
3. 100-μL Glass microsyringe for HPLC sample injection (Hamilton, Reno, NV).
4. Solvent A: 56:42:2 isopropanol/hexane/water (Sigma).
5. Solvent B: 54:41:10 isopropanol/hexane/40 n*M* ammonium acetate (Sigma).
6. Programmable automated gradient maker (low-pressure mixing LPH-600, Shimadzu).
7. Spectrofluorometer (e.g., Shimadzu RF-5301).
8. Spectrophotometer (e.g., Shimadzu UV/VIS 160U).

2.5. Determination of Total Lipid Phosphorus

1. Cell culture disposable glass tubes (Fisher).
2. Evaporation apparatus.
3. $HClO_4$ (Aldrich, Milwaukee, WI).
4. Heating apparatus to achieve 170–180°C. (Troemner 501 hotplate with aluminum block test tube holders, Thorofare, NJ, or equivalent).
5. 4.2% Sodium molybdate (ACS grade or higher; Sigma) in 1:3 5 *M* HCl/0.2% malachite green (ACS grade or higher; Sigma).
6. 1.5% Tween-20 (Sigma).
7. Spectrophotometer.
8. NaH_2PO_4 (Sigma).

2.6. Determination of Inorganic Phosphorus Content of Specific Phospholipid Classes

1. Obtain a set of phospholipid standards: cardiolipin (CL), phosphatidylcholine (PC), phosphatidyl-ethanoloamine (PE), phosphatidylinositol (PS), sphingomyelin, diphosphatidylglycerol, and lysophosphatidylcholine (Avanti Polar Lipids, Alabaster, AL).
2. 5 × 5-cm Whatman silica G thin-layer chromatography plates (Whatman, Clifton, NJ).
3. Chromatography chambers (e.g., 10-cm Latch-Lid Chromatotank, Thomas Scientific, Swedesboro, NJ).

4. 65:25:5 chloroform/methanol/28% ammonium hydroxide (HPLC grade; Sigma).
5. Appropriate "forced air blower" (e.g., Norelco Hair Dryer).
6. 50:20:10:10:5 chloroform/acetone/methanol/glacial acetic acid/water (all HPLC grade; Sigma).
7. Iodine crystals (Sigma).
8. 13 × 100-mm Borosilicate glass tubes (Fisher).
9. 70% Perchloric acid (ACS grade; Sigma).
10. Heating apparatus to achieve 170–180°C and 90–100°C.
11. 2.5% Sodium molybdate (Sigma).
12. 10% Ascorbic acid (Sigma).
13. Tabletop centrifuge.
14. Spectrophotometer.

3. Methods

3.1. Preparation of cis-PnA/hSA Complex

1. Dissolve cis-PnA in DMSO to a final concentration of 20 mg/mL.
2. Add 1.8 µmol *cis*-PnA in 25 µL to 50 mg hSA (760 nmol) in 1 mL of PBS.
3. Incubate this reaction mixture for 30 min at room temperature, then filter (0.45 mm). Aliquot solution, and store frozen at −80°C until use.

3.2. Metabolic Labeling of Cells With cis-PnA

1. Obtain cells from cultures in late log phase growth, and determine cell number and viability using trypan blue exclusion and a hemacytometer.
2. Wash suspension cells twice with centrifugation (400*g*, 10 min) in incubation medium, and then resuspend to a density of 1×10^6/mL. Similarly, rinse monolayer cultures with two changes of incubation medium, and then add 10 mL (for a 75-cm^2 flask) or 3 mL incubation medium (for a 3.5-cm-diameter well of a 6-well plate; *see* **Note 3**).
3. Add *cis*-PnA/hSA complex to a final concentration of 1–5 µg/mL, and incubate for 2 h at 37°C in a tissue culture incubator (*see* **Note 4**).
4. Wash labeled cells once with incubation medium containing 0.5 mg/mL fatty acid-free-hSA, and again without hSA.
5. Resuspend cell pellets or monolayers in a medium appropriate to apply an apoptotic (or other) stimulus, and incubate for desired times prior to lipid extractions (*see* **Notes 5** and **6**).

3.3. Lipid Extraction

1. Obtain approx 1×10^6 cells, wash once in PBS, and resuspend or scrape in 1 mL PBS (*see* **Note 7**).
2. Centrifuge cell suspensions (400*g*, 10 min), resuspend in 3 mL methanol containing 0.1 mg butylated hydroxytoluene, mix with 3 mL chloroform, then place under nitrogen atmosphere on ice in the dark for 1 h. Add 0.1 mL of 0.1 *M* NaCl to each sample, and vortex vigorously.
3. Collect the bottom chloroform layer after separation by centrifugation (1500*g*, 5 min), and evaporate to dryness under oxygen-free N$_2$.
4. Dissolve the resultant lipid film in 0.2 mL 4:3:0.16 (v/v/v) isopropanol/hexane/water.

3.4. HPLC Resolution of Phospholipid Classes

1. Prepare a dilution series of *cis*-PnA solutions for generation of standard curve (1, 2, 4, 6, 8, and 10 ng/100 µL prepared in 4:3:0.16 [v/v/v] isopropanol/hexane/water).

2. Apply a 100-μL sample of lipid extract to the injector port of an HPLC apparatus equipped with a 5-μm Supelcosil LC-Si column (4.6 × 250 mm) equilibrated with 1:9 solvent A: solvent B (*see* **Note 8**).

3. Elute the column using a preprogrammed automated gradient maker for 3 min with a linear gradient from 10% solvent B to 37% solvent B, then 3–15 min with isocratic 37% solvent B, 15–23 min with a linear gradient to 100% solvent B, and finally 23–45 min with isocratic solvent B. Apply the mobile phase at a flow rate of 1 mL/min.

4. Monitor the column effluent simultaneously for *cis*-PnA fluorescence at emission wavelength 420 nm after excitation at 324 nm, as well as absorbance at 205 nm for total lipids (*see* **Note 9** and **Fig. 1**).

5. Determine the *cis*-PnA content of each phospholipid class by calculating the fluorescent peak area using EZChrom software and comparison with the standard curve constructed using various amounts *cis*-PnA alone.

6. Normalize the amount of *cis*-PnA fluorescence in each individual phospholipid class to the amount of inorganic phosphorous (Pi) contained in the total lipid extract (relative PnA oxidation), as well as the Pi content of the individual phospholipid class (specific PnA oxidation) determined from parallel high-performance thin-layer chromatography (HP-TLC) plates (*see* **Subheadings 3.5.** and **3.6.** below).

Figure 1 shows representative chromatograms of *cis*-PnA–labeled phospholipids obtained from control Jurkat cells (top tracing) and cells treated with anti-Fas antibody for 2 h to induce apoptosis (bottom tracing). It is clear that Fas-mediated apoptosis is associated with specific loss of fluorescence in the peak corresponding to PS, while sparing the oxidation of the major phospholipids PE and PC. Significant oxidation of PI was also observed with this nonoxidant stimulus, a finding that mirrors our earlier observation with paraquat-induced apoptosis in 32D cells (*2*). Since both PS and PI are anionic phospholipids, negative charge may, in part, direct the selective oxidation of specific phospholipid species.

3.5. Determination of Total and Specific Lipid Phosphorus

1. Prepare a dilution series of NaH_2PO_4 of four to six concentrations between 1 and 10 nmol to generate a standard curve.

2. Pipet 50-μL aliquots of lipid extracts into test tubes, and evaporate the solvent to dryness under oxygen-free N_2.

3. Add 50 μL of $HClO_4$ to the dried samples, and incubate for 20 min at 170–180°C.

4. Prepare a stock solution of 200 mM NaH_2PO_4 in water. To generate a standard curve, pipet 100, 60, 40, 20, and 10 μL into separate tubes in duplicate, corresponding to 10, 6, 4, 2, and 1 nmol phosphate. Add water to yield a final volume of 4 mL.

5. After allowing the samples to cool, add 0.4 mL of water to each tube followed by 2 mL sodium molybdate-malachite green reagent solution and 80 μL of 1.5% Tween-20.

6. Shake the tubes immediately to stabilize the developed color, and quantify at 660 nm in a spectrophotometer.

7. Determine Pi content by comparison with the linear standard curve. Fluorescence can be normalized to the total amount of lipid phosphorus in each sample for determination of relative content of *cis*-PnA in each phospholipid class.

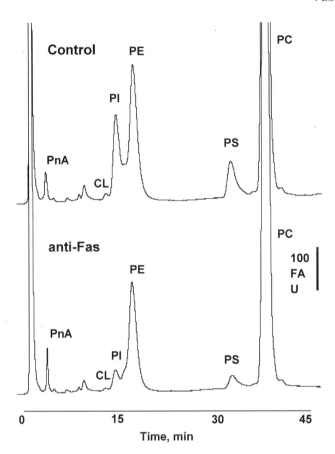

Fig. 1. HPLC chromatograms of *cis*-PnA-labeled phospholipids derived from control (top tracing) and anti-Fas–treated Jurkat cells (bottom tracing). CL, cardiolipin; PC, phosphatidylcholine; PE, phosphatidylethanoloamine; PI, inorganic phosphorus; PnA, parinaric acid; PS, phosphatidylserine.

3.6. Determination of Pi Content of Specific Phospholipid Classes

1. Activate HP-TLC plates by heating for 20 min at 120°C to remove all traces of H_2O.
2. Spot 20-μL aliquots of lipid extracts onto Whatman silica G TLC plates (5 × 5 cm), and allow to air-dry.
3. Spot similar preparations of phospholipid standards for comparison with experimental samples (e.g., 2.5 mg each per phospholipid).
4. Perform 2D HP-TLC by development of the spotted TLC plate(s) in the first dimension using 65:25:5 (v/v/v) chloroform/methanol/28% ammonium hydroxide. After removing the first solvent using a forced air blower, the TLC plate is rotated 90° and developed in the second dimension with 50:20:10:10:5 (v/v/v/v/v) chloroform/acetone/methanol/glacial acetic acid/water.

5. Place the plate in a chromatographic tank containing approx 0.5 g iodine crystals until dark spots corresponding to resolved lipids are observed. The length of time required depends on the age and amount of iodine crystals. Identify specific phospholipid classes by comparison with migration of authentic phospholipid standards (*see* **ref.** *3* for a typical migration pattern of cellular phospholipids). Scrape the spots corresponding to specific phospholipid classes from the plates, and transfer them to 13 × 100-mm borosilicate disposable glass tubes.
6. Add 125 mL of 70% perchloric acid to each silica gel sample, and heat to 175–180°C.
7. After cooling, add 825 μL of H_2O to each tube, followed by 125 μL 2.5% sodium molybdate, followed by 125 μL 10% ascorbic acid. Vortex immediately, and then heat to 90–100°C.
8. After cooling, clarify samples by centrifugation at 1000*g* for 5–10 min, and measure the absorbance of the supernatant at 797 nm. The Pi content of the samples is derived from comparison with the standard curve constructed with known amounts of NaH_2PO_4 (from **Subheading 3.5., step 1**).

4. Notes

1. The purity of each batch of *cis*-PnA is determined by UV spectroscopy using the molar extinction $e_{304\ nm\ (EtOH)} = 80 \times 10^3/mM/cm$.
2. Suspension cells ($7–10 \times 10^5$ cells per mL) or monolayer cells (70–80% confluence) can be used. The number of cells and wells/dishes required depends on the number of desired experimental points. Cell number and viability for monolayer cultures can be obtained after trypsinization of parallel plates or wells set up identically to those for *cis*-PnA assay. Lipids derived from approx 1×10^6 cells provide enough material designated for a single sample subjected to HPLC and fluorescent quantification.
3. We originally utilized L1210 buffer (115 m*M* NaCl, 5 m*M* KCl, 1 m*M* $MgCl_2$, 5 m*M* NaH_2PO_4, 10 m*M* glucose, and 25 m*M* HEPES, pH 7.4) but have found that other medium formulations such as RPMI-1640 and KGM-2 (keratinocyte growth medium) are compatible with incorporation of *cis*-PnA, provided they are utilized in the absence of fetal calf serum and phenol red.
4. It is necessary to derive the appropriate *cis*-PnA concentration empirically for each cell line to achieve maximal metabolic incorporation, while minimizing any potential toxicity of *cis*-PnA.
5. Some knowledge of the time-course and conditions for apoptosis is useful in designing the experiment. We usually restrict our incubations to no more than 2 h. The study of certain stimuli with prolonged induction of apoptosis, such as growth factor withdrawal, may be problematic given the confounding factors of basal spontaneous oxidation of *cis*-PnA and the continuing synthesis of new unlabeled phospholipids. Most stimuli that we have applied have an observable apoptotic response (changes in nuclear morphology, DNA fragmentation) in about 4–8 h and show selective PS oxidation within 2 h.
6. Media formulation may be important, as the presence of serum or other defined growth factors may be required to prevent apoptosis in the control untreated cells. For example, when using the interleukin-3 (IL-3)-dependent cell line 32D, we utilized media containing 10% media preconditioned by WeHi 3B cells as a source of IL-3.
7. Cells can be stored at –80°C at this point until lipid extraction.
8. We have also found a 5-mm (4.5 × 250-mm) Microsorb-MV column from Rainin (Woburn, MA) to be suitable.
9. It is strongly recommended that each laboratory calibrate the migration of specific phospholipid classes using purified authenticated standards.

References

1. Ritov, V. B., Banni, S., Yalowich, J. C., et al. (1996) Non-random peroxidation of different classes of membrane phospholipids in live cells detected by metabolically integrated *cis*-parinaric acid. *Biochim. Biophys. Acta* **1283,** 127–149.
2. Fabisiak, J. P., Kagan, V. E., Ritov, V. B., Johnson, D. E., and Lazo, J. S. (1997) Bcl-2 inhibits selective oxidation and externalization of phosphatidylserine during paraquat-induced apoptosis. *Am. J. Physiol. (Cell Physiol.)* **272,** C675–C684.
3. Fabisiak, J. P., Tyurina, Y. Y., Tyurin, V. A., Lazo, J. S., and Kagan, V. E. (1998) Random versus selective membrane oxidation in apoptosis: role of phosphatidylserine. *Biochemistry* **37,** 13781–13790.
4. Kagan, V. E., Gleiss, B., Tyurina, Y. Y., et al. (2002) A role of oxidative stress in apoptosis: oxidation and externalization of phosphatidylserine is required for macrophage clearance of cells undergoing Fas-mediated apoptosis. *J. Immunol.* **169,** 487–499.
5. Matsura, T., Serinkan, B. F., Jiang, J., and Kagan, V. E. (2002) Phosphatidylserine peroxidation/externalization during staurosporine-induced apoptosis in HL-60 cells. *FEBS Lett.* **524,** 25–30.

37

Quantitative Method of Measuring Phosphatidylserine Externalization During Apoptosis Using Electron Paramagnetic Resonance Spectroscopy and Annexin-Conjugated Iron

James P. Fabisiak, Grigory G. Borisenko, and Valerian E. Kagan

Summary

We present here the application of a novel assay that measures the absolute amount of phosphatidylserine (PS) externalized on the surface of cells. Although the assay is based on the same annexin binding principle as the fluorescent flow cytometry assay, we use paramagnetic iron as the ultimate reporter molecule, establishing a linear relationship between signal amplitude and amount of PS on the cell surface, allowing a quantitative assay of PS externalization over a wide dynamic range. The application of this technique, alone and in concert with the PS oxidation method presented in the previous chapter, will greatly aid in studying the mechanistic connection between lipid peroxidation and translocation events during apoptosis.

Key Words: Phospholipids; phosphatidylserine (PS); annexin V; electron paramagnetic resonance spectroscopy (EPR); apoptosis; oxidative stress; aminophospholipids.

1. Introduction

A characteristic of nearly all normal cells is the maintenance of an asymmetric distribution of phospholipids across cell membranes. Under normal conditions, phosphatidylcholine (PC) and sphingomyelin (SPH) are located primarily in the outer leaflet of plasma membrane, whereas aminophospholipids—phosphatidylethanolamine (PE) and phosphatidylserine (PS)—are found almost entirely in the inner leaflet (1). One of the hallmarks of apoptosis, however, is the translocation and externalization of PS (2), where it serves as a target for recognition and engulfment by phagocytic macrophages (3). Because externalized PS can bind the protein annexin V with high affinity in a Ca^{2+}-dependent manner, the use of fluorescently labeled annexin V has formed the basis for a widely used assay to enumerate apoptotic cells (4). However, this flow cytometric approach provides little information regarding the absolute amounts of PS appearing on the cell surface and does not report any structural modifications to the PS molecule that may be coincident with its externalization.

From: *Methods in Molecular Biology, vol. 291, Molecular Toxicology Protocols*
Edited by: P. Keohavong and S. G. Grant © Humana Press Inc., Totowa, NJ

Although it is clear that profound redistribution of membrane phospholipids accompanies apoptosis, the quantitative aspects of PS externalization have received little attention. The flow cytometric-based assay using the fluorescent-labeled cell-impermeable protein annexin V was designed to assess the number of apoptotic cells with externalized PS rather than quantify the amount of externalized PS available for annexin binding. Another approach involves chemical modification of aminophospholipids with cell-impermeable reagents for primary amines such as fluorescamine or trinitrobenzene sulfonic acid, followed by subsequent chromatographic separation of the modified PS and PE. This approach is time-consuming, lacks sensitivity, and requires ultimate lysis of the target cells. For this reason, we sought to develop a novel sensitive and specific quantitative assay for PS externalization on cell surfaces using annexin V-conjugated iron nanoparticles. These magnetic microbeads have been developed to isolate apoptotic cells physically from a mixed cell population by application of a magnetic field. We, however, exploited the paramagnetic properties of iron in order to quantify annexin V binding using electron paramagnetic resonance (EPR) spectroscopy. We have effectively used this approach to measure PS externalization on normal and apoptotic cells, as well as incorporation of exogenous PS into the plasma membrane. The amount of externalized PS on the surface of normal Jurkat and HL-60 cells is approx 1 pmol/10^6 cells. Treatment of Jurkat and HL-60 cells with camptothecin induces apoptosis with 240 pmol externalized PS/10^6 cells and 30 pmol PS/10^6 cells, respectively. Using naive cells with exogenously applied PS, it appears that only 20–40 pmol PS/10^6 cells is sufficient to trigger recognition and phagocytosis by macrophages.

2. Materials

2.1. Preparation of PS-Containing Liposomes

1. Phospholipids: 1-palmitoyl (C16:0)-2-arachidonyl (C20:4)-3-phosphatidylserine (PS) and phosphatidylcholine from brain (PC; Avanti Lipids, Alabaster, AL).
2. Chloroform (high-performance liquid chromatography [HPLC] grade; Sigma, St. Louis, MO).
3. 13 × 100-mm Borosilicate glass tubes (Fisher Scientific, Chicago, IL; or other appropriate disposable glass tubes).
4. Evaporation apparatus (e.g., Evap-O-Rac, Cole-Parmer, Chicago, IL).
5. Phosphate-buffered saline (PBS; Invitrogen, Gaithersburg, MD).
6. Vortex (e.g., Daigger Vortex Genie 2, Scientific Industries, Bohemia, NY).
7. Sonicator (e.g., Ultrasonic Homogenizer 4710, Cole-Parmer).
8. Microcentrifuge tubes (0.5–2 mL; Corning, Corning, NY).

2.2. Incorporation of PS Into Plasma Membrane

1. Cells of interest.
2. Incubation media: tissue culture media formulation usually used for maintenance of the cell line of interest (Invitrogen or ATCC, Manassas, VA).
3. Trypan blue (Sigma).
4. Hemocytometer.
5. Appropriate centrifuge (e.g. Centrifuge 5415 C, Brinkmann Instruments, Westbury, NY, equipped with Eppendorf tube rotor, ≤ 3000*g*).
6. PBS.

7. *N*-ethylmaleimide (NEM; Sigma).
8. Appropriate means of incubating cells and phospholipids at 37°C (e.g., Heraeus HERACell CO_2 Incubator, Kendro Laboratory Products, Newton, CT or TS-66518 AW-9 heated water bath, Precision Scientific, Chicago, IL).

2.3. HP-TLC Assay for Evaluation of Externalized PS by Labeling With Fluorescamine

1. Labeling buffer: 150 mM NaCl, 5 mM KCl, 1 mM MgCl$_2$, 2 mM CaCl$_2$, 5 mM NaHCO$_3$, 5 mM glucose, 20 mM HEPES, pH 8.0 (all components from Sigma).
2. Fluorescamine (ACS grade or higher; Sigma).
3. 40 mM Tris-HCl, pH 7.4.
4. Bio-Rad Fluor-S MultiImager (Hercules, CA) or other apparatus to allow UV visualization of fluorescamine-labeled PS on high-performance thin-layer liquid chromatography (HP-TLC) plates.

2.4. Annexin V-Microbead EPR Assay for Quantification of Externalized PS

1. Annexin V-microbead apoptosis detection kit and Basic microbeads (Miltenyi Biotech, Auburn, CA).
2. 0.1% Bovine serum albumin (BSA; fraction V, fatty acid-free; Sigma).
3. Gas-permeable Teflon tubing (Alpha Wire, Elizabeth, NJ).
4. Appropriate EPR quartz tube (e.g., Welmad Labglass, Buena, NJ).
5. JEOL RE1X EPR spectrometer (JEOL, Tokyo, Japan).

2.5. Annexin V-FITC Flow Cytometric Assay for Quantification of Cells With Externalized PS

1. Annexin V-microbead apoptosis detection kit and Basic microbeads (Miltenyi Biotech).
2. Propidium iodide (PI; Oncogene, Boston, MA).
3. Annexin V-fluorescein isothiocyanate (FITC; Oncogene).
4. Flow cytometer (e.g., Becton Dickinson FACScan, BD Biosciences, San Jose, CA).

3. Methods

Relative PS externalization on the cell surface can be simply determined by labeling cells with annexin V-microbeads followed by analysis by EPR spectroscopy. To establish the absolute amounts of PS$_{ext}$, however, one needs to prepare cells with known amounts of PS$_{ext}$ on their surface and calibrate the resultant EPR signal of annexin V-microbeads. To this end, cells are coincubated with PC/PS liposomes to incorporate various amounts of PS into the plasma membrane. To ensure that all exogenous PS remains on the cell surface, the cells are pretreated with NEM, a thiol-specific reagent shown to poison the PS-internalizing activity of aminophospholipid translocase metabolically *(5)*. PS-enriched cells are then analyzed by both EPR-based annexin–iron bead assay and by HP-TLC assay of surface PS derivatized with fluorescamine to create a calibration curve of EPR signal vs amount of PS$_{ext}$. Finally, the traditional annexin V-FITC flow cytometry assay can be applied for discriminating and quantifying cells with high and low levels of externalized PS, so that the amount of PS$_{ext}$ obtained by EPR-based assay can be recalculated per number of cells that externalize high levels of PS.

3.1. Preparation of PS-Containing Liposomes (see Note 1)

1. Dissolve purified phospholipids (PC and PS) in chloroform (100 mM final concentration). Frozen stocks can stored at $-80°C$ for at least 2 mo.
2. Make small unilamellar liposomes by making a 1:1 mix of the PC and PS stocks in a glass tube by adding 2.52 µmol (25.2 µL) of each phospholipid stock (2.4 µmol are required for analysis of fluorescamine-labeled PS by HP-TLC, and 0.12 µmol are required for EPR assay).
3. Evaporate chloroform from the liposome preparations under a stream of compressed nitrogen.
4. Add 5.0 mL PBS for a final concentration of 1 mM total lipids, and then mix the lipid mixture by vortexing vigorously (*see* **Note 2**).
5. Sonicate liposomes five times for 30 s on ice using a microtip and 20% output.
6. Prepare aliquots of liposomes in the following concentrations: 1 mM, 750 µM, 500 µM, 250 µM, 125 µM. (Concentrations in aliquots are fivefold greater than final concentration in solution with cells.) The total volume of each aliquot should be at least 1.68 mL (1.6 mL for HP-TLC and 0.08 mL for the EPR assay; *see* **Note 3**).

3.2. Incorporation of PS Into Plasma Membrane

1. Obtain cells from cultures in late log phase growth, and determine cell number and viability using trypan blue exclusion and a hemacytometer.
2. Wash suspension cells or harvested monolayer culture cells (method appropriate to cell type) twice with centrifugation (1000g) in incubation medium, and then resuspend in PBS at a density of 6.25×10^6 cells/mL The number of cells required for one series of measurements for a complete calibration curve is 252×10^6 cells (249×10^6 for HP-TLC and 12×10^6 for the EPR assay (*see* **Note 4**).
3. Treat cells with 10–50 µM NEM for 5 min at 37°C to inhibit aminophospholipid translocase activity (*see* **Note 5**).
4. To incorporate phospholipids into plasma membrane of cells, incubate cells with the indicated amounts (25, 50, 100, 150, and 200 µM) of the PS-containing liposomes (4 parts of cell solution to 1 part liposomes, prepared as described in **Subheading 3.1.**, **step 6**) for 30 min at 37°C. Sample volume for each experimental point is 8.4 mL (8 mL for HP-TLC and 0.4 mL for the EPR assay).
5. Remove unincorporated liposomes by washing cells twice with 1 mL PBS and centrifugation for 1000g for 5 min.

3.3. HP-TLC Assay for Evaluation of Externalized PS by Labeling With Fluorescamine

1. Resuspend 4×10^7 cells in 2 mL labeling buffer. Add 2 µL of 200 mM fluorescamine dissolved in dimethylsulfoxide (DMSO) to a final concentration of 200 µM, and agitate cells gently for 15 s. Add 3 mL of 40 mM Tris-HCl, pH 7.4.
2. Centrifuge cells (1000g for 5 min), and extract lipids (*see* Chap. 36, Subheading 3.3., steps 2–4).
3. Separate specific phospholipid classes using HP-TLC (*see* Chap. 36, Subheading 3.4.).
4. Localize fluorescamine-modified PS (mPS) on an HP-TLC plate by exposure to UV light using a Fluor-S MultiImager. Unmodified phospholipids can be localized by visible light after exposure of HP-TLC plates to iodine vapor (*see* Chap. 36, Subheading 3.4.). The identities of specific phospholipid species are determined by comparison with purified standards.

5. Determine the inorganic phosphorus (Pi) content of the externalized and nonexternalized PS (*see* Chap. 36, Subheadings 3.5. and 3.6.).

3.4. Annexin V-Microbead EPR Assay for Quantification of Externalized PS

1. Obtain cells from cultures in late log phase growth, and determine cell number and viability using trypan blue exclusion and a hemacytometer.
2. Wash suspension cells or harvested monolayer culture cells (method appropriate to cell type) twice with centrifugation ($1000g$) in incubation medium, and then wash 2×10^6 cells twice in 1 mL 1X Binding Buffer (from the annexin V-microbead kit).
3. Resuspend cells in 40 µL of Binding Buffer, and incubate with 10 µL of annexin V-microbead solution or equivalent amount of Basic beads for 5 min (*see* **Note 6**).
4. Wash cells twice with 1 mL Binding Buffer ($1000g$ for 5 min) to remove unbound annexin V-microbeads, and resuspend in 50 µL of Binding Buffer for EPR assay (*see* **Note 7**).
5. EPR measurements can be performed in gas-permeable Teflon tubing. Fill the tube with 50 µL of sample, and place in an EPR quartz tube and then in an EPR resonator (*see* **Note 8**).
6. Determine the amplitude of the PS-specific EPR signal as the difference between the EPR signals from annexin V-microbeads and Basic beads (**Fig. 1**).
7. Construct a calibration curve of PS-specific EPR signal amplitude vs Pi from fluorescamine-modified PS to find the relationship between EPR signal amplitude and amount of PS on cell surface (**Fig. 2**).

Figure 1 shows the EPR spectra from Jurkat cells labeled with annexin V-microbeads or Basic microbeads without annexin. **Figure 1A** represents untreated cells; **Fig. 1B** represents cells preincubated with PC/PS liposomes (0.3 mM phospholipids to saturate external membrane leaflet with PS); and **Fig. 1C** represents cells treated with camptothecin (50 mM) for 3 h to induce apoptosis. Cells then were labeled with annexin V-beads (thin line). Parallel samples were also incubated with Basic beads (bold line) to control for nonspecific binding of iron microbeads. EPR spectroscopy was performed on 2×10^6 cells/sample. EPR spectra of paramagentic iron from microbeads were recorded as described in **Note 8**.

Figure 2 shows the positive correlation between the PS-specific EPR signal amplitude and the fluorescamine-modified PS amount from Jurkat cells. PS was incorporated into the external bilayer of the plasma membrane by coincubation with liposomes prepared as described in **Subheading 3.2.** Note the linear relationship between the amount of PS incorporated on the surface of cells as measured by fluorescamine modification and the amount detected by binding of paramagnetic iron/annexin V microbeads.

3.5. Annexin V-FITC Flow Cytometric Assay for Quantification of Cells With Externalized PS

1. Centrifuge 0.5×10^6 cells at $1000g$ for 5 min, and resuspend in 1 mL of Binding Buffer.
2. Incubate the cell suspension with annexin V-FITC (1 µg/mL final concentration) and PI (5 µg/mL) in the dark for 5 min at room temperature.
3. Analyze labeled cell samples by flow cytometry. Gate out low fluorescent debris and necrotic cells prior to analysis (*see* **Note 9**). Collect 10,000 "events" (or "cell equivalents") per sample to analyze the annexin V-FITC–positive and PI-negative populations, which represent the apoptotic cells expressing PS on the external cell surface.

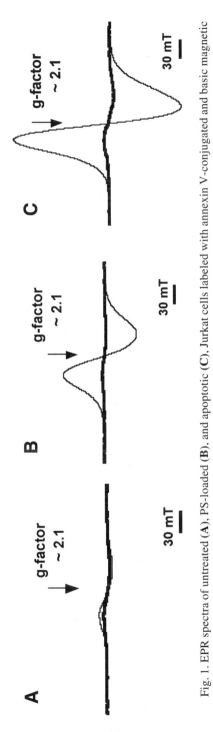

Fig. 1. EPR spectra of untreated (**A**), PS-loaded (**B**), and apoptotic (**C**), Jurkat cells labeled with annexin V-conjugated and basic magnetic microbeads.

462

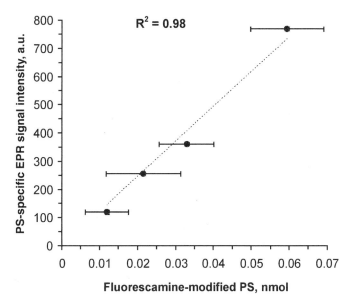

Fig. 2. Linear relationship between amount of external PS incorporated into plasma membrane and EPR signal measured with annexin V-magnetic microbeads in Jurkat cells.

4. Recalculate the amount of externalized PS obtained by the EPR-based assay per number of annexin V-FITC–positive cells based on the cytometric analysis.

4. Notes

1. Volumes and amounts given for the preparation of liposomes and incorporation into cells correspond to those necessary to construct a 6-point standard curve comparing EPR signal intensity and externalized PS measured by fluorescamine. Over 90% of the required liposomes are necessary for the fluorescamine determination by HP-TLC, and hence volumes of reagents can be significantly reduced after the relationship between EPR signal and lipid content is determined in the investigator's own laboratory. Once this standard curve is obtained, analysis of experimental samples can proceed by comparison with liposome-loaded cells measured by EPR alone.

2. During liposome preparation, make sure that all dry phospholipids are moved into the water phase.

3. Solutions of small unilamellar liposomes are translucent compared with a cloudy suspension characteristic of multilamellar liposomes. The PS-containing liposomes should be used immediately after preparation to avoid their oxidation.

4. Precautions should be taken to preserve cell viability during this assay, because the presence of endogenous externalized PS from apoptotic/necrotic cells will bias the standard curve. In addition, the EPR signal from nonspecific Basic beads alone is negatively correlated with the number of necrotic cells, suggesting that nonspecific binding of iron microbeads is increased in dead or dying cells. Cell viability can be ascertained using trypan blue exclusion before and after liposome incorporation and should be 95% or greater.

5. The optimum concentration of NEM for effective inhibition of aminophospholipid translocase should be determined empirically for each cell line using the NBD-PS internalization assay described in detail by McIntyre and Sleight *(6)*.

6. Before use, the annexin V-microbeads supplied with the kit should be washed on the magnetic column with 0.1% BSA solution to remove sodium azide and unbound annexin V as follows. Place separation column in the magnet for separation. Apply 0.5 mL of BSA solution on top of the column, and let the solution run through (do not let the column dry). Then apply microbeads solution (not more than 0.5 mL) onto the column, and allow the solution to flow through. Wash column twice with BSA solution. To remove microbeads from the column, add a volume of BSA solution equal to that originally applied to column. Immediately remove column from the magnet and flush out microbeads into the collection tube using the plunger. The volume of microbead solution collected, as well as the EPR signal intensity from the solution, should be equal to that of the initial solution of microbeads.

7. Do not keep cells on ice after labeling with annexin V-microbeads. This may cause precipitation of microbeads and lead to erroneous results. For best results, utilize annexin V-microbeads and Basic microbeads kits within 6 mo because nonspecific binding of annexin V-microbeads and Basic microbeads increases over time.

8. EPR spectra are recorded at room temperature under the following settings: 10 mW microwave power; 9.445 GHz microwave frequency; 300 mT center field; 150 mT sweep width; 2 mT field modulation; ×100 – ×1000 gain range; 0.3 s time constant; 1 min time scan.

9. First, use forward scattering (FSC) and side scattering (SSC) corrections to gate out cell debris, which have significantly lower FSC and SSC signals than live cells. Then set channel FL1 (530/30-nm bandpass filter) to collect annexin V-FITC fluorescence signal and channel FL3 (>650-nm long-pass filter) to collect PI fluorescence. Use untreated cells that possess nominal FL1 and FL3 signals to set threshold on channel FL1 for cells not expressing PS on the surface (annexin V-FITC–negative cells) and threshold on Fl3 for live cells (PI-negative cells). Collect 10,000 events per sample of cells of interest. Annexin V- and PI-positive cells can be arbitrarily defined as events that possess 50-fold greater signal intensity than the modal intensity of Fl1 and Fl3 channels, respectively, observed in a negative control viable nonapoptotic cell population.

References

1. Op Den Kamp, J. A. F. (1979) Lipid asymmetry in membranes. *Ann. Rev. Biochem.* **48**, 47–71.

2. Martin, S. J., Reutelingsperger, C. P. M., McGahon, A. J., et al. (1995) Early redistribution of plasma membrane phosphatidylserine is a general feature of apoptosis regardless of the initiating stimulus: inhibition by overexpression of Bcl-2 and Abl. *J. Exp. Med.* **182**, 1545–1556.

3. Fadok, V. A., Bratton, D. L., Frasch, S. C., Warner, M. L., and Henson, P. M. (1998) The role of phosphatidylserine in recognition of apoptotic cells by phagocytes. *Cell Death Differ.* **5**, 551–562.

4. Vermes, I., Haanen, C., Steffens-Nakken, H., and Reutelingsperger, C. A. (1995) A novel assay for apoptosis. Flow cytometric detection of phosphatidylserine expression on early apoptotic cells using fluorescein labelled Annexin V. *Immunol. Methods* **184**, 39–51.

5. Kagan, V. E., Gleiss, B., Tyurina, Y. Y., et al. (2002) A role of oxidative stress in apoptosis: oxidation and externalization of phosphatidylserine is required for macrophage clearance of cells undergoing Fas-mediated apoptosis. *J. Immunol.* **169**, 487–499.

6. McIntyre, J. C. and Sleight, R. G. (1991) Fluorescence assay for phospholipid membrane asymmetry. *Biochemistry* **30**, 11819–11827.

38

Detection of Programmed Cell Death in Cells Exposed to Genotoxic Agents Using a Caspase Activation Assay

Michael E. Gehring and Patrick P. Koty

Summary

Many environmental toxins cause DNA damage. Cells that have sustained significant DNA damage must attempt to repair the damage prior to replication, in which aberrant base incorporation can result in an irreversible mutation. If a cell cannot repair the damage, however, it may commit suicide through a genetically regulated programmed cell death (PCD) pathway. Crucial to the ultimate execution of PCD is a family of cysteine proteases called caspases. Activation of these enzymes occurs late in the PCD pathway, when a cell can no longer avoid cell death, but earlier than other PCD markers, such as morphological changes or DNA fragmentation. This protocol details a method for using fluorochrome-conjugated caspase inhibitors for the detection of activated caspases in intact cells using fluorescent microscopy.

Key Words: Apoptosis; programmed cell death (PCD); caspase; caspase inhibitor; fluorescence DNA damage; genotoxic agent.

1. Introduction

Every day we are exposed to a variety of toxic environmental and occupational agents. Some are inhaled, such as particulate toxins including asbestos and diesel exhaust, which generate reactive oxygen species that can damage the body (*1*), and some are ingested in over-the-counter remedies such as toremifene or doxycycline (*2*). Most toxins that are known or suspected carcinogens are genotoxic, meaning they directly damage DNA (*3*), even at low doses (*4*). Normally, the cell repairs such damage prior to DNA replication, but when it cannot adequately repair the damage, the cell is genetically programmed to halt replication and commit suicide. This outcome arises through a regulated pathway(s) called programmed cell death (PCD).

PCD is often associated with distinct morphological changes that distinguish it from a necrotic death. Necrosis typically involves many cells and occurs in response to a severe insult to the cell, such as cytotoxicity, hypoxia, or depletion of ATP. These severe conditions result in the dramatic release of the cellular contents into the inter-cellular space, causing an inflammatory response. PCD, on the other hand, signals a

From: *Methods in Molecular Biology, vol. 291, Molecular Toxicology Protocols*
Edited by: P. Keohavong and S. G. Grant © Humana Press Inc., Totowa, NJ

single damaged cell to enter a series of genetically regulated steps that culminate in the removal of the cell without releasing the cytoplasmic contents, thus avoiding any inflammatory response. During this process, the chromatin condenses and is subsequently digested into fragments in an organized manner, unlike necrosis, in which the DNA is digested in an apparently random pattern. The surface of the cell then retracts, breaking cell contact with its neighbors, followed by cellular blebbing. The cellular contents, including the now fragmented genome, are sequestered into small "apoptotic bodies," which are then phagocytosed by neighboring cells or macrophages and finally digested (for review, *see* **ref. 5**).

Maintaining normal genetic regulation of PCD is crucial for an organism's fitness and survival. Any change in the rate of PCD in either direction, even subtle changes, can manifest as a life-threatening disease. Excessive PCD contributes to several human diseases, including the neurodegenerative diseases named for Parkinson *(6)* and Alzheimer *(7)*. Decreased rates of PCD, on the other hand, are observed in diseases such as autoimmune diabetes, local self-reactive disorder, and cancer (for review, *see* **ref. 8**). Although some individuals inherit a higher susceptibility to these disorders, most are theorized to arise from a lifetime of exposure to a variety of known and unknown toxins.

There are two major pathways of PCD, which are usually distinct but may have overlapping signals. One pathway is regulated through receptors on the plasma membrane known as *death receptors* and include the tumor necrosis factor receptor (TNFR) family, such as Fas, TNFR1, DR3/WSL and TNF-related apoptosis-inducing ligand (TRAIL)/Apo-2L (for review, *see* **ref. 9**). These receptors respond to ligands presented by other cells or to toxins that mimic these ligands. The absence of a ligand, in particular growth factors, can also trigger a PCD signal of this type. When a PCD signal occurs in a receptor-based PCD pathway, the death receptor forms a death-inducing signal complex (DISC), which in turn activates additional downstream signals. The other major PCD pathway is mediated by the mitochondria and can be triggered by the inability to repair DNA damage caused by ionizing radiation or genotoxic effects, metabolic or cell cycle perturbation, or free radicals (for review, *see* **ref. 9**). This pathway is partially regulated through homo- and heterodimerization of PCD inducers, such as Bax and Bid, and inhibitors, such as Bcl-2 and Bcl-xL. These proteins are sequestered to the outer mitochondrial membrane and control the intracellular regulation of cytochrome *c* (for review, *see* **ref. 5**). Homodimerization of PCD inhibitors prevents the release of cytochrome *c*, whereas heterodimerization of PCD inducers with PCD inhibitors allows the release of cytochrome *c* from the mitochondria into the cytosol, irreversibly committing the cell to the PCD pathway *(10–13)*. Regardless of whether a receptor- or mitochondrial-based pathway is initiated, both involve the activation of a family of proteins called caspases that results in the morphological and physiological changes characteristic of PCD, including DNA fragmentation, surface blebbing, and the eventual formation of apoptotic bodies (for review, *see* **ref. 9**).

Caspases are a family of highly conserved enzymes that are expressed in organisms from worms to humans. There are currently 14 known mammalian caspases, 8 of which have been shown to be crucial in human PCD pathways. Caspases are catalytically inactive cysteine proteases that are cleaved to reveal a recognition sequence, producing a proteolytically active protein. These enzymes are functionally categorized as initiators, which include caspases-2, -8, -9, and -10, and effectors, which include caspases-3, -6, and -7. Initiators are characterized by a large prodomain (>90 residues), which is important to their function after undergoing autocleavage. Effectors, on the other hand, have small prodomains, between 20 and 30 residues, which are not required for the active protein to function. Each caspase contains a unique four-residue recognition sequence, which is used to specifically target substrates particular for the given caspase. Currently, a wide range of synthetic substrates have been developed that use these recognition sequences to target and covalently bind to the caspase proteins, permanently inactivating them. Given the unique nature of the recognition sequences, inhibitor substrates can target individual caspases, or they may target broad groups of caspases, using a binding sequence compatible with multiple caspases (for review, *see* **refs. *13*** and ***14***).

Clearly, caspases are a critical, if not essential, feature of the PCD pathway and appear to serve as a point of convergence of the PCD signal transduction pathways necessary for the execution of death. For this reason, the activation of caspases is a very good marker for PCD induction. Caspase activation detection also has advantages over other assays for PCD induction, such as cell viability or DNA fragmentation, since it detects events earlier in the PCD pathway and does not overlap with necrosis. Detecting morphological changes associated with PCD, which, if they do occur, are typically late events during PCD, is usually labor-intensive and limited to analyzing a small number of cells. On the other hand, caspase activation analysis can detect most cells undergoing PCD and can utilize flow cytometry, fluorescent spectrophotometry, or microscopy in which large numbers of cells can be easily and accurately assayed (for review, *see* **ref. *15***).

Caspase activation can be detected using either cellular lysates or intact cells. Cell lysates can be used to detect pro- or cleaved-caspases or their cleaved substrates using Western blot analysis. Quantification of caspase activation can also be performed on cell lysates using caspase substrates that are conjugated to chromophores or fluorochromes and detected spectrophotometrically on a microplate reader (for review, *see* **ref. *15***). Although assays using cell lysates can easily process a large number of cells, their limitations include antibody nonspecificity, inability to determine the number of cells undergoing PCD, and difficulty in identifying specific activated caspases owing to overlapping substrates. Intact cells can be analyzed using immunogenic staining against active caspases, conjugated-substrate cleavage, or fluorescent inhibitors that target either specific or nonspecific (pan) caspase active sites (*16*). Although there are some disadvantages to using intact cells, such as the inability to determine the amount of caspase activation within a specific cell or the potential of nonspecificity of antibodies, the advantages far outweigh these limitations. Using these assays for intact cells, the exact number of cells undergoing PCD can be determined at a given timepoint, small to large cell numbers can be easily analyzed, and analysis can utilize either a fluorescence or laser confocal microscope or a flow cytometer. For a more complete analysis of cells undergoing PCD, the use of fluorescent-conjugated inhibitors of activated caspases (an early PCD event) can be combined with nuclear staining to detect morphological changes (apoptotic bodies, a late PCD event) and analyzed simultaneously using darkfield microscopy.

The following protocol describes how to detect simultaneously caspase activation (using a pan or specific fluorescent-conjugated caspase inhibitor) and morphological changes associated with the induction of PCD using darkfield microscopy.

2. Materials

2.1. Cell Culturing and Genotoxic Exposure

1. Sterile 24-well tissue culture plates (*see* **Note 1**).
2. Sterile medium with supplements appropriate for cells of choice (e.g., RPMI-1640 supplemented with fetal bovine serum [FBS]).
3. Genotoxic agent to be tested.

2.2. Solutions

1. Caspase detection kit (e.g., Carboxyfluorescein Caspase Detection Kit, Cell Technology, Minneapolis, MN, or CaspaTag Kit, Intergen Company, Norcross, GA; *see* **Note 2**), which contains:
   a. Lyophilized carboxyfluorescein-benzyloxycarbonyl-valyl–alanyl-aspartic acid-fluoromethyl ketone (FAM-VAD-FMK) pan-caspase inhibitor (light-sensitive; store in the dark).
   b. Hoechst 33342 stain stock solution (200 μg/mL). **Caution:** possible mutagen, handle with care, using gloves and a mask.
   c. 10X Wash buffer. **Caution:** contains sodium azide, which is harmful if absorbed through skin; handle with care, using gloves (*see* **Note 3**).
   d. 10X Fixative solution. **Caution:** contains paraformaldehyde, which is toxic; handle with care, using gloves and a mask.
   e. Store kit at 4°C.
2. Sterile dimethylsulfoxide (DMSO). **Caution:** DMSO is toxic. Handle with care, using gloves and a mask.
3. Sterile cell culture grade 1X phosphate-buffered saline (PBS): 1.06 mM KH_2PO_4, 154 mM NaCl, 2.71 mM Na_2PO_4, pH 7.4.
4. Sterile deionized water.

2.3. Cell Labeling and Counterstaining

1. Sterile small-bore transfer pipets.
2. Sterile serum-free tissue culture medium appropriate for cell type of interest (e.g., RPMI-1640).
3. Hoechst 33342 stain stock solution (200 μg/mL; included in kit).
4. Sterile 15-mL polypropylene conical centrifuge tubes.

2.4. Cell Trypsinization and Fixation

1. Sterile cell culture grade 1X trypsin-EDTA: 0.05% trypsin, 0.53 mM EDTA.
2. FBS-enriched medium appropriate for cell type of interest (10–25% FBS, depending on cell type).
3. Sterile small-bore transfer pipets.
4. Lint- and dye-free tissues (e.g., Kimwipes, Merk, Roswell, GA).
5. 10X stock fixative (included in kit).

2.5. Microscopic Slide Preparation

1. Glass microscope slides, precleaned, untreated, $25 \times 75 \times 1$ mm.
2. Sterile 1X PBS.
3. Mounting medium (e.g., Cytoseal 60, Stephens Scientific, Kalamazoo, MI).
4. Glass cover slips, $25 \times 50 \times 1$ mm.
5. Coplin jar.

2.6. Fluorescence Microscopy Analysis

1. Fluorescence microscope with suitable light source (e.g., mercury or xenon arc lamp) and 35-mm or CCD camera for documentation.
2. Filter cubes compatible with carboxyfluorescein (e.g., bandpass filter, excitation 490 nm, emission 520 nm) and Hoechst 33342 staining (e.g., UV filter, excitation 365 nm, emission 480 nm; *see* **Note 4**).

3. Methods

3.1. Cell Culturing and Genotoxic Exposure

1. Seed an appropriate number of cells into a sterile 24-well tissue culture plate. Allow cells to adhere and grow for 24 h (*see* **Note 5**).
2. Expose cells to the genotoxic agent for the desired time-points according to your specific protocol.

3.2. Solutions (see Note 6)

1. Reconstitute lyophilized FAM-VAD-FMK inhibitor in 50 µL sterile DMSO (150X stock solution). The chemical is light-sensitive, so work in the dark. Mix well by gently swirling the bottle until inhibitor is completely dissolved (*see* **Note 7**).
2. Prepare an appropriate amount of 30X FAM-VAD-FMK inhibitor working solution by adding 4 parts sterile 1X PBS to 1 part 150X FAM-VAD-FMK inhibitor stock solution (*see* **Note 8**).
3. Prepare an appropriate amount (approx 4.5 mL/well for 24-well tissue culture plates) of 1X working wash buffer by diluting 10X stock wash buffer in a 1:10 ratio with deionized water (*see* **Note 9**).
4. Prewarm 1X working wash buffer at 37°C until use.
5. Prepare 1X FAM-VAD-FMK inhibitor solution by mixing 10 µL 30X FAM-VAD-FMK inhibitor working solution with 300 µL serum-free medium (310 µL of 1X FAM-VAD-FMK inhibitor/medium solution/well for 24-well tissue culture plates).

3.3. Cell Labeling and Counterstaining

1. Carefully remove the medium after genotoxic exposure, using a small-bore pipet so as not to collect detached cells, and discard medium (*see* **Note 10**).
2. Add 310 µL 1X FAM-VAD-FMK inhibitor/serum-free medium solution to each well. Incubate for 1 h at 37°C in a humidified atmosphere with 5% CO_2.
3. Add 1.5 µL Hoechst 33342 stock stain solution to each well, mix well by gently swirling plate, and incubate for 5 min at 37°C in a humidified atmosphere with 5% CO_2 (*see* **Note 11**).
4. Carefully remove the medium from each well using a small-bore pipet, and save in a labeled sterile 15-mL conical centrifuge tube.

3.4. Cell Trypsinization and Fixation

1. Add 0.5 mL of 0.5X trypsin-EDTA to each well, and incubate for 5 min at 37°C in a humidified atmosphere with 5% CO_2 (*see* **Note 12**).
2. Ensure that all cells are detached (*see* **Note 13**). Using a small-bore pipet, transfer cells to the 15-mL conical tube containing the previously removed medium.
3. Add 1 mL of FBS-enriched medium to each well, swirl plates gently to collect remaining cells in solution, and transfer medium to a 15-mL conical tube containing the previously removed medium and trypsin solution. Discard plates (*see* **Note 14**).
4. Centrifuge (100*g*) for 5 min at room temperature.
5. Carefully remove and discard the supernatant. Gently resuspend the cell pellet in 2 mL of 1X wash buffer.
6. Centrifuge (100*g*) for 5 min at room temperature.
7. Repeat **steps 5** and **6**.
8. Carefully remove and discard the supernatant. Briefly drain the tubes by inversion on a lint- and dye-free tissue to ensure that any remaining wash buffer has been removed, but do not allow the cells to dry out (*see* **Note 15**). Gently resuspend the pellet by pipeting in 100 µL of 1X wash buffer.
9. Add 10 µL of 10X stock fixative solution to each tube. Mix by gently swirling tubes and incubate for 15 min at room temperature.

3.5. Microscopic Slide Preparation (see Note 16)

1. Pipet cells in the wash buffer/fixative solution (110 µL) onto microscopic slides appropriately labeled and spread evenly, avoiding creating bubbles (*see* **Note 17**).
2. Dry slides on a flat surface (approx 30 min to 1 h), checking periodically to ensure even solution distribution (*see* **Note 18**).
3. Carefully wash cells once in 50 mL 1X PBS in a Coplin jar for 5 min.
4. Drain off excess liquid, and allow slides to air-dry briefly (2–3 min).
5. Add 3 drops of mounting medium, and place on a cover slip, trying to avoid bubbles. Allow slides to dry overnight in the dark at room temperature.

3.6. Fluorescence Microscopy Analysis

1. Analyze the slides using a fluorescent microscope with the appropriate bandpass and UV filters to observe caspase activation (either green or red, depending on which fluorescently labeled substrate is used) and Hoechst 33342 stain (blue). Cells should be analyzed on the basis of presence of caspase signal and presence of apoptotic bodies, as apparent from counterstaining. Although the number of cells needed to be analyzed will differ, depending on individual goals, counts of at least 500 cells per condition should be used to obtain reasonable power in statistical analysis (*see* **Note 19**).

4. Notes

1. Alternative tissue culture plates (i.e., 96-well or 12-well) or microscopic chamber slides can be used. However, reaction volumes must be adjusted accordingly.
2. Although we typically use a pan-caspase peptide inhibitor, specific peptide inhibitors for caspases-1, -2, -3, -6, -8, -9, and -10 are available and compatible with this protocol. In addition, caspase-3 and pan-caspase peptides conjugated to sulforhodamine (SR) are commercially available (Sulforhodamine Caspase Detection Kit, Cell Technology; CaspaTag Kit, Intergen Company).

3. **Caution:** sodium azide can react with lead- and copper-containing sink drains, forming explosive compounds. Use large volumes of water when disposing of excess wash buffer down the sink drain.

4. The SR-conjugated peptides require a filter cube with an excitation of 550 nm and emission of 595 nm (e.g., DAPI/FITC/Texas Red triple filter, Chroma Technology, Battleboro, VT).

5. Confluent growth may prevent exposure of some cells to the peptide inhibitor, resulting in uneven staining and inaccurate analysis. If one is using nonadherent cells, this protocol may be carried out in tubes rather than plates with a cell density of 10^6 cells/mL.

6. The FAM and SR fluorescent-conjugated peptide inhibitors and Hoechst 33342 are extremely sensitive to light. Avoid direct exposure to light, as this will result in photobleaching. All sample processing, incubations, and microscopic analysis should be performed in the dark.

7. Any unused 150X FAM-VAD-FMK inhibitor stock solution should be aliquoted into appropriate volumes, stored in the dark, and desiccated at –20°C. Repeated freeze-thaw of the 150X FAM-VAD-FMK inhibitor stock solution will result in substrate degradation.

8. Only prepare enough 30X FAM-VAD-FMK inhibitor working solution for the number of wells to be analyzed. A 30X FAM-VAD-FMK inhibitor working solution cannot be stored, and any remaining unused 30 X FAM-VAD-FMK inhibitor working solution must be discarded.

9. A precipitate may form in the 10X stock wash buffer when it is stored at 4°C. Therefore, incubate the 10X stock wash buffer at 37°C for 30 min prior to use, or until precipitation is completely dissolved.

10. If detached cells are collected in the medium, the medium can be centrifuged (100g) and the supernatant discarded. The cell pellet can then be resuspended in the 310 µL 1X FAM-VAD-FMK inhibitor/serum-free medium solution from the appropriate wells from **Subheading 3.3.**, **step 4** and added back to the appropriate well. Recovering these detached cells is important, since many may be undergoing PCD.

11. Proper mixing after the addition of the Hoechst 33342 stain is critical for even fluorescence of the entire cell population.

12. Incubation in trypsin may be increased from 5 to 10 min if necessary to detach all adherent cells.

13. Tap plates gently but firmly against the palm to knock cells loose. Visual inspection is preferable, because light microscopy will cause photobleaching of the cells. However, because analysis of all cells is critical, inspection using an inverted light microscope may be necessary, although exposure to light should be minimized.

14. The use of FBS-enriched medium is necessary to stop the trypsin activity.

15. Removing any excess wash buffer is important, as failure to do so will increase the volume spread on the microscope slide. This may result in an increased drying time and increased background fluorescence.

16. An alternative to air-drying the fixed cells onto the microscope slides is to use a cytospin. After incubation with fixative, follow the cytospin protocol for spinning cells onto slides. Be sure to determine an appropriate cell concentration prior to performing this caspase activation assay, as too high or low a concentration will make the subsequent microscopic analysis more difficult, if not impossible.

17. When spreading the solution onto the slides, it is important not to force air out of the pipet tip, as this will create bubbles. When dry, these bubbles will result in rings of high background and disrupt the even distribution of cells.

18. Slides should be dried on a completely level surface, as any incline will create pooling in one area of the slide, leading to high background and uneven cell distribution. It may be useful to check on the slides periodically as they dry and respread the solution on the slide as needed.

19. High background signal for the caspase staining may indicate insufficient washing of the cells. If counterstaining is weak, extend the incubation time with Hoechst 33342 to 10 min. If counterstaining is too strong, shorten the incubation time as needed.

References

1. Schins, R. P. (2002) Mechanisms of genotoxicity of particles and fibers. *Inhal. Toxicol.* **14,** 57–78.

2. Snyder, R. D. and Green, J. W. (2001) A review of the genotoxicity of marketed pharmaceuticals. *Mutat. Res.* **488,** 151–169.

3. Weisburger, J. H. (2001) Antimutagenesis and anticarcinogenesis from the past to the future. *Mutat. Res.* **480–481,** 23–35.

4. Zito, R. (2001) Low doses and thresholds in genotoxicity: from theories to experiments. *J. Exp. Clin. Cancer Res.* **20,** 315–325.

5. Lincz, L. F. (1998) Decipher the apoptotic pathway: all roads lead to death. *Immunol. Cell Biol.* **76,** 1–19.

6. Jenner, P. and Olanow, C. W. (1996) Oxidative stress and the pathogenesis of Parkinson's disease. *Neurology* **47,** 161–170.

7. Paradis, E., Douillard, H., Koutroumanis, M., Gooryer, C., and LeBlanc, A. (1996) Amyloid beta peptide of Alzheimer's disease downregulates bcl-2 and upregulates bax expression in human neurons. *J. Neurosci.* **16,** 7533–7539.

8. Hetts, S. W. (1998) To die or not to die: an overview of apoptosis and its role in disease. *JAMA* **279,** 300–307.

9. Zimmerman, K. C., Bonzon, C., and Green, D. R. (2001) The machinery of programmed cell death. *Pharmacol. Ther.* **92,** 57–70.

10. Zou, H., Henzel, J., Lui, X., Lutschg, A., and Wang, X. (1997) Apaf-1, a human protein homologous to *C. elegans* CED-4, participates in cytochrome c-dependent activation of caspase-3. *Cell* **90,** 405–413.

11. Li, P., Nijhawan, D., Budihardjo, I., et al. (1997) Cytochrome c and dATP-dependent formation of Apaf-1/caspase-9 complex initiates an apoptotic protease cascade. *Cell* **91,** 479–489.

12. Cai, J., Yang, J., and Jones, D. P. (1998) Mitochondrial control of apoptosis: the role of cytochrome c. *Biochim. Biophys. Acta* **1366,** 139–149.

13. Shi, Y. (2002) Mechanisms of caspase activation and inhibition during apoptosis. *Mol. Cell* **9,** 459–470.

14. Earnshaw, W. C., Martins, L. M., and Kaufmann, S. H. (1999) Mammalian caspases: structure, activation, substrates and functions during apoptosis. *Annu. Rev. Biochem.* **68,** 383–424.

15. McCarthy, N. J. and Evan, G. I. (1998) Methods for detecting and quantifying apoptosis, *Curr. Top. Dev. Biol.* **36,** 259–278.

16. Köhler, C., Orrenius, S., and Zhivotovsky, B. (2002) Evaluation of caspase activity in apoptotic cells. *J. Immunol. Methods* **265,** 97–110.

Index